TIDY'S
MASSAGE AND
REMEDIAL EXERCISES
IN MEDICAL AND SURGICAL CONDITIONS

EDITED AND REVISED BY

J. O. WALE, C.S.M.M.G., M.E., L.E.T., Teacher's Certificate

Formerly Physiotherapist-in-Charge, Neurological Section,
Physiotherapy Department, St. Thomas's Hospital

ELEVENTH EDITION

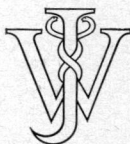

BRISTOL: JOHN WRIGHT & SONS LTD.
1973

© JOHN WRIGHT & SONS LTD., 1968

First edition, 1932
Second edition, 1934
Third edition, 1937
Fourth edition, 1939
Fifth edition, 1941
Sixth edition, 1944
Reprinted, 1945
Seventh edition, 1947
Eighth edition, 1949
Ninth edition, 1952
Tenth edition, 1961
Eleventh edition, 1968
Reprinted, 1973

This book is available in Braille.

ISBN 0 7236 0203 4

PRINTED IN GREAT BRITAIN BY JOHN WRIGHT AND SONS LTD.,
AT THE STONEBRIDGE PRESS, BRISTOL

PREFACE TO THE ELEVENTH EDITION

IN her preface to the first edition, Miss Tidy said that with regard to treatment her aim had been to provide most detail where others provided least. After much consideration I felt there to be such a variety of methods surrounding so many forms of treatment today, that a general textbook could not deal with them in sufficient detail. A thorough understanding of anatomy and physiology in health, as well as in disease, is essential if the student is to appreciate that the various methods employed are all directed to one end. It has therefore been my aim to concentrate on the basic principles of physical treatment in relation to the pathology, and the medical and surgical techniques employed. As in the ninth edition, orthodox and less orthodox methods are included and their rationale explained, but it is felt that the detailed application of the treatments practised in the various teaching hospitals should be left to the individual teachers in the school. In this way it seems to me that the purpose of Miss Tidy's original work can best be maintained, and it is my sincere hope that it will continue to be of value in the teaching and practice of physiotherapy.

Some of the chapters have been considerably condensed. The two chapters dealing with specific fractures have been joined to form one complete chapter, omitting many of the detailed treatments described in earlier editions but retaining the basic principles of the various surgical techniques employed and the principles of physical treatment relating to them. The chapters on postural deformities, constitutional diseases, and abdominal and pelvic conditions have been considerably reduced. The chapter on functional nervous diseases has been omitted completely, together with the section dealing with diseases of the blood, and many of the tables and lists of exercises. The sections dealing with prolapsed intervertebral disk lesions and fibrositis have been brought forward to Chapter IV, under joint and muscle injuries, respectively, and Pott's disease is now included under disease of bone.

New material includes the nature and causes of disease, and further details of inflammation and natural defences in Chapter I. In Chapter V the section on amputations has been revised to conform with modern practice and I offer my most grateful thanks to Dr. I. Curwen and Miss M. Lynch of Queen Mary's Hospital, Roehampton, for all their help and advice. In Chapter IX a description of experimental work on disseminated sclerosis is given and for this my thanks are due to Mrs. A. Potter, formerly of the Churchill Hospital, Oxford. The chapter on diseases of the heart has been divided into medical and surgical conditions and I would like to thank Miss J. Morris and Miss E. Hamilton of the Hammersmith Hospital, and Mrs. Kalaugher, *née* Thring, formerly of St. Thomas's Hospital, for arranging visits, explaining treatments, and correcting manuscripts. I imposed on a great deal of their time, and I am deeply indebted to them.

Many of the illustrations have been redrawn and some are new. For help with the latter I am indebted to the publishers of *Physiotherapy, The Nursing Times, Lower Limb Amputation* by W. Humm, and *Essentials of Orthopaedics* by P. Wiles, for permission to reprint from their published works.

Finally, my thanks are again given to Miss R. Wootton, Queen Alexandra's Hospital, East Grinstead, for her continued interest and help with burns, and to Miss Elphick and the staff of St. Thomas's Hospital for their invaluable help and inexhaustible patience.

J. O. WALE.

Alverstoke, Hants.
July, 1968.

FROM THE PREFACE TO THE FIRST EDITION

SOME years ago it occurred to me that although there were many excellent books on massage and exercises, there was none that was quite suitable as a text-book for senior students, for those recently qualified, or for junior teachers in training for the Chartered Society's examination. There were various good elementary text-books, and there were advanced works like Dr. Mennell's *Massage: its Principles and Practice*; but the former type did not seem to me to contain sufficient information for students preparing for the Conjoint Examination, while, in order to profit by the latter, a far more extensive background of knowledge and experience was necessary than would be possessed by any medical gymnast at the beginning of her career. It was in the hope of in some measure supplying this want that the present work was written.

The book makes no claim to originality. It has been my object merely to give an account of various modern methods of treatment, and to indicate, as far as possible, where further information about them can be obtained. At the same time I have personally tested most of these forms of treatment.

I have made little or no attempt to describe special massage manipulations, partly because the illustrations necessary to make such description effective would have taken up more space than could be spared, and partly because this has already been done most fully and beautifully by Dr. Mennell in his book on massage, as well as in other works on the subject. I have been careful to use only such terms as are contained in the Society's syllabus, or such as would be understood by every medical gymnast. When advising *passive movements*, I have tried in every case to make it quite clear whether *relaxed* movements (the only *true* passive movements) or *forced* movements are to be used, since the term ' passive movement ' has been a fruitful source of misunderstanding in the past.

In describing the various treatments, I have paid considerably more attention to some subjects than to others. My aim has been, in fact, to provide most details where other books provided least. I have, for instance, given fairly full notes on the treatment of fractures, and have tried to suggest approximate dates on which to begin the movements, guided by my own experience and that of others, and by the study of the works

v

of many authorities. As regards other conditions—scoliosis, for example —almost too much information is available. It is impossible even to summarize all the different systems of treatment. In such cases, therefore, I have tried to point out the general principles on which treatment should be based, leaving my readers to work these out in practice, with the assistance of the lectures and demonstrations which the C.S.M.M.G. is so generous in providing for its members.

NOEL M. TIDY.

Great Missenden,
October, 1932.

CONTENTS

MASSAGE AND REMEDIAL EXERCISES

IN MEDICAL AND SURGICAL CONDITIONS

CHAPTER I

PHYSIOTHERAPY: GENERAL CONSIDERATIONS

Role of physiotherapy—Principal body structures and their requirements for health—Nature and causes of disease—Natural defences—Inflammation—Immunity—Effects of inflammation on body structures—Principles of treatment—Methods and effects.

BEFORE considering the conditions met with in physiotherapy and the various methods of treatment, it is well to consider what the term implies. Today, with the great advances which have been made in medicine, both in the diagnostic and therapeutic fields, it is essential that all who deal with the patient on his road to recovery should be equipped with a clear understanding of the treatment which they offer. Particularly is this so in physiotherapy. Because of the pressure of modern life and the vast increase in the number of patients referred for treatment, accurate selection from a complex range of methods is necessary if the patient is to receive maximum benefit in the minimum time and with the least disruption of his daily life.

The Role of Physiotherapy.—Physiotherapy—"treatment by physical means". Perhaps too much stress is laid on the various physical means, and insufficient attention paid to what the term 'therapy' implies. The dictionary gives the definition "tending to the cure of disease". In physiotherapy the words 'tending to' are apt. All too often the condition is such that cure, in its true sense of complete restoration of full function, is not possible. It is the job of the physiotherapist to rehabilitate—"Restore to rights, privileges, reputation". In other words, to bring the patient to the point where he can again take his place as an independent member of society. From a patient's point of view his body must obey his will. He must be able to move freely and painlessly. It is largely failure in this that brings him to the Physiotherapy Department, and it is mainly with the re-education of movement that the physiotherapist is concerned. It is not within the province of this book to discuss the mechanics of movement; but without a thorough understanding of this field no physiotherapist can play her full part in Therapeutic Medicine. It is, however, relevant to consider briefly what governs efficient functioning of the body.

Principal Body Structures and their Requirements for Health.—Basically the body consists of fibrous or lymphoid connective tissue, from which the supporting tissues such as bone and cartilage, and the highly specialized muscles, nervous tissue, and skin, develop.* For perfect health these tissues depend on the metabolic interchange of fluids, both intracellular and extracellular. The blood-stream is of vital importance, since it constitutes one of the main defences against

---

* See 'Histology of Body Tissues', Gillison.

infection, as well as being the medium through which the necessary tissue-fluid interchange is effected, the nutritive and gaseous requirements of the body being supplied and waste products eliminated. Since the gaseous interchange ultimately depends upon external respiration, the respiratory system must also be efficient. For effortless movement joints must be mobile and muscles strong, but the key to precision movement lies in the accurate reception and interpretation of impulses throughout the central and peripheral nervous systems. It is to the nervous system that the body looks for smooth co-ordination and control.

The requirements for perfect bodily health and function may be summarized as follows: One must have (1) Efficient circulatory and respiratory systems; (2) Healthy bone and joint structures; (3) Strong but supple soft tissues; (4) Perfect central and peripheral nervous systems.

The adequate maintenance of tissue-fluid interchange keeps the tissues in working order; the nervous system allows them to work. Thus all the major systems and structures of the body are functionally closely interrelated and failure on the part of one may have far-reaching effects.

What then can go wrong? In general terms the answer is *disease*, i.e., a pathological condition of the tissues, of which the causes fall into five main groups:—

1. *Infection*: Conditions caused by invading micro-organisms known as *bacteria*, e.g., the common cold; anterior poliomyelitis; tuberculosis. An infective condition may be *acute*, or *chronic*, and the organism may be highly virulent or low grade.

2. *Trauma*: Conditions caused by *injury*, e.g., violence leading to fracture; or exposure to harmful agents, e.g., extreme temperatures, chemical or radiological substances.

3. *Degeneration*: Conditions caused by *degenerative changes* in the tissues. These may be due to "wear and tear", or senility, as in osteo-arthritis; the result of trauma as in hemiplegia; or the result of acute or chronic infection as in anterior poliomyelitis, or tabes dorsalis.

4. *Regeneration*: Conditions caused by new growths or *neoplasms*, which may be benign or malignant, e.g., lipoma, carcinoma.

5. *Congenital*: Conditions caused by some defective development in utero, leading to underdevelopment of certain tissues, e.g., congenital deformities such as congenital dislocation of the hip; or spastic conditions such as spastic quadriplegia.

Infection.—In this chapter we will deal only with infection, since *bacteria are one of the chief sources of human disease, and since the reaction to infection is the fundamental inflammatory reaction common to all forms of disease*.

Bacteria.—These are living organisms which exist all round us: in the air we breathe; in the soil; in the animate and inanimate objects with which we are in daily contact. They fall into two main groups; *pathogenic* and *non-pathogenic*. The pathogenic bacteria are those which cause disease and they sub-divide into four main groups: *bacilli*; *cocci*; *spirochaetes* and *protozoa*; and *viruses*.

Bacilli.—These are rod-shaped organisms into which category falls the tubercle bacillus.

Cocci.—These are small spherical organisms such as the streptococcus and staphylococcus.

Spirochaetes and **Protozoa.**—These are small unicellular organisms responsible for a great range of diseases, amongst which are dysentery, malaria, and syphilis.

Viruses.—These organisms are so minute that they are invisible under normal microscopy. Again they are responsible for a great many infections, amongst which are influenza, the common cold, and anterior poliomyelitis.

There are many differing strains of the various types of bacteria and they exhibit different patterns of life and infection. Some are *specific* in that they attack a certain type of tissue only (A.P.M. virus). Some require oxygen for the propagation of life. Some are destroyed by heat, others by cold—the vagaries are legion—*but all produce a uniform response in human tissues, an inflammatory reaction.* Before dealing with inflammation in detail, however, we should briefly consider the ways in which bacteria gain access to the tissues, and the natural defences of the body.

Methods of Entry and Body Defence.—As has been said, we are in daily contact with bacteria and there are three main methods of entry to the body:—

1. *Direct Contact or Contagion*: i.e., by touching an infected body or object. In this case entry is via the skin, through the pores or hair follicles (we are all familiar with styes and 'pimples'); or through an abrasion.

2. *Inhalation*: Bacteria are breathed in and gain access to the tissues via the respiratory tract, e.g., the common cold or the tubercle bacillus.

3. *Ingestion*: Bacteria are taken in with our food and reach the tissues via the digestive tract, e.g., food poisoning or, again, tubercle.

Normally the skin provides an adequate external defence against infection, being the great protective cover for the tissues, though the pores and hair follicles provide openings for bacterial entry as will any dissolution in the surface. *However, the main defence mechanism of the body lies in the reticulo-endothelial system* —the *leucocytes* (white blood corpuscles) found in the blood-stream itself and in the areas of lymphoid tissue found throughout the body (tonsils and adenoids, lymph glands and areas of lymphoid tissue found in the digestive tract).

Some of the lymphocytes, the *neutrophils* and *monocytes*, are *phagocytic*, i.e., capable of ingesting dead cells and bacteria. They are found in the lymphoid tissue and the blood-stream and are free to migrate. Others, the *lymphocytes*, are responsible for long-term defence and immunity through the production of *antitoxins*. *It is on the reticulo-endothelial system, therefore, that the body relies once infection has occurred.*

Inflammation.—Inflammation may be defined as *the reaction of body tissues to any irritant*, which, as we have seen, may be bacterial, traumatic, degenerative, or regenerative. *It is important that the student should realize that the response to any pathological stimulus will be an inflammatory one initially, since this is the body's chief defence and repair mechanism.* At times her work will be directed towards producing an inflammatory reaction in order to promote healing, and at others, and in far the greater number of cases, to mitigating the effects of such a reaction. She should, therefore, be fully conversant with the processes involved. The basic physiological changes are the same whether the reaction is local or general, so we will deal first with an acute local inflammatory reaction of bacterial origin.

Signs and Symptoms.—Everyone is familiar with the signs and symptoms of an acute local inflammation, such as an infected scratch or a cold, and they can be summarized as follows:—

1. *Redness*: Or in lay terms, the area is 'inflamed'.

2. *Heat*: This will vary with the type and degree of inflammation. In the case of an infected scratch, the surrounding area will feel hot and may throb. In the case of a cold there will be a general rise in temperature.

3. *Swelling*: In the case of the scratch this may, or may not, be visible. In the case of a cold it manifests itself in a feeling of congestion in the throat and nose.

4. *Pain*: This is caused by pressure on nerve-endings in the area.

5. *Loss of Function*: Again this will vary with the type and degree of infection and may, or may not, be appreciated by the patient. In the case of the scratch there will probably be little or no effect. In the case of the cold, respiration is impeded.

Physiological Changes.—Once bacteria have gained access to the tissues, the following changes take place:—

1. *Capillary Dilatation* (*Redness and Heat*): This leads to an increased blood-supply to the area and to increased permeability of the vessel walls.

2. *Extravasation of Tissue Fluid* (*Swelling*): Tissue fluid seeps out into the surrounding tissues. The nature of the exudate varies according to the condition but it frequently contains a high degree of fibrinogen.

3. *Clustering of Leucocytes on Vessel Walls.*

4. *Migration of Leucocytes from the Vessels into the Tissues.*

This increased metabolic activity gives rise to a general rise in temperature if the infection is fairly widespread, or if the organism is a virulent one. At the same time activity in the lymphoid tissue will be manifest in swollen glands near the focus of infection, e.g., the cervical glands in the case of a cold.

Termination of Inflammation.—These events having taken place, a 'battle' ensues between the reticulo-endothelial cells and the invading organism, and the inflammatory reaction ends in one of two ways:—

1. *Resolution*: In this method the invading organisms are completely destroyed and ingested by the reticulo-endothelial cells. The tissues then return to normal. In some cases, e.g., the infectious diseases of childhood such as measles, the *lymphocytes*, together with the *plasma proteins* build up substances called *antibodies*, which are reabsorbed into the blood-stream and render the patient immune, or partially immune, to subsequent attack.

2. *Suppuration*: In certain types of infection the invading organism is a *pyogenic* one, i.e., the resulting debris of inflammatory exudate and dead cells liquefies and turns to pus, e.g., a stye. The pus has to discharge before healing occurs by resolution.

General Inflammation.—If either, or both, the general health and circulation of the patient is poor, and particularly if the organism is a virulent one, it may gain access to the blood-stream. Travelling via the lymphatic system, it then gives rise to *general septicæmia*. If the organism is a pyogenic one, or if pus gains access to the blood-stream, boils or abscesses will occur in other parts of the body. The condition is then known as *pyæmia*.

In both cases the signs and symptoms are the same as those of local inflammation but of greater intensity, and the patient feels and is very ill, though antibiotics have done much to lessen the gravity of these conditions.

Chronic Inflammation.—This may be the result of an acute inflammatory reaction, in which the patient's resistance is poor and the reticulo-endothelial system is unable to control the invading organism effectively, e.g., infection by the tubercle bacillus. On the other hand, it may be the result of a low-grade infection from the beginning, e.g., rheumatoid arthritis or syphilis. Chronic inflammatory conditions generally follow a progressive course and may be characterized by periods of sudden acute flare-up, followed by periods of relative quiescence.

Immunity.—Before closing this section on disease and inflammation, a word should be said about immunity. It has already been mentioned that once contact has been made with certain infections, a degree of immunity can be built up through the production of antibodies. Such immunity is called *acquired immunity*. Nor is it necessary that disease should actually occur before such immunity is gained. We are probably all in contact with the tubercle bacillus at some time in our lives, but we do not all become victims of tuberculosis. A newborn child gains a certain amount of immunity from its mother during fœtal life, which is designed to protect it through its first few months until it can begin to build up its own resistance.

Besides natural immunity, it is now possible to give immunity by artificial means, either passively by *immunization* or actively by *vaccination*.

1. *Immunization*: This is passive, in that serum containing the required antibodies is injected into the human body, e.g., anti-tetantus, diphtheria, and whooping-cough (the 'triple' injection now given to babies in the first few months of life).

2. *Vaccination*: This is active, in that bacteria of an allied disease, e.g., cow-pox for small-pox, are introduced into the body to allow the natural processes of immunity to be triggered off.

The Effects of Inflammation on Body Structures.—It was stated at the beginning of the section on inflammation that, besides being a defence mechanism, inflammation was also the main *repair* mechanism. The daily processes of metabolism are designed to maintain the integrity of the tissues *but, following major traumatic or pathological intervention, the tissues are capable of only limited regeneration.* There are two methods of repair, by *homogenous tissue* or by *scar tissue*.

1. *Repair by Homogenous Tissue*: The inflammatory reaction leads to the formation of new cells and the tissues are again restored to normal, e.g., superficial cuts. There may or may not be suppuration. Homogenous repair will occur in bone, fibrous tissue, and epidermal structures. The more highly specialized tissues such as muscles and nervous tissue degenerate, in that they repair by scar tissue.

2. *Repair by Scar Tissue*: The inflammatory reaction leads to the formation of fibrous tissue which takes the place of the original tissue, e.g., deep cuts which reach the dermis. Because of this area of scarring, function is lost to some extent. Again, there may or may not be suppuration.

Let us now consider the effects of inflammation on the main body structures but first let it be said that *wherever a lesion occurs there must be a local hyperæmia,* since the inflammatory reaction leading to repair springs from the blood-stream. Failure in this leads to delay in healing.

The Structural System.—As stated above, bone repairs by homogenous tissue.

The Cardiovascular System.—If an inflammatory reaction occurs in any part of this system degenerative changes result. The overall effect of these changes is a diminution in circulation which may be local or general. Tissues deprived of blood become devitalized and this may have serious and far-reaching effects. Not only do waste products accumulate as a result of decreased metabolism, but any or all of the following trophic changes may occur:—

1. The *skin* becomes dry and papery. It breaks easily and provides an entry for micro-organisms. Since the blood-supply is poor, infection can set in and, once established, healing will be slow and prolonged. If the organism is a virulent one there is grave danger of a rapid spread of infection.

2. *Fibrous tissue* thickens and contracts, restricting movement.

3. *Muscle power* is diminished since the extra oxygen required for activity is not available. In addition waste products accumulate and have a further deleterious effect. If the ischæmia is prolonged the fibres will atrophy in time, and the special properties of muscle will be lost.

4. *Nervous tissue* atrophies. In time the cells die and the fibres fibrose. Eventually both become necrotic.

Since the cardiovascular system is the life-line of the body it is essential, for health or healing, that an adequate circulation is maintained.

The Respiratory System.—An inflammatory reaction in any part of the respiratory system leads to a certain degree of hypoventilation. Although the cardiovascular system may be normal, metabolic processes cannot be carried out adequately if ventilation is poor, for oxygenation will be inadequate and carbon dioxide will accumulate. It is therefore useless to have an effective cardiovascular system if ventilation is defective and vice versa.

Fibrous Soft Tissues.—Fibrous tissue being the basic body structure, it is also the principal repair tissue. Its response to inflammation is prolific regeneration.

The danger inherent in this natural repair lies in the fact that fibrin is required for it, and excess fibrin leads to the formation of adhesions. Adhesions are thin strong fibrous strands which stretch between structures and bind them to neighbouring structures. This leads to considerable restriction in movement, and to painful movement. Once adhesions form, contractures and deformities can ensue. *In all cases of inflammation in the fibrous tissues, it is essential that the fibrinous exudate is kept within limits compatible with health.*

Musculature.—Since muscles are basically soft tissues and since they are encased in fibrous tissue, an inflammatory reaction in muscles can also give rise to adhesions. If the fibres are cut or ruptured scarring follows. Either of these results leads to restricted activity and diminished power.

The Nervous Systems.—An inflammatory reaction in any part of the central nervous system results in irrevocable degenerative changes. Since the central nervous system controls all muscle and joint activity the results are serious and often diffuse. Any or all of the following symptoms may exist:—

1. *Paralysis*: This may be flaccid or spastic. From it contractures and deformity may result.

2. *Incoordination*: This can range from slight clumsiness to complete ataxia.

3. *Altered Sensation*: This may range from hypo-æsthesia to complete anæsthesia, or it may take the form of hyperæsthesia.

The effect of an inflammatory reaction in the peripheral nervous system depends on the site and degree of damage. The peripheral nerves are capable of limited regeneration, but a peripheral nerve lesion results in a period of muscular paralysis. If the lesion lies in the anterior horn cells, the cells of origin of the nerve-fibres and therefore of muscle action, the result is degeneration. The muscle-fibres supplied by the affected cells are denervated and their function is lost.

The autonomic nervous system is capable of regeneration.

The Skin.—Epidermal structures will regenerate following inflammation. If the dermal structures are involved and the epidermis is destroyed, scarring will result. With other vital organs the physiotherapist is not directly concerned.

PRINCIPLES OF TREATMENT

The ultimate aim of physiotherapy is the *restoration of the fullest functional activity possible*.

From the preceding consideration of the requirements for health and function, certain principles emerge of vital importance in the rehabilitation of a patient. These may be summarized as follows.

Circulation and Tissue-fluid Interchange must be Maintained or Increased.—This will be necessary in the interests of healing, in order to alleviate symptoms, or in the interests of general tissue health. By stimulating circulation and metabolic interchange locally it is possible to promote healing in cases where this is required, and at the same time minimize the risk of adhesions by the absorption of excess inflammatory exudate; to disperse metabolic waste products, or œdema, thereby reducing pain and limitation of movement due to pressure or toxins; to combat the effects of inactivity and thereby reduce the risk of trophic changes or disuse atrophy; to prepare muscles for work and to maintain unaffected tissues in a healthy, functional state. *Whatever may be the underlying reason, this principle is of paramount importance in physiotherapy.*

Joint Mobility must be Maintained or Increased.—For ease of movement joints must be as mobile as possible. When joints are affected attempts must be made to relieve the condition and to gain a wider range of movement. This may involve the use of splints and appliances, or even operative treatment in severe cases. *It should be remembered that any interference in joint mobility will throw strain on unaffected joints and this endangers their health and function.* It may therefore be necessary to treat unaffected as well as affected areas and muscle power must not be neglected.

Muscle Power must be Maintained and Increased.—Joint mobility and muscle power are closely interrelated, joint range depending on muscle power to a large extent. If the muscle is weak it cannot move the joint through its full range. If the joint is allowed to fall into disuse changes may occur in its structure which further limit its range. If this happens extra effort is required to produce joint movement which, in its weakened state, the muscle cannot give. *In any case of weak musculature joint range must be maintained whilst muscle power is being built up.* It may be necessary to train muscles to take over from affected muscles, or to share their work. In some cases it is necessary to give specific muscle training in order to enable the patient to use mechanical aids or appliances. *In any form of muscle re-education the importance of the anterior horn cells must never be forgotten.*

Respiration must be Adequate.—Tissue ventilation being of such importance it may be necessary to assist respiration, not only in specific chest conditions, but in the interests of the patient's general health.

Specific Symptoms must be Relieved as far as Possible.—Symptoms vary with the condition. Such things as pain, œdema, and spasticity must be relieved where possible since, besides gravely incapacitating the patient, they can reduce metabolism and restrict muscle and joint activity.

Complications must be Prevented.—Again, these vary with the condition but the possibility of trophic change, the formation of adhesions, contractures, sepsis, thrombosis, and chest conditions should be taken into account and steps taken to reduce their risk.

General Health may need Improvement.—This applies particularly in chronic conditions, in infective conditions, and in the case of elderly patients. In all cases, however, the general condition of the patient should be considered when a treatment scheme is being prepared. Where it is considered beneficial, steps should be taken to improve the general health.

The Use and Care of Aids and Appliances.—Where any form of aid or appliance is to be used it is the province of the physiotherapist to instruct the patient in its use and maintenance. It may also be her job to make and repair them.

In general the principles of maintaining circulation and tissue-fluid interchange, and maintaining joint mobility and muscle power apply in almost every case treated by physiotherapy. They are in fact the guiding principles of physiotherapy. The other principles are applicable or not, depending on the condition.

METHODS OF TREATMENT AND THEIR EFFECTS

Before concluding this chapter it seems appropriate to give a brief résumé of the various methods of treatment and their effects.

Massage.—Although the various techniques produce slightly different effects, the overall effects only need be considered here, since a massage treatment would rarely, if ever, be confined to the use of one technique. Firstly, the sensory nerve-endings in the skin may be stimulated or sedated, the latter assisting both local and general relaxation. Secondly, a local hyperæmic effect may be produced, either directly through the stimulation of sensory nerve-endings, or indirectly through slight cellular damage leading to the liberation of H-substance. Both these effects result in arteriole dilatation. Thirdly, venous and lymphatic return is given mechanical assistance by alternate pressure and relaxation. Fourthly, the skin and subcutaneous tissues are moved. This has a stretching and softening effect, particularly on fibrous tissue.

Exercise.—The movement of muscles and joints has a mechanical pumping effect which assists venous and lymphatic return. Also by keeping cortical pathways open the pattern of movement is not forgotten. Mobility and range of movement can be increased by all forms of movement. Passive movements can stretch, and therefore soften, fibrous structures. Resisted movement will build up muscle power. Balance and co-ordination can be improved. If generalized and of sufficient vigour, the general circulatory rate can be raised through the effect of exercise on the heart.

Electrical Treatment.—By means of electrical equipment heat is administered, ultra-violet radiation given, artificial exercise induced, and drugs driven in.

The administration of heat has a sedatory effect on nerve-endings, thereby inducing local and general relaxation. A local hyperæmia can be induced and a general increase in circulation and metabolism may sometimes be produced.

Ultra-violet radiation can be used locally for its effect on the skin, or generally for its effect on metabolism.

Artificial exercise, having the effects of joint and muscle activation, can be given by the use of the faradic current. Interrupted direct current can be used to prevent disuse atrophy in denervated tissue, and the sinusoidal current stimulates circulation through its effect on sensory nerve-endings and also through the mechanical effect of muscle contraction and relaxation.

In addition to its use for the ionization of specific drugs the direct current may be used to sedate or stimulate sensory nerve-endings, and through the latter to produce an increase in circulation. It may also be used for its phoretic effect, general ionic interchange in the tissues being brought about in the area treated. For detailed effects of electrotherapy the student should refer to a standard text-book on electrotherapy.

In this chapter an attempt has been made to provide a background for more detailed study of diseases and their various methods of treatment. *It is important that every physiotherapist should be fully aware of the interdependence of all the body structures and appreciate the danger to other structures inherent in failure on the part of one.* By drawing attention to this it is hoped that the student will more clearly understand that, although physiotherapy covers such a wide field, and individual cases create individual problems, certain factors are common to all. The main basic principles apply to all cases, and the varying methods of treatment lead to one end.

CHAPTER II

FRACTURES: GENERAL CONSIDERATIONS

Varieties—Causes—Displacement—General symptoms—Healing—Complications—Principles treatment.

THE physiotherapist, as we well know, is required to deal with many different forms of injury. Cases of fracture, dislocation, sprain, rupture of muscle, or nerve lesions are numerous in our hospital departments and amongst our private patients.

A fracture has been defined as *the interruption of the continuity of a bone.* This interruption, however, may be complete or incomplete. The varieties, causes, and symptoms are briefly summarized below. For further details, specific text-books should be consulted.*

Varieties.—Fractures may be classified as follows:—

INCOMPLETE.—(1) *Greenstick*; in which the bone is bent, and broken only part of the way through its shaft; this type is found only in children. (2) *Fissured*; consisting of a mere split of the bone without displacement of the fragments. (3) *Perforating*; in which there is a hole such as is made by a bullet. (4) *Depressed*; saucer- or gutter-shaped depressions, usually seen in fractures of the skull.

COMPLETE.—(1) *Simple*; in which the skin is intact. This is sometimes called a 'closed' fracture. (2) *Impacted*; in which the broken bone-ends are driven into each other. (3) *Comminuted*; in which the bone is splintered, or broken into several pieces. (4) *Compound*; in which the broken bone has pierced the skin. This is sometimes called an 'open' fracture, and there is grave danger of infection. (5) *Complicated*; in which there is injury to some organ or important structure in the neighbourhood of the fracture.

SEPARATION OF AN EPIPHYSIS. This occurs in young people before the bones are completely ossified.

Causes.—Fractures may be *traumatic* or *spontaneous.*

TRAUMATIC FRACTURES are those due to violence. In these fractures the bone is normal and the causative force maximal. The force causing a fracture may consist of: (1) *Direct violence,* as when the arm or leg is broken by a wheel passing over it, or by a blow. (2) *Indirect violence,* in which case the force is transmitted to the bone through some other part of the body, as when the clavicle is broken by a fall on the hand, or the tibia and fibula by a fall on the feet. (3) *Muscular action,* as in fracture of the patella due to a sudden contraction of the quadriceps extensors.

SPONTANEOUS FRACTURES are always of pathological origin. Local or general disease causes the bone to be unduly brittle, and to fracture with minimal traumatic force.

Displacement.—Fractures may be transverse, oblique, or spiral in form. Transverse fractures are generally the result of direct violence and are accompanied by a great deal of soft-tissue damage. Spiral and oblique fractures generally result from indirect violence, and soft-tissue damage is often slight.

---

* E.g., R. Watson-Jones, *Fractures and Other Bone and Joint Injuries*; J. G. Bonnin, *Fractures and Related Injuries*; L. Böhler, *The Treatment of Fractures*; G. Perkins, *Fractures and Dislocations*.

The displacement of the fragments may consist of: (*a*) *Lateral displacement.* (*b*) *Angulation,* in which the fragments form an angle with each other instead of being in a line. (*c*) *Overlapping,* resulting in shortening of the bone. (*d*) *Rotation,* or twisting of the distal fragment. (*Fig.* 1.)

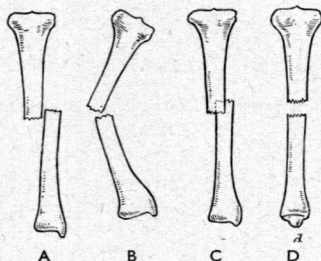

Fig. 1.—Types of displacement in fractures. A, Lateral displacement; B, Angulation; C, Overlapping; D, Rotation.

General Symptoms.—The symptoms of fracture at the time of injury, or shortly after are:—

1. *Unnatural Mobility.*
2. *Crepitus:* Grating between the broken bone ends.
3. *Deformity, Pain, and Loss of Function:* This is due to a *protective reflex* designed to keep the fragments in position. The muscles immediately go into spasm, which varies directly with the degree of mobility of the bone-ends. It soon disappears once the limb is supported and mobilized and is, therefore, rarely seen in the physiotherapy department.
4. *Œdema (swelling):* This may be intense, extending over a great part of the injured limb. It will persist for some time but should gradually subside as the fracture unites.

Healing.—When a bone is broken, swelling takes place within twenty-four hours. This is partly due to hæmorrhage into the tissues, and partly to slowing of the venous circulation, with increased exudation of lymph.

Between the broken bone-ends a clot, or *hæmatoma,* forms. This organizes and into this soft mass grow new blood-vessels. The new tissue is formed not only between the bone-ends but also outside them, beneath the periosteum. The space where the medullary cavity of the bone would be is also filled up by granulation tissue, the whole forming a rubbery mass. The bone-ends become rarified and calcium is laid down in the granulation tissue. This new substance is known as *callus* and the fracture is said to be clinically united at the end of this stage, i.e., the bone-ends move as one, *but they are not yet strong enough to withstand stress.* (*Fig.* 2 A–D.)

When union by callus is complete, a process resembling the normal ossification of bone occurs. *Osteoblasts* bring about a deposit of bone salts in the soft tissue, gradually hardening it. *Osteoclasts* then pass into the new bone, hollowing out cavities and making its structure less dense. The medullary cavity is reproduced, and the marrow-cells reappear. This process is known as 'consolidation' or 'bony union' (*Fig.* 2 E). Finally, remodelling of the new bone takes place.

TIME NEEDED TO OBTAIN UNION.—This varies in the different bones, depending on the thickness of the bone, the richness of its blood-supply, and the amount of separation between the fragments. Spiral or oblique fractures generally unite before transverse fractures and the upper extremity before the lower extremity. The time needed for union also depends on which part of the bone is injured. The blood-supply near joints is good, so that fractures in these regions unite more quickly than those of the shafts of bones. The time factor varies in different individuals, the age of the patient being an important point.

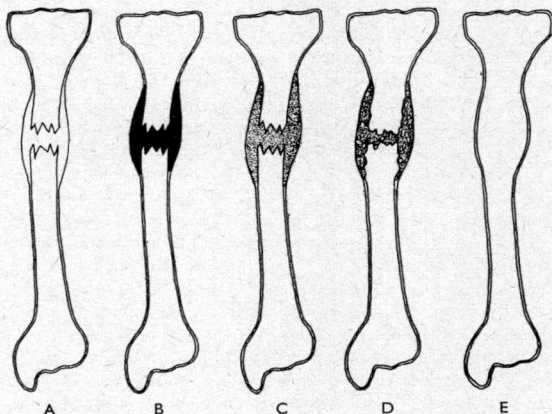

Fig. 2.—Showing method of fracture repair. A, Fracture of bone and stripping of periosteum; B, Hæmatoma at fracture site; C, Granulation tissue; D, Callus formation; E, Consolidation.

Fractures unite more quickly in children than in adults, and may take much longer in elderly patients. Professor Perkins gives the following table for approximate dates in adults:—

	Upper Limb		Lower Limb	
	Union	Consolidation	Union	Consolidation
Spiral fracture	3 weeks	6 weeks	6 weeks	12 weeks
Transverse fracture	6 weeks	12 weeks	12 weeks	24 weeks

DELAYED UNION AND NON-UNION.—These are terms used to denote respectively that union is taking longer than is usual, and that callus has failed to form (that is to say, *it is only a fibrous union*). Delayed union often results in non-union.

Delayed union may be due to some general disease, such as severe anæmia, syphilis, etc.; to some local disease of the bone, e.g., osteomyelitis; or to sepsis in the bone or surrounding tissues. Union will also be delayed if the blood-supply to one fragment is impaired, since the power of the non-vascular fragment to lay down callus is limited. If the blood-supply of both fragments is impaired the time required for union will be considerably longer. If one fragment is completely deprived of its blood-supply it can take no part in the repair of the fracture, and finally dies. This is known as '*avascular bone necrosis*'. The living fragment can lay down tissue which invades and ultimately replaces the dead portion—but this process is very slow indeed.★

Non-union may be due to the same causes as delayed union; to extensive loss of bone substance as in a gunshot wound; to the fact that muscular or ligamentous fibres have become interposed between the fragments; to lack of immobility at the fracture site; or to too great disparity between the bone-ends.

★ Watson-Jones, *Fractures and Other Bone and Joint Injuries.*

Complications.—

INJURIES TO JOINTS.—The fracture may extend into a joint, the movements of which may be seriously restricted by imperfect replacement of the fragments. Although the surgeon aims at exact anatomical alinement, it is not always possible, particularly if the joint surface is disrupted and in such cases movement may help to mould the surfaces and regain joint congruity. Joints may also be impaired by excessive callus formation; or by the formation of adhesions. A condition known as *traumatic arthritis* is then established and this may lead to osteo-arthritis, following on the traumatic arthritis due to the injury.

INJURIES TO THE SKIN, in compound fractures. In these cases, bacteria may enter and infect the wound, unless proper precautions are taken. *Because of this danger a skin wound takes precedence over the fracture.* Sometimes temporary treatment only is given to the fracture until the wound is healed.

ADHESIONS: PERSISTENT ŒDEMA.—Œdema is brought about by the liberation of histamine from the injured tissues. This causes the neighbouring capillaries to dilate, thus increasing the flow of blood to the affected part, and slowing the circulation in this area. The walls of the vessels become more permeable and fluid passes out into the tissue spaces. If excessive it can prevent treatment of the fracture, temporary measures only being possible. This sero-fibrinous exudate lays down fibrin, forming dense bands which may impair the mobility of joints, producing stiffness, with pain at the limit of movement. In the early stage of an injury the swelling is soft, but later, when some of the fluid part of the exudate has been absorbed, it may, if it persists, become harder and more resistant, pitting deeply on pressure. In severe cases, especially in the lower extremity, the whole limb may remain permanently enlarged and the muscle-tone of the limb is lowered. The patient may complain of a feeling of weight in the limb, or of fatigue. It is, therefore, essential to disperse œdema as quickly as possible.

Persistent œdema may be caused by recurrent injury, e.g., too early or too forcible movement of an injured joint (or of the joint nearest the fracture) whether by injudicious treatment by a physiotherapist, or by the patient's own indiscretion; by functional inactivity which produces circulatory stasis, e.g., if the knee is immobilized and no movements of hip or foot are given to maintain the circulation of the leg; infection in or near the joint or joints; or injury to the vessels of the limb (for thrombosis, *see below*). *Recurrent œdema* is a condition in which œdema gradually comes on after the limb has been dependent for some time. It is brought about by the action of gravity on a limb with poor muscle tone, and is noticed when a patient begins to walk after a lower-limb fracture. To combat this it is advisable to accustom the patient to dependent limbs by letting him sit on the side of the bed for gradually increasing periods, before beginning to stand or walk, and to use his muscles by going through the motions of walking, even though he may be non-weight-bearing. (*See* Shadow-walking, p. 48.)

INJURIES TO BLOOD-VESSELS.—These consist of: (1) *Hæmorrhage*, due to tearing of large vessels. (2) *Blocking of a Large Artery.* If such a vessel be *partially* occluded, the result is ischæmic contracture (*see* pp. 25–7); if it be *completely* blocked, in such a position as to cut off practically the whole blood-supply of the limb, the result is mortification (gangrene). Either of these conditions may also be caused by over-tight bandages, by improperly applied splints or plaster, or compression of an artery by bone fragments. (3) *Thrombosis* (*see* Chapter XIX) of veins in the neighbourhood of the fracture. This is manifested by the sudden development of cramp-like pain in the part, by an increase in swelling, and by marked tenderness along the line of the affected vein. Anything that appears to be abnormal in the circulatory condition of the injured limb must be reported immediately to the surgeon. In cases of suspected thrombosis, all treatment must be stopped.

INJURIES TO MUSCLE.—Fibres may be torn or ruptured as a result of the injury ; or a condition known as myositis ossificans occur. (*See* pp. 24–5.)

INJURIES TO NERVES.—A nerve may have been injured at the time the fracture occurred, in which case symptoms appear at once. If the nerve is actually severed, there will be immediate paralysis and anæsthesia of the parts supplied by it. The surgeon will at once suture the nerve.

A deep-lying nerve may become involved in forming callus, or compressed by displaced bone; if this is so, the symptoms develop gradually. It is the duty of the physiotherapist to notice and report them.

DELAYED UNION AND NON-UNION.—These have already been discussed.

PRINCIPLES OF TREATMENT

The aims of the surgeon and of those who co-operate with him in the treatment of fracture are, firstly, to obtain accurate anatomical alinement in order to promote good repair; and, secondly, to restore perfect function to the limb. It is therefore essential that the physiotherapist understands fully the principles of the surgeon's treatment as well as her own.

All fractures are now X-rayed as a matter of routine and the X-rays are later used to ascertain whether reduction has been maintained, how union is progressing, whether internal fixation is holding, or whether a bone-graft has taken. The physiotherapist should make a point of seeing the plates of the case she is treating.

Principles of Treatment by the Surgeon.—While the soft callus is forming the fragments of the bone are *hyperæmic*, owing to the inflammatory reaction which takes place as the result of the injury. This leads to *decalcification* of the fragments, because the calcium in the bone is carried away by the increased blood-flow. During the consolidation period, i.e., the hardening of the callus, the bone-ends become *ischæmic*, that is to say their blood-supply becomes greatly reduced; the calcium accumulates, and the bone is said to be *recalcified*. "Hyperæmia of bone is always accompanied by decalcification, and ischæmia by sclerosis" (Watson-Jones). Now a certain degree of inflammatory reaction and consequent hyperæmia is necessary for callus formation; but it should not be excessive, or continue for long, otherwise too much calcium will be lost. A small amount of movement at the site of a fracture in the recent stage promotes callus formation by increasing the inflammatory reaction, but if this small amount is exceeded various unfortunate results will follow. In certain parts, e.g., near the elbow, a very large amount of callus may be formed, which will later ossify and block the joint, while dense fibrous adhesions may be laid down which will further limit mobility. If, however, the movement between the fragments is continuous or excessive, the bones may unite very slowly or even fail to unite at all. Professor Perkins states, "If the young repair material is stretched it ends up as a pliable scar, if it is compressed it ends up as rigid bone. One should therefore, during the mending of a fracture, encourage everything that compresses the embryonic callus, and discourage anything that stretches it."* He lists factors which contribute to compression as muscle tone, voluntary muscle action, and weight-bearing. Factors contributing to stretching are traction, hinging, and rotation.

To further these ends there are three great principles of treatment: (1) Reduction; (2) Fixation; (3) Protection.

REDUCTION.—This is undertaken to regain perfect alinement of the fragments. If there is no displacement, or if the fragments are impacted, there is

---

* G. Perkins, *Fractures and Dislocations.*

usually no need for reduction. Reduction may be Closed, i.e., by manipulation under anæsthetic, or Open, i.e., performed by open operation.

FIXATION.—This is designed to maintain reduction, and to prevent any harmful stress until union has occurred.

Methods of Fixation.—The old or classic treatment of fractures after reduction consisted of splinting and fixation of the whole limb until union was firm. This ensured a good *anatomical* result, but since the joints had in the meantime become stiff and the muscles wasted, the *functional* result often left much to be desired. Today the surgeon does not resort to more extensive fixation than is necessary to ensure immobilization of the site of the fracture. No joints which can safely be left free are included in the plaster; and in these free joints movement is encouraged. Static contractions are taught where joints are immobilized.

Fixation may take the form of External splintage, Internal splintage, and Traction.

External splintage: This includes plaster-of-Paris casts, or slabs; apparatus, such as a Thomas's splint; strapping or bandages which hold the fracture site. Sometimes a sling is the only form of support.

Internal splintage: This is applied by open operation, the fragments being fixed together by steel or silver plates, screws, or nails. Sometimes the fragments are sutured with wire or catgut, or they may be pegged together with pegs of bone (*Figs.* 3–5). Many surgeons use some form of external splintage as well until union has occurred. Others believe that internal fixation gives sufficient support.

These operative measures may be employed initially, or following delayed union or non-union.

Traction: This combines reduction with fixation and is used particularly for overlap. In the upper limb gravity exerts sufficient force. In the lower limb apparatus must be used, *see* pp. 33, 34.

PROTECTION.—Even though union has occurred *the fracture cannot withstand stress until consolidation is established.* It is necessary therefore to protect the fracture if it is likely to be subjected to a rotation strain, a hinging strain, or to traction by muscle action, such as occurs at the elbow or knee.

Methods of Protection.—In the upper limb slings, plaster slabs, or suitably padded malleable wire or metal splints are used. In the lower limb plaster slabs, walking plasters, calipers, irons, and crutches are commonly used.

The method of fixation selected by the surgeon and the amount of physical treatment allowed depend entirely on his views. The importance of preventing joint stiffness and muscle atrophy is widely recognized, and it is generally accepted that certain fractures do not require any fixation. Such fractures are treated as soft-tissue injuries, stress being laid on preventing adhesions. They include fractures without displacement; some fractures in non-weight-bearing bones; some fractures which are impacted; and some minor fractures in weight-bearing bones.

In fractures with gross displacement, or where muscle action or weight-bearing would lead to strain, fixation and protection will be required. All free joints must be moved assiduously, however, and static contractions are allowed in the immobilized muscle groups *provided they do not strain the fracture site.*

If the fracture extends into a joint perfect alinement must be achieved if possible, and, once obtained, maintained until union. Full fixation, however, leads to joint stiffness and traction may be used to overcome this difficulty. If reduction is not possible many surgeons advocate early movement to help moulding of the fragments, and to prevent gross stiffness.

Some surgeons use splintage extensively, others use it sparingly, but *whatever views the surgeon may hold the principles of physical treatment remain the same.*

Principles of Physical Treatment.—These are very simple. In order to assist repair and help to restore function the physiotherapist must ensure three things: (1) Circulation must be adequate for the formation of callus. (2) Joint mobility and muscle power must be maintained. (3) Nothing must be allowed to occur which could delay or prevent healing.

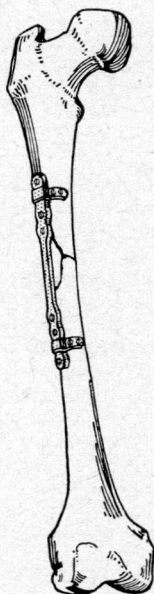

Fig. 4.—Treatment of fracture by wiring. In the upper figure the wire is loose and the fragments are not adjusted; this leads to chafing, delayed union, and secondary sepsis. In the lower figure are shown exact restitution, tight twisting, and efficient fixation.

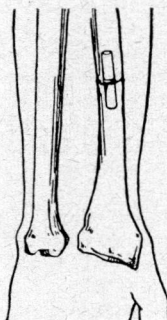

Fig. 3.—Fracture of shaft of femur treated by plating.

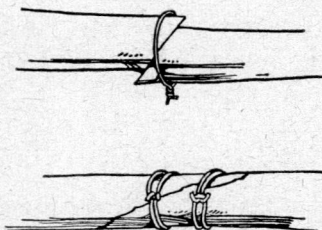

Fig. 5.—Treatment of fractured radius by intramedullary peg.

By satisfying these requirements the formation of bone tissue will be assisted and the risk of complications greatly reduced. Passive movements and active assisted movement may be used to regain mobility *but no forced movement should ever be given.*

Radiant Heat, Infra-red Radiation, or *Short-wave Diathermy* may be used to improve the circulation, decrease pain, and prepare the way for active movement.

CHAPTER III

FRACTURES OF THE UPPER AND LOWER EXTREMITY, PELVIS, AND SPINE

General principles of physical treatment—Fractures of upper extremity—Fixation and support—Outline of principle fractures—Myositis ossificans—Volkmann's ischæmic contracture—Fractures of lower extremity—Outline of principal fractures—Re-education in walking—Fractures of spine and skull.

General Principles of Physical Treatment.—

The physical treatment of fractures falls into two categories; *treatment during immobilization* and *final rehabilitation* following immobilization. In both stages the *principal role of the physiotherapist is to care for the soft tissues and by so doing, assist the process of union and the return to full function.*

Although she is not directly concerned with the actual bone repair she must be scrupulously careful to avoid anything which might delay repair or lead to non-union. No movement may be given which could cause this, and no apparatus should be interfered with. If removal of apparatus is allowed for treatment it must be correctly reapplied and the fracture site carefully supported whilst it is off. Any softening of a plaster or similar damage which might allow unwanted movement must be repaired. In addition she must watch for any possible complications and report any untoward signs. In cases of fractures in the lower limb special techniques of walking will have to be taught.

Treatment during Immobilization.—The aims of physical treatment may be summarized as follows:—

1. *To assist the maintenance of an adequate circulation,* particularly by relieving spasm, pain, and œdema if present.

An adequate circulation is essential if a hæmatoma is to form; if the undamaged tissues are to remain healthy, and trophic changes be avoided; and if adhesions are to be prevented.

It has been said in Chapter II that as soon as the fracture occurs the muscles go into protective spasm, and since the fibres cause pressure on vessels, blood-flow tends to be impeded. Although the initial spasm disappears on reduction, pain, which may persist for some time, also induces a form of protective spasm which may impede circulation. Œdema is another factor which may contribute to a diminished blood-supply. If it is allowed to persist the results referred to on p. 12 will become established. It is therefore essential to relieve pain, spasm, and œdema as soon as possible, not only for the patient's comfort, but also in the interests of the repair processes.

2. *To maintain joint mobility and muscle power* and thereby prevent adhesions and disuse atrophy. Both must be maintained in all free joints, and muscle power as far as possible in immobilized joints, if the patient is to be restored to full functional activity as soon as possible. It should be remembered that the fact that part of the limb is immobilized tends to have an adverse effect on circulation, since it reduces muscle and joint activity.

3. *To teach any special techniques that may be required.*

4. *To care for and maintain any appliances or apparatus* and to teach the patient to care for them.

5. *To watch for complications*, particularly nerve lesions, ischaemic conditions, myositis ossificans, thrombosis, and skin infections.

Physical Methods.—These include Massage and Movement and Electrical treatment.

Methods of treatment may be summed up as follows:—

Massage is not often used during the early stages. In the lower limb, particularly, it is often impossible because of the inaccessibility of the part and there is also the risk that it may disturb the repair processes and lead to non-union. It can, however, materially add to the patient's comfort by reducing swelling and relieving tension and pain in the muscles—particularly those proximal to the fracture site. If given for this purpose it should be of a sedative nature, gentle and rhythmical, great care being exercised near the fracture site, *the site itself being rigorously avoided.* Massage is sometimes ordered by the surgeon, *before* the application of plaster in order to reduce swelling, but this is not usual.

Movements: All joints other than those fixed by the plaster must be *exercised freely and frequently.* This is especially important in the case of the hand and fingers and of the foot and toes, or whilst lying in bed with apparatus attached to the lower limb. Slings or pulleys may often be usefully employed in such treatment.★

It is extremely important to see that a correct gait is taught when a plaster or appliance is worn. Apart from the fact that bad habits are easily formed but only broken with difficulty, an incorrect gait throws strain on the joints. This inevitably causes trauma, which can give rise to arthritic changes if it is allowed to persist.

It is most important that the normal amount of dorsiflexion of the ankle should be maintained, not only to prevent stiffness, but to assist venous return through the mechanical action afforded by contraction of the muscles, particularly those in the calf.

The patella, if not enclosed in plaster, should be kept mobile by means of *passive movements.* An adherent patella may be one of the worst factors of a stiff knee. It should be moved laterally and, if possible, up and down as well.

Those joints which must be fixed in order to retain the fragments in position can only be moved after the period of immobilization is ended; but it is generally possible to exercise the muscles by means of static contractions, e.g., quadriceps contractions when the knee is fixed, or gluteal contractions in an injury near the hip. Static contractions not only help to prevent disuse atrophy and keep cortical pathways alert, but by contracting fibres against the pressure of the plaster a slight impetus is given to venous and lymphatic return by alterations in pressure. This helps to reduce œdema. The bone-ends also tend to become compressed.

Any postural faults must be corrected. Some patients tend to develop these whilst wearing a sling or plaster. It should be remembered that fractures of the lower extremity may involve long periods in bed; also, many of the patients are elderly. A general scheme of exercises may need to be included in the treatment. To this end pulleys and slings fixed over the patient's bed are helpful.

In any muscle re-education the importance of the anterior horn cells should not be forgotten and proprioceptive facilitation should be given by placing the hands on the surface in the direction of movement, slight traction being given and where possible the muscle being put on the stretch, *but in cases of fracture the two*

★ *See* Olive F. Guthrie-Smith, *Rehabilitation, Re-education, and Remedial Exercises.* This book should be studied by all interested in rehabilitation of the injured. Full accounts are given of suspension, pulley, and spring therapy, as well as of other special methods of re-education. *See also* J. C. H. Colson, *Rehabilitation of the Injured,* Vol. II, Chapters IX–XI.

latter should never be attempted if there is the slightest danger of straining the callus.

Electrical Treatment.—

Faradism is sometimes applied while the limb is still immobilized, in order to obtain muscle contractions, without causing a movement in any joint.

Heat is invaluable in relieving pain and muscle spasm. It will also assist circulation and help fluid absorption. Infra-red radiation, radiant heat, and short-wave diathermy may all be used.

Light.—Ultra-violet light may be given in cases where there is an infected wound.

Some form of recreational therapy is valuable during a long period of recumbency. It may be necessary to train certain muscle groups for the use of aids or appliances, e.g., the use of crutches and re-education in walking.

Treatment after Immobilization.—The aim now is final rehabilitation. The accent is on movement at this stage. Following removal of the plaster there will be a certain amount of residual stiffness, and *full mobility must be regained in all previously immobilized or restricted joints.* The patient may need re-education in the correct use of the limb, since stiffness can lead to the development of some bad muscular habit or abnormal joint movement, e.g., he may compensate for stiffness in the humeroscapular articulation by movement in the sternoclavicular and acromioclavicular joints; or replace true abduction by the deltoid and supraspinatus by elevation and rotation of the scapula, using the trapezius and other elevator muscles. It should be stressed that *before any re-education of a limb is undertaken an assessment of movement in the sound limb should be made to discover the normal range, since this varies with the individual.*

Because of the long immobilization period in fractures of the lower limb, there is a greater need for intensive rehabilitation. There is often more residual stiffness, and since the glutei and quadriceps waste quickly and considerably, despite measures taken to counteract the effect of inactivity, their power must be fully regained.

When considering any form of maintenance of power or re-education of the quadriceps *it is important to remember the action of vastus medialis in achieving the last degree of extension necessary to a stable knee.* In this respect it is well to remember the associated action required of vastus medialis to stabilize the tibia during resisted contraction of the tibialis anterior. By making use of *this* associated action it is possible to assist the re-education of vastus medialis, though the muscle itself may be immobilized.

Spring-resistance exercises have been found very helpful, and can be adapted to the requirements of any patient—though it must be remembered that the resistance of a spring is always weakest at the beginning of a movement and strongest at its end, which, from an exercise point of view, is incorrect. (*See* Chapter XXIII.)

Heat may be given to assist circulation, and to relieve pain. Besides the forms used during immobilization, wax baths and immersion in warm water will be found invaluable since the whole area or joint surface can be treated.

Massage is often required and should be deep and vigorous, frictions being given around the joint. If the skin is very dry lanoline or oil massage will improve its condition.

Movement: *Passive movements* may be required to regain mobility, and may be followed by *active assisted movements* but *forced movements should never be given, unless expressly ordered by the surgeon in charge of the case. Resisted exercises and free mobility exercises* must be given to build up muscle power and regain mobility. In the case of the lower limb, it is usual to leave the patient free in bed for a week or two, in order to regain range and power. *Faradism* may be given in the later stages to help in the restoration of power *but it must never be allowed to take the place of voluntary movement.* If posture has been checked it should cause no anxiety at this stage.

The patient should return as soon as possible to his or her habitual occupation. Treatment is often combined with occupational therapy and if necessary the rehabilitation may be completed at a special Occupational Therapy Centre. Such occupations as rug-making, weaving, basket-making, leather work, etc., are taught, while if the patient can never hope to use his hands for the work he was doing before his accident, he should be trained for some other trade or occupation in which he can take an interest.

FRACTURES OF THE UPPER EXTREMITY

Splinting and Support.—Most fractures of the upper extremity are now put up in plaster-of-Paris or merely supported in a sling, but internal splintage is also frequently used. The physiotherapist should be familiar with all forms of slings or similar supports and should be able to bandage into place securely, comfortably, and without constricting the circulation, any splint with which she may be confronted.

It has been seen in the previous chapter that the *time* for which the supporting apparatus is retained in any particular case varies according to the nature and severity of the injury, the age and constitution of the patient, the evidence of union supplied by the X-rays, and the views of the surgeon in charge of the case. Only approximate dates for its removal can therefore be given in the text.

THE CLAVICLE

The clavicle is most commonly fractured at about the middle of the shaft, or at the junction of its middle and outer third, generally due to a fall on the hand; that is, to indirect violence. It is fractured far less frequently at the acromial extremity, and less often still at the sternal extremity. The clavicle being a highly vascular bone, union occurs in two to three weeks. Callus forms in excess and results in a noticeable bony lump over the fracture site.

The outer fragment is depressed by the weight of the arm, and carried forward and inward; the inner fragment is held firmly in place by the rhomboid ligament.

Fixation is achieved by bandages which brace the shoulders back—the commonest method being the 'handkerchief method' (*Fig.* 6). A large arm sling is usually worn as well. Both can generally be discarded in 2 weeks, though the sling may be continued for a further week.

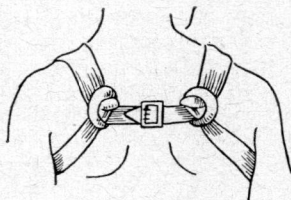

Fig. 6.—'Handkerchief' method of supporting a fracture of the shaft of the clavicle.

From the point of view of physiotherapy this fracture is treated mainly as a soft-tissue injury. In some hospitals the physiotherapist is only asked to adjust the braces. Where physiotherapy is ordered it is chiefly directed towards regaining full shoulder movement as soon as possible. There is no danger of displacement occurring and full mobility should be regained in a week.

In cases where it is desirable that there should be no excess callus formation or sign of deformity (e.g., in models), the patient lies flat in bed with a sand-bag between her shoulders, the arm being kept in slight abduction or by the side. The patient remains in this position for 3 weeks, no movement of the shoulder being allowed.

The clavicle may also be fractured at the acromial and sternal extremities but these are rare. Treatment is similar to that for the shaft but progress is usually a little quicker.

THE SCAPULA

The body of the scapula is usually the part injured. Fractures of the neck, acromion process, and glenoid cavity are rare. Scapular fractures are usually caused by direct violence. Displacement is very slight as a rule, because of the support afforded to the fragments by the large number of muscles attached to the scapula. For this reason fixation is not usually required. The arm is supported in a large arm sling for one to two weeks, depending on the surgeon's views.

There is little or no danger of displacement and it is essential to restore shoulder mobility as soon as possible to prevent adhesions forming. If allowed to form, they will be very strong and disabling, and will probably necessitate manipulation under an anæsthetic. Even so, the result is not always entirely satisfactory. *Movements* will be given to all joints of the arm and shoulder as for fracture of the clavicle. Full range of movement in the shoulder-joint should be regained in about 10 days, but treatment must continue until this is achieved.

For Kabat techniques for use on the shoulder-joint *see* pp. 130, 131.

THE HUMERUS

The humerus may be fractured at so many different levels that it is impossible to consider all the injuries. At the upper extremity, fractures involve the neck or great tuberosity. The shaft may be fractured at its upper, middle, or lower third, while at the lower extremity we meet with supracondylar fracture, T- or Y-shaped fracture into the elbow-joint, fractures of either condyle, and separated lower epiphyses. We shall deal briefly with fracture of the neck, of the middle third of the shaft, and fractures round the elbow-joint.

Fractures of the Upper Extremity of the Humerus

These fractures are commonly seen in elderly women, and are usually caused by a fall on an outstretched arm, i.e., indirect violence. There are three common fractures in this region. Various classifications are adopted by various surgeons. Watson-Jones classifies them as: (1) *Contusion crack fractures*, with a contusion of the great tuberosity, and a crack across the neck, generally without displacement (*Fig.* 7 A). (2) *Adduction fractures*, high in the neck, with slight outward angulation of fragments and impaction on the inner side, limiting abduction (*Fig.* 7 B). (3) *Abduction fractures*, with inward angulation, generally slight, and impaction on the outer side, always accompanied by fracture of the great tuberosity (*Fig.* 7 C). Greater degrees of displacement than those shown in the diagram may occur. The fracture may be unimpacted, and the great tuberosity is sometimes, though rarely, fractured alone.

The important factor from the point of view of treatment is whether or not the fragments are impacted. If the fracture is impacted there is generally no need for reduction or fixation and, bearing in mind the age of the patient, it is essential to prevent adhesions forming in the joint. From the nature of the displacement there will be residual limitation of joint range, but in the elderly patient this is not usually a great handicap. Where there is separation of the fragments the treatment depends on the surgeon's views. Some surgeons treat such cases by reduction and fixation; others treat them by early movement.

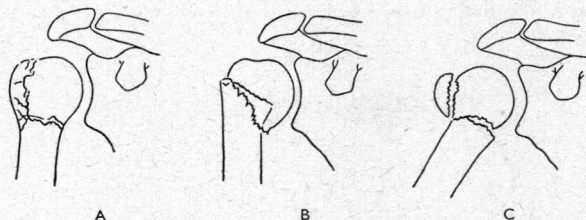

Fig. 7.—Fractures of the neck of the humerus. A, Contusion crack fracture; B, Adduction fracture; C, Abduction fracture.

IMPACTED FRACTURES

There is no need for reduction or fixation, but the arm is supported in a sling for about a week. It is important to remember that elderly patients are very liable to be considerably shocked, and that strange situations fluster and confuse them. They need time to adjust themselves and to gain confidence. On the other hand, these patients should be made to understand that their recovery depends as much on their own efforts as those of the physiotherapist.

The patients are most comfortably treated in the half-lying position, or sitting with the arm comfortably supported. The full-lying position is often precluded by the condition of the heart or lungs. There is a great deal of bruising over the shoulder and down the arm and there may be considerable accompanying effusion. Heat and massage may be usefully employed to disperse fluid, to soothe the patient, and to make her more comfortable. Massage should be gentle and rhythmical and should include the whole arm and shoulder region. Great care must be taken around the fracture site, the actual site being avoided. *Shoulder movements* should be given as for a fractured clavicle and the use of the fingers, hand, and forearm must be encouraged. Later when all movements can be performed actively, pulleys, slings, free mobility exercises, and resisted movements can be given to increase range and power, but full range should not be expected.

UNIMPACTED FRACTURES

Adduction Fractures (see Fig. 7 B)

Here the *upper fragment* is *abducted* by the supraspinatus, the *lower* fragment *adducted* by the pectoralis major, etc.

The treatment adopted will depend on the surgeon. Any of the following may be used: (1) No fixation, the arm being supported in a sling for 7–10 days. Shoulder movements are given from the beginning. (2) After closed reduction, the arm is supported in a sling for 3 weeks, by which time the callus is firm enough to splint the fracture. No shoulder movements are allowed for 3 weeks. (3) Following closed reduction the arm is supported in a plaster spica, with the arm in abduction and the hand near the mouth, or on an abduction frame. All free joints must be exercised and static contractions taught to immobilized muscles. Full mobility must be regained after immobilization.

Abduction Fractures (see Fig. 7 C)

The *upper* fragment is not abducted in these cases; the *lower* fragment is abducted by the deltoid. Methods of treatment depend entirely on the surgeon's views. Those who advocate *early movement* support the arm in a sling and allow shoulder movements from the beginning. During shoulder movements the fracture site must be carefully supported, and the weight of the arm taken. (*See* Fig. 8.) Those who follow more *conservative lines* allow no shoulder movements for 3 weeks.

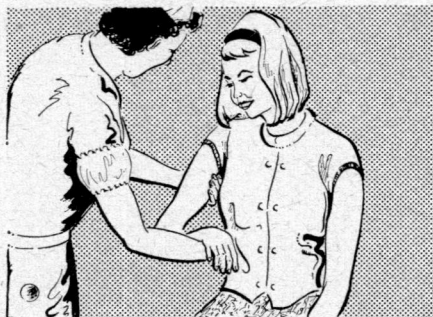

Fig. 8.—Showing the operator's method of support while giving movements to a case of fractured upper extremity of humerus. The same grasp may be used for a dislocated shoulder, with stronger upward pressure in the axilla.

COMPLICATIONS.—Dislocation of the shoulder, involvement of the axillary vessels or the circumflex nerve, or, more rarely, of the radial (musculospiral) nerve may accompany any fracture of the upper extremity of the humerus. (For treatment *see* Chapter XII.)

Fracture of the Shaft of the Humerus

This may be caused by direct or indirect violence and the fracture may be at any level. The typical fractures are: (*a*) Fracture of upper third, below the surgical neck; (*b*) Fracture of the middle third, above or below the insertion of the deltoid; (*c*) Fracture of the lower third (supracondylar fracture). (*See* Fractures around the Elbow-joint.)

FRACTURE OF THE MIDDLE THIRD OF THE SHAFT

The cause may be direct or indirect violence, the fracture line accordingly being transverse or spiral. A transverse fracture is considered here. Spiral fractures will be treated similarly but union will occur in 3 weeks, and treatment is therefore progressed more quickly.

The displacement is lateral, with overlapping of the fragments. If the fracture is *above the level of insertion of the deltoid*, the upper fragment is drawn inwards by the adductors; if *below* this level, it is drawn outwards (abducted) by the deltoid, while the lower fragment is drawn upwards by the combined action of the triceps, biceps, and coracobrachialis (*Fig.* 9).

Methods of fixation are many and varied ranging from internal fixation, some form of plaster cast or splint, or sling alone and, again, depend on the surgeon's views. Immobilization will be continued until *union* in 6 weeks but, since *consolidation* will not occur for another 6 weeks, some form of protection will be required after immobilization. Throughout the elbow must be flexed to 90° whether in plaster or by sling alone.

Physical treatment will depend on the method of fixation used and on the surgeon's wishes, but *no abduction of the shoulder should be given for 3 weeks.* When it is allowed, the fracture site should be well supported.

COMPLICATIONS.—*Delayed union* or *non-union*, often due to some fibres of the triceps being caught between the broken ends of the bone. *Injury to the radial (musculospiral) nerve,* either at the time of fracture, or, more often, by its involvement in the forming callus. In the first case symptoms appear at once, or almost at once; in the second, about 10 days after the accident. They must be reported at once to the surgeon in charge of the case.

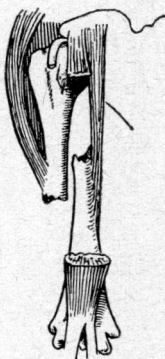

Fig. 9.—Displacement in fracture of middle of shaft of humerus.

Treatment of Delayed Union.—The shoulder and elbow are generally immobilized in plaster for 5 or 6 months. Movements of the fingers and wrist must be practised assiduously; the shoulder and elbow are exercised when the fixation period is ended.

Treatment of Non-union.—This is not a very common complication, but if union is long delayed, or does not take place at all, special treatment is needed. If the patient is suffering from any general or local disease, he will receive appropriate medical attention, but the trouble is more often due to interposition of muscular fibres between the fragments, to failure to immobilize them adequately or failure to prevent strain on the site of fracture. One of the following operations may be performed: (1) Excision of fibrous tissue and roughening of the bone-ends. (2) Beck's bone drilling. A number of holes are drilled in both bone-ends. This sets up an inflammatory reaction and promotes callus formation at the line of fracture. The arm is then put in plaster, and treated as a recent fracture. (3) Introduction of an intramedullary bone-peg. (4) Bone-grafting. (5) The last two methods combined.

Radial nerve injury. For treatment *see* Chapter XII.

FRACTURES AROUND THE ELBOW-JOINT

Fractures in the region of the elbow-joint include supracondylar fracture; T- or Y-shaped fracture into the joint; fractures of the olecranon and head or neck of radius. They need very careful handling *and certain principles are common to all.* Because of the danger to vital structures in the region, either due to the initial injury, to pressure, or to injudicious movement, and because of the danger of myosotis ossificans, the patient should be seen daily for a week. Careful watch must be kept for any danger signals, and any adverse symptoms reported immediately.

Following reduction the arm is put into flexion and supination (*see Fig.* 10), the degree depending on the views of the surgeon. Because of swelling, the desired amount may have to be obtained gradually during the first week. Once it is obtained it is maintained until union. *No elbow movements are allowed* during the period of fixation, with the possible exception of rotation in the forearm

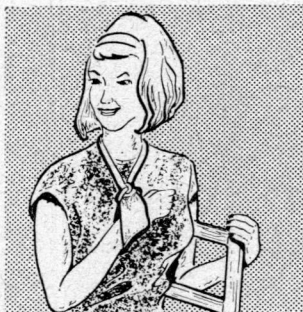

Fig. 10.—'Collar-and-cuff' method of support. The hand can be kept in supination by means of adhesive strapping.

If there is any danger of displacement, shoulder movements should only be allowed in a very small range and with the assistance of gravity, but the fingers, hand, and wrist must be exercised constantly. Protection is usually required until consolidation. If, however, the radiographs show good progress elbow movements may be given and the sling is gradually lowered before this. It is of vital importance that the ability to gain full flexion is maintained. *Any decrease in range, or any limitation of movement must be reported at once.* When the sling can be discarded progression is made in the form of increased activity.

Danger Signals.—Watch must be kept for the following signs: *Any exacerbation of pain; any limitation of range; any spasm of biceps.* These may indicate myositis ossificans, or Volkmann's ischaemic contracture. If the only sign is limitation of range, the arm is usually rested in the original position for 24 hours. If range is still limited it is treated for myositis ossificans.

COMPLICATIONS.—

1. *Myositis ossificans.*
2. *Volkmann's ischæmic contracture.*
3. An *ulnar* or *median nerve involvement* at the time of injury, or during healing.

For treatment *see* Chapter XII.

Myositis Ossificans

This, in the first place, consists of ossification of the hæmatoma which forms beneath the periosteum. Injudicious movement, or insecure fixation of the fracture in the early stages, may lead to loosening and dissipation of this ossifying mass, so that, instead of remaining fixed to the bone, it may impinge upon or penetrate other structures, and may thus seriously interfere with the movements of the joint. The condition is always a possibility after injuries in the region of the elbow, and it may occur in other parts also, e.g., around the hip after fractures or dislocations, or involving the quadriceps in injuries to the knee-joint. Its aetiology is not well understood. In fact, the term 'myositis ossificans' has been used to cover several different conditions. These include:* (1) New bone formed in the neighbourhood of displaced bony or cartilaginous fragments, e.g., in comminuted fractures. (2) Widespread formation of new bone in tissues involved in the hæmatoma of a fracture (*see* p. 10). (3) Small scattered areas of bone in muscular tissues some way from the fracture. True myositis ossificans is an *acute inflammatory* condition, in which new bone is laid down in the region of a fracture. A common site is the brachialis muscle after an elbow injury, or occasionally the supinator in a fracture of the head of the radius. Bone-cells escape into these muscles, and in due time ossify. What exactly happens to cause the condition is not clear. There may be a local excess of calcium in the tissues, and true myositis ossificans may be due to vasomotor changes. Contributing factors may be: (1) Insecure fixation of the joint, or fixation in an unsuitable position, i.e., with insufficient flexion and supination. It has been known to occur as the result of a patient wearing an internal angular splint after removal of the head of the radius following a fracture. (2) Too early, or too vigorous, movement of the elbow or radio-ulnar joint, or too heavy massage in the vicinity. The subject can be studied in the work referred to below, or in other works on fractures.

What is important to us as physiotherapists is *to realize that any damage to a muscle in the vicinity of a fracture of the elbow may result in that muscle becoming the seat of one or other form of 'myositis ossificans', and that any injudicious movement causing further injury in that area increases that possibility.*

Symptoms.—
In the early stages: (1) Increase of pain; (2) Decrease of mobility; (3) Local tenderness; (4) Local œdema. *Later*, as soon as definite ossification begins, the X-rays will reveal the presence of bone in the muscle, and at this stage the mass can be often felt with the fingers. In some cases, there are no acute symptoms, and the only sign is a decreasing range of movement.

Treatment.—In suspected cases the affected area should be rested and the elbow put in flexion and supination, maintained by a 'collar-and-cuff' or a sling. No movements should be given to the elbow or radio-ulnar joints for 14 to 21 days in most cases.

If this unfortunate complication *has* arisen, the only safe form of treatment is to rest the part completely, keeping the elbow fixed in flexion and supination for many months (possibly six), in hopes that the surplus bone will be absorbed. If this treatment is successful, active movements may be encouraged when the fixation apparatus is removed. In the opinion of some surgeons, slighter (painless) cases may be left free, but the patient must avoid heavy work, and *no attempt must be made either by the physiotherapist or the patient himself to stretch the elbow forcibly.* He should be cautioned not to carry heavy weights.

Sometimes, if the mass of bone is not absorbed and the movements of the joint are greatly impaired the surgeon decides to remove the bone. The operation does not as a rule take place until some months have elapsed, so that ossification may be complete and the risk of recurrence minimized. Even so, there is a great tendency for the surplus bone to re-form, as the periosteum must of necessity be injured again at the operation. In slighter cases, the disability is often not serious enough to require surgical interference.

Volkmann's Ischæmic Contracture

This condition is much more common in the forearm and hand than elsewhere. It consists of a contracture of muscles, together with nerve injury, and is due to

* J. C. Bonnin, *Fractures and Related Injuries*, Chapter VI.

occlusion of the arteries and veins in the limb. It is commonest in children, generally in those under 12 years of age, though it may occur in adults. The exact aetiology is unknown, but it appears that a focus of irritation is set up in the musculature of the artery. This leads to a contraction of the vessel and stoppage of the blood-supply. It probably spreads to collateral vessels so that both main and subsidiary vessels are occluded. There is a temporary stoppage of both arterial and venous circulation in the area (a complete stoppage would cause gangrene). The actual cause of the irritable focus is unknown but it may be: (1) *Pressure on the vessels* by splints, or tight bandages, particularly in the region of the elbow; (2) *Injury to the brachial arteries* at the time of the fracture; (3) *Latent disease in the vessel*.

Pathological Changes are found in the muscles, nerves, and skin. Nervous tissue is highly susceptible to oxygen lack. It quickly dies and becomes fibrosed. Next the muscles degenerate and die, their place being taken by fibrous tissue. (In severe cases nerves and muscles are seen as a mat of fibrous tissue.) Later trophic changes appear in the skin (*see* p. 5).

At the time of onset there is *severe and increasing pain*. This is the only constant factor. Any, all, or none of the following symptoms may be present: (1) The hand and fingers become swollen and discoloured—first red, then blue— and blebs (blisters) appear; (2) Absence of the radial pulse; (3) Spasm of muscles, in which case the limb has a hard 'woody' feeling; (4) Loss of muscle extensibility. A very short time (3–4 hours only) suffices for irreparable harm to be done.

Within 24 hours the condition of Volkmann's ischæmic contracture will be present. The arm is held with the elbow flexed; the forearm pronated; the wrist flexed and the hand clawed. That is to say the metacarpophalangeal joint is hyperextended and the fingers are flexed. The fingers can only be straightened if the wrist is fully flexed. The flexor tendons stand out like whip-cords. There is no pulse and motor and sensory activity is lost. Ultimately, if nothing is done, gangrene will occur.

Prophylactic Treatment.—Great care should be taken in applying splints, bandages, or plaster, especially in children. They must not be too tight anywhere. If swelling is still present, or likely to be present later, allowance must be made for it. If a short anterior forearm splint, or plaster, has been applied, the physiotherapist should see that its upper end does not press on the structures at the bend of the elbow. In any case of elbow fracture the following procedure should be observed:—

1. Following the application of splints or bandages the radial pulse should be taken at the wrist, and its strength compared with that in the opposite limb. The finger should be pressed on the patient's hand, so as to whiten the part, and the operator should see if the blood returns immediately on removal of the pressure. If there is the least doubt the splint or bandage should be removed and reapplied. It is far better do do so needlessly than to risk such serious harm to the patient.

2. No *child* ought to be allowed to leave hospital for at least twenty-four hours after his fracture has been splinted or put into plaster for the first time. In any case, the patient, or his parents, should be warned to report *immediately* to his doctor if there should be—*at any time*—any sign of pain, œdema, or discoloration.

3. If any such signs are noticed, the physiotherapist should let the doctor know at once, and pending his arrival the bandages, splints, or plaster must be removed.

Treatment in Suspected Cases.—Heat should be applied to the other limbs and trunk to promote general vasodilatation (Adams).* A radiograph should be

---

* *Outline of Fractures*, Chapter V.

taken to establish the alinement of the fracture. If it is displaced it must be reduced at once. If the circulation has not improved within an hour the brachial artery is explored (Bonnin). If the vessel is kinked it will be freed; if punctured or thrombosed, the injured part may be removed, and the two ends sutured, or an arterial graft inserted.

Post-operative Treatment: The mobility regained at the operation must be maintained. Passive and active assisted movements should be given to the fingers, hand, wrist, and forearm, and muscle power must be built up in the flexor and extensor groups. Faradism may be used to stimulate individual muscles if the nerve is conducting, or interrupted direct current if there is no nerve conduction. Sinusoidal or whirlpool baths may also be used. Provided the unaffected arm is used as a control, short-wave diathermy using a longitudinal field, or contrast baths, may also be applied. Massage as described for treatment of established cases may be given effectively.

The prognosis is not good in established cases, but a substantial improvement can often be obtained by splinting, the following Robert Jones method or some variant of it being used.

First Position.—The wrist and metacarpophalangeal joints are fully flexed, and the interphalangeal joints are extended. The fingers are separately splinted in this position.

Second Position.—A splint reaching to the wrist is applied over the finger-splints, the metacarpophalangeal joint being now extended. The wrist is still flexed.

Third Position.—A splint is put on over the others from finger-tips to elbow. It is gradually altered as the wrist is brought from flexion to hyperextension, the final position being maintained for some weeks.

A similar result may be obtained by means of successive plasters.

The hand may be massaged whenever the splints or plaster are removed for alteration, and the arm and forearm should be treated daily. The extensors of the wrist may receive stimulating massage, *but the flexor aspect of the forearm must be treated with gentleness*, kneading—with the palm of the hand or with the fingers—and effleurage being the best movements. It is well to soak the patient's arm in hot water before treatment, in order to soften the tissues. The whirlpool bath, if available, is better still. The heat of the water must be carefully regulated, as the patient's sensation may be subnormal or absent. *Passive* and *active movements* to elbow and shoulder must not be neglected. Extension of the elbow and supination of the forearm are important, as these movements are limited. (The existence of the original injury—fracture or dislocation—may, of course, have to be considered in the early stages.) When the splints are removed, stretching manipulations and active movements may be given, e.g., in the early stage when the interphalangeal joints have been splinted in extension, but the metacarpophalangeal joints are still flexed, passive and active extension are given to the latter.

T-shaped and Y-shaped Fractures into the Joint

These occur in adults, but not in children. They are the result of direct violence. The lower fragment is displaced *forward*, and the line of fracture runs down into the joint. The displacement is generally gross. Because the joint is affected many surgeons allow movement at the elbow from the beginning. If plaster is used static contractions should be given. If a sling only is used movement will be encouraged to regain congruity. Full movement in the joint is rarely recovered.

FRACTURES OF THE FOREARM BONES

Fractures may occur in the ulna or radius alone (though the latter is rare); or, more commonly, in both bones. The ulna fractures most easily in the lower one-third, the radius in the upper one-third. When a fracture occurs in both bones, the fracture line is, therefore, spiral.

Fractures of the radius result in *supination of the upper fragment* and *pronation of the lower fragment*. It is vitally important that accurate reduction is maintained, otherwise there may be *cross-union* (union of ulna with radius) in the case of fracture of both bones; or faulty union leading to *interference with the movement of the radius round the ulna*, in cases of fracture of the radius alone. For this reason many surgeons treat these fractures by internal fixation. Even so, *any rotational strain must be avoided until consolidation is well established* (6–12 weeks) and for this reason some form of plaster is also used. It will include the elbow and wrist, but the degree of flexion at the elbow and dorsiflexion at the wrist will depend on the surgeon's views.

It is important to maintain full mobility of the shoulder and hand during immobilization. Static contractions of the flexors and extensors of the wrist should be taught *but any rotational stress must be rigorously avoided.*

Colles's Fracture

This is one of the most common fractures seen in our departments and occurs most frequently in middle-aged and elderly women. It is generally the result of a fall on the outstretched hand, with the wrist extended—that is, of indirect violence. The fracture is a transverse one through the lowest inch of the radius, sometimes accompanied by a breaking off of the styloid process of the ulna. If this process is not broken, the internal lateral ligament is badly wrenched or torn. The lower fragment is displaced and rotated backwards, displaced radially and rotated radially, and displaced upwards (Slesinger). This displacement causes the typical 'dinner-fork deformity' (*Fig.* 11). The hand is also displaced, with the lower fragment of the radius, to the outer side. The fracture is often an impacted one, and is sometimes comminuted.

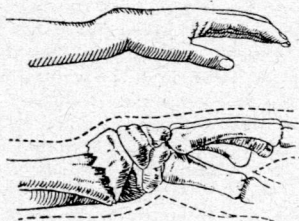

Fig. 11.—'Dinner-fork' deformity and displacement in Colles's fracture.

The wrist-joint is the seat of traumatic arthritis, and an intense synovitis of the sheaths of the flexor tendons is always present; occasionally those of the extensors are affected as well, though in a less acute degree. The wrist and hand are generally much swollen at first, and very painful. Bruising may extend well up the forearm, or even into the upper arm. There is a particularly tender point over the internal lateral ligament.

The sooner the displacement is reduced, the better are the prospects of obtaining a correct position of the lower fragment. If this remains displaced slightly backwards, as is sometimes the case, flexion will be limited, and the grip weak. Also a certain amount of visible deformity will remain.

The fracture is reduced and put up in plaster for 3–6 weeks, according to the severity of the injury, with the wrist in ulnar deviation and slight flexion. The plaster extends from just below the elbow to behind the metacarpal heads. It must not come too far up the palm of the hand, because the fingers, as well as the elbow and shoulder, must be left free. Exercises are given during this period to all free joints. Shoulder movements must be practised assiduously since *any latent damage to the shoulder can lead to serious incapacity if it is overlooked and the joint stiffens* (*see below*). In addition, full movements of the fingers and thumb, and flexion and extension of the elbow must be practised. The last-named are important, since stiffness of the fingers is very difficult to overcome once it develops. Following union the plaster is discarded and the arm may be left free.

When the plaster is removed ordinary hand and wrist exercises as for an old fracture are begun, the chief difficulty being *pronation* and *supination*. Again, wax baths or treatment in warm water help to reduce stiffness. Massage, including finger kneadings around the wrist and fingers, may also help to restore mobility.

COMPLICATIONS.—(1) *Accompanying injury to the shoulder*, consisting of a bruising of the cartilage. Pain arises in the shoulder two or three weeks after injury. (2) *Median neuritis*, with tingling and numbness of the fingers, and sometimes acute pain, as well as weakness of the thumb muscles. (3) *Rupture of the tendon of the extensor longus pollicis*, with loss of extension of the last phalanx of the thumb, produced by fraying of the tendon over the backwardly displaced lower fragment of the radius. This may not occur until 1–2 months after the fracture. (4) *Sudeck's atrophy*: The hand becomes painful, cold, and blue. The cause is unknown. It recovers spontaneously, but it may take up to 2 years.

Treatment of Complications.—If there has been considerable damage to the shoulder as well it may require specific treatment. Heat and massage may be necessary in addition to movenemts and active exercise. Sometimes treatment for a rotor cuff lesion may be necessary (*see* Chapter IV). Rupture of the extensor longus pollicis is treated by operation, the tendon of extensor indicis being transferred to the distal end of the extensor of the thumb. As soon as the plaster is removed, active movements may begin, *but no strong stretching should be given for at least 6 weeks.* Sudeck's atrophy may be treated by active exercise, but *no forced movement should be given.* Heat may prove helpful, though it sometimes aggravates the condition.

BONES OF THE WRIST AND HAND

Fracture of the Scaphoid

This is a troublesome injury, which can be most disabling if not adequately treated. Unless the fracture is efficiently immobilized until bony union has taken place, the fragments may fail to unite or a fibrous union only form between them. Pain may persist, arthritis may develop in the wrist-joint and permanent weakness may be the final result.

The scaphoid is the only carpal bone commonly fractured. It is generally broken across the middle or 'waist' by a fall on the wrist; but the tuberosity or the proximal end may also be broken. A fracture of the proximal end is the most troublesome type, since the poor blood-supply to this fragment may cause it to degenerate (*see* p. 11). (*Fig. 12.*)

There is pain and tenderness in the 'anatomical snuff-box', which takes a long time to disappear entirely. All movements of the wrist are painful, but especially abduction, and there is pain on pressure on the thenar eminence.

Treatment.—Fixation is achieved by plaster from just below the elbow to the metacarpal heads, with *the wrists in dorsiflexion, and slight adduction.* Some surgeons fix the thumb, others leave it free. If fixed, it should be in *abduction* and *opposition.* The *time* of fixation varies according to the nature of the injury,

The plaster may be retained for about 3 weeks if the tuberosity only is broken, and 6–8 weeks for the 'waist' fracture, while for the fracture of the small proximal fragment anything from 3 to 12 months may be required. The wrist is examined by X-rays at intervals, and the plaster is not removed till there is definite evidence of union. If the patient's hand feels weak and painful after removal of the plaster, it will probably be reapplied for a further period. If the plaster becomes loose during the immobilization period, it will be removed and reapplied. Physical treatment is similar to that for Colles's fracture.

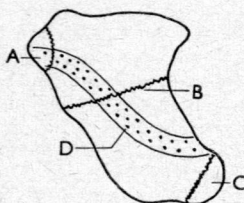

Fig. 12.—Fractured scaphoid sites of fracture. A, Tubercle; B, Waist; C, Proximal pole —it will be noticed that in this case the fragment is cut off from the area of the vascular foramina, hence the non-union at this site; D, Line of vascular foramina.

If the fracture fails to unite after adequate immobilization the bone may be *drilled* (*see* p. 23) to set up an inflammatory reaction and so promote healing, or the surgeon may insert a *bone-graft.* If the proximal fragment becomes necrotic, the fragment, or the whole bone, may be removed. Otherwise osteo-arthritis of the wrist and intercarpal joints will develop. The prognosis after this operation is not very good, and subsequent movement is rarely complete. If arthritis of the wrist and carpal joints has supervened, *arthrodesis* of the wrist is necessary. The joint is fixed in about 15 to 20 degrees of dorsiflexion (Watson-Jones). The carpal joints are also fixed, but the inferior radio-ulnar articulation must be left mobile to preserve pronation and supination. Following any of these procedures the wrist is immobilized for a period varying according to the operation performed. Physical treatment follows ordinary lines except in the case of arthrodesis of the wrist, when, naturally, no movement in this joint must be attempted.

Fractures of the other carpal bones are rare, except of the triquetral. Fractures of this bone are treated on similar lines to fractures of the scaphoid.

Fractures of the Hand and Fingers

Fractures of the hand and fingers involve the metacarpal and phalangeal bones. They result from direct violence—often of a crushing nature. They need very careful treatment, because *any stiffness or deformity will be very disabling.* Watson-Jones* emphasizes the following points with regard to finger injuries: The injured finger must be immobilized. The patient will then be willing to move the other fingers and so prevent them from becoming stiff. He must be encouraged to exercise them in full range, perseveringly, and many times a day. No finger except the injured one should be fixed. *It should be immobilized in flexion,* since, otherwise, stiffness is almost inevitable and deformity may be increased; moreover, a finger stiff in extension prevents flexion movements of the other fingers. When the fixation period is over, the injured finger must be exercised, *but its joints must never be forcibly stretched.* A garter splint applied to the damaged finger and a sound finger will assist flexion, as movement of the sound finger

* *Fractures and Other Bone and Joint Injuries.*

automatically results in movement of the damaged one. (*See Fig.* 13.) Fractures of the phalanges must be reduced and retained in the correct position with special care, because "angulation limits movement, and unreduced displacement may injure flexor tendons, obstruct their movements, or produce adhesions".

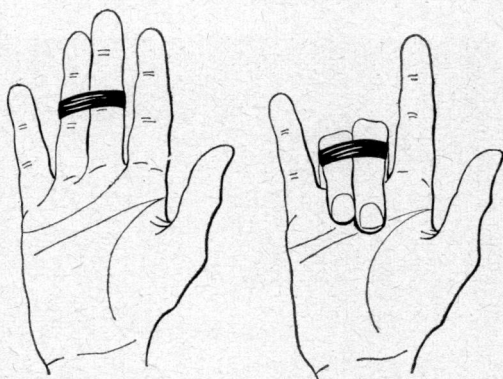

Fig. 13.—Garter splint applied to sound and damaged fingers to assist movement of latter.

CRUSHING INJURIES.—These are severe injuries with much soft-tissue damage, which result from accidents in industry and on the roads. In most of these injuries any fractures sustained take second place. Infection must be avoided wherever possible, or, if present, its spread prevented. Careful physical treatment is started as soon as possible after surgical treatment, in 3 or 5 days if possible, and follows the lines of that given for sutures and grafts (*see* Chapter V). *The important thing is to prevent œdema and adhesions, and to regain the fullest possible function.*

FRACTURES OF THE LOWER EXTREMITY

The bones of the lower limb are mainly weight-bearing ones, *therefore fixation and protection are required in most fractures.* In addition, there is often a great deal of displacement, and *traction* is often used to overcome this. This may be achieved by means of special splints, sometimes combined with weights and pulleys (Thomas splint, etc.), by skeletal traction, or by strapping. In some cases, a simple plaster gives sufficient support. Many of the splints used are modifications of the well-known Thomas type. Others, such as the Braun and Böhler splints, cannot be described in detail here, but illustrations and descriptions of those and many other types can be found in any modern work on fractures.★ *Fig.* 14 shows Böhler's modification of the Braun splint applied. *Protection* is given in the form of ambulatory plasters, or walking calipers. These are sometimes worn before union has occurred, so that the patient can get about as soon as possible. In some cases a plaster back slab or gaiter affords sufficient protection. In other cases T-straps and irons may be used.

During the immobilization period physical treatment follows the same principles as for fractures of the upper extremity, but, because the period of immobilization is of necessity longer, *the prevention of adhesions and of disuse atrophy is of even greater importance.* Pressure sores must be avoided.

★ E.g., Böhler, *The Treatment of Fractures*; Watson-Jones, *Fractures and Other Bone and Joint Injuries*; J. G. Bonnin, *Fractures and Related Injuries.*

Heat can be given to any accessible region to relieve pain and to help in the maintenance of circulation. Massage can also be given to any accessible part of the limb. It does not, of course, act as a substitute for active movement but, by improving the local circulation, it reduces swelling, helps to keep up the nutrition of the muscles, and contributes much to the patient's comfort.

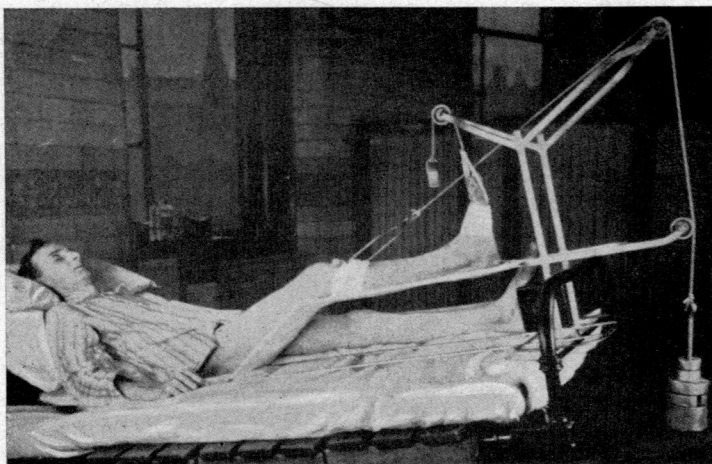

Fig. 14.—Supracondylar fracture of the femur treated in the Böhler-Braun splint.

As was seen in Chapter II, care must be taken to prevent the development of œdema in the leg when the patient resumes the upright position. To begin with, the limb must not be kept vertical for too long at a time, and if the fixation or protection allows, it is well to accustom the patient to dependent limbs by letting him sit with his legs over the side of the bed for gradually increasing periods, before attempting to stand. The time taken over this can also be used to give simple balancing exercises which will also help to prepare him for the resumption of an upright posture. Before he is allowed to take weight on the limb, he should be prepared for walking by means of suitable exercises without weight. If at any stage he walks on axillary crutches, he should be instructed in their correct use, taking the weight of his body on the hands and not in the axillæ. If the patient is able, with crutches, to take *some* weight on the injured as well as the sound leg, he should at first put the crutches and the injured limb to the ground simultaneously, and then move the sound limb forward; later he must be taught to move leg and crutch forward alternately.* It is not advisable to use *one* crutch or stick. When beginning to walk without support, he must be taught to do so correctly and without limping. Attention must be paid to the maintenance or recovery of correct posture.

THE FEMUR

As in the humerus, the femur may fracture at (1) *The neck*; (2) *The shaft* (upper, middle, or lower third); (3) *The lower extremity*, involving the knee-joint. But first it is necessary to say something about the splinting of these fractures.

* For details of Re-education in walking, and of Crutch walking, *see* pp. 49, 50.

It is essential, in almost all cases of fracture of the femur, to apply *traction* to the injured limb, in order to correct any overlapping of the bones and consequent shortening of the leg. *Traction must be maintained until union is firm*, otherwise re-displacement may be brought about by the pull of the powerful muscles of the thigh.

In applying traction to a limb, it is necessary that there should be some fixed point from which the stretching force can act—that is, as well as traction there must be *counter-traction*. This counter-traction is obtained in various ways in the different types of traction apparatus.

1. *The Thomas splint* is, in one or more of its forms, familiar to all. The simplest variety consists of a leather-covered ring, which should fit accurately round the upper part of the thigh, lying close below the tuberosity of the ischium. From this ring two side-bars pass downwards and are joined at their lower ends by a notched cross-piece. The limb is supported in the splint by flannel slings stretched between the side-bars. Two bands are affixed to the sides of the limb by means of circular strips of adhesive plaster or by some similar method. Below the level of the foot these bands are fastened to a flat piece of wood, or 'spreader', which in its turn is attached to the cross-piece at the end of the splint. Sometimes, instead of being attached directly to the end of the splint, the bands are fixed to a sliding bar placed across it. This may be drawn down by means of a screw connected to the end bar of the splint, so that the amount of traction can be increased at will (*Fig.* 15). The pressure of the ring against the ischial tuberosity provides the counter-traction. The end of the splint rests on a block or sand-bag, so that the leg is kept clear of the bed, or the leg is slung from a beam overhead. This form of splint is often used for children and young people. In adults the traction is more often applied by means of a weight and pulley. The more elaborate forms of the application of traction cannot be described here. Many of these, like the *Hodgen splint*, use the weight of the patient's body as counter-traction by raising the foot of the bed six inches, or more, on wooden blocks. This obviates the necessity of the ring pressing on the ischial tuberosity, and thus avoids the danger to the patient's skin from friction in that region. The hip may be kept more or less flexed according to the height at which it is slung from the bed. If it is to be abducted, the overhead beam is placed diagonally across the bed. In the Hodgen splint, and in some varieties of the Thomas splint, the knee is slightly flexed. The same is true of Braun's and Böhler's splints. Splints which maintain abduction of both hips are also used.

2. *Skeletal Traction.*—Instead of fastening the leg to the end of the splint, or direct to a weight and pulley apparatus, by adhesive strapping, bandages, etc., the traction is carried out by means of a steel rod taken right through the lower extremity of the femur, or through the tibial tubercle (*Fig.* 20). The varieties most commonly used are those known as the *Kirschner wire* and *Steinmann's pin*. These methods have the advantage of leaving the knee free, so that it can be moved from the beginning, and subsequent stiffness in the joint be avoided. *Counter-traction* is provided by the patient's body-weight, *the foot of the bed being raised* 1 *in. for every pound weight applied.* Thus a traction force of 20 lb. will require a 20-in. elevation of the bed.

3. '*Gallows*' splint for small children (up to 4 years). Both legs are slung up vertically, at right angles to the trunk, by means of strapping and cords to a bar over the child's bed. The weight of the body exerts the traction. Simple skin traction, avoiding the 'gallows' position, can also be used on children.

These splints often have a footpiece so arranged that the foot is kept at a right angle with the leg. Great care must be taken in restoring to its correct position any part of the apparatus which has been removed for treatment.

2

No weights must ever be removed or allowed to assume a position in which they cease to exert a traction force, e.g., resting on the foot of the bed. The care of the patient's skin is the responsibility of the physiotherapist, and this needs special attention in cases where counter-traction is obtained by pressure on the tuberosity of the ischium. The skin should be drawn upwards or downwards from under the ring, so that the same part does not always receive the pressure.

OTHER METHODS OF FIXATION.—

Plaster.—This usually takes the form of a complete plaster cast extending from the groin to the heads of the metatarsals.

Ambulatory plasters are used to support the site of the fracture, and enable the patient to walk without putting weight on it. In walking plasters the heel is thickened by additional layers of plaster, by a walking iron or metal stirrup, by sponge-rubber pads, etc. Transfixion pins may be incorporated in the plaster.

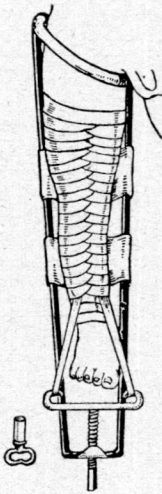

Fig. 15.—Fracture of femur treated by Thomas splint.

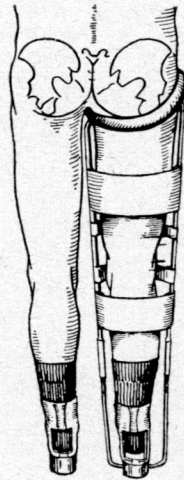

Fig. 16.—The walking caliper splint.

PROTECTION OF THE FEMUR.—

1. *Walking Plasters.*—Described above.

2. *The Walking Caliper.*—This may be used in preference to an ambulatory plaster when it is considered advisable for the patient to walk, but when union of the bone is not sufficiently strong to allow of the weight of the body being safely transmitted through the injured limb to the ground. The walking caliper resembles a Thomas splint, but the ends of the side-bars, instead of being joined by a cross-piece, are inserted into the sides of the heel of the boot (*Fig.* 16). They are of sufficient length to keep the patient's heel at least ¾ in. above the upper surface of the heel of the boot. Thus the body-weight is transmitted from the ischial tuberosity to the ring of the splint on which it rests, and thence down the side-bars through the heel of the boot to the ground. The injured leg, therefore, hangs free within the splint. The heel of the boot of the sound leg should also be raised ¾ in.

Fractures of the Neck of the Femur

Fractures in this region may take place high in the neck close to the head, or low down near the trochanters. The former corresponds to what is often called a 'subcapital' or 'transcervical' fracture, the latter to an 'intertrochanteric' fracture. The transcervical fracture is most common in elderly women and takes place as the result of indirect violence, generally of a trivial character. These fractures can further be classified as *abduction* and *adduction* fractures. The former is always an impacted fracture. In the latter union is difficult to obtain because this fracture is intracapsular, and the blood-supply to the upper fragment may be impaired. Internal fixation is therefore often employed. The intertrochanteric fracture occurs most frequently in working men of middle age, and is usually caused by direct violence, e.g., a blow on the great trochanter.

ABDUCTION TRANSCERVICAL FRACTURE.—This is generally the result of a fall on the great trochanter. The fracture is always at a high level. *The lower fragment is rotated outward.* It is invariably impacted and any attempt to take weight on the leg impacts it further, because the line of the fracture is nearly horizontal, i.e., almost at right angles to the direction of pressure of the body-weight (*Fig. 17 A*). Therefore this fracture does not tend to become displaced and unites quickly in about 7 or 8 weeks.

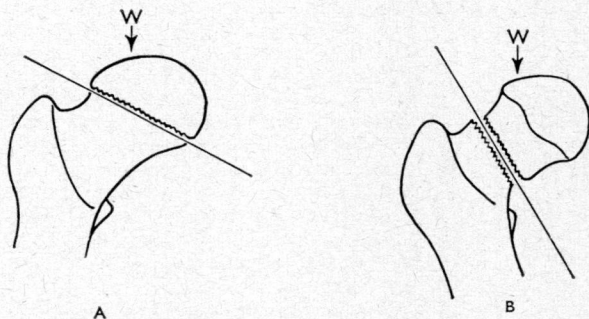

Fig. 17.—Fractures of femoral neck. A, Horizontal line of fracture in abduction transcervical fracture; the arrow indicates the direction of the body-weight, tending to cause impaction of the fragments. B, Vertical line of fracture in adduction transcervical fracture; the weight tends to produce further slipping of the upper fragments on the lower.

Since weight-bearing tends to increase the impaction, and therefore to assist union, these fractures are usually treated without fixation. If, however, there is any possibility of disimpaction, fixation is given in the form of a Smith-Petersen nail. Protection, as such, is not required but the patient will walk with sticks or crutches to begin with. Although, technically, there is no bar to the patient taking weight immediately it is usual to allow the patient to remain in bed for a varying period, depending on the surgeon's views. In cases without fixation some surgeons allow the patient to get up and to take weight as soon as she can lift the leg off the bed and circumduct it. Others prefer to keep the patient in bed for 2–3 weeks. Similarly, following nailing some surgeons allow weight-bearing at once, others only allow partial weight-bearing until union occurs. The patient should be completely restored to normal by the end of three months.

From the point of view of physiotherapy, since the aim is to get the patient up as soon as possible, the accent should be on movement. Whilst the patient is in bed a general scheme of exercises should be given, to reduce the risk of any complications arising. Vigorous foot and knee movements must be practised and particular attention paid to the quadriceps extensors and abductors of the injured hip. Gentle resistance should be given to the *abductors* in particular, since they must be strong enough to allow weight-transference when the patient walks again.

Crutch Walking.—Whether or not the patient is allowed to bear weight fully, it is essential to see that she takes even steps when she first begins to walk with crutches or sticks. Re-education in walking may be required when the crutches or sticks are discarded.

ADDUCTION TRANSCERVICAL FRACTURE AND INTERTROCHANTERIC FRACTURE.— The fracture line is more vertical than in the abduction transcervical fracture. The displacement is common to both transcervical and intertrochanteric fractures. The lower fragment is *adducted, displaced upwards*, and *rotated outwards*. The pain and disability at the time of the accident are severe. The external rotation is marked. The movements are very limited, and there is some degree of shortening. The degree of shortening is clinically the only distinguishing feature, it being greater in the intertrochanteric than in the transcervical fracture. Since the line of fracture in these cases is nearly vertical (*Fig.* 17 B), weight-bearing tends to increase the displacement, and union does not take place so easily as in abduction fractures.

Unless the patient is unsuitable for operative treatment an open reduction is carried out and the fracture fixed internally by the Smith-Petersen nail.

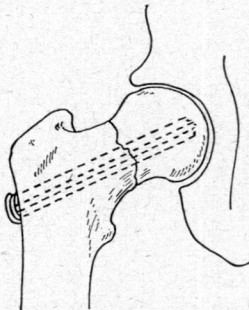

Fig. 18.—The Smith-Petersen nail.

This operation consists of the insertion of a three-flanged stainless-steel nail through the great trochanter and neck, into the head of the bone (*Fig.* 18). The three flanges prevent the nail from rotating. The hip-joint is not opened, and the operation can be done under spinal anæsthesia. Sometimes a bone-graft, taken from the patient's tibia, or consisting of part of the fibula, is inserted above the nail. Some surgeons like to prevent external rotation of the hip following the nailing operation. A slipper with a piece of wood fixed to the sole is sometimes used to prevent this.

The patient must not take full weight on the limb until the fracture is consolidated in about 6 months. Protection is therefore given by means of a walking caliper or crutches alone. Opinions vary as to whether or not partial weight-bearing can be allowed, and the physiotherapists must follow the surgeon's instructions regarding this. If allowed, it can usually begin in 2–3 months.

Knee and *foot* exercises should be given at once, and flexion of the former should be full in about a week. The patient should practise contractions of the quadriceps and of the gluteal and abdominal muscles. Since crutches are to be used, specific exercises should be given to strengthen the *triceps* and the *latissimus dorsi*. A general scheme of exercises should also be included in the treatment.

Shadow-walking should be practised until weight-bearing is allowed (*see* p. 50). In this way a stiff hip and knee can be avoided. If a weight-relieving caliper is in use this is not possible, and mobilizing exercises will be required when the caliper is discarded. When the patient actually begins to take weight on the injured leg, his standing and walking should be most carefully supervised. This is a matter which is often disregarded. *After an injury to the lower extremity every patient tends to evert his foot; everyone is a potential victim of flat-foot.* This fact cannot be too much emphasized. If necessary, the boot should be raised on the inner side.

For *re-education in walking, see* pp. 49, 50.

COMPLICATIONS.—Sometimes the operation is not successful, and union does not take place. The neck of the femur may be absorbed, the nail may extrude, and the fragments become displaced. Other operations may then be attempted—various forms of osteotomy, arthrodesis, or arthroplasty.* These cannot be described here. The treatment is similar to that given above, but must be undertaken in close co-operation with the surgeon. *Arthrodesis* needs a long period of immobilization in plaster.

TREATMENT OF OLD AND WEAK PATIENTS.—Elderly patients are not kept in bed longer than is absolutely necessary owing to their liability to develop hypostatic lung troubles, pressure sores, and cystitis. It used to be considered that a surgical operation was impracticable in their case, but Watson-Jones has pointed out that age is not in itself a contra-indication of operation, and since the introduction of the nailing operation which can be performed without causing much shock, the prospect for these patients is a great deal better. Only a very few are really unsuitable for operation. Such patients may be treated by traction but many surgeons feel that as this necessitates a long period in bed, it is better to treat the fracture as a simple abduction transcervical fracture. They therefore allow the patient to walk, with the help of crutches, believing that the resultant deformity, namely slight shortening of the leg, is preferable to the risk of prolonged immobilization in the elderly patient.

INTERTROCHANTERIC FRACTURE

Reduction and fixation can be achieved by means of traction. For skeletal traction the pin or wire is passed through the tibial tubercle. A force of 20 lb. is required. Traction must be maintained for 12 weeks. Protection in the form of crutches is required for a further 12 weeks until consolidation occurs. To obviate the lengthy mobilization period attendant on traction fixation, operative treatment is often preferred. Besides the nailing operation described above a plate is screwed to the lateral aspect of the femur. Thereafter treatment follows the lines of an adduction transcervical fracture.

For treatment during traction *see* pp. 39, 40.

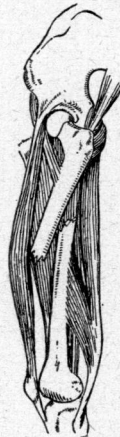

Fig. 19.—Displacement in fracture of middle of shaft of femur.

Fractures of the Shaft of the Femur

These fractures are generally the result of severe violence. They may occur at any part of the shaft, and be of any kind—transverse, oblique, spiral, or comminuted. *The displacement is usually marked, and there may be injuries to the soft tissues as well as to the bone.*

UPPER THIRD

The upper fragment is *flexed* by the psoas and iliacus, *abducted* by the glutei, and *outwardly rotated* by the short muscles attached to the great trochanter; *the lower fragment* is *adducted* and *drawn upwards.* The hip is put in flexion and abduction, and traction applied by means of special splints, or by skeletal means. Physical treatment is the same as for fracture of the middle third.

---

* See J. C. Adams, *Outline of Fractures*, Chapter VI.

MIDDLE THIRD

The upper fragment is *flexed* by the iliopsoas, and *drawn inward* by the adductors; *the lower* fragment is *tilted backwards* by the lower part of adductor magnus, and *drawn upwards* by the hamstrings and rectus femoris. There is generally a good deal of overlapping, with marked shortening of the leg (*Fig.* 19).

If traction is the selected method of fixation it must be continued for at least 12 weeks. A pillow or sling should be placed under the thigh to preserve the anterior bow of the femur. *Protection* is given by a walking caliper, by plaster, or crutches alone.

Heat may be given to any accessible parts of the limb from the beginning, but most surgeons prefer that no massage be given at all. Passive movements of the patella are essential if the knee cannot be moved actively. Active movements of

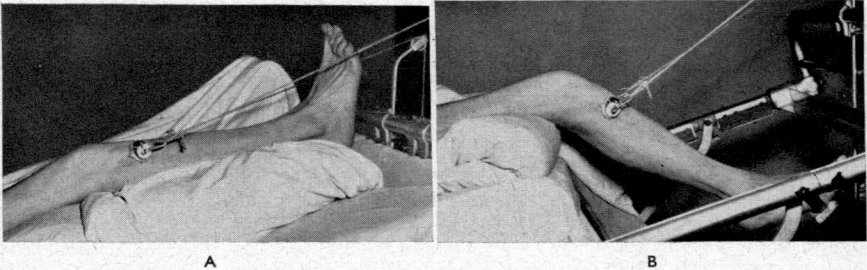

A   B

Fig. 20.—Fractured shaft of femur treated by skeletal traction. A, Patient on split bed. Pillow under knee to preserve forward bow of femur. B, Bottom half of bed removed for flexion exercises.

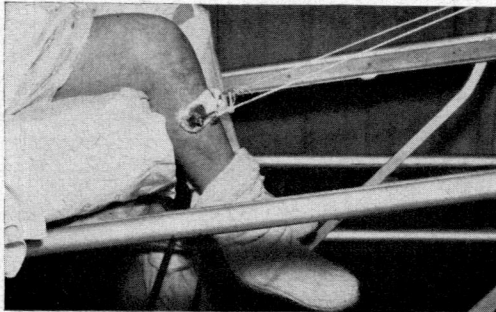

Fig. 21.—Degree of flexion which can be expected when patient is treated on split bed.

the toes, ankle, and foot must be practised assiduously. If the apparatus permits knee movements, these should be given. For ease of knee movements a split bed (*Fig.* 20 A, B) is invaluable. In this way full movement can be achieved, as the split bed allows complete removal of the lower half during treatment (*Fig.* 21). Some of the special splints are hinged to allow knee movements, but if the bed is not of the split type the degree of range obtainable is necessarily limited. *Knee flexion will not be attempted until control of the quadriceps is achieved*, i.e., the patient can straight-leg raise. Until this is possible the quadriceps cannot control the femur eccentrically during flexion of the knee and delayed union or non-union would result. *It will be found that straight-leg raising is not achieved until union is firm enough to splint the fracture naturally*, i.e., in 2–3 weeks, when fibrous union is established. Static contractions of glutei and quadriceps must be practised and abdominal contractions, arm movements, and a general scheme of exercises taught. An overhead rope is helpful as it allows the patient to lift himself up the bed and to change his position in the bed. For treatment after removal of apparatus *see* pp. 18, 49, 50, and 63.

Because the traction method means a lengthy period in hospital, internal fixation is often used. For this the Küntscher nail is used. This is a long nail, almost the length of the shaft of the femur, which is driven through the great trochanter and down the shaft (*Fig.* 22). Post-operative treatment is the same as for adduction trans-cervical fracture, in that the patient is allowed up once control of the limb is regained, full or partial weight-bearing being allowed according to the surgeon's wishes.

Fractures Round the Knee-joint

These are similar to fractures round the elbow-joint and include *supracondylar fracture* (lower third femur); T-*shaped fracture into the joint*; *fracture of the head of the tibia*; and *fracture of the patella.*

In all fractures involving the knee-joint there will be gross effusion. *It is of vital importance that adhesions are prevented and that full range, strength, and control of the joint is regained wherever possible.*

Since all these fractures involve an articular surface the treatment of choice, from the physiotherapist's point of view, is one which allows early movement, while

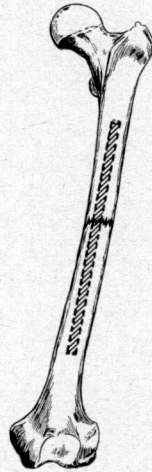

Fig. 22.—Fractured shaft of femur treated by Kuntchner nail.

maintaining reduction. This can be achieved by traction, and fortunately this method is widely adopted nowadays.

If plaster fixation is employed it will extend from the groin to the metatarsal heads. Some surgeons allow the plaster to be bi-valved in about 4–6 weeks, so that movements of knee and ankle can be given. *Protection* will be required until *consolidation*, but it is usual to allow a *gradual* resumption of weight-bearing once union has occurred.

COMPLICATIONS.—

1. *Involvement of nerves and/or vessels.*—In supracondylar fractures the medial and lateral popliteal nerves or popliteal artery may be compressed. In fracture of the tibia involving the joint, the posterior tibial nerve or vessels may be damaged. This may lead to ischæmic contracture.

2. *Non-union.*—If this happens an intra-medullary nail; a plate; bone-graft or screws will be employed. Following this the supports used are the same as for those fractures where the bones are set without operation but they have to be retained longer, since any strain on the ununited bone may loosen the screws. The patient will have to remain in bed for a longer period and will be obliged to wear a walking caliper, or use crutches, for many months.

Physical treatment is on the same lines as for the other cases. The knee should be moved as early as the surgeon will allow, otherwise the long course of fixation produces that terrible stiffness of this joint which is the despair of the unfortunate physiotherapist who is given the case some months after injury. The scar needs proper care (*see* pp. 92, 93).

THE PATELLA

Stellate Fracture; Crack Fracture; Comminuted Fracture without Separation of Fragments

These fractures are caused by direct violence, such as a fall or blow on the knee. The stellate form consists of cracks radiating outwards from the centre of the bone. *The important factor is whether or not there is rupture of the ligamentum patellæ*, since this governs whether or not the fragments are displaced (*Fig.* 23 A).

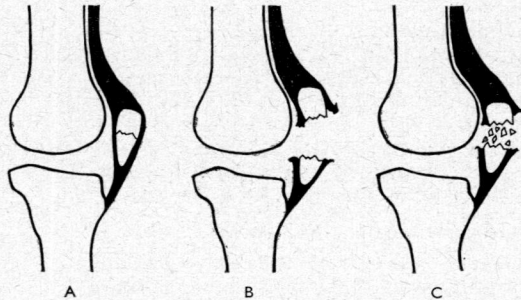

Fig. 23.—A, Crack fracture, ligamentum patellæ intact, no displacement. B, Rupture of ligamentum patellæ, separation of fragments. C, Comminuted fracture with displacement of fragments.

Fractures without displacement: There is gross effusion but since there is no displacement the injury is treated as a simple case of synovitis. The leg is put up with the knee in full extension, or just short of full extension, on a posterior plaster splint, or complete plaster from thigh to ankle, for 14 to 21 days. Walking is allowed at once, or in a few days. (The knee is sometimes aspirated, and the leg allowed to rest on a splint until the swelling subsides before being put in plaster.) There is no need for any further protection once the plaster is discarded. Some surgeons do not immobilize the knee at all. The patient remains in bed until he can hold the knee extended against resistance. He is then allowed to get up and walk.★

Exercises for the hip, ankle and toes, and quadriceps contractions are given from the beginning. *Knee movements* begin when the plaster is removed in 2 or 3 weeks. They must be given carefully at first and gradually increased in range. If the patient is on a back splint this can be removed for treatment and knee movements given, if the surgeon allows. Faradism under pressure may be given to the quadriceps in the early stages, to help dispersal of fluid. Later faradism may be used to help regain power, *but it should be combined with active contraction.*

Fracture with Separation of Fragments

These are much more serious injuries, resulting from muscular action—that is, of a sudden and strong contraction of the quadriceps whilst the knee is flexing, generally made by the patient in order to save himself from falling. The ligamentum patellæ, as well as the bone, is torn across. Therefore the *upper fragment* is *drawn up* for a considerable distance *by the quadriceps*, leaving a gap of from ½ in. to 1 in. between itself and the lower fragment (*Fig.* 23 B, C). The torn fibres of the

---

★ G. Perkins, *Fractures and Dislocations.*

ligament may interpose themselves between the broken parts and prevent bony union from taking place, even if the fragments can be brought and kept together. In fact, unless an operation is performed, fibrous union is the rule. If the gap is wide, this is a serious matter, as the extra inch or so let into the quadriceps tendon prevents these muscles from locking the knee firmly in extension, and the patient complains of its 'giving way under him'. There is always much swelling—the patella seems to lie in a bag of fluid and the gap between the fragments can easily be felt.

In nearly all cases, except those in which the patient is too old or too delicate, these fractures are treated by open operations, since it is essential to repair the torn ligament as well as the bone. One of the following is performed:—

1. SUTURE.—The upper and lower fragments are fastened together by a screw driven vertically upwards through the patella. The ligamentum patellæ is sutured with catgut.

2. EXCISION.—The whole patella is removed, and the quadriceps expansion sutured. The former method is generally used for transverse fractures in patients under 40, unless the fragments cannot be replaced in such a way as to leave the articular surface quite smooth, since an irregular surface would cause osteo-arthritis later on. In older patients (and those with comminuted fractures), excision is generally the choice, because the long immobilization period that most surgeons prefer after suture is liable to result in permanent limitation of knee movement.

> The advocates of excision, in any case, claim that it avoids osteo-arthritis of the knee, does away with the necessity for fixation, and enables the patient to exercise the knee at once, thus preserving its mobility. Other authorities maintain that among other disadvantages, the removal of the patella brings about friction between the ligamentum patellæ and the patella, thus damaging the joint.

The opinions of surgeons differ very much with regard to post-operative treatment. Some treat the case in much the same way, whether the patella has been sutured or excised. Others insist on a long immobilization period after *suture*, and only apply a bandage over wool after *excision*. Most surgeons advocate quadriceps contractions from the beginning, others allow them after about 7 days. *Flexion and extension of the knee* can be given in small range when the stitches have been removed, but must, of course, be discontinued if a walking plaster is applied.

Some surgeons prefer to immobilize the knee in a fixed plaster for 2 months. In this case, intensive knee exercises must be carried out when it is removed.

THE TIBIA

Fracture of the Shaft of the Tibia

The commonest site of fracture is between the middle and lower thirds of the bone. The injury may be the result of direct violence, producing a transverse fracture; or of indirect violence, causing one of the oblique or spiral type.

Displacement is slight as a rule, and there is no shortening if the fibula is not broken. There may be angulation, or slight rotation in the oblique fractures. Fractures of the shafts of the tibia and fibula are often compound, the subcutaneous bone-ends being driven through the skin, and are therefore liable to become infected. Skin and subcutaneous tissue damage is of great significance in the treatment of compound fractures. (*See* pp. 9, 11, 12, 44, 91.) The knee is generally put up in slight flexion, with the ankle dorsiflexed, and is retained in position by some form of plaster fixation. Internal fixation is frequently used, but plaster fixation is also required. *Protection is needed until consolidation* in another 12 weeks, and is afforded by a walking caliper, a walking plaster, or a plaster gaiter. Provided reduction is good, partial weight-bearing is usually allowed after 2–3 weeks. Some surgeons allow partial weight-bearing at once.

TIBIA AND FIBULA
Fracture of Shafts of Both Bones

This fracture is common in adults, particularly as a result of road accidents. It may be due to *direct* or *indirect violence*. In children it is generally caused by direct violence, such as being run over. This produces a transverse fracture of both bones at the same level (*Fig.* 24). There is generally much lateral displacement, and angulation may be very marked. The fracture is often compound, the broken end of the tibia protruding through the skin, or the soft tissues being severely damaged at the time of the accident.

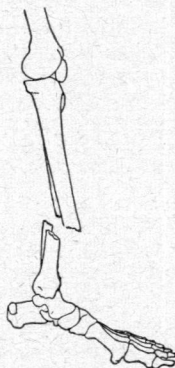

In fractures produced by indirect violence each bone gives way at its weakest part, *the tibia at the junction of its middle and lower third, and the fibula near its upper end.* The fractures are spiral or oblique. There is a good deal of overlapping, and rotation of the lower fragments is often considerable. Swelling in these fractures may be very great. This has to be taken into account when plaster is applied. A split plaster is often used to begin with, a complete, skin-tight, cast being put on when the swelling subsides.

Cases with Slight Displacement.—The leg may be in a posterior plaster, supported on a *Braun's splint* for about 14 to 21 days, or a complete plaster may be applied from the beginning. A *walking plaster is worn until union* in about 12 weeks from the date of injury. For fractures in the upper third of the leg it extends above the knee; for those in the lower third, only to the knee. *Protection* is provided, if required, by a plaster gaiter, extending from below the knee to above the ankle, or by elastoplast, etc.

Fig. 24.—Fracture of tibia and fibula.

Cases with Serious Displacement.—There is overlapping and angulation and this fracture is a difficult one to reduce. Traction will ensure alinement, but will not maintain it unless the traction force is such that non-union is inevitable. The knee is slightly flexed, and traction is applied by means of a wire or pin through the calcaneum, or from the lower end of the tibia. It is usual to apply a complete plaster as soon as alinement is stable. Some surgeons allow this to be a walking plaster, others maintain traction for a few more weeks, with the leg in the plaster cast, until firm consolidation occurs in about 6 months from the date of injury. Some form of *protection*, either the walking plaster, a gaiter, or elastoplast, must be worn. Some of these fractures are very slow in uniting, and may require even longer fixation than is described above.

Cases with Skin and Tissue Damage.—The nature and extent of the soft-tissue damage depends to a large extent on the traumatic force.* Infection leads to non-union. If, therefore, there is any risk of infection, a wound toilet is performed immediately. Any dead or devitalized tissue is excised and skin-grafts applied if necessary. *Temporary measures are applied for the fracture until the skin condition permits full treatment.* Skeletal traction is applied

---

* G. Perkins, *Fractures and Dislocations*, pp. 309–10.

through the os calcis but the weight must not be excessive. In all cases of fracture of both bones it is usual to give 10-lb. traction and a 10-in. raise. During the traction period routine physiotherapy is given. Treatment may be required for the wound (*see* Chapter V, p. 92). As soon as the state of the skin allows a complete plaster is applied and treatment continues as for a simple fracture. Should infection occur *after* the application of a plaster, the area must be exposed to allow drainage, and in order to treat the condition. To this end the plaster is usually removed and traction applied until healing occurs. In some cases a window may be cut out over the affected area, but this is rarely as satisfactory.

If the fragments cannot otherwise be got into correct position, the case is treated by open operation, the fragments of the tibia being fixed into place by a plate, wire bands, a bone-peg, or one or two screws transfixing the tibial fragments. The fibula is not plated. *Post-operative Treatment* is on the same lines as described above but the support must be even more carefully maintained.

COMPLICATIONS.—The following complications may occur:—

1. *Non-union.*—This may be due to infection; speedy union of the fibula which prevents the tibial fragments impinging on one another; too much traction; or insufficient fixation. Whatever the cause, one or other of the forms of treatment described for cases of non-union will be applied. (*See* p. 23.)

2. *Osteomyelitis.*—This is an infective condition of the bone which leads to the formation of a sinus through which pus and, later, sequestra reach the surface. Immediate treatment provides free drainage through a window in the plaster. This must be retained until the sinus heals. The leg must be rested. For late treatment *see* Chapter VII, pp. 162–3.

3. *Œdema.*—This only occurs if the leg is not fully used during the immobilization period. By giving physical treatment and seeing that it is carried out daily this complication can be avoided. If it occurs treatment for œdema is required. (*See* p. 96.)

4. *Stiff Painful Foot.*—Again, if physiotherapy has been properly carried out this should be absent. However, owing to the long period of immobilization required, and the possible infection, it is seen fairly frequently after these fractures. Treatment is described in Chapter VI, pp. 127–9.

FRACTURES ROUND THE ANKLE-JOINT

The common fractures in this region are fractures involving the lower ends of the tibia and fibula, often associated with dislocation of the ankle. The fractures considered here are: *Fracture of the medial malleolus, Pott's fracture,* and *Dupuytren's fracture.* Because these fractures involve an articular surface the principles of restoration of accurate alinement and the regaining of full mobility will apply, *but in the case of the ankle it is important to remember that it plays an essential part in the correct distribution of weight throughout the body. Any alteration in this will throw a strain on other weight-bearing joints, and in particular will affect the mechanics of the foot.* Besides paying scrupulous attention to treatment of the ankle-joint, the strength of the intrinsic muscles of the foot must be maintained.

Fracture of the Medial Malleolus

This may occur either as the result of violent inversion or eversion of the foot. In the latter case the malleolus is torn off by the drag on the deltoid ligament, which may hold while the bone gives way. This fracture is not often serious and fixation, as such, is not usually required. Elastoplast strapping or a light walking plaster is worn for support for 3–4 weeks and it is treated as a soft-tissue injury. It may be combined with a Pott's fracture and this makes it a serious injury.

Pott's Fracture

(Abduction or external rotation and adduction fractures, and fracture-dislocations of the ankle and foot)

As this heading implies, many fractures are included under the term 'Pott's fracture'.* They are caused by a violent eversion, or inversion, of the foot. The physical treatment being the same for all types, we will consider the abduction fracture. This consists of an oblique fracture of the fibula just above the inferior tibio-fibular articulation. It may be combined with either rupture of the deltoid ligament, or fracture of the medial malleolus (*Fig.* 25). It is caused by *indirect violence*—that is, by a violent eversion of the foot.

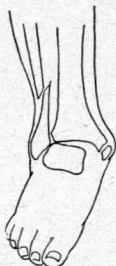

Three types of abduction fracture are recognized:—

1. *First degree abduction fracture*, in which there is no displacement, the deltoid ligament not being ruptured.

2. *Second degree abduction fracture* (the typical 'Pott's fracture'), in which the foot is displaced *outwards*. The deltoid ligament is torn, or the medial malleolus fractured, by the violent eversion strain. Hence the ankle-joint becomes insecure, the talus no longer being held firmly between the lower ends of the tibia and fibula.

Fig. 25.—Pott's fracture. Second degree abduction fracture.

3. *Third degree abduction fracture*, in which the displacement of the foot is *outward* and *backward*. The posterior margin of the tibia is fractured, and usually the medial malleolus, as well as the fibula. In this type dorsiflexion of the ankle is limited. In the severer types of abduction fracture there is much swelling and pain, with traumatic arthritis of the ankle-joint.

COMPLICATION.—Flat or weak foot may be a late complication if care is not taken to prevent this. In serious injuries there may be inevitable joint stiffness, leading later to arthritic changes.

First Degree Abduction Fracture

This is virtually treated as a sprained ankle. Fixation as such is not required and it is treated as a soft-tissue injury, the ankle being supported by adhesive strapping or a light walking plaster.

Second Degree Abduction Fracture

This fracture is easily reduced by closed manipulation, and the reduction can be maintained by a well-moulded plaster cast extending from below the knee to the metatarsal heads. A rocker is usually incorporated so that the patient can walk. Owing to swelling, a succession of plasters may have to be put on before a tight enough fit can be obtained to allow safe weight bearing. Some surgeons do not allow the patient to walk for 2–3 weeks, others allow walking quite early, i.e., during the first week. The plaster is retained for 8–10 weeks, when union should have occurred. Elastoplast, or some similar type of support, may be applied for a few weeks after this. A valgus wedge (*see* p. 260) is sometimes worn in the shoe. Treatment is basically the same as for any case immobilized by plaster. The patient must be taught to walk in the plaster without limping. This is not easy, and needs considerable skill and patience. When the plaster is removed full mobility must be regained and normal walking restored. All

---

* For a detailed description of fractures in the region of the ankle, *see* J. G. Bonnin, *Fractures and Related Injuries*, G. Perkins, *Fractures and Dislocations*, and other standard works on fractures.

exercises for flat-foot must be practised assiduously. Faradic foot baths may be a useful adjunct (*see* p. 314).

THIRD DEGREE ABDUCTION FRACTURE

All surgeons emphasize the extreme importance of correct reduction of this fracture, *since the weight-bearing function of the ankle is very gravely impaired.*

Fixation is achieved by a *plaster* cast, retained throughout; or by *skeletal traction* (Kirschner wire through the os calcis) with or without plaster, followed by a *walking plaster.* The advantage of traction alone is that it allows mobility to be regained in the ankle-joint before the application of the walking plaster. This considerably reduces the risk of a stiff, painful foot and ankle after the fracture has healed. (Some surgeons make use of traction before the application of plaster for *a second degree fracture* for this reason, in which case it is maintained until full dorsiflexion is obtained, when a plaster cast is applied.) Protection may be given in the form of elastoplast, strapping, or a T-strap and iron, for a few weeks after removal of the plaster. If the fragment of the posterior margin of the tibia is large—which is rare—it may have to be fixed into position by a screw, treatment then following normal lines. Physical treatment follows the lines outlined above.

CASES IN WHICH THE JOINT SURFACE IS IRREPARABLY DAMAGED

Sometimes the injury is so severe that joint congruity is unobtainable. In such cases there will inevitably be structural changes leading to a painful arthritic condition. All that can be done is to encourage the fullest possible mobility in the joint. To this end traction is usually applied for the treatment of the fracture, to enable physical treatment to begin at once. *It is the physiotherapist's job to see that the foot and ankle are as mobile as possible, and that the functional activity of the foot is restored in the fullest possible measure.*

Dupuytren's Fracture

This fracture is due to a fall on the feet and is a very serious injury. *The interosseous ligament connecting the tibia and fibula is ruptured, and the talus is forced*

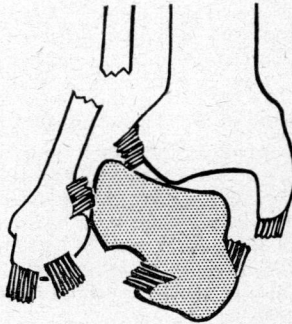

Fig. 26.—Medial, lateral, and interosseous ligaments ruptured. Talus displaced upward between inferior tibiofibular articulation.

up between the two bones. There may be fracture of the lower end of the fibula, or of the tibia, or of both bones (*Fig.* 26). The foot may be displaced backwards, inwards, or outwards, as well as upwards.

The methods of fixation are similar to those described for third degree abduction fracture but to begin with the foot may be put up in plantar flexion, which is gradually reduced in subsequent plasters. *Fixation* is maintained until union, and *protection* is required until consolidation. Physical treatment is the same as for third degree abduction fracture. The results may not be entirely satisfactory owing to the development of arthritis in the ankle.

If the displacement cannot be satisfactorily reduced by manipulation, an open operation will be necessary. The tibia and fibula are bolted together, or the loose fragments of bone are removed. *Post-operative treatment* is carried out on the usual lines. If osteo-arthritis of the ankle sets in, the surgeon may perform an arthrodesis of the ankle (*see* p. 211). *Post-operative treatment* consists of movements of the hip, knee, toes, and mid-tarsal joint but the *ankle* must not, of course, be mobilized. Re-education in walking is necessary.

THE BONES OF THE FOOT

Most important of these are fractures of *the talus* and of *the calcaneum* (os calcis). Fracture of any other tarsal bone is rare.

Fractures of the Talus

These are troublesome, but fortunately not very common, injuries. The cause is generally direct violence—a fall on the foot from a height. The *body* or the *neck* may be broken. These fractures are often associated with injury to, or dislocation of, other bones about the ankle. The ankle-joint itself may be dislocated, or the talus displaced. Fractures of the body must necessarily involve the ankle-joint and their treatment is not always completely successful, the foot often remaining weak and painful.

The fracture and dislocation are reduced, and the foot is put up in dorsiflexion or plantar-flexion (according to the nature of the displacement) in *plaster*, for from 6 to 12 weeks, depending on the severity of the injury. Some surgeons allow the plaster to be *bivalved* at about 6 weeks, so that exercises may be given to the ankle. In the case of a serious fracture-dislocation, an *ambulatory plaster* may be applied after about 8 weeks, or when the X-rays show firm union between the fragments. In a less severe case (e.g., fracture of the *neck*) without dislocation, a walking plaster is sometimes allowed from the outset. In cases where the talus has been completely shattered attempts can be made to remould the surfaces by early movement. Weight-bearing cannot, however, be allowed for 3 months. Physical treatment will follow the lines of any other fracture of the lower leg immobilized by plaster.

Fractures of the Calcaneum (Os Calcis)

Many types of fracture occur in this situation, varying in severity from simple fractures of a bony process, e.g., the internal tuberosity, to comminuted fractures of the body involving one or more of the articular facets of the subtalar joint. The commonest type is a fracture of the body involving the outer half of the posterior articular facet of the calcaneum. Such joint injuries may result in arthritis and, in consequence, in a foot which remains stiff and painful. As this type of fracture is nearly always caused by a fall from a height on to the feet, it is not unusual for both heels to be injured.

Treatment is similar to that for *Pott's fracture*, but the patient is not allowed to take weight for *at least* 12 weeks. If there is little hope of restoration of the joint surface, the emphasis must be on early and intensive movement of the joint. The patient's foot may not be normal for over a year or more, and in some cases pain, tenderness, and rigidity persist. The arches of the foot may be flattened, and should arthritis of the tarsal joints develop, spasmodic flat-foot may be a complication. Sometimes a lump of bone forms, which causes pain when weight is taken. A sorbo ring, which allows this bony mass to rest in its centre, often affords relief.

In cases where pain is persistent owing to arthritis of the subtalar and mid-tarsal joints, *arthrodesis* of these articulations may be necessary but the result is not always entirely satisfactory, the patient still complaining of pain in the heel. *Post-operatively no attempt should be made to obtain inversion or eversion.*

Fractures of the Metatarsal Bones

One or more of these bones may be broken, generally as the result of direct violence, such as crushing of the foot. *Injury of the first metatarsal is the most serious.* The fracture known as a 'march fracture' is a fissure fracture of the shaft of the second, third, or fourth metatarsal, and occurs most frequently in young soldiers who were leading a more or less sedentary life before joining the army.

Displacement is rarely marked, the worst feature of the injury being the damage to the anterior transverse arch of the foot. *This fact must be borne in mind, especially during the later stages of treatment.*

If there is no displacement a *walking plaster* is usually applied. If there is displacement, *traction* may be applied through the pulp of the toe and incorporated in the plaster. Routine physical treatment will be given during the immobilization period. When the plaster is removed *gentle mobilization of the foot and toes* is especially necessary. Foot drill and *flat-foot exercises should be practised* (*see* pp. 127 and 314–15). *Faradic foot baths* are useful, especially after march fractures, and re-education in walking will be required.

Fracture of the Phalanges

Fractures of the phalanges are treated similarly to those of the metatarsals.

Before closing this section on fractures of the lower extremity the importance, from a physiotherapist's point of view, of the following muscles or muscle groups should again be stressed: (1) *A strong gluteus medius is essential if the correct balance of the pelvis is to be maintained during weight-transference.* (2) *The quadriceps must be strong if the knee is to be really stable, particularly during flexion of a weight-bearing leg.* (3) *The intrinsic muscles of the foot are of paramount importance in the maintenance of the arches, and the mechanics of the foot.* In order, therefore, to fully rehabilitate a patient who has suffered injury to the lower limb, particular attention must be paid to the maintenance or restoration of power in these muscles.

CRUTCH WALKING

The following principles must be observed in all cases where crutches are used although the age of the patient, and the nature of the injury or disease from which he is suffering may necessitate certain adaptations.

PRINCIPLES OF CRUTCH WALKING.—

1. The crutches must be of the right height for the patient. *For full-length crutches* a measurement should be taken from the anterior fold of the axilla to the medial malleolus. This allows for the extra distance from malleolus to the ground and ensures that the top of the crutch comes well below the axilla when in use. *Elbow crutches* should be measured from the point of the elbow to the ground.

2. The patient must be able to *take his weight on the crutches by pressing down on his extended arm and hands in the case of full-length crutches, and by means of the forearm in elbow crutches.* The ability to do this depends largely on the *triceps* and *the depressors of the shoulder girdle.* Specific exercises to strengthen these muscles may be required before crutches can be used.

3. Before getting up, the patient should sit over the side of the bed. This enables him to become accustomed to the erect position, and to dependent limbs. Balancing exercises can be given in this position if required.

4. Postural muscles must be strong, *particularly the gluteus medius* since it is responsible for maintaining correct balance of the pelvis during weight transference.

5. Before any re-education of walking is undertaken, be it with crutches or otherwise, *posture must be correct*, i.e., head erect, shoulders level and braced, and hips and knees extended. *Care must be taken to see that the knees are not hyper-extended.*

6. When the patient is standing the crutches should be held at a slight angle outwards from the body and should be about 4 in. away from the feet (*Fig. 27*).

Full-length crutches must be gripped firmly to the body by means of the adductors of the shoulder, not by pressing the crutch up into the axilla.

7. Before attempting to walk the patient must learn to balance on the crutches, and *to take his full weight on them by pressing down on his arms and hands*. He must also be able to move the crutches forwards, backwards, and to the side.

8. He must be able to use the crutches to travel up and down stairs, steps, kerbs, etc.

9. When walking *he must take even steps and use the feet and legs correctly*.

METHODS OF CRUTCH WALKING.—There are two main types of crutch walking, weight-bearing and non-weight-bearing.

Weight-bearing Methods.—

1. The crutches and affected leg are moved forward together, the body-weight being taken on the sound leg meanwhile. The sound leg is then brought forward and *beyond* the crutches. This is in essence a normal gait, except that crutches are used as aids. The commands are, "Crutches and injured leg, and follow *through*" Stress must be laid on bringing the sound leg *beyond* the crutches. The patient instinctively brings the sound leg level with the injured leg, which, if not checked, results in a limping gait, which easily becomes a habit.

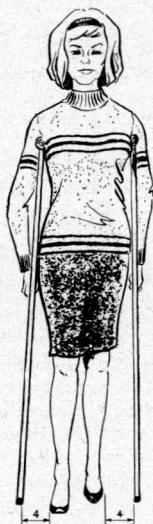

Fig. 27.—Correct position of crutches as in paragraph No. 6.

2. The crutches are moved forward alternately, at the same time as the opposite limb. The commands are, "Right crutch left leg, left crutch right leg". To begin with the patient may find it easier to move the crutch and then the legs, but as soon as possible, crutch and leg should move together.

The former method is most usually used in fractures and injuries where weight can be taken, the latter in certain neurological conditions. Sticks can be used instead of crutches when less support is required.

*Non-weight-bearing Methods.—*Both crutches are moved first. The patient then takes all his body-weight on the crutches and swings the leg or legs level with the crutches. *It is very important to see that this is done correctly, and that the patient does not lean on the crutches and drag the legs along the floor.*

SHADOW WALKING.—When the patient can take weight on one leg but not the other, as in fractures of the lower limb, *the correct pattern of walking should be maintained*. That is to say the injured limb is put through the flexion and extension motions, although it is not actually put to the ground, or weight taken on it. The patient does not find this easy, and patience is required in teaching shadow walking.

SUMMARY OF ERRORS AND FAULTS TO BE CORRECTED.—

1. Uneven steps.
2. Bringing the foot beyond or behind the crutches.

3. Resting on full-length crutches with the head of the crutch pressing into the axilla.

4. Faulty posture, in particular flexion or hyper-extension of the hips.

5. External rotation of the hip, and/or pivoting on the foot. This is very tempting to the patient, and must be checked before it becomes a habit.

6. Failure to use the leg and foot correctly. The leg is held stiffly and the foot 'plonked' on the ground.

RE-EDUCATION IN WALKING

This is most important in *all* fractures of the lower extremity, since the wasting and loss of tone of the leg muscles, however slight, causes the foot to fall into the position of *weakness*—that is, into *eversion*. This leads to collapse of the arches, or at all events, to a 'weak foot', with pain, diminished mobility, and loss of the 'spring' in walking. In Pott's or Dupuytren's fracture, this disastrous result will inevitably follow the injury unless proper measures are taken to prevent it, since apart from the general weakening of muscles, the structures on the inner side of the foot—especially the *deltoid ligament, one of the most important supports of the longitudinal arch through its connection with the 'spring' ligament, and the tibiales anterior and posterior*—are wrenched by the accident, the ligament being possibly torn right across.

Dr. Mennell pointed out the supreme importance of regaining the correct *co-ordination* necessary for walking. Weakness of any muscle or group of muscles, from whatever cause, will interfere with this co-ordination, not only because these muscles contract with lessened force, but because the latent period between the reception of the nerve stimulus by the muscle, and its resultant contraction is lengthened, so that it no longer acts in time with the healthy muscles, the latent period of which is normal.

Exercises to re-establish co-ordination should begin some time before it is safe for the patient to take the weight of his body on the injured limb. All the movements of leg and foot required in walking can be practised without standing on the leg at all. Every physiotherapist should read Dr. Mennell's chapter on re-education in walking in which he described and classified these 'exercises without weight', which are so valuable at the stage of recovery after fractures, or other conditions of injury or weakness.* Most of these exercises are now used everywhere, and have been found most successful.

EXERCISES BEFORE THE PATIENT IS ALLOWED TO WALK.—These consist of Leg-swinging, Knee-bending and -stretching, Foot-bending and -stretching (heel- and toe-raising) and Foot-inversion.

Knee-swinging (sitting on a high table). This is also a mobility exercise; but the patient should swing not only the injured leg but the sound one as well, and they should be swung *alternately*, not together. Later, he should combine the forward swing of the leg with dorsiflexion of the ankle, and the backward swing with plantar-flexion. *Knee-bending* and *-stretching*+*Foot-bending* and *-stretching* may be done combined as above, with resistance to the knee movements.

Alternate heel-raising is practised, the patient sitting on a stool; and then *Alternate toe-raising* (dorsiflexion of the ankle), in the same position. *Heel-* and *toe-raising* follows. This consists of dorsiflexion of one foot at the same time as plantar-flexion of the other. Inversion of both feet together must also be practised, as well as flexion and extension of the toes.

THE TAKING OF WEIGHT.—The patient is at first allowed some support, e.g., he may stand between parallel bars, or between two chairs. He has now to be

---

* *Physical Treatment by Movement, Manipulation and Massage*, Chapter XXI.

taught the correct method of taking steps. He stands with the feet together, and both pointing straight forward (close-standing). He then moves the *injured foot forward in a straight line, and places the heel on the ground. The heel of the sound foot is then raised, the weight transferred to the injured one, the front of which is brought down. The weight is to be taken on the outer border of the foot, and the toes are to be pressed firmly on the ground.* Then the sound foot is brought up alongside it, and the forward step is repeated with the injured foot. After this has been done several times, *the process is reversed,* the sound foot is moved forward, and the heel of the injured (back) foot raised, the weight of the body being brought over the forward leg. The injured foot is then carried forward *past* the sound foot, and the heel placed on the ground as above. The support is now gradually withdrawn.

After this, *heel-and-toe walking* along a line is practised. The patient should be carefully supervised, and no incorrect step allowed. *Eversion of the foot must be guarded against all the time,* and the patient must not be allowed to acquire a limp—a habit which, once contracted, is most difficult to eradicate.

Ordinary leg exercises are now undertaken, not forgetting those suitable for flat-foot; also exercises for any joint or joints in which the movements are not complete.

ERRORS IN WALKING.—Whether from muscular weakness; failure in co-ordination; pain, or the fear of pain; stiffness; or because he has acquired certain abnormal habits of walking during a period in plaster, there are various errors into which the patient is liable to fall. He may *hold the hip or knee stiffly,* though the actual mobility in these joints may not be seriously impaired. He may *hyper-extend the knee.* He may *rotate the leg outward,* especially after fractures of the upper end of the femur, *tilt the pelvis laterally,* or *swing the spine towards the sound side.* He may *rotate the pelvis forward on the injured side instead of flexing the hip.* He may *hold the ankle stiffly,* and fail to lift the heel from the ground, or "push off with the toes". *He may evert* or, less commonly, *invert the foot,* or develop a very troublesome limp by *taking steps of unequal length* (being afraid to retain weight on the injured limb), or by *moving the injured limb more slowly than the sound one.* All these faults must be guarded against, or corrected if they have already occurred. Adequate training during the period of "exercises without weight" will prevent some of them. Others must be dealt with as they arise.

N.B.—*Hyperextension of the knees in walking* may be corrected by making the patient walk with bent knees "as he would do if he were under a low roof" (Colson).

THE PELVIS

The majority of pelvic fractures are caused by direct violence, e.g., by falls or blows, or, in the case of the severer forms, by crushing. Apart from the shock sustained by the patient at the time of the accident, or from damage to pelvic organs, the injury is rarely dangerous and displacement is often not marked, because of the support afforded to the bone by the numerous muscles and ligaments attached to its surface.

The pelvic ring may be described as consisting of two segments: *the anterior or pubic portion, which protects the pelvic organs,* and serves for the attachment of the muscles of the lower extremity, and the *posterolateral or iliac portion, through which the weight of the body is transmitted to the legs.* An isolated fracture in either segment, e.g., of the ascending ramus of the pubis or the body of the ilium, is not as a rule serious (unless complicated by injury to organs), and there is little displacement. The same is true of double or even multiple fractures in the anterior or pubic segment, *provided there is no fracture or dislocation in the iliac segment.* But if there are two or more fractures or dislocations, at least one in each segment, e.g., unilateral fracture of the ascending and descending rami of pubis, with fracture of the ilium near the sacro-iliac joint (or dislocation of this joint), the displacement may be considerable. It is brought about both by the causative force and by the pull of the muscles passing from the spine to the pelvis or femur. (*See Fig.* 28.)

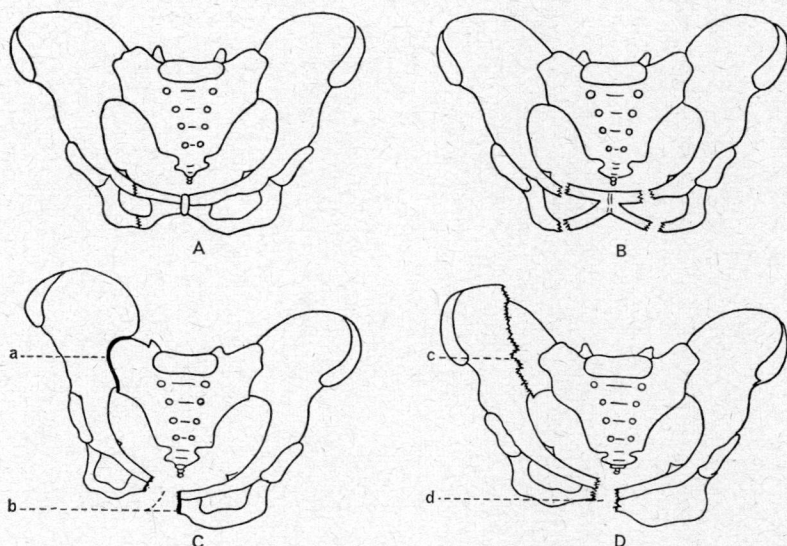

Fig. 28.—Fractures and dislocations of the pelvis. A, Unilateral fracture of both pubic rami—no displacement. B, Bilateral fracture of both pubic rami—slight displacement. C, Injury in both portions of the pelvis: a, Dislocation of sacro-iliac articulation; b, Dislocation of symphysis pubis—marked displacement, outward swing of injured half of pelvis. D, Injury in both portions of pelvis: c, Fracture of ala of ilium; d, Separation of symphysis pubis—marked upward and outward displacement.

INJURIES TO INDIVIDUAL BONES AND ISOLATED INJURIES TO THE PELVIC RING

For fractures with little displacement, complete immobilization is not necessary. In many cases the patient lies in bed until he can lift his leg off the bed. He is then allowed to get up and to walk, taking full weight. Sometimes a pelvic sling is used to support the pelvis during the period of recumbency.

AT LEAST ONE INJURY IN EACH PORTION
(Iliac and Pubic)

In fractures with displacement and shortening of a limb, *fixation* is required. This may take the form of a *plaster spica* extending from *the lumbar region to below the knee*, with the legs in slight abduction; or *traction*, applied to both legs but with greater weight on the injured one, the pelvis being supported by a sling. Fixation is maintained for about 12 weeks, though it may sometimes be discarded earlier in cases on traction. Physical treatment follows the basic principles and re-education in walking will be necessary when weight-bearing is allowed.

COMPLICATED FRACTURES

These generally involve injuries to the bladder or urethra, and operations will have to be performed for their repair. The surgeon will decide when physical treatment may begin.

THE SPINE

Fracture or dislocation of the vertebræ may take place in any region of the spinal column. *Transverse processes, spinous processes,* or *bodies of vertebræ* may be broken (*Fig.* 29).

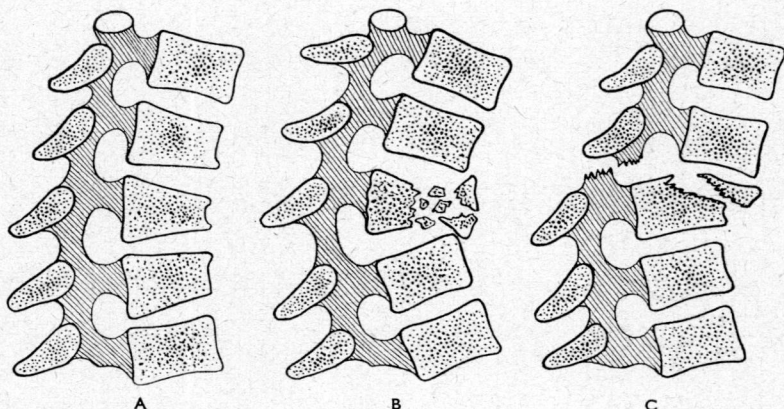

Fig. 29.—Three types of crush fracture of the spine: A, Wedging of one or more vertebral bodies; B, Comminuted fracture of a vertebral body; C, Fracture-dislocation.

The important factor in any serious fracture of the vertebrae is *whether or not the spinal cord is damaged.* If there has been damage to the cord there will be some form of paraplegia (*see* p. 53). *In cases where there are neurological signs the state of the cord takes precedence over the fracture.* In some cases the neurological symptoms are transitory, in others they are permanent.* In such cases treatment is directed towards *assisting regeneration of the cord,* if possible, by reducing any displacement and immobilizing the spine, and to *alleviating the paraplegia* by preventing such complications as bed-sores, bladder infections, and contractures.

Fractures of *transverse and spinous processes* are generally treated with strapping or a light plaster jacket for a month or two. *Back exercises* should be given during this period and *intensive mobility and strengthening exercises* after immobilization.

Fractures of the *vertebral bodies without cord injury* are treated with plaster fixation for periods of 3–9 months, depending on the site and nature of the injury. Besides the importance of maintaining the strength and tone of the back extensors, *breathing exercises* are particularly important during immobilization, specially *diaphragmatic breathing.* If the patient shows signs of respiratory difficulty an 'abdominal window' may be cut in the plaster, which allows for free excursions of the abdominal wall. Breathing may also be practised in conjunction with arm exercises.

Nowadays many surgeons consider that it is unnecessary to fix the vertebral column in this way, since the prolonged immobilization leads to adhesions and considerable weakening of the back muscles. Professor Perkins states "Of the miners who return to the coal face those not treated in plaster outnumber those treated in plaster by two to one." Surgeons who hold these views keep the patient

---

* G. Perkins, *Fractures and Dislocations,* pp. 79–81.

in bed but allow active exercises to strengthen the sacrospinalis muscle (erector spinæ) and the short muscles of the deeper layers.

Fractures in the cervical region are dangerous lesions because of possible injury to the spinal cord, though they are not nearly so often fatal as is generally supposed. In fractures where there is dislocation, *traction as well as plaster fixation* is usually required.

PARAPLEGIA

This is a possible complication of a lesion in any region of the spine. A cervical lesion, if the patient survives, may produce a diplegia (*see* p. 188). The nature and extent of the paralysis varies according to the site and severity of the lesion, and may thus be spastic or flaccid, or partly one and partly the other. In injuries of the cord itself, recovery is unlikely to be complete unless the symptoms are only due to pressure, but the cauda equina is capable of regeneration. The subject is too large to be treated here in detail, but the student should consult the table on page 234 for the symptoms liable to occur as the result of lesions at various levels. For treatment, the sections on the treatment of *spastic paralysis*, and *flaccid paralysis* (Chapter IX) will give the general principles. No case of paralysis of this kind should be considered hopeless until a very long period has elapsed.

FRACTURES OF THE RIBS

These are generally caused by direct violence. The break usually occurs near the angle. Displacement is rare, the only dangerous complication being injury to the lung or pleura by the extremity of a fragment. The ribs unite spontaneously, but the affected side of the thorax is often strapped for about a week or so. This relieves the patient, even if not strictly necessary. The only form of physical treatment required consists of breathing exercises, either before or after the strapping is removed, to ensure full use of the thorax and expansion of the lung. Heat and massage of the affected side of the thorax sometimes adds to the patient's comfort.

FRACTURES OF THE SKULL

Treatment is not usually required. The patient may experience difficulty in balancing, or suffer from dizziness when he gets up. Exercises may therefore be required to overcome this. (*See* Chapter XXII, pp. 470–1.)

CHAPTER IV

JOINT AND MUSCLE INJURIES

Joint injuries. Dislocations. I. Dislocations of the upper extremity. II. Dislocations of the lower extremity. III. Sacro-iliac strain. IV. Prolapsed intervertebral disk. V. Sprains: Sprained wrist—Sprained ankle—Sprained back. VI. Injury of muscles and their tendons—Tennis elbow—Rupture of calf muscles—Fibrositis.

JOINT INJURIES

JOINT injuries, other than fractures into joint surfaces and/or fracture dislocations, include dislocations, subluxations, sprains, and strains.

A *dislocation* or *luxation*, is a condition in which the articular surfaces of the bones forming a joint are completely displaced from each other by violence—generally indirect—and remain so displaced. A *subluxation* is one in which the joint surfaces remain partially displaced from each other. A *sprain* is one in which the surfaces, though separated from each other by violence, return of themselves to their normal position. A *strain* is one in which the structures are not stretched beyond their normal limits of elastic recovery.

All these conditions, if due to trauma, are accompanied by more or less severe stretching or tearing of the structures in, or surrounding, the joint. There may be partial or complete rupture of ligaments, in which case at least 6 weeks will be needed for repair since their blood-supply is poor. Muscles, tendons, synovial sheaths or membranes, and cartilage may also be injured. There is generally extravasation of blood from the injured vessels of the structures, causing *contusion* (bruising). It should be remembered that the exudation from an inflammatory reaction in a joint capsule will be a *serofibrinous one and this enhances the risk of adhesions*. The results, in the more serious traumas, may be arthritis, myositis, and possibly tenosynovitis.

DISLOCATIONS

SYMPTOMS.—

At the Time of Injury.—(1) There is intense, sickening pain, worse than that of a fracture; the patient is often conscious of a tearing sensation different from the sensation of breaking or snapping of a bone. The pain is less severe later (unless the displaced bone is pressing on a nerve). (2) There is deformity of the limb. (3) The joint is fixed. (4) The function of the limb is lost.

Later.—(1) Dull, aching pain, increasing on movement. (2) Swelling of the limb, and all the signs of acute inflammation. (3) Bruising appears after a few days. It is variable in extent.

Principles of Treatment.—The principles of treatment can be summarized as follows:—

1. REDUCTION of the displacement so that the joint surfaces are again in apposition. Because muscles respond to injury by protective spasm, an anæsthetic is required to allow sufficient relaxation for reduction to be achieved, but unlike fractures, in which reduction must be maintained by fixation, a dislocated joint is usually stable once reduction has been carried out. The muscles should provide adequate splintage and protection from further injury in most cases, and fixation, as such, is not required.

2. REST, to enable the inflammatory reaction to die down and the damaged structures to heal or return to normal. There are two schools of thought regarding this. Some surgeons feel that the only way to ensure adequate rest is by immobilization for some weeks. They therefore immobilize the joint as in cases of fracture. It should be stressed, however, that *this is done for the structures round the joint,* rather than for the bony injury as is the case in fractures. Other surgeons feel that since the muscles will splint the joint, early movement is to be encouraged, *provided it is carefully given.* This reduces the risk of adhesions and inevitable loss of muscle power which follows when joints are immobilized.

3. REHABILITATION.—The main responsibility for this lies with the physiotherapist. The principles of physical treatment are basically the same as for fractures, *the prevention of adhesions and disuse atrophy being of prime importance.* Pain and swelling must be relieved. All free joints must be exercised, and static contractions should be taught as for fractures, if the joint is immobilized. After immobilization, full mobility and strength must be regained.

COMPLICATIONS.—These are similar to those found in conjunction with fractures. As in fractures, *adhesions* and *disuse atrophy* are liable to occur if treatment is neglected or incorrectly carried out.

INJURIES TO BONES.—(1) *Fracture-dislocations,* in which a bone is broken, as well as joint surfaces displaced, e.g., Pott's fracture, or a fracture of the neck or shaft of the humerus with dislocation of the shoulder. In any case of dislocation complicated by fracture, there may be a risk of skin damage and infection if the fracture is a comminuted one. (2) *Injury to the periosteum*: Inflammation in that membrane causes an out-throwing of osteoblasts, which may impede the movements of the joint or lodge in the nearest muscles. (There is a risk of myositis ossificans in the brachialis anterior in a case of dislocated elbow.)

RECURRENCE.—Certain dislocations, especially those of the shoulder-joint and the temporomandibular-joint, are liable to recur.

INJURIES TO NERVES, causing paresis or paralysis; e.g., the circumflex nerve may be injured in dislocation of the shoulder, or the ulnar nerve in dislocation of the elbow.

INJURIES TO MUSCLE.—Severe dislocations can be accompanied by considerable muscle damage such as rupture, or partial rupture, of fibres or tendons. Before movement becomes full and painless the muscles must recover, and this may delay ultimate recovery for several months.

INJURIES TO BLOOD-VESSELS; similar to those occurring in fractures (*see* p. 12), hæmorrhage, ischæmia, or gangrene.

I. DISLOCATIONS OF THE UPPER EXTREMITY

ACROMIOCLAVICULAR JOINT

This is usually the result of direct violence, a blow or a fall on the shoulder. The clavicle is displaced upwards. In a *subluxation, the conoid and trapezoid ligaments are intact,* and the displacement slight; in a *dislocation* (luxation), *these ligaments are torn,* and the displacement is greater.

Treatment.—It is easy to replace the bones in their correct position, but difficult to keep them there while the ligaments heal, since the weight of the arm drags the scapula downwards away from the clavicle. Some form of strapping, such as *Robert Jones strapping* (*Fig.* 30) may be applied. This consists of a length of 4-in. strapping, applied from below the inferior angle of the scapula behind, over a pad close to the root of the neck, down in front of the arm and under the elbow, a pad of felt being interposed between it and the skin, up behind the arm and over the pad near the neck, and finally across the chest to just beneath the nipple of the sound side (Bonnin), or just beyond the midline of the chest. Strapping must be retained for 4–6 weeks and the disadvantage is that it limits activity, both from the point of view of daily living and of treatment. Also, however skilfully treated, some slight deformity may remain. To overcome these disadvantages *surgical treatment* may be used. The acromion process and clavicle are held together by means of a steel wire or pin. This is retained for 6 weeks, after which it is removed. Following this method of treatment a full range of movement can be given, there being no fear of re-displacement. *Elevation* should be given through flexion to begin with, but all movements should be full by the end of a week or 10 days. (In subluxation a sling only may be worn for a few days, though some surgeons may apply strapping for 2 or 3 weeks.)

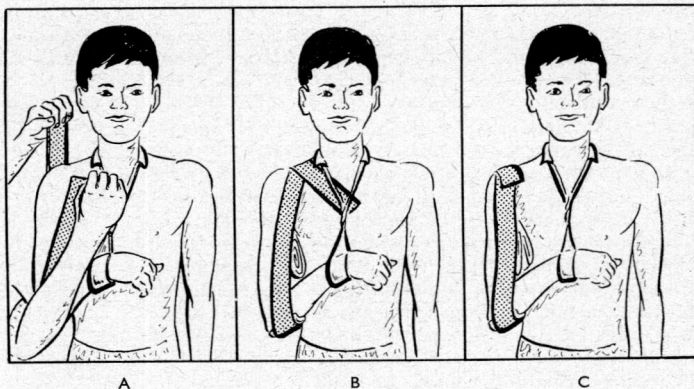

A   B   C

Fig. 30.—Robert Jones strapping for acromioclavicular dislocations.

A, Applying the strapping so that the humerus and scapula are elevated and the clavicle full down; B, Correctly strapped; C, Incorrectly strapped—reduction is only stable if the strapping lies over the clavicle itself and not over the point of the shoulder.

If strapping is used *shoulder movements* will not be allowed until it is discarded. They should begin with shoulder shrugging (*elevation*) and internal and external rotation of the humeroscapular joint *with the arm in adduction*. Flexion and extension are then added. *Abduction* must be progressed gradually and when it reaches 90°, internal and external rotation may be given in the abducted position (gleno-humeral joint). *Heat* and *massage* may be given from the beginning, the *deltoid* and *pectoralis major* receiving particular attention. Massage should be gentle to begin with, gradually becoming deeper and more stimulating.

Whether shoulder movements are given early or late, the elbow should be supported, as in clavicular fractures, during the early stages.

SHOULDER

This is the commonest of all dislocations, and one that every physiotherapist will certainly be required to treat at some time. The shoulder may be dislocated by direct or indirect violence, i.e., by a fall or a blow on the joint itself, or by a fall on the outstretched hand causing a violent abduction of the arm. The latter form of violence is the commoner cause.

DISPLACEMENT.—Four kinds of displacement are recognized:—

SUBCORACOID.—*The humeral head passes forwards and downwards* and comes to lie below and external to the coracoid process. This is the commonest form of dislocation and the one we will deal with here.

SUBCLAVICULAR.—Occasionally it passes still further inwards and lies below the clavicle, though this is rare.

SUBGLENOID.—*The head of the humerus passes out through the lower part of capsule and remains beneath the glenoid cavity, resting on the axillary border of the scapula.* This form is not very common. Though the humerus must pass through this position, it rarely remains there.

SUBSPINOUS.—In this case *the humeral head is driven backwards and downwards into the infraspinous fossa, where it lies below the spine of the scapula.* This form also is rare, the long head of the triceps usually preventing the bone from passing in this direction.

Subcoracoid Dislocation

Intense pain is felt at the time of the accident. The shoulder is flattened on top and the acromion process is prominent, making the contour appear angular instead of rounded. The elbow cannot be brought to the side, and the axis of the arm is oblique instead of vertical (*Fig.* 31). The usual symptoms resulting from a dislocation are present; there is often much pain and swelling, and sometimes extensive bruising. *Adhesions are very liable to form* and are most crippling; hence the necessity of early movement, especially in elderly people.

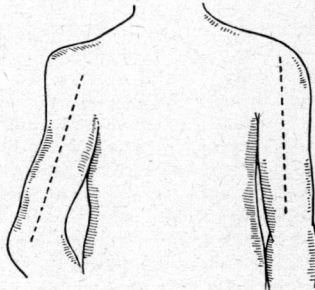

Fig. 31.—Diagram to show flattening and angulation of shoulder and direction of axis of arm in dislocation of subcoracoid type.

Treatment.—*The arm may be bandaged to the side with the elbow supported, so as to prevent any abduction and hold the head of the humerus in contact with the glenoid cavity.* The bandage is put on under the patient's clothes. It is worn for a few days, then replaced by a large arm sling, which must be kept taut beneath the elbow. Frequently a sling alone is worn under the clothes for a few days. Some surgeons use merely a *collar-and-cuff sling*, with a wool pad in the axilla, for 3 weeks from the outset. The support is maintained for about 3 weeks or a month, and the patient must not on any account remove his sling, or interfere with the bandage without permission.

An abduction splint or similar apparatus is sometimes used to maintain the arm in various degrees of abduction. It is claimed, by its supporters, that adhesions are less troublesome if the arm is supported in this position.

AVERAGE SCHEME OF PHYSICAL TREATMENT.—For the first few days physical treatment consists of *heat, massage,* and *active exercises* of fingers, wrist, elbow, and radio-ulnar joints. The elbow movements are most important, as it is essential *that the tendon of the long head of the biceps, passing as it does through the shoulder-joint, should not be allowed to adhere to its own sheath or to any surrounding structures.*

The arm should be supported on a table of sufficient height to keep the elbow pressed upward and prevent the humerus from being dragged out of the glenoid fossa, yet low enough for the arm to be kept close to the side and not abducted.

To begin with *massage* should take the form of gentle stroking and light effleurage to the whole arm and shoulder. By the 2nd or 3rd day careful kneading can be added. *Shoulder movements* are not usually given before the 3rd day, beginning with *flexion* and *extension* in small range. Support should be given as for fracture of the head of the humerus (*see Fig.* 8, p. 22). *Internal* and *external rotation* are first given *with the arm in adduction*. *Abduction* can usually begin about the 5th day, starting with *circumduction*. Support should be given by the hand under the axilla pressing in an upward direction, in order to support the head of the humerus, and prevent any risk of it again making its way out through the still weakened capsule. The grasp is similar to that for a fractured surgical neck.

Abduction should have reached 90° by about the 7th or 8th day and *elevation* should then progress through abduction. From the 10th or 12th day *internal* and *external rotation* can be given *with the arm in abduction but these movements should never be forced*. (For the subcoracoid form of dislocation, give internal rotation first, and later external rotation. For the subspinous, reverse the order.)

Once the support is discarded the emphasis is on *the restoration of full mobility and power*.

Full elevation and rotational movements, *particularly internal rotation*, are usually those which the patient finds most difficult. Carefully selected home exercises should always be taught.

The arm should be normal in about 5 to 6 weeks if both the operator *and* the patient have done their best. Elderly patients are sometimes difficult to manage, and the physiotherapist is often unduly alarmed about the possibility of redislocation. It *is* a possibility, but as Dr. Mennell remarked, "It is safer to administer movement freely during the first week after dislocation than during the third, if the joint has been immobilized meanwhile." If early active movement is not given, the muscles which, as observed above, *are the main support of the joint*, become weak and wasted, and when attempts are made to stretch or break down the adhesions which have meanwhile formed, disaster may easily occur.

Kabat techniques (*see* pp. 130–1) can be used from the beginning, the techniques used being those of the *isometric group*. Before attempting this method of treatment in any case of recent injury, the student must be thoroughly conversant with the underlying principles, as well as the techniques themselves, otherwise she may cause more harm than good.

COMPLICATIONS.—

FRACTURE of the great tuberosity, or surgical neck of the humerus.

RUPTURE OF THE SUPRASPINATUS TENDON, which is torn away from its point of attachment to the head of the humerus (for symptoms, *see* p. 80). Other tendons of the short muscles round the shoulder may also be torn.

INJURY TO THE CIRCUMFLEX NERVE.—*This is a not uncommon occurrence* and a watch should be kept for it. It should be reported at once. The physiotherapist should take care to see that the deltoid really does contract. If there is any doubt about it, the sensation in the skin over the muscle should be tested, and the surgeon should be consulted.

A lesion of the circumflex nerve in a shoulder injury is much more easily missed than is an ulnar lesion in an elbow injury, since the patient may be able to perform weak abduction with the supraspinatus, the nerve-supply of which is probably intact. The physiotherapist should, therefore, be on the alert for this. A slight circumflex injury is often the cause of a belated recovery from this accident. If it is not discovered in time, the nerve, which may have been only bruised or concussed, will partially or completely recover, but in the meantime, the deltoid will have wasted and the joint become stiff.

RECURRENCE OF DISLOCATION.—*This happens more frequently in the shoulder than in any other joint.* It calls for special treatment (*see below*).

TREATMENT OF COMPLICATIONS.—

Fracture of Humerus (see p. 20) *or Avulsion of Supraspinatus Tendon.*— If there is displacement of bone, or the supraspinatus is torn away from the humerus, the arm may be placed in some degree of abduction. Open operation is sometimes necessary to replace the humeral head in the glenoid cavity, to fix the great tuberosity in position, or to re-attach the supraspinatus tendon to the humerus.

Circumflex Injury.—The difficulty in this case is the impossibility of any but the weakest *active* abduction. The treatment is much as usual, but the arm must not be kept down at the side unsupported until the deltoid is sufficiently recovered to exercise its function. Passive, or almost passive, abduction and elevation must be given, with very careful support. The patient should be treated in the lying position. Electrical treatment may be required. (*See also* CIRCUMFLEX PARALYSIS, Chapter XII.)

RECURRENT DISLOCATION.—This is sometimes treated by the *wearing of an appliance to prevent abduction of the arm beyond the danger point* (about 70°). Since, however, this considerably limits activity, an *open operation* is more usually performed.

Many different operations have been performed for the relief of this condition. The Bankart and Putti-Platt operations are the most frequently used at the present time.

Bankart Operation.—The capsular ligament is re-attached to the anterior margin of the glenoid cavity.

Putti-Platt Operation.*—The subscapularis is shortened to limit outward rotation.

Post-operative treatment is directed towards strengthening the arm and shoulder muscles. Massage may be given for the first 3 weeks, with active movements of distal joints. *Shoulder movements* will not be given until the muscles have had time to heal, i.e., after about 3—4 weeks.

N.B.—The rare posterior dislocation can be treated similarly to the anterior one or in abduction and external rotation on an abduction frame, in which case the arm can be slowly lowered to the side after 2 or 3 weeks. In this type of case, re-dislocation tends to take place when the arm is *adducted* or *internally rotated.*

ELBOW

The displacements which occur in the region of the elbow and superior radio-ulnar articulations are: (1) *Dislocation of both radius and ulna.* (2) *Dislocation of the radius alone.*

1. Dislocation of Radius and Ulna from the Humeral Articular Surfaces
(*True Dislocation of the Elbow-joint*)

This is caused by a fall on the elbow or hand, i.e., forced extension of the elbow. The dislocation may be *forward, backward, lateral,* or even *divergent,* the olecranon being displaced backwards, and the head of the radius forwards. By far the most common type is *posterior* dislocation. The radius and ulna are displaced backwards and upwards behind the humerus, the anterior ligament being stretched or torn, and the coronoid process often fractured as well. The elbow is held in

---

* *See* "Rehabilitation following Surgical Repair of Shoulder Dislocation", *Physiotherapy, Lond.,* March, 1959.

slight flexion and cannot be moved. Pronation and supination are limited. The lower extremity of the humerus can be felt at the front of the bend of the elbow, or below it. The back of the elbow projects, the projection being formed by the olecranon process, and the elbow appears broadened from behind.

Treatment.—The elbow is generally put up in flexion and supination, as for fractures near the elbow-joint, for 2 to 3 weeks, but sometimes this is only continued for 10 days. After 3 weeks it is substituted for a *low sling*.

While this dislocation, unlike that of the shoulder, is very unlikely to recur and therefore early movement would seem to be indicated, the possibility of myositis ossificans has to be considered, even if no fracture complicates the injury. For this reason movements are not usually given for 7 to 10 days, although some surgeons may allow them before this. Others prefer to keep the arm immobilized for 2 to 3 weeks. The author has, personally, never known any harm to result from careful movements, given in small range at an early period, but the arm should certainly be kept in the flexed position for at least a fortnight, after which great care must be taken not to lose the full flexion which has thus been preserved. The maintenance of this position, as in other injuries of the elbow, fulfils the threefold purpose of assisting the anti-gravity muscles, preventing limitation of the movement which is most difficult to regain if lost, and eliminating the danger of myositis.

Heat and massage may be given as for dislocation of the shoulder, together with active exercises for fingers, wrist, and shoulders, within the limits imposed by the support. *Care must be taken to see that radial deviation of the wrist does not become pronation.* The latter must not be allowed until the 7th day and it must be carefully supervised. Extension can begin around the 8th or 9th day. From about the 3rd or 4th week the range of movement can gradually be increased.

The same rules apply to dislocations of the elbow as apply to fractures. *No elbow movement should be forced, and the physiotherapist must be careful to see that the ability to flex the elbow to its full extent is maintained.* Strong exercises can be added later if necessary but hanging by the hands or the carrying of heavy weights are not allowed.

COMPLICATIONS.—These are similar to those accompanying fractures in this region.

ISCHÆMIC CONTRACTURE (*see* pp. 25–7).

MYOSITIS OSSIFICANS may occur even if no bones are broken. The cause is not understood, but it may be that the periosteum is so much torn that it becomes the seat of considerable inflammation; hence its activity is increased, and it throws out numerous bone-cells. If the coronoid process or the internal condyle is fractured, this danger is even greater (*see* pp. 23–5).

INVOLVEMENT OF THE ULNAR NERVE, or occasionally of other nerves (*see* Chapter XII).

CUBITUS VALGUS OR VARUS, abnormal increase or decrease of the carrying angle.

2. Dislocation of Radius alone

The radius may be displaced *forwards* or *downwards*.

DISPLACEMENT FORWARDS

The radius lies in the radial depression above the capitellum. The bone can be felt to be displaced. The patient can neither flex nor extend the elbow, though he can pronate and partially supinate the forearm.

Treatment.—The arm is supported in a *collar and cuff* or *sling* with the arm well flexed for 2 to 3 weeks. After this period the sling is worn for another 10 to 14 days, the arm being gradually lowered from the almost fully flexed position to a right angle. This is a much less serious injury than dislocation of both bones; there is no danger of myositis ossificans, though all injuries to the elbow-joint are best approached with caution. Movements can therefore begin earlier and all elbow movements can be given on about the 5th day. Some surgeons allow them from the beginning.

DISPLACEMENT DOWNWARDS

This is the 'pulled elbow' of small children, generally caused by the child's falling when being held by the hand. The radius is drawn out of the orbicular ligament. The child can bend and straighten the elbow but cannot fully supinate the forearm. The elbow is painful, and the child does not use the arm. Reduction is easy and treatment is rarely required. If ordered, it consists mainly of persuading the child to use the arm again.

WRIST

This is a rare accident, of which not much need be said. The dislocation, when it does occur, is more often a *posterior* than an *anterior* one, and is not infrequently complicated by a fracture of the radius into the joint. If there is no fracture, the condition is generally treated as a severe sprain, the wrist being bandaged and the arm placed in a sling. Movements of fingers and wrist are given from the beginning. If the dislocation is complicated by a fracture, the wrist will either be put in *plaster* in dorsiflexion, or on a short *cock-up splint* for 2 to 3 weeks.

THUMB

Dislocation of the thumb usually occurs at the *carpometacarpal* or *metacarpophalangeal joints*. In the first of these the metacarpal bone is displaced *outwards and backwards on the trapezium*; in the second, there is *backward displacement of the phalanx on the metacarpal*, caused by violent hyperextension of the thumb (Page and Bristow). The former is the more serious accident, because of the importance of the movements which take place in the saddle-joint—flexion, extension, abduction, adduction, and opposition. The joint is supported by plaster or strapping. It is maintained for a fortnight, after which active movements are given.

II. DISLOCATIONS OF THE LOWER EXTREMITY

HIP

(For CONGENITAL DISLOCATION, *see* Chapter XV.)

Traumatic dislocation is rare because of the great stability of the joint and the strength of the iliofemoral ligament, fracture of the bone, i.e., of the neck of the femur, being far more common. Only very great violence, such as occurs in road, rail, or mining accidents, produces an injury of this kind. The damage may consist of a *simple* dislocation, with tearing of the lower part of the capsule, or of a more severe and *complicated* lesion, with rupture of the iliofemoral ligament and fracture of the acetabulum. The displacement may be *anterior* or *posterior*. In either type, *the head of the femur passes out of the joint through the lower part of the capsule*, and then either *forward* or *backward*, the latter direction being the more common.

Posterior Dislocation takes place when the thigh is *adducted, inwardly rotated*, and *flexed*, the patient generally being in a stooping position. The femoral head passes out of the lower and back part of the capsule, and then up on to the dorsum ilii. The hip is slightly adducted, rotated inwards and slightly flexed. The mobility of the joint is lessened and the limb, before reduction, is rigidly fixed by spasm of all the thigh muscles. There is *apparent shortening of the leg, the great trochanter being above Nelaton's line*. This displacement is therefore similar to the congenital variety.

Complications.—(1) Injury to the sciatic nerve: (2) Myositis ossificans; (3) Fracture of the femoral neck or necrosis of the femoral head.

Anterior Dislocation occurs while the leg is *abducted* and *externally rotated*. The leg is slightly abducted and outwardly rotated, with the foot in eversion. *There is no apparent shortening as a rule* and the displaced head may be felt in the groin.

Complications: Injury to the femoral artery.

Treatment.—Recurrence is very improbable, therefore early movements are indicated and the patient will not be long disabled. Support is not required in a simple dislocation as a rule. The patient remains in bed for about a fortnight, or until he has regained control of the hip, i.e., he can straight-leg raise and move the limb in the air. He is then allowed to get up and walk. Some surgeons put the thigh and pelvis in plaster for 3 to 5 weeks, the patient walking in a week with the plaster still on. Others prefer to immobilize the hip in plaster for varying periods, or to keep the patient in bed for a few weeks, and then apply a plaster spica for walking for another few weeks.

Heat, massage, and active movements can be given from the beginning, the movements being in small range at first and gradually increased. Assistance will be needed at first, and *care should be taken with regard to the movements which predispose the dislocation*. As this injury involves a weight-bearing joint, the foot, ankle, and knee must not be neglected. The limb should be *normal* in 5 to 6 weeks.

Complicated Dislocation, with Rupture of the Iliofemoral Ligament and Fracture of the Acetabulum

This is a very serious injury. In such injuries the support really constitutes fixation. The limb is either put up in full normal abduction in *a plaster spica including both hips*; or *traction* is applied, the leg being kept in abduction.

Physical treatment follows the lines of treatment for any fracture immobilized in plaster or on traction. When the fixation is removed, gentle movements may be given. When the patient begins to walk re-education will be very necessary. It is impossible to give dates for movements, etc., in the case of an injury of this kind. It must be carefully treated in co-operation with the surgeon.

DISLOCATION OR INJURY OF THE KNEE

Injuries to the knee-joint include a great number and variety of different conditions. The ones considered here are those most often seen in the physiotherapy department: (1) *Dislocated knee*. (2) *Dislocated patella*. (3) *Slipped semilunar cartilage*. (4) *Injury to the medial ligament without displacement of the cartilage*.

1. Dislocated Knee

Dislocation pure and simple is rare: almost invariably there is damage to the bones as well. The spine of the tibia may be broken off, or one or both of the cruciate ligaments ruptured, as well as part of the capsule. *Dislocation* may occur anteriorly, posteriorly, or laterally. *Lateral subluxation* is more common, one or other of the lateral ligaments being damaged in the process.

The injury is a very serious one, since, *unless the cruciate ligaments heal well and firmly, the knee will always be unstable*. For this reason the joint is invariably immobilized for a long period, support in this case again being virtually *fixation*. Six weeks at least are necessary for the complete repair of ligaments and in such a joint as the knee, *which depends for its stability on the ligaments rather than on the conformation of its bony surfaces*, it is well to allow a little extra time. Even after 6 or 8 weeks some form of *protection* may be required for weight-bearing. This must hold the knee extended until the muscles regain sufficient strength to stabilize the joint.

Treatment.—The knee is put in extension, either in *plaster* or on a *back-splint*, for about 2 months, after which a *walking caliper* or *plaster* is provided. If a Thomas splint is used the knee is kept in extension for about a fortnight. After this a walking plaster is applied from groin to toes, with the knee in 10° of flexion and weight-bearing is allowed in 3 to 4 weeks. A knee plaster or support may have to be worn for 4 to 6 months in all, from the time of injury, before free movements and weight-bearing can be permitted (Bonnin).*

Because of the lengthy period of immobilization *it is essential to prevent disuse atrophy of muscles*, particularly the *flexors* and *extensors* of the knee. Not only is there the danger of an instable joint through weak musculature affecting the locking mechanisms of the knee, but disuse further decreases the circulation. *The more sluggish the circulation, the greater the tissue-fluid exudation and the high fibrin content in the joint.* The formation of adhesions in the knee-joint can be a most crippling condition. Heat and massage may be given from the beginning, if the apparatus permits, to assist the circulation and to relieve pain and swelling, special attention being paid to the quadriceps. Movements should begin as soon as possible. Some surgeons allow these at once, as the plaster prevents excess movement; others do not permit them during the first week or 10 days. *Static contractions of the flexors and calf muscles must be given during the period of immobilization* and, if possible, *lateral movements of the patella*. If the anterior ligament has been severely injured quadriceps contractions may be postponed for 3 weeks or so. Faradism (graduated contractions) may be given after the third week, *but no movement should be allowed to take place in the joint*. If a full-length plaster has been worn the knee must be mobilized gradually and carefully after its removal.

Operations are sometimes performed for the repair of the medial or lateral ligament (tibial or fibular collateral). This is done with stainless-steel wire; it is followed by immobilization in a walking plaster for about 2 months. Longer immobilization is required for rupture of the cruciate ligaments but they are not generally treated by operation.

2. Dislocated Patella

This, again, is a rare accident without accompanying bony and muscular injury. Knock-knee and weakness, or paralysis, of the quadriceps are predisposing causes. Certain patients show deficient development of the external condyle of the femur, or of the knee-joint, causing the patella to slip outwards easily. In all these cases the dislocation is liable to recur constantly. The displacement is almost always outward. The patella can be felt to be out of place. There is not much swelling as a rule, but there may be severe pain at the time of the accident.

Treatment.—The knee is supported for 10 to 14 days (it may be for a longer or shorter period, according to the severity of the injury), with a compression bandage to keep down effusion and hold the bone in place, but weight-bearing is usually allowed from the beginning, or as soon as the patient can straight-leg raise. *Physical treatment* usually begins at once, but some surgeons prefer to delay this for 2–3 days or even a week. Heat and massage are often precluded by the compression bandage, and in any case emphasis should really be laid on the

* *Fractures and Related Injuries*, Chapter XXXV.

strength of the *quadriceps*. *Static contractions* are given as soon as the surgeon allows and *faradism* for these muscles is also indicated.

Cases in which there is imperfect development of the external condyle are sometimes dealt with by *open operation*, the front of the condyle being brought farther forward by the insertion of a bone-graft into a wedge-shaped incision on its outer surface. Various operations are also performed on the quadriceps tendon, in order to give its pull a more inward direction.★

3. Slipped Semilunar Cartilage

ANATOMICAL POINTS.—The position and attachments of the structures which take part in the formation of the knee-joint should always be kept well in mind while treating any injury to that joint, or in its neighbourhood; in fact, *accurate anatomical knowledge is necessary in order to ensure success.* If there are internal derangements such as slipped or torn cartilages, the following points especially should be remembered:—

THE MEDIAL SEMILUNAR CARTILAGE (OR MENISCUS).—(1) The under-surface of the cartilage is not attached to the head of the tibia. (2) Its anterior extremity is attached to the front of the tibia by the coronary ligament; its posterior part is firmly adherent to the deepest fibres of the medial ligament, which is much nearer to the back than to the front of the joint. Between these two points— the anterior extremity and the point corresponding to the anterior margin of the medial ligament—the attachment of the cartilage is much less firm. Consequently *the anterior portion is less fixed than the posterior, and is more liable to become displaced.* A tear of the cartilage may occur at the junction of the anterior and posterior parts, or it may be torn longitudinally down its centre, producing what is known as the 'bucket-handle' type of injury (*see Fig.* 32). It then gets

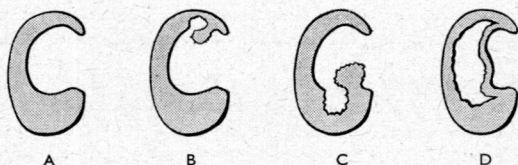

Fig. 32.—A, Normal cartilage; B, Anterior tear; C, Posterior tear; D, 'Bucket-handle' tear—the dotted line represents the line of tear.

between the bony surfaces in such a way as to prevent complete extension of the knee. Because of its attachments to the coronary and medial ligaments, some surgeons believe that a force strong enough to tear the cartilage will automatically strain the coronary ligament and may also damage the medial ligament.

THE LATERAL SEMILUNAR CARTILAGE (OR MENISCUS) owing to its greater breadth and firmer attachments, is less subject to injury than that on the inner side. Moreover, the firm pressure between tibia and femur on the outer side of the knee (the weight of the body being transmitted through the lateral condyle and tuberosity) tends to keep it in place.

THE CRUCIATE LIGAMENTS.—*On the cruciate ligaments the stability of the knee largely depends.* If both are injured, the knee hyperextends, and there is abnormal lateral mobility. If the anterior one alone suffers, the tibia can be moved backwards and forwards on the femur, especially in the flexed position. In either case the knee is rendered weak and undependable, and is liable to give way when weight is placed on it.

★ Jones and Lovett (1905), *J. orthoped. Surg.*, **3**, 34.

THE SYNOVIAL MEMBRANE need not be described in detail here. Its great extent and the existence of its many processes should be borne in mind. Some of the latter are liable to injury by being nipped between the bones when the joint is moved. An intense synovitis generally develops, with great effusion into the knee, when any injury of the joint takes place.

THE INFRAPATELLAR PAD OF FAT, which has a process extending over the medial semilunar cartilage, lies behind the patella, between the ligamentum patellæ and the synovial membrane. This also may be nipped or otherwise injured.

MOVEMENTS OF THE KNEE.—These are familiar to us, but a few points need emphasizing in order to understand the cause of this injury, which is an *outward* twist of the knee when it is in a *semi-flexed* position. It may either be a violent *outward* rotation of the *tibia on the femur* with the thigh fixed, or an *inward* rotation of *the femur* or *the tibia* with the leg fixed.

1. *The 'screw-home'* movement at the end of extension, i.e., the outward rotation of the tibia on the femur just before extension is complete. If this movement does not take place, and extension is therefore incomplete, the knee is not 'locked', and remains insecure.

2. *The rotatory movement* which takes place when the knee is in semiflexion, and the cruciates therefore relaxed. It occurs between the semilunar cartilages and the head of the tibia. Internal rotation of the tibia is limited by the anterior cruciate ligament and the crossing of the two cruciates. External rotation is limited only by the medial ligament—*the cruciates being uncrossed in this position.* Hence the danger in outward rotation of the flexed knee; the joint is 'opened' on the inner side, so that the medial semilunar cartilage is held less firmly in position, between the femur and the tibia. While movement is taking place between the cartilage and the tibia the drag on the medial ligament further tends to pull the cartilage from its attachment.

SYMPTOMS.—The knee is locked in slight flexion and the patient cannot extend it fully. Sometimes the loss of extension is so slight that it is only the 'screw-home' that is absent. This, however, may interfere gravely with the stability of the knee. Symptoms of traumatic synovitis appear (*see* pp. 134–5) and there is pain at the inner side and front of the knee. In neglected cases arthritic changes are generally found, and the patient suffers from 'giving of the knee', or locking of the joint. The displacement is liable to recur.

HEALING OF THE CARTILAGE.—Repair of cartilage is very slow, because of its poor blood-supply. In serious lesions healing may not take place at all. In these, therefore, as well as in recurrent displacements, it is generally considered better to remove the damaged cartilage rather than trust to the possibility of healing (Timbrell Fisher).

Treatment.—Sometimes spontaneous reduction occurs and the only requirement is physical treatment for the ligamentous strain. Most cases, however, require reduction, and possibly operative treatment at a later date.

Reduction is carried out under anæsthetic and should be followed by physical treatment. After reduction, a crêpe bandage is put on, or an ordinary gauze bandage firmly applied over several layers of cotton-wool. This serves the double purpose of affording support and checking effusion. Sometimes a short splint is kept behind the knee for a few days to immobilize it while the injured ligaments and tendons heal. Occasionally, the joint is completely immobilized for 3–4 weeks, or even longer. *Massage* can be given from the beginning. At first it should consist principally of effleurage of the thigh, to reduce the swelling, but rhythmic kneading and squeeze kneading may also be included. Gentle but firm finger kneadings round the joint can be added on the second or third day and the ligaments treated with frictions (*Fig.* 33). The large extent of the medial ligament should be taken into consideration, and frictions carried well down over the shaft of the tibia.

Massage of the lower leg is less important, but should not be omitted, because swelling often appears round the ankle. *Faradism* is often ordered, graduated contractions of the quadriceps being given. It serves both to reduce swelling (particularly if given under pressure, i.e., in this case with the bandage on) and also to keep up the strength of these muscles.

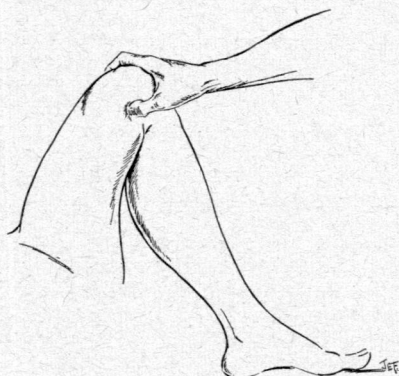

Fig. 33.—Transverse friction to the medial collateral ligament during knee flexion. Note that the physiotherapist's thumb moves the ligament to and fro, in imitation of its normal behaviour. (*By kind permission of Dr. J. Cyriax.*)

Active movements are given from the beginning, or at latest after two or three days. *Quadriceps contractions* should be taught, and assiduously practised by the patient, this being a form of exercise which he can do by himself, even if wearing a back splint. *Flexion* of the knee can also be performed. It is easiest if the patient sits on the edge of his couch or bed, and the knee is gently allowed to flex. The operator carefully supports the knee throughout and ensures that no rotation of the leg takes place, especially lateral rotation. The patient then extends the knee with the operator's assistance.

The patient is generally allowed to walk in a few days, and it is most important to see that he does so correctly. *If he everts his foot, he may easily 'turn his ankle', and in so doing twist the knee outward, and redisplace the cartilage.* He should be taught the foot-drill (*see* pp. 49 and 50) and required to practise it for himself. At the same time ordinary leg exercises should be given. Any exercise which does not produce lateral rotation of the knee while the patient has his weight on the limb is suitable. In about 3 weeks he may try medial and lateral rotation of the knee while in the sitting position, *but lateral rotation should never be forced.* The exercises must be graduated according to the patient's condition and strength. He should be warned to be careful when walking for the first few weeks, lest there should be a repetition of the original accident. He should ultimately, however, if young and strong, progress to vigorous exercise and a scheme of *progressive weight resistance* is often included in the treatment (*see* p. 68). If the cartilage slips out again, operation will be necessary.

MENISCECTOMY.—In cases where the injury to the cartilage is very severe, if it has slipped more than once, or if the knee cannot be entirely straightened by manipulation, *an open operation* is performed. The joint is opened with most careful precautions as regards asepsis, the medial ligament being preserved intact.

The anterior part—if this only is displaced or injured—or the whole cartilage is removed. The incision is generally a curved one on the inner side of the joint. A bandage is applied firmly over a thick dressing of cotton-wool.

Pre-operative Treatment.—This may be ordered for the purpose of decreasing the fluid in the joint, and keeping up the strength of the quadriceps. The patient may be kept in bed, or on a couch, for a few days with the knee bandaged. The treatment consists of massage, especially of the thigh, faradism (graduated contractions and possibly faradism under pressure), and voluntary quadriceps contractions.

Another form of pre-operative treatment which may be requested is *provocative treatment*. A patient may give a history of repeated 'locking' of the knee, there being no effusion or other positive symptoms. A torn cartilage is suspected, but before subjecting the patient to an operation the surgeon may send him to a physiotherapist for a scheme of exercises designed to displace a torn cartilage. Such exercises must be very strong and, in compliance with the anatomical points noted above, *make use of body-weight on a flexed and externally rotating knee*, e.g., Cossack dance movements; Hopping on one flexed knee, the other being held extended; Balance walking on a form incorporating movements which flex the knee and rotate the body on it.

Post-operative Treatment.—The patient is kept in bed for a few days after the operation. Heat and massage can be given from the beginning but are rarely required. *Active movements* are given to hip, foot, ankles, and toes. *Quadriceps contractions* are usually given from the beginning but may be delayed until the 3rd day. The stitches are removed 7 to 10 days after the operation and *active movements* of the knee should then begin. If the stitches are removed at the later date—10 days—*slight* flexion and extension may be started on the 7th day. *Flexion* should be in small range and with due precautions regarding the scar and stitches.

Once the stitches are removed movements progress fairly quickly. The patient is usually allowed to walk *with the support of crutches or sticks in 14 days or less*. A week later he should be able to walk *without sticks*, though a crêpe bandage is worn to support the knee. Meanwhile exercises are given to restore full flexion of the knee, and to strengthen the quadriceps. *Strong resisted exercises for the quadriceps* and re-education in walking complete the treatment. *Faradism* is a useful adjunct after the operation as well as before it.

4. Injury to the Medial Ligament without Displacement of the Cartilage

ANATOMY.—This ligament consists of superficial and deep fibres. The superficial set are attached above to the medial epicondyle of the femur, and below to the medial condyle of the tibia, and to the surface of the shaft of that bone for about two inches. The deep set connect the lower part of the medial condyle of the femur with the margin of the upper extremity of the tibia. It is usually these deep fibres that are injured, most often at their attachment to the tibia.

There is no locking of the joint. The principal symptom is pain on the inner side of the knee on certain movements: (a) when the foot is everted; (b) when the medial ligament is passively stretched, or when pressure is exerted over it.

Treatment.—These injuries are treated in much the same way as the slipped cartilages which have been replaced for the first time or which have merely required massage and exercises without manipulation. In severer cases the knee is rested for a time—2 to 3 weeks—and treatment by massage and exercise begins when this period is over. Again the *most important factor is the building up of a really strong group of quadriceps muscles*, as in any other injury to the knee.

Dr. Cyriax's Method.—Dr. Cyriax advocates treatment by deep transverse frictions alone, followed by active movements in the acute stage, and by forced passive movements in the chronic stage.* It must be stressed that Dr. Cyriax's methods of treatment for joint and muscle injuries make use of skilled techniques which should only be performed by those adequately trained in their use.

PROGRESSIVE RESISTANCE EXERCISE.—The outstanding names in connexion with this technique are McQueen, and Delorme and Watkins The method of treatment is based on the physiological fact that *muscle strength is increased by a resistance which demands maximal effort* and that *the contraction is greater following stretching of the muscle-fibres.* Broadly speaking the patient lifts a given weight thirty times, usually in three sessions of ten lifts each. The maximum weight which the patient can lift ten times in succession without a break is taken as the criterion. Say the patient's maximum load is 10 lb.: In order to hypertrophy muscle McQueen advocates the following programme: three sets of ten lifts each using maximum load throughout, i.e., 1st set, 10 lb. × 10; 2nd set, 10 lb. × 10; 3rd set, 10 lb. × 10, with a 2-minute rest between each. Delorme and Watkins advocate the following lifts: three sets of ten lifts each using $\frac{1}{2}$, $\frac{3}{4}$, and full load respectively, i.e., 1st set, 5 lb. × 10; 2nd set, $7\frac{1}{2}$ lb. × 10; 3rd set, 10 lb. × 10, again with a 2-minute rest between each. Thereafter the load is increased according to the patient's strength. The maximal load must always be used, however. Details of adaptations and modifications cannot be given here. For further details *see* J. M. Piercy, "Progressive Resistance Exercise", *Physiotherapy, Lond.,* September, 1959, and J. L. Rudd, "Moderate Resistance Exercises", *Physiotherapy, Lond.,* May 1960.

DISLOCATED ANKLE

A very rare injury without accompanying fracture. For treatment *see* Pott's fracture (pp. 44–5).

III. SACRO-ILIAC STRAIN

The sacro-iliac articulation may be attacked by tuberculosis, or some other form of infective arthritis. With these cases we have little to do. Those with which we are concerned constitute *strains* and *subluxations* of the joint, rather than dislocations.

ANATOMY.—The joint is that between the articular surfaces of the sacrum and ilium. The bones are connected by the anterior sacro-iliac ligament, composed of a number of thin fibrous bands, and the much stronger posterior sacro-iliac ligament. This joint was once classed among the *amphiarthroses,* or *cartilaginous* joints: but it is now described as a *diarthrosis,* or *synovial* joint, since it has been discovered that it has normally far more movement than was previously supposed. In addition to this, during pregnancy the ligaments become much relaxed, and after childbirth they tighten again while the uterus is in process of involution. In the erect posture the weight of the body falls on the sacro-iliac joints, and if their ligaments are not sufficiently strong, they give way and subluxation occurs. Incorrect posture naturally increases the strain by tipping the pelvis too far back or too far forward. If a gravid uterus is added to this the strain is increased. The *causes* of these 'strains' or subluxations are, therefore: (1) Habitual poor posture, particularly in a position of lordosis. (2) Pregnancy. (3) Weak musculature following pregnancy. (4) Strain or injury while the patient is bending forward, particularly when carrying a heavy weight. (It is more probable, however, that this results in herniation of an intra-articular disk.)

---

* *See* James Cyriax, *Textbook of Orthopædic Medicine,* Vol. II.

The ilium may be displaced forwards on the sacrum, or the sacrum forward on the ilium, the latter being most common after childbirth. In either case, the displacement may be unilateral or bilateral.

There is pain over one or both sacro-iliac joints, or in the lumbar region. In some cases there is a feeling of instability which is sometimes so marked as to react on the nervous system and set up neurotic symptoms. The pain is a dull ache, with occasional short knife-like stabs. It is worst when the patients sits or lies with the normal lumbar curve obliterated; or in positions which put a strain on the joint, such as are taken in going up or down stairs. There may be referred pain in the gluteal region or abdomen. Pain is felt on pressure over the posterior superior spines of the ilium, which lie directly behind the joint.

Treatment.—In some cases of mere *strain*, strapping applied round the pelvis affords relief and by relieving this strain, and the consequent muscle spasm, leads to recovery. The patient may wear a belt of some kind, but more commonly a band of adhesive plaster is applied round the pelvis. The plaster is about four inches wide, and is put on just below the iliac crests. It generally consists of two strips, one at the back and one at the front. The posterior strip is applied first, and extends across the back to about two inches in front of the anterior superior iliac spines. This should be put on with the patient standing. The anterior strip stretches across the abdomen, its ends overlapping those of the posterior strip, and extending two or three inches behind the anterior superior spines. The patient should lie down during the application of this strip, so that the abdominal organs may be relieved of the pull of gravity, and the strapping may thus be put on in such a way as to hold them in this position when she stands upright. If actually displaced, the articular surfaces are put back into correct position under an anæsthetic.

Physical Treatment should begin as soon as possible after manipulation, e.g., on the evening of the same day. The patient should be treated by a dose of radiant heat or infra-red radiation (15 to 20 minutes), then the joints should be moved passively. With the patient in crook-lying, the knees should be flexed on to the chest; after this, first one and then the other hip should be abducted as fully as possible, the knee being semi-flexed and the pelvis supported on the opposite side. The trunk should next be rotated. The patient then turns over into the prone position and the hips and lumbar spine are extended, the physiotherapist placing one hand on the sacrum and lifting the legs backward with the other. (The help of a second operator is advisable for this movement, especially in the case of a heavy patient.) These are the movements performed during the operation and it is a great advantage for the physiotherapist to have been present during the surgeon's manipulation. She will then know exactly how he wishes the movements to be given, and what degree of mobility she may expect to obtain in the patient's joints. Before leaving the patient, the adhesive strapping is applied. Some surgeons do not strap the pelvis *after* manipulation, but rely on the strengthening of the muscles by exercises to provide the necessary support for the joint.

The next day *heat* and *gentle massage* is given to the back and hips. As soon as possible *active movements* are added, e.g., Prone-lying Alternate leg-backward-raising, progressing to Prone-lying Back-raising; and Heave-grasp-lying 2-Knee-updrawing-and-lowering. Treatment by radiant heat may be continued as long as pain is present. Later the glutei and lumbar muscles should be treated with vigorous effleurage and kneading, and deep frictions be given round the joint.

Exercise should be chosen to strengthen the abdominal and back muscles, mobilize the hip and sacro-iliac joints, and teach correct posture. They are given at first in lying or prone-lying, later in standing. *Instruction in the maintenance of the correct pelvic tilt is all-important* (pp. 342, 344).

IV. PROLAPSED INTERVERTEBRAL DISK

ANATOMY AND PATHOLOGY.—The intervertebral disk consists of two parts, an outer, the *annulus fibrosus*, composed of fibrous tissue and fibro-cartilage, and an inner, the *nucleus pulposus*, composed of a soft, pulpy, highly elastic substance. The disks are attached to the thin layers of hyalin cartilage which cover the upper and lower surfaces of the vertebræ. It is possible for the whole disk to be displaced, but a much commoner condition is *a rupture of the annulus fibrosus*, due to injury, strain, or degeneration. In some cases *a fragmented portion of the annulus fibrosus becomes dislodged* in much the same way as does a torn meniscus, and causes pressure on a nerve. This may cause neuralgia or neuritis. In other cases there is *a protrusion of the nucleus pulposus through the ruptured annulus fibrosus.* The prolapsed nucleus pulposus may pass *downwards* into the spongy tissue of the body of the vertebra below, or it may protrude *posterolaterally* into the vertebral canal, through, or to one side, of the posterior longitudinal ligament which is attached to the posterior surfaces of the bodies of all the vertebræ from the axis to the sacrum (*Fig.* 34). In the former cases it will cause

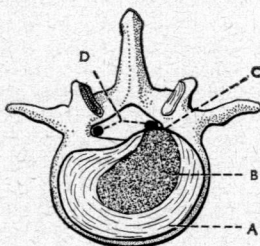

Fig. 34.—Lumbar vertebra and intervertebral disk. A, Annulus fibrosus; B, Nucleus pulposus; C, Protrusion of nucleus pulposus through rupture of annulus fibrosus causing pressure on nerve; D, Nerve trunks in vertebral foramen.

backache but not sciatica. In the latter case it compresses one of the lumbar or sacral nerve-roots passing out towards the intervertebral foramen through which it leaves the canal. The disk between lumbar 4 and 5, and that between lumbar 5 and the sacrum are most often affected, compressing respectively the 4th lumbar and the 1st sacral nerve-roots, both of which enter into the composition of the sciatic nerve.

SYMPTOMS.—In the early stages, there is *pain in the back*, of the type generally described as 'lumbago'. This occurs when the annulus fibrosus is torn, but the protrusion of the nucleus pulposus has not yet occurred, or is only beginning.* The extensor muscles of the back go into protective spasm to prevent any further pressure on the nerve. *This limits flexion of the spine* and may produce *lordosis.* Flexion, side-flexion, and rotation may be both limited and painful. If protrusion of the nucleus pulposus follows, or as it continues, the pressure on the nerve-root increases, and the *typical sciatic pain develops down the back of the thigh.* It is often made worse if the patient coughs or sneezes. There may be *parœsthesia* ('pins and needles') in the feet, or areas of *hyperœsthesia* in the distribution of the affected nerve-root. Radiologically, the space between the two vertebræ now becomes widened. The normal lumbar lordosis disappears, and its place may be taken by a *lumbar kyphosis. Scoliosis* may also develop, as described on p. 274. In long-standing cases *the muscles supplied by the affected nerve-root may become*

---

* It should be noted that protrusion of the nucleus pulposus does not always follow.

atrophied and weakened. The *ankle-jerk may be absent* if S.1 is compressed. *Lasègue's Sign* (*see* p. 275) is present.

Treatment.—Many varied methods of treatment are in use today, but authorities agree that *rest* is an essential part of treatment. This may be achieved by: (1) *Rest in bed* until the acute symptoms have died down (3 weeks or so). (2) *Plaster jacket* similar to that used after fracture of a lumbar vertebra. The spine may be in full hyperextension, or slight extension only, depending on the views of the physician or surgeon in charge of the case. This opens the disk spaces, and keeps them open, relieving pressure on the disks and avoiding stretching of the nerve-roots. The jacket is retained until the condition is well settled (usually at least 3 months, often more). Other methods of treatment include: (1) *Manipulation,* with or without anæsthetic. (2) *Traction* to the lumbar spine applied by means of a special couch. The traction may be used alone or may be followed by manipulation. (3) *Open operation.* Laminectomy (removal of all or part of the vertebral lamina) with excision of the protruding part of the nucleus pulposus, and as much of this structure as possible from the interior of the disk.

PHYSICAL TREATMENT OF PATIENTS IN PLASTER OR ON BED-REST.—Most forms of physical treatment other than exercises are precluded by the plaster, but if the patient is merely on bed-rest *heat* and *massage* may be given for the relief of pain and spasm. However, the primary aim of treatment is to strengthen the back muscles and lessen the chance of recurrence. In either case *extension exercises* are essential. They may begin at once, or, for patients in plaster, as soon as it is dry. To begin with, they should be simple, e.g., Prone-lying Head-raising; Prone-lying Alternate leg-raising; lying Back-arching so that only the head and buttocks rest on the bed (Gervis). Progressions are made in Prone-lying in the following way: First by raising head and shoulders together; then by raising head and shoulders and both legs. From this progression the lever may be increased by (*a*) placing the hands behind the neck, and (*b*) holding them in elevation (this is a very strong progression indeed). As the condition improves prone-kneeling may be taken as a variation in the starting position. From this position Alternate Leg-lifting backwards, Alternate Arm-lifting, and Alternate Arm- and Leg-lifting can be given.

General Exercises.—Respiratory exercises are important, since breathing will be hampered by the plaster to some extent. General arm and head exercises may be included to keep the muscles in good condition, and pulleys and springs are useful if available. If abdominal exercises are required they should be confined to abdominal contractions. A programme of gradually progressive exercises is continued after the plaster is removed, or the patient is allowed up. Whilst general exercises may be included in the scheme, *the accent must be on specific exercises to strengthen the back muscles, and the extensors in particular.* Postural correction should receive attention. The patient should guard against assuming a bad posture with the spine in flexion, as in modern arm-chairs or car seats (Gervis) and should be taught how to lift objects with the spine in extension. Many patients are advised to wear a corset to give support, and to act as a deterrent to further attacks by limiting flexion.

Flexion of the spine is a very controversial point. Many authorities do not allow it at all, believing that the flexed spine constitutes a weakened position, and that to encourage the patient to adopt it is courting disaster. Others allow it in the belief that full spinal mobility is necessary for the nutrition and health of the cartilage. They hold that if flexion is disallowed, degenerative changes, which may enhance a tendency to disk protrusion, are liable to occur. Even so, they feel that flexion should be avoided for some weeks, and that it must then be introduced with caution.

PHYSICAL TREATMENT AFTER MANIPULATIVE REDUCTION OR TRACTION.—These patients are treated on much the same lines as above. They should be dealt with in close co-operation with the manipulative surgeon.

Dr. Cyriax's Method.—The rationale of Dr. Cyriax's method of treatment cannot be discussed here.* His treatments include *manipulative techniques* (generally applied in the case of lesions of the annulus fibrosus), *traction*, and *epidural injections*. He also advocates the use of plaster jackets and corsets for support and protection, and lays great stress on the avoidance of flexion of the spine.

PHYSIOTHERAPY FOR PATIENTS TREATED BY OPERATION.—The patient is kept in bed for a period varying from 4 to 21 days according to the opinion of the surgeon. The aims of treatment are *to strengthen the trunk muscles*, especially those of the lumbar spine, and *extension exercises should still take first place. Flexion* of the spine will depend on the surgeon's views. It should not in any case be given for $3\frac{1}{2}$–4 weeks and should then be introduced gradually and with discretion. Pain at the site of the operation, backache, and possibly sciatic pain due to drag on the already irritated nerve, might result from neglect of this precaution. Treatment will begin when the surgeon sanctions it (usually from the 3rd to the 5th day after the operation), but breathing exercises, quadriceps contractions, and foot and ankle exercises may be given immediately. The stitches will be removed about the 10th or 12th day. Until the stitches are removed, treatment will consist of gentle breathing exercises, static contractions of the quadriceps, and foot and ankle exercises. Specific exercises for the back should be given but are confined to gentle head raising and turning, shoulder bracing and gluteal contractions, given in prone-lying. After the stitches have been removed progression can be made along the lines indicated for patients in plaster. The physiotherapist will naturally take into consideration the age, health, and physique of the patient when planning any treatment scheme. It is usual for patients to return to sedentary or light work in about 4 to 5 weeks. A patient doing heavy work is usually required to wait 8 to 12 weeks before returning.

V. SPRAINS

Confusion sometimes arises as to the different degrees of ligamentous injury. Briefly, a *strain* is an injury to a ligament which does not stretch it beyond its normal limits of elastic recovery (Bonnin). No fibres are ruptured. There is some local pain and swelling, and possibly a small amount of effusion into the joint concerned. A *sprain* is caused by a more violent stretching which ruptures some of the ligamentous fibres within its outer sheath, so that the ligament is slightly lengthened, but although there is more swelling, pain, and limitation of movement than in a strain, there is little or no hæmorrhage. *In neither of these injuries is there displacement, or instability of the joint*, although, as already stated at the beginning of the chapter, in a sprain the joint surfaces parted initially. They do not, however, remain displaced. There is no deformity. The joint can be moved, though movement causes pain. Other symptoms are similar to those present in dislocations, but less marked. The pain, though severe at the time of injury, later consists of a dull ache and only becomes sharp on movement which put the injured structures on the stretch.

The treatment of sprains is not difficult and all are dealt with on the same lines. It would be superfluous to describe in detail the treatment of every joint which may possibly be sprained. The three commonest sprains—those of the wrist, ankle, and back—will be described here.

---

* For Dr. Cyriax's method of manipulation, *see* his *Text-book of Orthopædic Medicine*, Vol. II The pathology of disk lesions in lumbago and sciatica is dealt with in Vol. I of the same work.

Principles of Treatment.—Since there is an acute inflammatory reaction round the joint a certain amount of rest is necessary to allow this to die down. Some form of support is therefore given. Since, however, there is rarely more than partial rupture of ligaments and tendons it need not be extensive and can usually be discarded in a week or so. As with any inflammatory condition there is a risk of adhesions forming, particularly since the injured structures are fibrous tissue, and it is essential to prevent this. Full mobility must be restored as quickly as possible. *The principal aims of physical treatment* can, therefore, be summarized as: (1) *The prevention of adhesions.* It is necessary to prevent organization of the highly fibrinous inflammatory exudate, by preventing or reducing swelling and encouraging early movements. (2) *The relief of pain.* Pain precludes movement as the patient is unwilling to incur pain by using the joint and this increases the risk of adhesions. (3) *The restoration of full mobility and muscle power* as soon as possible. This is very important. If the muscles are not returned to full strength they may be unable to prevent recurrence of the injury and the patient will have a joint which 'gives'.

Heat, massage, prolonged anodal galvanism, and passive and active exercises are all used in the treatment of sprains.

Note on early passive movement and deep massage in recent articular sprains.— Dr. James Cyriax* states that "contrary to general belief, deep massage and passive movements are the mainstay of treatment during the early stage of articular sprains. The present insistence on active movement alone greatly retards recovery at some joints. Some ligaments, e.g., the coronary ligaments at the knee, can be kept adequately moving only by the physiotherapist's finger." He points out that the movements between bone and ligament are the same during a passive movement as during an active movement, *but the range of passive movement is always greater in a sprained joint than that of an active movement.* Moreover, passive movements prevent the formation of adhesions. Of passive movements, in which he includes deep massage and gentle forced movements, he says, "The movements must not be so forcible as to overstretch those fibrils that are gaining longitudinal attachment within the healing breach; nor should they be so gentle as to fail to disengage those fibrils that are gaining abnormal transverse adherence. A safe rule is to push movements to the point of discomfort, but not of pain." He does not, of course, discount the value of active movements.

In chronic sprains, besides mobilization under a general or local anæsthetic or a local analgesia produced by heat and deep massage, he advocates deep transverse frictions,† which move the ligaments to and fro over the bone, thinning out the scar tissue and breaking down the transverse adhesions in its substance. Forced movements are given to free adhesions about the joint, followed by active movements, first free and then resisted.

SPRAINED WRIST

This may be caused by violent wrenching of the wrist in any direction, though the most usual is *forward* or *backward* into *forced flexion* or *extension*. Under the term 'sprained wrist' are included all degrees of injuries, from the most trivial to the really serious. Which ligaments and muscles are injured depends, of course, on the direction of the causative force. Violent extension will cause wrenching of the anterior radiocarpal ligament and the flexor muscles, and

* James Cyriax, *Text-book of Orthopædic Medicine*, Vol. I, p. 31.
† For a description of these techniques, *see* Dr. Cyriax, *Text-book of Orthopædic Medicine*, Vol. II: also the article by Jennifer Hickling on 'Soft Tissue Lesions; Localization and Deep Massage", *Physiotherapy, Lond.*, May, 1957.

probably tenosynovitis of their sheaths; violent flexion will produce similar damage to the structures on the posterior aspect. The medial or lateral radio-carpal ligaments (ulnar or radial collateral) are occasionally injured, or some of the small ligaments between the carpal bones, especially that between the lunate and capitate bones.* A tender spot will be found over the torn ligament. In a bad sprain there may be a good deal of swelling, extending some way up the forearm.

Treatment.—Generally a firm bandage over cotton-wool, or strapping, gives adequate support but occasionally a splint of some kind is prescribed. If possible a sling should be avoided as it tends to 'invalid' the patient. If, however, it is felt that the patient is likely to do too much with the wrist and hand, a sling is advisable. Cold compresses or evaporating lotions may be applied. Hot or cold applications, whichever affords most relief, or contrast bathing may be advised for home use.

PHYSICAL TREATMENT.—If the patient is seen immediately after injury *prolonged anodal galvanism* is helpful in the treatment of sprains, the anaphoretic effect being used to prevent or reduce swelling. It may be continued on the 2nd and 3rd day but should not be required after that. A relatively large anode is wrapped round the joint, the smaller cathode being placed near the main lymph-glands, in this case on the shoulder or upper arm. A current of very low intensity ($\frac{1}{2}$–1 mA. per sq. in.) should be passed for as long a duration as practicable, i.e., 1–1$\frac{1}{2}$ hr. at least.

Heat and massage should be given for the relief of pain and swelling. If anodal galvanism is given heat treatment is usually delayed for the first few days, it being superfluous in conjunction with electrical treatment. Radiant heat, infra-red radiation, short-wave diathermy, and wax baths are all suitable. If swelling is diffuse, massage should include the whole arm. Particular attention should be paid to the fingers and hand, finger kneadings and frictions being used. Finger kneadings and deep frictions should be given to the wrist-joint as soon as the patient can tolerate them. For deep transverse frictions the affected ligament should be put on a slight stretch. Full use of the hand must be encouraged. Full flexion and extension of the fingers must be practised as this assists in the dispersal of fluid. *Relaxed passive movements and active assisted wrist movements* should be given to begin with, progression to free and resisted exercises being made as soon as possible. Movements should be full and pain-free in 7–14 days. If, however, there is any residual stiffness, deep transverse frictions and passive stretchings should be given to the joint. Careful forced passive movements may be required.

SPRAINED ANKLE

This is really a sprain of the *mid-tarsal* and *talocalcaneal* (subtaloid) *joints* as well as of the *ankle joint*. It is generally caused by 'turning over the ankle', that is, by a violent inversion of the foot—the same force that sometimes fractures the internal malleolus. The patient generally falls down when the accident occurs, and in severe sprains is unable to walk without pain. The lateral ligament is partially or completely ruptured, and there may be damage to the small liga-ments on the outer side of the foot. The *peronei* and *extensor brevis digitorum* are wrenched. The swelling may be very considerable over the foot and round the ankle, and may extend some way up the leg.

Treatment.—As a result of the large amount of exudation adhesions are very liable to form, and unless properly treated the patient's foot may remain stiff and painful for a long time. It is essential therefore to check effusion as soon as possible and to keep the foot mobile. The foot should be bandaged in *dorsiflexion*

---

* *See* James Cyriax, *Text-book of Orthopædic Medicine*, Vol. I, Chapter XIII.

and eversion. Zinc oxide strapping or elastoplast afford the best support, but a crêpe or elastonet bandage can be used. *The bandage should start behind the metatarsal heads and extend well above the ankle-joint* to avoid an œdematous pouching above the bandage. It is also very important to see that adequate support is given over the lateral malleolus to avoid a pocket of œdema there. If the bandage is started on the medial side, the foot is pulled into eversion by the turns of the bandage.

PHYSICAL TREATMENT follows the same lines as that of the wrist-joint. If prolonged anodal galvanism is used the anode should include the dorsum of the foot as well as the ankle-joint. Particular attention must be given to the dorsum of the foot and around the malleoli and tendo Achillis, when massage is given. When giving frictions to the lateral ligament, the foot should be in slight inversion and plantar flexion. *It is very important to exercise the intrinsic muscles of the foot, particular attention being given to lumbrical action.* The peronei must also be adequately strengthened. Faradic foot baths can be given when the support is discarded.

RE-EDUCATION OF WALKING is essential, and should begin on the 1st day. The physiotherapist must see that the weight of the body is correctly taken on the foot in standing and in walking, i.e., *through the calcaneum to the base of the 5th metatarsal and across the heads of the metatarsals.* The hip, knee, ankle, and toes must be used correctly when steps are taken, and the steps must be even.

Some doctors prefer to defer the more active treatment for a few days or a week, and may advise the use of a stick or sticks. The author feels, however, that the best results are obtained by early movement and use of the limb, but the patient should not stand for too long at a time. He should be advised to rest the foot on a stool when he is sitting down.

SPRAINED BACK

This is really a muscle rather than a joint injury, and consists of stretching or tearing of some part of the erector spinæ, or of some muscle of the 5th layer. It may occur while at play, or may merely be the result of a false step, the patient having contracted his muscles over-strongly in order to avoid a fall. It is often quite a slight injury, but may cause a good deal of trouble if it does not receive attention from the beginning. It is not uncommon, however, for a functional element to become superimposed on the organic trouble.

Treatment.—

PHYSICAL TREATMENT.—*Heat* and *massage* should be given from the beginning. Massage should consist of firm kneading and effleurage to check and disperse effusion, with finger kneading and frictions along the spine. The treatment may be given in prone-lying or in lean-sitting, whichever the patient finds most comfortable and relaxing. The patient should come for treatment as soon after the accident as possible, because if the effusion is allowed to organize and form adhesions there may be pain and disability for months afterwards. *Extension exercises,* both free and with resistance, should be given to strengthen the back muscles and a general scheme of trunk exercises should be included in the treatment. There is no need to limit flexion as in disk lesions. Constant current may be used for the relief of pain; and various forms of ionization such as histamine, novocain, and iodine can be used to produce analgesia or a fibrolytic effect.

VI. INJURY OF MUSCLES AND THEIR TENDONS

Under this heading are included inflammatory conditions in muscle-fibres, connective tissue, tendons, and synovial sheaths; also rupture of actual muscle-fibres, tendons, and aponeuroses.

INFLAMMATORY CONDITIONS include: (1) *Myositis*, which is inflammation of the muscle tissue itself. (2) *Fibrositis*, which covers inflammation of connective tissue, whether between muscles or in their substance. (3) *Tendinitis*, which is inflammation in the tendon itself. It may occur at the junction of the tendon with the periosteum of the bone to which it is attached, or in the substance of the tendon itself. (4) *Tenosynovitis and Tenovaginitis*, which is an inflammatory condition of a synovial sheath. The sheath of the tendon (where it possesses one) as well as the tendon itself, may be the seat of the trouble. The surfaces of the sheath and the tendon may be roughened, causing crepitus and pain where they glide on one another (tenosynovitis), or the primary lesion may be in the sheath itself, which is inflamed and thickened (tenovaginitis). There is no crepitus in this type of injury. Inflammatory conditions can be caused by any of the following. (1) *Trauma*. We have already seen that forces which cause fractures, dislocations and sprains affect soft tissues in the area, as well as the bones of joint surfaces. (2) *Strain*. This may be traumatic or may result from prolonged overuse, or altered mechanics, of a muscle or tendon. (3) *Fatigue*. This leads to an accumulation of waste products which give rise to an inflammatory reaction. (4) *Certain rheumatic conditions*. These again lead to cumulative waste products and result in inflammation.

RUPTURE of muscle-fibres, tendons, or aponeuroses may be *partial* or *complete*. Repair is by white-fibrous scar tissue. This results in a certain amount of loss of elasticity in muscle which may or may not seriously incapacitate the patient. Complete or partial ruptures are the result of traumatic forces. In some fractures a spur of callus forms beneath a tendon and the constant play of the tendon over this causes it to rupture. It should be noted that this constitutes a form of trauma.

The general symptoms of muscle or tendon injuries are consistent with an inflammatory reaction. There is *pain* in the affected area, increased by pressure or on movement, *aching, swelling*, and *altered consistency*. Tendons feel spongy and there is crepitus. Muscles may feel soft and inelastic, or hard and firm, nodules sometimes being palpable. There is *loss of function* in the limb where the inflammation is present, both because of the loss of power in the inflamed muscles, and because the pain inhibits movement. The commonest complication of these conditions is pressure on nerves in the vicinity, giving rise to cramp, tremor, or neuralgia.

Principles of Treatment.—These are similar to those of any joint injury. It should be realized that while muscle or tendon injuries of traumatic origin are usually seen in the acute stage, i.e., immediately after the injury, those of non-traumatic origin are often insidious in onset, and may not be seen until the condition has become a chronic one. We must therefore consider the principles of treatment in acute and chronic cases.

IN THE ACUTE STAGE rest is needed to allow the inflammatory reaction to die down. The highly fibrinous inflammatory exudate must be absorbed in order to prevent adhesions from forming, and full function must be restored. This means the maintenance or restoration of mobility and strength, and for this to be achieved pain must first be relieved. Rest will be achieved by providing some form of support. Heat, massage, and electrical treatments will assist the absorption of fluid and the relief of pain. Passive and active movements will restore function.

IN THE CHRONIC STAGE adhesions and scarring will have occurred, with resultant loss of function. Mobility must be regained and muscle power built up. Heat and massage will relieve pain but the most important treatment consists of *deep massage to soften and stretch adhesions and scar tissue, followed by active exercises*, free and resisted. Forced passive movements may be necessary.

With myositis we have little to do. Here, suffice it to say that vague unidentified muscular pains will be treated conservatively with heat, massage, and exercises, and in some cases by electrotherapy. Tenosynovitis and Tenovaginitis are dealt with in Chapter VII. Here we shall consider lesions of supraspinatus, tennis elbow, rupture of muscle-fibres in the calf, and fibrositis. The first three are primarily inflammatory conditions resulting from trauma. The latter is an inflammatory condition of unknown origin. Similar injuries can happen to other muscles in the body but follow the same general principles.

LESIONS OF THE SUPRASPINATUS TENDON

ANATOMY AND PHYSIOLOGY.—The student will remember that, in the ball-and-socket joint of the shoulder, the head of the humerus is much larger in extent than the glenoid cavity and the capsule very loose, especially at its inner side. Its main support consists of the tendons of the surrounding short muscles, sometimes known collectively as the *tendinous* or *rotator cuff* of the shoulder. At the upper part of this cuff lies the tendon of the supraspinatus. When the arm is by the side of the body, the greater tuberosity, to which the *supraspinatus, infraspinatus,* and *teres minor* are attached, is at the same level as the upper part of the articular surface of the humeral head (which lies beneath the acromion). The greater tuberosity lies beyond the tip of the acromion process. When the arm is abducted the tuberosity passes upwards and inwards beneath the acromion, the humeral head sliding downwards on the glenoid, the movement being facilitated by the presence beneath the acromion of a large bursa (the *subacromial* or *subdeltoid bursa*). The tendons attached to the tuberosity, in particular the supraspinatus, now lie between it and the acromion, and are compressed between these bones. As the arm is raised still higher, the tuberosity is carried further inwards, so that the tendons no longer lie between the bony processes. This fact explains why *inflammatory lesions of these muscles exhibit a painful mid-arc of abduction from about 60° to 120°.* It is obvious that, if there is swelling in any of these tendons, part of the movement during which they are pressed against the acromion will give rise to severe pain.

TYPES OF LESION.—The supraspinatus may become the seat of an acute or chronic *tendinitis,* the commonest site being its *teno-periosteal junction.* The tendinitis is occasioned by strain and may be accompanied by partial rupture of fibres. In elderly patients the inflammatory reaction may involve all the muscles of the "rotator cuff". Another form of lesion is *complete rupture* of all the fibres. In young people these lesions result from severe trauma. As people grow older, the supraspinatus tendon becomes the site of progressive degeneration (Jenkins), probably owing to repeated minor injuries and the compression of the tendon between the bones. Being, therefore, weakened, and its power of recovery after injury impaired, it is particularly liable to partial or complete rupture. In such cases the direct cause is often trivial in nature.

Supraspinatus Tendinitis With or Without Partial Rupture of the Tendon

As has been said, this lesion may be due to a slight or severe accident, or to repeated small strains. The patient usually feels a sharp pain which tends to increase, particularly at night. It often radiates to the deltoid insertion. There is localized tenderness over the anterior aspect of the shoulder-joint. The patient is able to elevate the arm in spite of the pain, *which will be intense in the mid-arc of movement.* Abduction up to 60° may be painless and there may be a fair range of movement in the stooping position, with the arm hanging free. *The patient shrugs the shoulder whilst abducting the arm.* Subdeltoid bursitis is often a complication. In neglected cases, especially in the elderly, dense adhesions may form and movement become permanently limited.

Treatment.—Early treatment is essential in the interests of restoring full function. The arm may be put up on a splint in abduction (90°) and outward rotation (45°), or simply rested in a sling.

Heat can be given in the form of infra-red irradiation, radiant heat, or short-wave diathermy. The patient should be in a relaxed and comfortable posture, with the arm and shoulder well supported. Heat sometimes aggravates the condition, in which case it must be discontinued.

MOVEMENTS.—Opinions vary as to the type of early movement advisable. Some authorities consider that the early movements should be completely relaxed *passive movements*, given once or twice daily within the limits of pain. They believe that this prevents the formation of adhesions, whilst causing no irritation to the damaged tendon (Jenkins).* The patient is treated in the lying position. The physiotherapist, carefully supporting the arm and shoulder, carries the arm gently and smoothly into abduction, at the same time rotating it outwards. She stops as soon as pain is felt, *and keeps within the limits of pain when repeating the movement.* Gradually the range is increased. The movements must never, at this stage, be carried beyond the limits of pain, either by the operator or by the patient himself, and he must be careful to avoid such movements at home. When inflammation has subsided (but not before) *active movements* are added, to stretch adhesions and restore the strength of the muscles. Such exercises as the following may be given:—

1. *Suspension Exercises or Pool Therapy.*—In this way a greater range of movement is possible as gravity is eliminated. Special attention is paid to abduction and external movements.

2. *Pulley Exercises.*—An overhead pulley is arranged so that one arm helps the other.

3. *Roller Towel Exercises.*—This is a useful substitute if a pulley is unobtainable. For external rotation it is used as in drying the back.

4. *Stooping Exercises.*—The patient bends forward until the trunk is parallel with the floor; he may rest the hand or forearm of the sound side on a table or chair-back. He swings the injured arm in circles, backwards and forwards, outwards and inwards, gradually increasing the range of movement.

5. *'Crawling up the Wall'.*—(a) Facing the wall, for elevation and outward rotation through flexion; (b) Injured side to the wall, for elevation and outward rotation through abduction.

6. *Kabat Techniques.*—Treatment being similar to that indicated for dislocated shoulder.

Later, general shoulder exercises can be practised and resistance added, but this must be used with discretion, especially in the case of elderly patients.

Other authorities advocate free and resisted *active* movements as soon as possible, resistance being designed to hypertrophy the other muscles of the rotator cuff in order to compensate for the weakness of supraspinatus, and here the Kabat system can be employed with advantage. Sometimes the full range of forced passive movements may be included in the treatment once the acute stage has subsided. Injections of novocain, or some other local anæsthetic, are sometimes given before treatment.

'Rotator cuff' lesions may be treated by either of these methods but treatment often increases the pain and loss of function and the shoulder gradually becomes 'frozen'. Spontaneous recovery occurs in eighteen months to two years, and many authorities prefer to treat the patients by local analgesia alone until recovery takes place.

---

* S. Aubrey Jenkins, "Periarticular Lesions of the Shoulder", *Physiotherapy, Lond.*, May, 1951. For early active movement, *see* P. Wiles and Watson-Jones, *Fractures and Other Bone and Joint Injuries.*

MANIPULATION.—If the adhesions cannot be stretched by the patient's own efforts, or by ordinary forced movements, the shoulder may be manipulated under an anæsthetic. *After-treatment* consists of daily vigorous exercises to maintain and increase the range of shoulder movement. These must be carried out in spite of discomfort or pain.

DR. CYRIAX'S METHOD.—Deep transverse frictions are given over the tendon, the patient half-lying on a low couch. The arm is held in *extension, adduction, and internal rotation* by placing the patient's hand behind his back (*Fig.* 35).

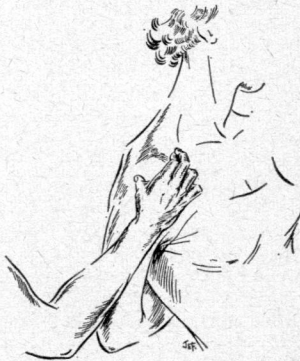

Fig. 35.—Transverse friction to the supraspinatus tendon. The physiotherapist's finger passes across the tendon which lies in the sagittal plane because of full medial rotation of the humerus. (*Figs.* 35–6 *by kind permission of Dr. J. Cyriax.*)

The physiotherapist sits facing the patient. The position of *extension brings the tendon forwards in front of the acromion,* and that of *adduction draws the distal extremity outwards beyond the acromion.* The tendon now lies well in front of, and just lateral to, the anterior extremity of the acromion process. The physiotherapist identifies both this point and the greater tuberosity of the humerus. In the groove palpable between the two bones the tendon of the supraspinatus muscle can be clearly palpated (Cyriax).* Dr. Cyriax recommends about a quarter of an hour's friction twice a week, and considers that two to six weeks' treatment is generally required to effect a cure. *It is essential that the tendon should be accurately located.*

This is a most valuable treatment and many physiotherapists use it in conjunction with active (or passive and active) movements.

Calcified Deposits in the Supraspinatus Tendon

Sometimes calcified deposits form in the tendon. These may cause no symptoms and only be discovered accidentally. Symptoms arise when the deposit impinges on the floor of the subacromial bursa which may become inflamed. Their onset may be sudden or gradual. The patient sometimes complains of aching of the shoulder and there is tenderness over the affected area. Abduction is painful in the mid-arc (*see* p. 77), active movement being more limited than passive. Sometimes the calcified deposit ruptures into the bursa, in which case the pain ceases and does not recur, the chalky material being absorbed. If the condition persists and symptoms are present, operative treatment is recommended.

---

* James Cyriax, *Text-book of Orthopædic Medicine*, Vol. II, pp. 8, 114; also *Recent Advances in Physical Medicine*, edited by Francis Bach, Chapter VI (contributed by Dr. Cyriax).

Complete Rupture of the Tendon

This injury is caused by a fall on the shoulder or on the outstretched hand; or by a slip when lifting a heavy object. The patient feels a sharp pain, which gets rapidly worse, and is intolerable by night time. The pain may be referred to the neck or down the arm to the hand (Wiles). Abduction cannot be initiated actively; full, or almost full, passive movement is possible but it causes pain, especially in the mid-arc. The symptoms diminish with rest, but return if work is attempted. The pain is always worse at night. The subdeltoid bursa becomes inflamed, much thickened, and distended with fluid.

Treatment.—If the rupture is complete, i.e., if *all* fibres have given way, an operation is necessary. The tendon is repaired, and the arm supported in abduction (90°), flexion (60°), and outward rotation (45°). The plaster is not removed until active elevation of the arm is possible (about 6 to 9 weeks), but after 3 weeks the upper part of the plaster covering the arm may be removed, so that movements can be practised. When the splint is finally removed, full mobility must be regained by active exercises.

The *prognosis* is fair if the operation is carried out a few days after injury, but bad if it is delayed (Wiles). To avoid operative treatment the remaining muscles can be hypertrophied, to compensate for the loss of supraspinatus.

If in spite of all other treatment the pain persists, owing to continued tendinitis, or a ruptured tendon that does not heal—the surgeon may decide on removal of the acromion process (Acromionectomy). This does away with compression of the tendon between the acromion and the tuberosity during abduction. *Heat* and *massage* can be given as soon as the wound is healed, if the area is painful. Care should be taken when administering heat treatment because the top of the shoulder may be anæsthetic, owing to severance of the superficial nerves of the cervical plexus. *Graduated active movements*, with assistance at first, form the major part of physical treatment.

Infraspinatus Tendinitis

The infraspinatus may also suffer traumatic inflammation. Similar treatment to that described for supraspinatus lesions will be given. In order to give accurate deep frictions as advocated by Dr. Cyriax the tendon must be brought

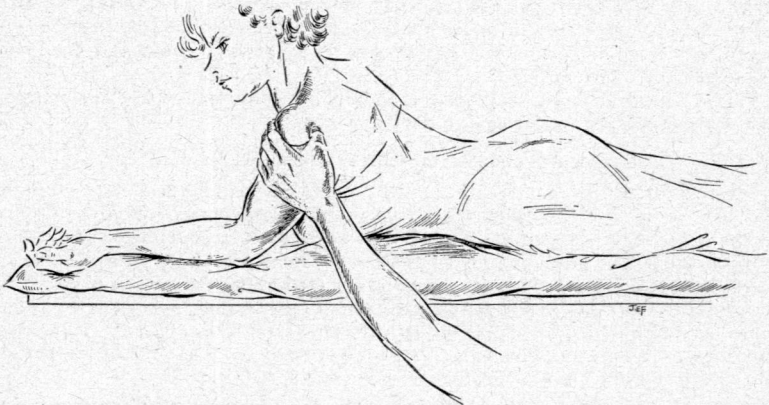

Fig. 36.—Transverse friction to the infraspinatus tendon. Flexion, adduction, and lateral rotation of the humerus have brought the tendon to an easily accessible position.

into an accessible position. This is done by putting the arm into *flexion, adduction,* and *lateral rotation* (*Fig.* 36).

TENNIS ELBOW

This is primarily a condition of muscular overstrain, due to the playing of tennis or some other game, or to over-indulgence in some strenuous occupation producing strain of the muscles near the elbow, especially of those acting on the superior radio-ulnar joint, or of the muscles arising from the common extensor tendon. The use of too heavy a racket, or of any other tool or implement too large or heavy for the user, may be responsible for the trouble. The onset is nearly always gradual.

PATHOLOGY.—Many different accounts have been given of this injury and there appear to be several types of lesion which occur. Romer describes three types:—

1. A *myositis* or *fibrositis* of the muscles round the elbow, the result of the constant jerking of the muscles at their origin on the internal and external condyles, the muscles from the external condyle and supracondylar ridge being most affected. The *brachioradialis* is the chief sufferer, since it is dragged upon when taking 'back-handers' in tennis.

2. A *periostitis* in the region of the external condyle, probably caused by the actual tearing of some muscle-fibre from its periosteal attachment.

3. *A synovitis or, later an arthritis,* of the superior radio-ulnar joint, possibly with injury to the orbicular ligament.

These types may be combined, but are also frequently seen alone.

While agreeing with Romer in his classification many authorities assert that the muscle chiefly affected is the *extensor carpi radialis brevis.* Watson-Jones states that it is incomplete rupture of the fibres of the common extensor tendon and of extensor carpi radialis brevis which causes pain and that complete rupture releases the strain, relieving symptoms and allowing the muscle to heal: hence the success of various operations for bursitis, etc., which include division of the common extensor tendon, or its dissection from the external condyle. Dr. Cyriax describes four main types of lesion: (1) A tear at the tenoperiosteal junction of the common extensor tendon and the lateral epicondyle of the humerus. (2) A tear at the junction of the common extensor tendon and the radial extensor bellies, particularly that of extensor carpi radialis. (3) A tear at the origin of the extensor carpi radialis longus. (4) A tear in the muscle belly of extensores carpi radialis.

To summarize, we can say that the lesion may be *tenoperiosteal, tendinous* or *musculotendinous.* It is important that the student should realize that *active movement causes repeated break-down in the formation of scar tissue which subsequently prolongs the inflammatory reaction and leads to the formation of adhesions.* These adhesions cause pain and restriction of movement.

SIGNS AND SYMPTOMS.—

1. Pain and aching in the region of the elbow, often radiating down the arm to the wrist.

2. The grip becomes weak.

3. Resisted extension of the wrist and resisted radial deviation of the wrist are painful.

4. There may be an acutely tender spot, which gives rise to a burning sensation when pressure is applied. This is a helpful aid to localization of the lesion.

5. There may or may not be swelling and tenderness over the head of the radius, with pain on pronation and supination. These signs usually indicate a synovitis or arthritis.

Tendinous or Musculotendinous Type

Treatment.—The opinions of physicians and surgeons upon this matter differ to such an extent that it is impossible to dogmatize on the subject. Some cases have been successfully treated by manipulation, others by various open operations, but the patient must give up, if possible, the activity or occupation causing the injury. From the point of view of physiotherapy the primary aims are the *relief of pain* and the *prevention, or softening, of adhesions. Heat* and *massage* are given for the relief of pain. Infra-red radiation, radiant heat, and short-wave diathermy are all suitable. To begin with massage will consist of gentle effleurage and kneading, but as the acute stage dies down finger kneadings and frictions can be added and the depth of the manipulations increased. Relaxed *passive movements* may be given, but they should be combined with gentle *active movements* from the beginning. In 2–3 weeks active exercises can usually begin.

ELECTRICAL TREATMENT.—Anodal galvanism, ultrasonics, and various forms of ionization can be used for an analgesic or fibrolytic effect.

INJECTIONS.—Hydrocortisone and novocain can be injected into the site, again for their fibrolytic or analgesic effect.

DR. CYRIAX'S METHODS.—For *tendinous* or *musculotendinous* lesions Dr. Cyriax recommends localized deep transverse friction. Treatment is given for 15–20 minutes at a time and is not combined with any other form of treatment. For the *tenoperiosteal* type of lesion he gives deep transverse frictions to produce analgesia before manipulation. For the manipulation the wrist is held fully flexed, with the elbow in semi-flexion. The elbow is then sharply extended.* The manipulation is most easily performed with the arm in *abduction* and *internal rotation.*

Arthritic Type

Treatment.—These cases require a much longer period of rest until pain on movement has disappeared. *Massage* and *movements* are given as above, but the external condyle in the periostitic type, and the region of the radio-ulnar joint in the arthritic type, should be avoided during massage. Movements are delayed for 2–3 weeks and active exercises are not allowed under a month.

Dr. Cyriax does not treat the arthritic type by his methods. Some people feel that the periosteal type of lesion should be treated similarly to an arthritic type, i.e., by prolonged rest and very gentle physical treatment. In some cases a splint is applied to keep the wrist in dorsiflexion until the pain is no longer present on movement.

RUPTURE OF MUSCLE-FIBRES IN THE CALF

TYPES OF LESION.—These include rupture of some fibres of the gastrocnemius and rupture of the Achilles tendon. There is diversity of opinion as to whether the tendon of plantaris ruptures, or whether a so-called 'rupture' is in reality a rupture of gastrocnemius.

A sudden strong contraction of the calf muscles while standing on tip-toe causes the injury. There is severe pain at the moment of the accident, the patient often thinking he has received a blow on the leg. This is followed by weakness in the action of plantar-flexion and there is pain on dorsiflexion of the ankle.

Rupture of the Gastrocnemius and/or Plantaris Tendon

Treatment.—A good deal of difference of opinion exists with regard to the best way of treating this injury. Probably the best thing is for the patient to use the leg rather than rest it, or to rest it only for about 24 hours in cases of minor injury. Whether the patient is to rest in more severe injuries and for how long depends

---

* Dr. Cyriax, *Text-book of Orthopædic Medicine*, Vol. II, p, 144.

entirely on the severity of the injury and the views of the physician or surgeon in charge of the case. In some cases, a few days will probably suffice; in other cases, the patient may have to keep off his feet for a week or so. The principles of physical treatment are basically the same as in other muscle and tendon injuries.

Dr. Mennell pointed out the importance in this, and in all cases of rupture of muscle-fibres, of *checking effusion*, which will otherwise organize and lead to the formation of thickenings and adhesions in the muscle. To this end *heat* and *massage* should be given daily if possible. *Prolonged anodal galvanism* is also valuable in the first few days. Strapping, applied vertically down the leg, with short transverse pieces crossing it, or a bandage over cotton-wool, should be applied. *Gentle active movements* should be given as soon as possible, though some defer these for a few days in very severe cases. Later when all inflammation has subsided, *vigorous massage* and *exercises* are indicated. The physiotherapist must see that there is full range of dorsiflexion in the ankle. If it is limited, *forced passive movements* may be required.

Dr. Cyriax, who considers that these minor lesions in the calf are *always* due to rupture of a few fibres of the gastrocnemius (and not to a ruptured plantaris) treats them by local anæsthesia, followed by deep friction the next day. Massage should be given for 20 minutes, followed by exercises, three times a week. These should be off-weight to begin with. The heel of the shoe should be raised, by means of a felt or cork heel inside the shoe.

RUPTURE OF THE ACHILLES TENDON

Treatment.—This is often a more serious injury. Again, opinions vary as to treatment. Some surgeons or physicians secure the foot in moderate plantar-flexion, either by a splint or by means of a bandage. No movements in the direction of dorsiflexion are given for 2–3 weeks, and no stretching movements for 4 to 5 weeks. Otherwise treatment is on the same lines as for slighter injuries. The patient will not be allowed to walk for 6 or 7 weeks. *Careful re-education in correct walking is essential.* In cases of partial rupture some physicians believe in early movement, often combined with deep massage from the beginning.

FIBROSITIS

(Non-articular Rheumatism; Acute or Chronic Muscular Rheumatism)

The term 'fibrositis' is an ambiguous one. Does it exist at all except as a secondary condition? If it does, what is it? and what causes it? Of what do the 'nodules' consist? There are as many opinions as there are authorities on the subject! The general medical text-book usually gives a list of possible explanations and cautiously leave it at that. Dr. Cyriax* says it does not exist as a primary condition. Dr. Copeman† thinks it does. Dr. Duthie‡ remarks that "it is probable that there is no single explanation for all cases diagnosed as non-articular rheumatism, but that a variety of causes may result in a similar clinical picture". He points out, however, that it is now recognized that *the majority of cases of brachial neuralgia, acute lumbago, and sciatica are due to degenerative changes in the intervertebral disks and the posterior spinal articulations*, which lead to compression or irritation of the posterior nerve-roots. There is no doubt that a thorough examination by a specialist is advisable in all cases of obstinate fibrositis, in order to ascertain whether in fact any lesion is present in a joint, muscle, or nerve. Whatever the cause or nature of this condition may be, it is certainly very

---

* *Text-book of Orthopædic Medicine*, Vol. I.
† *Text-book of Rheumatic Diseases*, Chapter XV.
‡ Sir Stanley Davidson, *Principles and Practice of Medicine*, Chapter on Chronic Rheumatic Disease.

common and there are very few people who have not suffered from it, in some form or other, in the course of their lives. The *actual cause*—as stated above—is obscure; but certain factors *predispose* to it, or precipitate an attack. These are:—

1. *Cold*, generally local chilling, such as sitting in a draught, which results in 'stiff neck'.

2. *Physical fatigue or muscle overstrain*, resulting in pain and stiffness, e.g., lumbago other than that caused by a disk lesion. (An actual 'strain' may be accompanied by the rupture of a few muscle-fibres, and should probably be considered as a *myositis*.)

3. *Injury to a muscle*, causing a fibrosis or scar which is painful when stretched.

4. *Bad posture*, generally giving rise to trouble in some region of the spine, especially in the lumbar region. Bad posture causes undue strain on certain muscles and ligaments. Scoliosis, kyphosis, round shoulders, and lordosis, or serious degrees of foot deformity (severe flat or everted foot, etc.) may all give rise to postural strain, and hence to pain in the affected structure. The psychological factor in some cases of bad posture should not be forgotten.

5. *Psychological Factors*.—It is now recognized that there is a psychogenic factor in many cases of fibrositis, especially in the chronic cases. Fibrositis does occur in anxiety neurosis or in various types of hysteria; but this factor may also be present in cases of fatigue, overstrain, or ill-health, which could not be actually classified as neurotic. It is difficult to distinguish between cause and effect in such patients—to know in fact whether the pain caused the anxiety, or the anxiety the pain; or whether the two interact on each other.

6. *Infection*.—A 'focus of infection' is not generally blamed nowadays, but it must be admitted that an occasional case does recover after the removal of infected tonsils or teeth. Some similar conditions, such as epidemic myalgia (Bornholm Disease), are believed to be due to a virus.

N.B.—Secondary fibrositis may be present in arthritis, spondylitis, deficiency diseases, etc.

PATHOLOGY.—

The Fibrositic Nodule.—This mysterious structure is present in most cases, though in some the tenderness is more diffuse. It has been explained in various ways. It used to be described as an inflammatory condition in muscular or fibrous tissue, but this theory has been abandoned by most authorities. The two most generally accepted opinions today are as follows:—

1. It is produced by a *herniation of lobules of fatty material through their covering fibrous septa*.—". . . The tender palpable 'fibrositic' nodules in a series of selected cases consist of tense œdematous lobules of deep fatty tissue which has pushed through a flaw in their fibrous covering membrane to a more superficial layer. The œdema appeared to be of non-inflammatory origin. In some cases these fat herniæ had developed a pedicle. This type of lesion usually occurs in the lumbar region and over the iliac crests and is manifested clinically by the presence of a tense tender nodule, pressure upon which reproduces the patient's pain. This must be differentiated from cases in which nodular thickening may be felt within an area of deep tenderness in which pressure, though painful, does not reproduce the pain of which the patient complains in its entirety." (Copeman.) Dr. Copeman adds that fat herniæ of this type can be reduced by deep massage, and may also be reduced spontaneously by muscular action, but that they more often end by becoming either adherent to surrounding structures, or partially strangulated, and so become irreducible and chronic. The reason why such herniation of fat occurs is obscure but it may possibly have an endocrine factor.

2. The other opinion is that the pain is *referred from a lesion elsewhere in the body, but within the same neural segment*,* for instance an injured ligament or

---

* In the area supplied by the same nerve that supplies the region in which the pain is felt.

intervertebral disk. The 'nodule' is thought to be produced by *local muscle spasm*, probably of reflex origin. Pressure on the site of the lesion or 'trigger area' causes renewed pain in the reflex area and an injection of a local anaesthetic at this point relieves it. (Nowadays many doctors use this method of treatment, without resource to physiotherapy.) The muscular fibres in spasm are said to have a diminished blood-supply and this ischæmia may be one cause of the pain. It is probable that both these views are correct and that 'fibrositis' is a generic term used to cover several different conditions. It has also been maintained that similar nodules occur in most middle-aged people. They do not generally cause symptoms and, of course, do not require treatment.

N.B.—Dr. Cyriax* says that "these nodules feel like fibrolipomata, the larger often being characteristically lobulated". He considers that they merely coincide with the onset of middle age, and have nothing to do with rheumatism or 'fibrositis'.

Acute Fibrositis.—The pain may be present in any part of the body in varying degrees of intensity and is often neuralgic in character. Stretching of the muscles is painful, as is pressure on the tender area. The patient may be completely incapacitated for the time being. Most acute cases clear up in 1–2 weeks,*† but some become chronic, especially if neglected in the early stages. There may be tender nodules or regions in the affected area.

Chronic Fibrositis.—The pain and aching is less severe, but still persists during movement and may be worse after rest. Stiffness in joints may develop because movement has been inhibited by pain. Fibrositis is not crippling like arthritis, but may cause much pain, discomfort and fatigue. The nodules are generally found in the tendons and aponeuroses of muscles, close to their attachments to bone.

Principles of Treatment.—In *acute cases* the principal aims of treatment are to relieve pain and spasm and to increase the local circulation. In *sub-acute* and *chronic cases* the main aim is to stretch and mobilize tissues and strengthen the muscles, though this cannot be fully achieved unless pain and spasm have been relieved. *Heat, massage,* and *exercises* are all used, the accent being on heat and massage in the former case and on massage and exercises in the latter.

The following are the commonest forms: (1) Lumbago; (2) Pleurodynia; (3) 'Stiff neck'.

Lumbago‡

In its acute form lumbago consists of severe pain in the lumbar or gluteal regions, especially localized to the area occupied by the *latissimus dorsi* and *erector spinæ*. Every movement causes pain, and the patient's gait becomes stiff and awkward. There may be a good deal of muscle spasm. It may be brought on by some known strain or chill, but in some cases it appears to come on without any ascertainable cause, though often *habitual strain* may be responsible, or at least the exciting cause.

Treatment.—

Acute Stage.—Rest in bed, or at least some degree of immobilization or support used always to be advised for this condition, since it was thought to be one of acute inflammation. This method is still sometimes adopted today but Dr. Copeman and many other authorities consider that analgesics should be given and only if these cannot be used immediately for any reason should the patient be kept in bed, or the part supported by strapping. *Heat,* in the form of radiant

---

* *Text-book of Orthopædic Medicine*, Vol. I.
† Disk lesions sometimes recover spontaneously with rest.
‡ This refers to cases due, or partly due, to strain, chill, or fatigue; not to those due to displaced disks, or other definite lesions.

heat, infra-red radiation, short-wave diathermy or the constant current, can all be used to increase the circulation, relieve congestion, and relax muscular spasm and if it can be tolerated gentle stretching, effleurage or kneading may be added. It should be noted that effleurage sometimes exacerbates the pain, in which case it is not given. Some doctors prefer that massage is delayed until the sub-acute stage in any case.

Sub-acute Stage.—*Heat* is continued and may precede, follow, or be given in conjunction with *massage*.★ The patient should be in the prone position, suitably supported by pillows, so that all the muscles, especially those in the affected area, may be as relaxed as possible. Very light and rhythmic stroking may, in some cases—but not all—promote relaxation. The massage should first be given above and below the affected area and the physiotherapist should approach the tenderest area gradually and with care. This preliminary massage is given to relieve congestion, increase circulation, obtain relaxation and, not least important, prepare the patient for the more specialized friction massage to follow. *Frictions* are added as soon as the patient can tolerate them. They are given to the 'trigger points' or nodules. These are often to be found along the outer border of the erector spinae, or in the region of the iliac crests or sacro-iliac joints. The frictions should be gradually deepened. If the nodules are fatty herniæ, this procedure should 'break up' or, at least, loosen them. The treatment usually concludes with a repetition of the kneading and effleurage in order to soothe any pain that has been caused.

Chronic (or Convalescent) Stage.—*Heat* is generally continued and as the patient recovers the massage becomes deeper and more vigorous. Frictions should be as strong and deep as possible to disperse any nodular or diffuse thickenings which can still be felt in the lumbar or gluteal muscles. *Exercises* should be introduced as soon as possible in the course of the treatment, both to preserve mobility, which may become limited by adhesions, and to improve the circulation and nutrition of the lumbar and gluteal muscles. Resisted exercises, which work the extensors of the spine in this region, should be given as soon as possible. Free extension exercises and 'straight' abdominal exercises which flex the spine and stretch its posterior ligaments and muscles, are also required, and side-bendings and trunk-rotations should be included.

Electrical Treatment.—Histamine ionization may be applied to one particularly painful spot, to act as a counter-irritant. Surged or labile faradism is sometimes given.

Pleurodynia

This consists of thickenings in the *pectoral muscles*, the *intercostals*, or the *serratus magnus*. It usually affects one side of the body only. The pain is felt most on *inspiration*. This affection often develops into intercostal neuralgia or even neuritis. It is sometimes mistaken for pleurisy—or pleurisy is mistaken for it. The latter condition, however, shows other signs and symptoms, which are not present in pleurodynia (*see* p. 392).

Treatment.—This consists of heat, massage, and breathing exercises and is similar to that described in the sub-acute and chronic stages of lumbago.

Stiff Neck

This condition is usually caused by inflammation in the *sternomastoid* and, sometimes, in other neck muscles. As a rule it clears up completely in a short time, but it must not be forgotten that this does not always happen and some

---

★ Dr. Copeman is of the opinion that this should not be given until after the patient has begun active movements, because he may tend to rely on it to effect his cure.

patients are left with impaired mobility, especially in the matter of rotation of the neck.

Treatment.—Is on the same lines as that described above but recovery may be expected in a shorter time.

CHRONIC FIBROSITIS

In certain cases, fibrositis does not start with an acute phase, but is 'chronic' from the beginning. In such conditions the nodules or thickenings are usually situated in the tendons and aponeuroses of muscles, close to their attachments to bone. A common example of this kind of chronic fibrositis is to be found in the ordinary, fibrositic, headache, or occipital neuralgia.

Fibrositic Headache

The headache is in the *occipital region. Pain* may also be present in *the shoulders* and there is *stiffness of the neck. Tenderness* and *thickenings* are found in the *cervical tendons and aponeuroses.* Occasionally the trouble spreads to the face, and there is tenderness in the areas supplied by branches of the *5th nerve,* especially at the points where they emerge through their respective bony foramina.

Treatment.—The condition is easiest to treat if the patient sits on a stool, places his elbows on a table, and supports his forehead on his hands. This support is most necessary in order to relax the *trapezius* and other *extensors of the neck.* If in bed, he must lie prone with pillows suitably arranged as for any back and neck massage. The operator stands behind the patient.

Massage and Movement.—The aims are to break up or loosen the thickenings, and to improve the local circulation. To this end massage will be of the deepest possible kind. If there is one definite painful point, massage should be concentrated on it.*

Treatment should begin with the *upper part of the back and the shoulders* and, as a preliminary measure, firm effleurage and deep kneadings are given. Strong frictions are next given to any thickenings which can be felt. These should be followed by a second series of deep kneadings and by strong effleurage.

Massage is next given to the *region of the neck.* Here the same series of movements are repeated, dealing with the upper fibres of the *trapezius.* Frictions will be given on either side of the ligamentum nuchæ, along the superior curved line, below the mastoid process, and over the top of the shoulder.

The physiotherapist should now change her own position so that she stands in front of the patient to treat the head. Any hairpins, combs, etc., must be removed. The best movements that can be used here are frictions but it is impossible to give them as deeply in this region as in the back and neck, since the epicranial aponeurosis lies over bone, and bruising of the nerves would be the result of too heavy work. Performed carefully, however, they bring great relief to the patient, who often asks that this part of the treatment be prolonged.

Finally, *passive and active movements* are given—the patient sitting upright. Head-rolling is the most useful passive movement. *Active exercises* should include Head-side-bending, Head-rotation, active Head-rolling, Head-extension, and Back-raising. Movements which stretch the affected muscles of the upper back and shoulders should also be included.

In a long-standing case, the treatment may need to be continued for some time. If a complete cure is obtained, the patient may well remain free of the trouble but if, on any subsequent occasion, he should again be attacked, prompt

---

* It must be realized, however, that many patients will not tolerate this deep work in the first few treatments.

treatment will generally succeed in cutting short the attack. Obese patients should reduce their weight.

Trigeminal Neuralgia due to Fibrositis

This condition must not be confused with a true neuritis of the trigeminal nerve, which is not suitable for treatment by massage. The painful points, as mentioned above, are found where the branches of the fifth nerve emerge on the face. The most common sites of pain are over the points of emergence of the supra-orbital and supratrochlear branches of the frontal division of the ophthalmic nerve. Other possible points may be: (1) At the emergence of the terminal branch of the superior maxillary (the infra-orbital) nerve, immediately below the eye; (2) At the emergence of the temporal branch of the orbital (temporo-malar) nerve (a branch of the superior maxillary) above the zygoma; (3) Occasion-ally at the emergence of the mental nerve (a branch of the inferior dental division of the inferior maxillary) (*Fig.* 37).

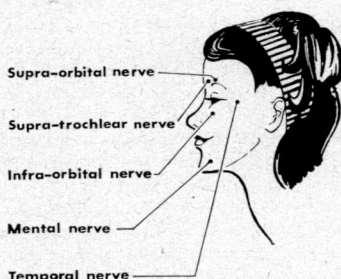

Supra-orbital nerve

Supra-trochlear nerve

Infra-orbital nerve

Mental nerve

Temporal nerve

Fig. 37.—Points of emergence of sensory nerves on the face, showing where pain is most commonly present in trigeminal neuralgia.

Treatment.*—This is best given in the lying or half-lying position, the patient's head being supported on a soft cushion. The physiotherapist should stand or sit at the side of the couch, facing her.

Massage for neuralgic pains in the face must perforce be much gentler than in other less sensitive regions. Only the area in the face where pain is present need be treated, but the cervical region, from which the trouble may stem, should also receive attention (*see* p. 87). Treatment of the face consists of very gentle stroking and frictions.

THE FOREHEAD.—Stroking should be performed with one hand, across the forehead and down to the temple, followed by gentle frictions over the frontal region, special attention being paid to the points of emergence of the *supra-orbital nerve* and the *supratrochlear nerve* (*Fig.* 37). After this the stroking movements should be repeated.

TEMPORAL REGION.—Stroking and frictions should be given in the manner described above, especially over the point of emergence of the *temporal nerve*.

REGION OF THE CHEEK.—Stroking is given to one or both sides of the face. The hands are placed lightly over the patient's eyes, the tips of the index fingers resting lightly on the forehead. The hand then passes downwards, the index fingers being drawn down between the eye and nose. The other fingers are slightly

---

* In view of the doubtful aetiology and pathology of fibrositis, it is difficult—if not impossible—to say why this treatment should be as effective as it is. It is retained here because it *is* effective.

raised so as not to press heavily on the eyes. The movement is continued *downwards and outwards* over the cheeks and the lower jaw. (This movement might really be classed as effleurage, because it follows more or less the course of the facial vein.) Frictions are given over the cheek, especially at the point where the *infra-orbital nerve* leaves the foramen of the same name.

THE MENTAL REGION is rarely affected. If pain is present here, the stroking should be from the mid-line of the chin, upwards toward the angle of the jaw, and frictions should be given over the point of emergence of the mental nerve through the mental foramen.

Electrical Treatment.—Calcium ionization (or some other analgesic) is sometimes ordered for the affected side of the face. A large active pad which covers the whole area should be used, the contours being padded with cotton-wool soaked in the ionizing solution.

CHAPTER V

WOUNDS AND SCARS: SUPPURATIVE CONDITIONS: BURNS AND SKIN-GRAFTS: AMPUTATIONS

I. Wounds and scars: Healing of wounds—Open wounds—Recently healed scars—Pain in healed scars. II. Suppurative conditions: Ulceration and infection—Varicose ulcers—Whitlows, boils, carbuncles, abscesses. III. Burns and skin-grafts—Burns of the hand—Burns of the face—Skin-grafts. IV. Amputation stumps: Lower limb amputations—Upper limb amputations.

I. WOUNDS AND SCARS

HAVING dealt with injuries affecting bones and joint structures, we come to another group of injuries affecting the skin and subcutaneous tissues.

WOUNDS.—A wound can be described as the "solution of continuity of tissue". They fall into three categories: (1) *Incisions*, in which the surface area exceeds the depth. These are caused by sharp instruments, and under this heading come surgical incisions as well as injuries such as knife-wounds. (2) *Lacerations*, in which the damage is extensive. There is jagged tearing of the skin and contusion of underlying tissues. They can result from shell splinters in warfare, from accidents in factories and on the roads, and injuries involving broken glass. (3) *Punctures*, in which the depth exceeds the surface area. They are again made by thin sharp instruments from without, e.g., the prong of a garden fork, or by fragments of bone from within.

HEALING OF WOUNDS.—A clean wound or incision in which the raw surfaces are in contact heals by *first intention*. Following a localized hyperæmia and inflammatory reaction, a very thin layer of fibrous tissue forms between the surfaces, uniting them to one another. The skin then grows over the wound and little or no trace of the injury remains.

Lacerations, and wounds with extensive skin loss, or incisions which gape open, heal by *second intention* or granulation. By this method healing occurs from the base of the wound. Again, an inflammatory reaction occurs, and a fibrinous clot forms at the base of the wound. Capillary loops and fibroblasts invade the clot and granulation tissue is formed. Healthy granulation tissue is characterized by raised red spots. The new tissue builds up from below and heals the wound. Fibrous tissue is laid down and a scar forms. While these changes are taking place the surface epithelial cells are increasing and in time new skin forms over the surface. It differs from normal skin in that its special properties are lost. It contains no sweat or sebaceous glands, nor do hair follicles appear in it. As soon as the scar tissue is fully formed the hyperæmia diminishes, leaving the part white in appearance. During this stage the new tissue begins to shrink. In some cases the contraction in the healed wound is so great as to interfere seriously with movement in the nearest joint (*see Fig.* 45, p. 103). The scar may, moreover, adhere to structures around it, such as muscle or bone. In extensive wounds this contraction of scar tissue may cut off the blood-supply from parts of the wound which are not fully repaired and so prevent their healing. If infection occurs in the wound it will heal by *suppuration*. The same events occur, the inflammatory reaction building up a strong wall of capillaries around the wound, thus separating the healthy tissues from the wound. Phagocytic cells leave the blood-stream and fight the invading organisms. The resultant debris liquefies and pus forms. When this has drained away and the wound surfaces are clean, healing occurs *by second intention*.

REQUIREMENTS FOR HEALING.—Certain factors are essential for both types of healing: (1) There must be an adequate inflammatory reaction for the formation of the clot and subsequent tissue growth. (2) The wound must be clean. (3) The delicate granulation tissue must not be subjected to damage or strain which might cause it to break down and delay repair. Injudicious movement which strains the wound can cause this, in the same way that it can delay fracture repairs. So can the careless removal of a dressing which has stuck to the wound, since in pulling it away, some of the capillaries become torn.

OPEN WOUNDS

Principles of Treatment.—When discussing the treatment of wounds, both surgical and physical principles must be considered.

SURGICAL TREATMENT.—From the surgeon's point of view the aims are to combat shock and to promote repair. The method he uses depends on the nature of the wound. Surgical incisions and incisional wounds require re-apposition of the surfaces, and this can be achieved by suture. The surfaces must also be clean. In these days of antibiotics it is usual to treat all such wounds prophylactically, applying an antibiotic in powder form, or incorporated in the dressing.

Lacerations present a different problem.

The treatment most often applied to such wounds at the present day is that associated with the name of Trueta,* though, of course, practised by many other surgeons.

When a patient is wounded, he needs, first of all, treatment for shock and hæmorrhage. After these, the next matter requiring attention is the condition of the wound itself. It has, in most cases, been contaminated by micro-organisms —the pyogenic bacteria, streptococcus or staphylococcus, or the bacteria of gas gangrene or tetanus. Later, these will tend to multiply in the wound and penetrate deeply into the tissues. It has been found that antiseptics, once freely used in treating wounds, injure the tissues more than the bacteria, and so lower their resistance to the invaders. The modern method consists in removing everything on which the bacteria can thrive—foreign bodies, damaged or devitalized tissues (except important nerves or blood-vessels), and raw surfaces. This drastic treatment is known as *débridement*, and is carried out as soon as the patient's condition and circumstances permit—if possible, within six to eight hours of the injury.† No stitches are put into the deep tissues, unless absolutely necessary, since they would act as foreign bodies; but the skin edges are sutured if they can be brought together. Otherwise the wound is left open and dressed or packed with plain sterile gauze or petroleum jelly in gauze. If a limb is the part affected, it is enclosed in plaster-of-Paris applied directly to the skin (sometimes it is lightly padded), so as to immobilize the wound. In some cases zinc ointment is applied to the skin before the plaster is put on, in order to avoid the occurrence of dermatitis, which may be caused by the discharge from the

---

* Dr. Joseph Trueta, *Treatment of War Wounds and Fractures*.
 † But it has now been found that a wound can be successfully treated later than this. This is partly due to the use of antibiotics, such as penicillin and sulphonamide. Débridement should not, however, be carried out after 24 hr., as infection will have set in by then, and besides enhancing the risk of surgical treatment will have instituted repair by suppuration.

wound. The plaster is not removed more often than is absolutely necessary. The discharge, if any, soaks into the plaster, and the consequent offensive odour may necessitate a change at intervals, but these intervals should be as long as possible. The plaster is removed when the wound is healed.

The patient will later require massage, mobilization of joints, exercises and occupational therapy to restore function. If there is danger of great contraction, as in extensive wounds, the limb will probably be splinted in such a way as to prevent it.

PHYSICAL TREATMENT.—The aims of physical treatment are: (1) *To assist the promotion of healing* by maintaining a good flow of blood to the part, by preventing infection, and by preserving the integrity of the new tissue. (2) *To prevent adhesions and contracture.* By fulfilling these aims much is done in the way of regaining the fullest functional activity after injuries. Steps may need to be taken later to perfect the restoration of mobility and function, however.

Treatment of Clean Open Wounds.—The essential factor in treatment is the increase of blood-flow to the part, provided that proper precautions are taken with regard to asepsis. If the wound is in the leg or arm, the whole limb may be treated.

PHYSICAL TREATMENT.—

GENERAL.—The wound should have been dressed and covered with a layer of gauze before the treatment is begun. The physiotherapist must be careful not to displace this in the course of her manipulations; it may be lightly strapped on if necessary, or fixed by a turn or two of bandage.

If massage is given the whole limb should receive effleurage and pétrissage, but the area of the wound must be given a wide margin. Heat can also be given, provided sensation is normal. The most suitable forms are short-wave diathermy for its intense circulatory effect, or infra-red radiation. The latter, besides increasing the circulation, has a drying effect which assists the formation of granulation tissue.

All joints of the limb should be moved passively and actively, provided no strain is put on the healing wound. If there is any doubt about this latter point, it is as well to leave the movements in the joints nearest the wound until the wound is exposed, so that their effect on it can be watched.

LOCAL.—The physiotherapist now scrubs her hands and soaks them in a weak disinfectant solution (e.g., 1 per cent lysol), not drying them unless she has a sterile towel; she then removes the dressing from the wound and replaces it with a small piece of sterile gauze cut to fit the raw surface of the wound exactly. Frictions and finger kneadings are then given, firmly but gently, round its edges, the pressure always being *inwards* towards the raw surface. Vibrations, performed with the finger-tips and in the same direction, may be added. If passive and active movements to the nearest joints have not been administered already, they can begin now, but if any drag on the wound results from such movements, the patient should be taught static contractions which do not move the joints at all. Both massage and passive movements help to prevent the formation of adhesions, as well as to improve the circulation. The physiotherapist again washes her hands, removes the temporary dressing, applies the ordinary one, and finally washes and disinfects her hands after she has finished with the case. A similar treatment is carried out in the case of burns.

ELECTRICAL TREATMENT.—First or second degree erythema doses of ultra-violet light can be given locally to stimulate epithelial growth. *Ultrasonics* can also be used.

Details of treatment of septic wounds and ulcers are given later in the chapter.

RECENTLY HEALED SCARS

Treatment.—It is a mistake to suppose that a scar requires no particular care just because the wound is actually closed. No movements which tend to separate the edges are permissible until the healing is quite firm—that is, until three to four weeks after the closing of the wound in the absence of sepsis. If there has been sepsis, the greatest care is necessary, as injudicious treatment may make it flare up again.

Any ordinary scar, however, can be dealt with quite successfully provided both patient and operator possess the gifts of patience and perseverance. The treatment will have to be long-continued and it cannot be hurried.

N.B.—Scars resulting from surgical operations rarely give trouble nowadays, owing to improved surgical technique. In cases of disfiguring scars plastic surgery may be undertaken.

MASSAGE is on the same lines as for open wounds, though the manipulations can be rather stronger. Very deep work is required for *old adherent scars*. Frictions should be given in such a way as to raise the scar from the under-lying tissues. Olive oil or lanoline is used in conjunction with massage to soften the scar.

MOVEMENTS (for firmly-healed scars).—Strong *passive movements* are given to the nearest joints to stretch the contracture, and are followed by *active movements*. The scar should be grasped by the operator while the patient contracts his muscles. Vigorous, free, home exercises should be practised. Splints are often applied for the purpose of preventing contracture, or of gradually stretching the tissues, if it has already taken place.

OTHER FORMS OF TREATMENT.—Whirlpool baths, if obtainable, help to soften the scar. Failing these, the part may be soaked in hot water, or wax baths given before massage. Electrical treatment such as ultrasonics or ionization with chlorine or iodine may be ordered for their fibrolytic effect. Cupping is also used, the alternate effect of suction and release serving to loosen the scar tissue and increase the blood-supply as well. Histamine, or renotin, by producing an artificial inflammatory reaction also helps to soften and stretch the tissues. The drug is administered to the tissues round the scar, *not to the scar itself.*

PAIN IN HEALED SCARS

CAUSE.—The pain may be due to: (1) Neuralgia or neuritis caused by the involvement of nerves in scar tissue; or (2) Venous congestion in deep scars.

Treatment.—In the first case, vibrations and frictions can be tried, also the forms of electrical treatment mentioned above, in order to loosen the nerve from its surroundings. Cupping is also used.

In the case of the large deep scar, Sir Robert Jones★ considered the pain to be due to venous congestion and irregularities of blood-pressure in the tissues below the surface, and that the remedy lies in the promotion of vascular activity. He therefore advised fairly free use of the affected limb, deep massage, hot applications to the part at night (to relieve pain and allow the patient to sleep), and *contrast baths*, which consist of plunging the limb alternately into cold and hot water for about 5 to 10 minutes. (On other parts of the body hot and cold sponges are applied in turn.) This treatment causes successive dilatation and constriction of the blood-vessels, so exercising the muscular fibres of their walls, and thus improving the circulatory condition of the part. If the scar is on a limb, sinusoidal baths can be given to improve circulation.

EXERCISES.—If required, these should be of the quick, rhythmic, swinging type, which tend to increase circulation and stretch tissues.

★ *Injuries to Bones and Joints.*

II. SUPPURATIVE CONDITIONS

Suppurative conditions fall into two categories: (1) Open wounds which ulcerate and become infected. (2) Infection in closed areas. We will deal with open wounds first.

ULCERATION AND INFECTION.—If, for some reason, the blood-supply is unable to provide an adequate inflammatory reaction following skin damage, *ulceration* will occur. This is in effect a reversal of the healing process. Because of the poor blood-supply, formerly healthy tissue becomes devitalized and eventually breaks down. The wound, therefore, instead of diminishing, increases in size. It may increase in surface area alone, or in depth *and* surface area, in which case an *ulcer* is said to have formed. If it increases in depth alone *a sinus* forms. Since the blood-supply is inadequate for healing it will also be unable to deal with infection; thus ulcers and sinuses are very liable to become infected.

SIGNS AND SYMPTOMS OF ULCERATION.—The wound becomes soggy and unhealthy looking. Such granulations as form are dull and purplish in colour, due to venous congestion in underlying tissues. The surrounds become œdematous. The wound is moist, and there is usually a copious serous discharge.

SIGNS AND SYMPTOMS OF INFECTION.—There will be a rise in temperature, both local and general, the degree of rise in general temperature depending on the patient's general health and the virulence of the infecting organism.

The skin round the wound will be swollen, red, and hot to the touch. There will be pain and throbbing in the region of the wound, which is made worse by warmth, e.g., in bed at night. The wound discharges. This may be mucopurulent to begin with, later becoming highly purulent; or highly purulent from the beginning. The nature of the discharge depends on the infecting organism. There may be a characteristic colour and odour. The granulation tissues become streaked with white or yellow patches.

PRINCIPLES OF TREATMENT.—In cases of ulceration and infection, treatment falls into two categories. There must be *local treatment* for the wound or ulcer but in addition, since the tissue resistance is poor, the *general health* must also be improved.

LOCAL TREATMENT.—The principles of treatment are basically the same as for cases of clean wounds, but infection must be controlled before healing can begin. An *artificial inflammatory reaction* must be produced, and rest assured, to prevent a spread of infection. An inflammatory reaction can be produced by means of massage and heat, the most suitable choice being short-wave diathermy, by erythema doses of ultra-violet irradiation, and in some cases by ionization with histamine. Infection is controlled by erythema doses of ultra-violet irradiation, using only the short antibiotic rays; by zinc ionization, and by antibiotic dressings.

Once infection has been controlled treatment is continued as for clean wounds.

GENERAL TREATMENT is given to raise the patient's general resistance. This includes rest, and attention to diet. If the reticulo-endothelial system is deficient, sectional ultra-violet irradiation is given daily, chiefly for its œsophylactic effect, for a week or ten days. Thereafter treatment is continued in the form of general irradiation.

These techniques of treatment can be adapted to all forms of infected wounds. It is only proposed to give details of treatment of varicose ulcers here.

VARICOSE ULCERS

These ulcers develop on the legs, particularly on the medial aspect of the lower third, because of œdema, congestion and devitalization of tissues arising from interference with venous return to the heart. Some injury—often a very slight one—breaks the weakened skin and the resultant ulcer becomes infected with micro-organisms. Because of the impaired circulation of the limb, the ulcer becomes *indolent*, that is, it fails to form healthy granulations, and consequently does not heal. The skin around the ulcer is *indurated* (hardened) and often discoloured (*see Fig.* 38 A). This induration is due to organization of œdema which, leading to interstitial fibrosis, further impedes the circulation in the region of the ulcer itself. Thus a vicious circle is established.

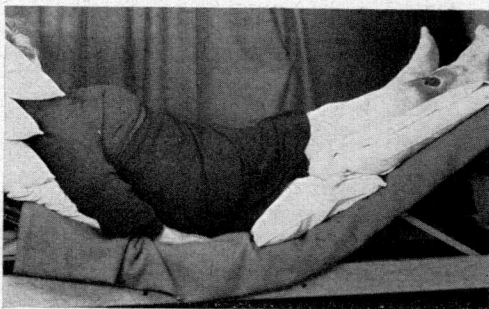

A

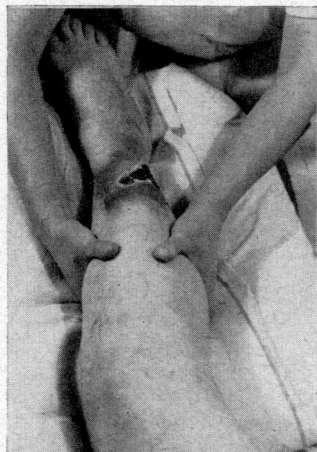

B

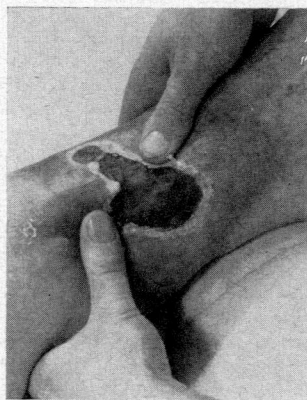

C

Fig. 38.—Massage in elevation for varicose ulcer. A, Patient lying with legs in elevation prior to massage. Note appearance of ulcer and surrounding area of discoloured skin. B, Squeezing kneading applied to proximal part of leg before massage is given to the actual ulcer. C, Finger-kneading around the ulcer itself. Note the sloping edges and the formation of healthy granulation tissue at the base of the ulcer, also dead flaking skin at the edge of the surrounding area with wide area of discoloration. (*Figs.* 38–43 *by kind permission of Miss A. E. Bartholomew.*)

Treatment.—

AIMS OF TREATMENT.—In addition to aims already set forth in the treatment of wounds, when dealing with varicose ulcers one must get rid of œdema in the whole limb in order to prevent venous and lymphatic stasis round the ulcer. The induration must be broken down and the tissues mobilized, as well as infection controlled and repair instituted.

METHODS OF TREATMENT.—Various methods of treatment are in use today:—

1. PROLONGED RECUMBENCY, WITH THE LIMB RAISED until healing takes place. This—though almost always successful—has obvious disadvantages, and it is rarely possible for the patient to be absent from work for the necessary length of time.

2. ZINC IONIZATION OR ULTRA-VIOLET IRRADIATION for the purpose of destroying micro-organisms, producing an inflammatory reaction and instituting repair. To destroy micro-organisms by ultra-violet light, local treatment with the Kromayer lamp (or mercury vapour lamp for large areas) should be designed to give a fourth degree, or double fourth degree erythema to the base, and a second or first degree erythema to the surrounds. As infection is controlled longer rays and first or second degree doses should be given to the whole, to produce epithelial growth.

3. HOT SALINE OR MAGNESIUM PADS applied for a week, with infra-red irradiation at 18 inches for 15 minutes until the local swelling has subsided. The ulcer and skin surrounding it are then treated by ultra-violet irradiation of sufficient intensity to give a second, third, or fourth degree erythema depending on the state of the tissues. A bandage of elastoplast or some similar elastic material is then put on to control œdema and give support to the limb. It extends from above the toes to the knee, including the heel. *The patient must not remove it.* It remains in place for one, two, or three weeks. The ultra-violet irradiation can be repeated between successive applications of the bandage. When the ulcer is healed, the patient should continue to wear an elastic stocking. While the ulcer is being dealt with. the varicose veins themselves should be receiving appropriate medical or surgical treatment (Dr. Myer Fisher★).

4. THE BISGAARD METHOD (modified).—This method is used at St. Thomas's Hospital and is based on that taught by Dr. Bisgaard of Denmark, the main difference being in the type of massage applied to the patient's leg and thigh.

Massage.—The patient lies with the leg raised (*Fig.* 38 A). Deep massage is given to the whole limb to reduce œdema and congestion, *beginning with the thigh and continuing down the limb*, the most effectual manipulations being slow deep effleurage and kneading as for any case of œdema (*Fig.* 38 B). Special attention should be paid to the sole of the foot, the instep, the region of the tendo Achillis, and the external and internal 'coulisses', that is, the grooves behind the malleoli.

The region of the ulcer is next treated with deep frictions to soften the induration, working inward towards the edges of the ulcer itself (*Fig.* 38 C). *The physiotherapist must persist with these manipulations, even though they cause pain.* The ulcer can also be moved from side to side, the physiotherapist placing her fingers on one side and her thumbs on the other, to free it from underlying tissues and improve the circulation to it. Zinc oxide ointment with 2 per cent menthol may be applied round the edges to increase the rate of granulation, the ulcer often being dressed with this ointment.

Tracing.—A record of progress should be made by means of tracing. For this a double layer of cellophane is laid over the ulcer and a tracing made. The layer in contact with the ulcer should be swabbed with ether before it touches the leg *and should be thrown away immediately after use.* The layer on which the tracing is made can then be kept for record purposes. *Figs.* 39 and 40 show a tracing being taken and a record of tracings kept over a 2-month period.

Application of Pressure.—This is applied for the purpose of reducing the œdema round the ulcer and in the limb generally.

★ *British Journal of Physical Medicine*, May–June, 1949.

A half-inch 'sorbo' pad, or gauze compress, is applied over the dressing, of a size corresponding to the ulcer and the œdematous area round it. It should remain in position day and night.

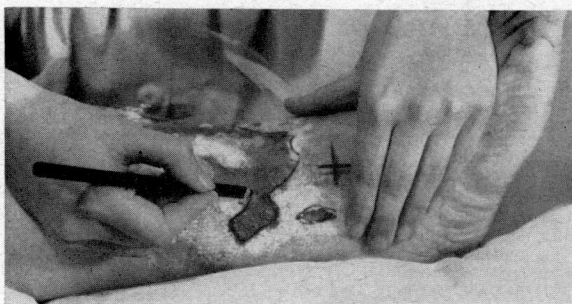

Fig. 39.—Tracing an ulcer.

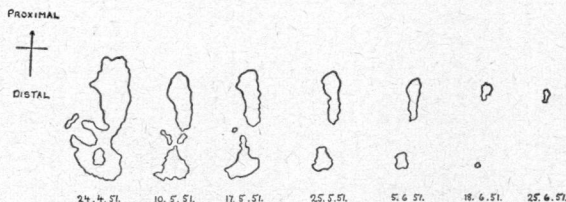

Fig. 40.—Record of tracings over 2-month period.

Wool or felt padding is placed in the grooves behind the malleoli and round the lower leg and foot. It is kept in position by a gauze bandage. Over this a bandage of elastic webbing (11 ft. long) is applied, a special technique being used to maintain even and continuous pressure (*Figs.* 41–43). It starts from under the inner side of the sole, is carried once straight round the foot, then *upward* and *outward* over the dorsum, round the back of the heel just above the point, *outwards* and *downwards* across the dorsum, under the sole and upwards (near the heel) across the bend of the ankle. *These two turns must be accurately applied in order to give the essential support and pressure round the tendo Achillis and malleoli.* It is thence continued as a simple spiral to just below the patella. (For further details, the student should consult the article on treatment of varicose ulcers by Miss A. Bartholomew in Dr. Cyriax's *Text-book of Orthopædic Medicine*, Vol. II, which gives a full and clear account of this treatment.)

Exercises.—Ankle exercises should be given, first with and then without the bandage, in order to improve circulation and help to mobilize the indurated tissues. Correct walking must also be taught and practised.

Home Treatment.—The patient should be taught to do his own treatment at home. He must learn to dress the ulcer, apply the pads and bandages, which (with the exception of that over the ulcer itself) are removed at night and put on again before rising in the morning, and carry out the massage as well as he can, especially the frictions round the ulcer. He must, however, remain under supervision and continue to attend the hospital department, or visit his private physiotherapist, as often as instructed.

4

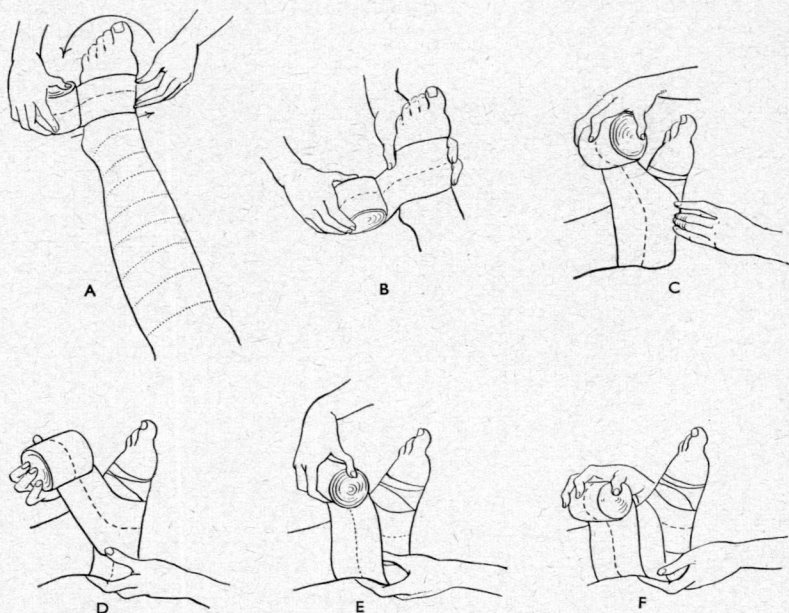

Fig. 41.—The Bisgaard bandage. A, The first turn; B, Beginning of the heel turn; C, Fixation of the heel turn; D, The stirrup turn; E, Holding the fixation of the stirrup turn; F, Bandaging up the leg.

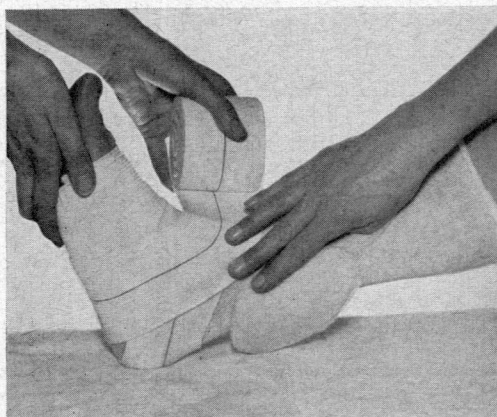

Fig. 42.—Application of the Bisgaard bandage over 'stock-inette' sock. The first important turn has been taken round the heel and the second is being applied. It is taken up the medial side of the foot to the malleolus before being continued over the ankle-joint. A felt pad is placed over the ulcer to provide pressure and encourage healing.

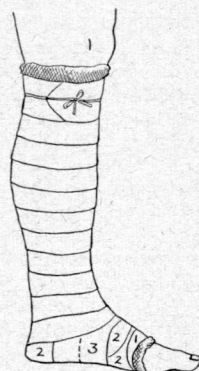

Fig. 43.—The completed Bisgaard bandage. 1, First turn; 2, Heel turn; 3, Stirrup turn.

The Bisgaard method of treatment can be combined with zinc ionization or ultra-violet irradiation as required. Ultrasonics, iodine or chlorine ionization, and histamine ionization can also be given to areas of induration following healing of the ulcer.

Whichever method of treatment is chosen, an elastic stocking should be worn for a considerable time, or even permanently, after its conclusion. Some patients prefer to retain the elastic bandage.

The same forms of treatment can be applied to indolent ulcers other than those caused by varicose veins.

WHITLOWS, BOILS, CARBUNCLES, AND ABSCESSES

Before closing this section on suppurative conditions, a little must be said about infections originating in closed areas. Such infections occurring in the skin and subcutaneous tissues commonly enter through a hair follicle or sebaceous gland. In some cases they result from blood or lymphatic spread. Although the principles and methods of treatment are similar in all these infections, the student must be quite clear as to the meaning of the various terms used to describe these conditions.

WHITLOW.—This denotes infection of a nail bed, most frequently seen on the fingers, although they can occur on the toes. There is considerable risk of the infection tracking to the fascial compartments of the hand and foot.

BOIL.—This denotes a localized infection of a hair follicle or sebaceous gland. If the resistance of the tissues is very good, spontaneous resolution may occur, the boil never becoming more than a hard, indurated spot. In most cases, however, pus forms and the dead cells form a hard central core. Eventually the accumulation of pus in a confined space stretches the skin until it bursts. This enables the pus to drain and once this is accomplished healing will occur. Common sites for boils are the back of the neck, the axilla, groin, and buttocks.

CARBUNCLE.—This differs from a boil in that several hair follicles or sebaceous glands are involved. The infection, instead of becoming localized, tracks through the subcutaneous connective tissue and several purulent spots, or 'heads', are manifest on the surface. At first drainage occurs through all these points, but in time the whole area becomes necrotic and breaks down. At the base of the resultant wound can be seen a thick, tacky slough, with stringy processes attached to the initial infective foci. As soon as this slough separates, healing will begin *but a carbuncle leaves a crater-like wound, which takes longer to heal than the wound left by a boil.*

ABSCESS.—This denotes an infection in a closed space, such as the axilla, chest, or pelvis. Treatments of thoracic and pelvic abscesses are given in the chapters dealing with chest and pelvic conditions.

SIGNS AND SYMPTOMS OF THE ABOVE CONDITIONS.—These are the same as for any bacterial inflammation, namely, a rise in local and general temperature, reddening and swelling of the skin, pain and throbbing locally. Later a 'head' forms and pus discharges.

Principles of Treatment.—

From the point of view of treatment three stages have to be considered: (1) The *acute stage*, in which the infection and inflammatory reactions are active. (2) The *subacute stage*, during which the inflammatory reaction and infection are dying down. (3) *The healing stage*.

In the *acute stage* rest is required since there is an active inflammatory reaction present. This is supplied by a sling in the case of axillary conditions, a sling and sometimes a splint in the case of finger and hand infections. Crutches or sticks are used in cases of groin or foot infections. Local strapping with elastoplast is often used in the case of septic conditions on the neck or buttocks. *It is essential at this stage to localize the infection and prevent the spread.* This is achieved by producing an artificial inflammatory reaction to assist the formation of a capillary barrier between the infected and the healthy tissues, and to combat the infection through the reticulo-endothelial cells and leucocytes. In order to localize the infection and assist inflammation, daily, or, ideally, twice daily, doses of short-wave diathermy are given. The field should be superficial and the dose just thermal. Three to five minutes' treatment are given at each session to begin with, progressing to ten-minute treatments. In order to stimulate an inflammatory reaction local second degree erythema doses of ultra-violet light can also be given. If the patient's general resistance is poor, first degree erythema doses of ultra-violet irradiation may be administered by sectional technique.

In the *subacute stage* rest is still required. Drainage must be promoted and the infection cleared up. If necessary the skin is opened to allow drainage. The affected area is cleaned with ether or cetracetamide and a sterile technique used. Short-wave diathermy is continued as before, but the dosage can begin with a 5- or 7-minute treatment per session. The time should not, however, exceed 10 minutes. If pain is increased the dosage should be cut, as this indicates a flaring of activity. The base of the open area should be given local fourth, or double fourth degree erythema doses and the surrounding areas a good first, or mild second degree erythema. This is to kill the infecting organisms and promote repair. Zinc ionization can also be given for the infection. Antibiotic fluffing and dressings are also used. Sectional irradiation is continued until all areas have received at least two treatments, after which the sectional technique is replaced by general ultra-violet irradiation for its tonic effect.

In the *healing stage* short-wave diathermy is tapered off. Fourth degree erythema doses to the base are replaced by first or second degree erythema doses to stimulate repair, and treatment is continued as for clean open wounds.

III. BURNS AND SKIN-GRAFTS

For practical purposes the important consideration in terms of treatment and eventual healing of burns is whether the burn is *partial skin thickness* or *full skin thickness.* However, three degrees of burns are commonly recognized:—

1. FIRST DEGREE, in which there is only *reddening of the skin* with no tissue destruction.

2. SECOND DEGREE, in which there is *blistering of the skin, and destruction of the top of the epidermis,* i.e., partial skin thickening. In these cases regeneration is possible since the dermis is intact.

3. THIRD DEGREE, in which there is *destruction of both epidermal and dermal layers,* i.e., full skin thickness. Here regeneration is not possible since the dermis, which is responsible for new skin growth, has been destroyed. A skin-graft will therefore be required. There is often damage to subcutaneous tissues as well. The skin is literally cooked. It looks brown and leathery or dead and white. It is the severer types of burns, of the second and third degree, that we are generally required to treat. Milder second degree burns may require treatment for stiffness arising from disinclination to move a painful area. They are most often burns of the hand, or sometimes of the face. The hands are particularly vulnerable since the patient instinctively uses them to protect the face.

TYPES OF BURNS.—Burns can be caused by any of the following causes: (1) *Flame burns.* These probably constitute the majority of burns seen in our departments. Epileptic patients are often victims of such burns, having fallen on to a fire during an epileptic fit; clothing may catch fire; or the wreckage of air or road disasters ignite. (2) *Scalds.* These are again common domestic burns sustained from hot liquids and steam. (3) *Electrical burns.* These are the result of earth shocks. (4) *Contact burns.* These occur in laundries and workshops, the patient being caught in a steam press, etc. (5) *Acid and chemical burns.* Again, these usually result from injury in factory or laboratory but the physiotherapy student should remember that such burns can occur from careless administration of direct-current treatments.

PATHOLOGY.—*The most important factor in any case of burn is shock.* In untreated, large-area burns, shock may ensue due to critical *reduction in blood volume,* extensive *loss* of *fluid* and to *pain.* With present-day methods of resuscitation, particularly fluid replacement, shock rarely becomes sufficiently severe to threaten life, but when facilities for fluid replacement are inadequate, e.g., battle casualties or in underdeveloped communities, early death may occur from shock in extensive burn injuries. In our community, wound infection of large-area burns constitutes the most serious threat to life. Infecting organisms may become resistant to antibiotics, leading to retardation of healing and failure of skin-grafting. If the infection cannot be controlled a massive infection will eventually occur leading to the patient's death.

SIGNS AND SYMPTOMS OF SHOCK.—(1) *Rapid, unsteady pulse,* an attempt being made to maintain the circulating blood-volume. (2) *Low blood-pressure,* due to collapse of the veins owing to the dilatation of their walls. (3) *Pale, cold skin.* (4) *Apathy.* (5) *Drowsiness.* (6) *Thirst* resulting from fluid loss.

FACTORS GOVERNING BURNS AND THEIR PROGNOSIS.—It is the *length of exposure,* rather than the temperature, which governs the depth and severity of a burn. The greater the skin destruction, the greater the tissue fluid loss and the less the chance of survival; 30–45 per cent total body surface destruction is usually fatal, though patients with as high as 78 per cent body surface destruction have survived. For purposes of assessment the legs each count as 18 per cent, the arms as 9 per cent, the back and front of the trunk as 18 per cent, the face and head as 9 per cent, and the perineum as 1 per cent. In addition, when estimating prognosis the following factors must be taken into account: (1) The age of the patient, the young being far better able to withstand shock than the elderly. (2) The patient's general health. (3) The delay between receiving treatment. As has been said, the sooner the patient is able to receive treatment for shock, the greater the chances of recovery. (4) Associated injuries, particularly damage to liver, kidneys, or cerebral hemispheres arising from the alteration in blood-pressure. (5) The depth of the burn. (6) The will to live. This is by no means the least important as the psychological effect of burns, and the fear of disfigurement, can be profound.

Principles of Medical and Surgical Treatment.—

The primary concern in any case of severe burn is to *counteract shock.* The secondary concern is the tissues themselves.

TREATMENT FOR SHOCK.—The aim is *to counteract the shock by maintaining the circulating blood-volume* by: (1) Administering analgesics to lessen the severity of the pain. The excruciating pain of severe burns lasts for 48 hr., and during this time analgesics will be required. (2) Replacing fluids. This is achieved by intravenous plasma drips. (3) Keeping the patient warm. *However, if the body is overheated the vessels dilate. Therefore if too great a heat is applied, far from raising blood-pressure, it will be still further reduced. This is an important factor in first aid.* The warmth of a blanket should be sufficient. (4) Maintaining a high calorific diet, rich in protein, vitamins, and iron. (5) Administering oxygen if the burn is deep enough to have destroyed the red blood-cells.

TREATMENT OF THE TISSUES.—The heat sterilizes the area—an effect which lasts for about 6 hr. Later than that infection must be prevented or controlled. In burns with full skin thickness loss the only possible means of repair is by skin-grafting. This can be done at once if the state of the tissues allows it, or may be delayed until the tissues are in a fit state for grafting.

Two methods of treatment are in common use today:—

1. *Treatment by Exposure* (*Fig. 44*).—This is excellent for small areas of the trunk or limbs, or for single limbs, but is less practicable for extensive burns, though in specialized burns centres, and units where ideal conditions pertain, this is the method of choice. The patient lies on a sterile sheet under a large body cradle, draped with a sterile sheet. The room temperature must be constant at

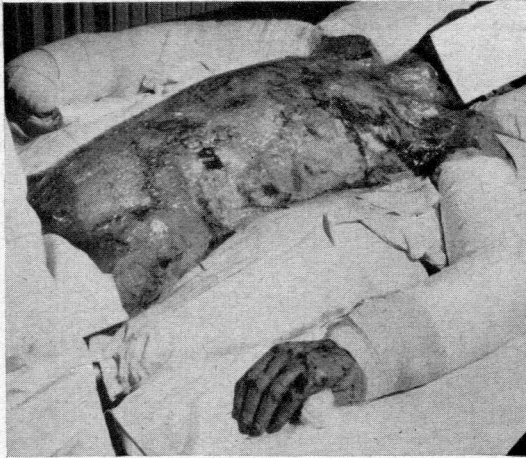

Fig. 44.—Severe third degree burns of trunk and hands. Trunk treated by exposure method. Arm treated by saline dressings.

80° F. The burns are sprayed with penicillin powder and antibiotics are administered. In 14–21 days the drying scabs and slough separate leaving a clean granulating surface ready for grafting.

2. *Treatment by Tulle Gras and Saline Dressings.*—One type of dressing consists of *sulphamezathine* powder, applied by means of an insufflator. The part is then covered with *tulle gras*, a sterilized material consisting of small-meshed curtain-net impregnated with soft paraffin and balsam of Peru. Over this a pad consisting of several layers of gauze wrung out in normal saline may be applied. The tulle gras does not stick to the wound, and so the newly forming skin is not disturbed when the dressings are changed, but in order to avoid any risk of injury to the delicate new tissues, it is best to soak off the dressings in the saline bath.

THE USE OF SALINE BATHS.—Immersion of the part in saline is invaluable in the treatment of burns, unless, of course, the exposure method is used. It can be used in grafted cases, and cases awaiting grafting. Dressings can be soaked off, thus relieving pain, and anxiety caused by the fear of pain. Physical treatment can begin early. The first saline bath and change of dressings is given 5 days after grafting, and physical treatment can then start. The soothing effect of the saline and the buoyancy of the water is of great assistance in the early days of restoration of movement. If saline is not used but movements are requested for grafted cases with the dressings still on, treatment cannot begin for 8 or 10 days for fear of friction causing the delicate skin to break down.

PRINCIPLES OF PHYSICAL TREATMENT.—The aims of physical treatment are threefold: (1) *To restore function.* (2) *To prevent skin hardening.* Burns are particularly liable to the formation of hard keloid scars, which besides disfiguring lead to contracture and deformity (*Fig.* 45). (3)*To minimize the degree of contracture.* There will inevitably be some shrinking of the scar tissue when burns repair naturally. This can lead to terrible contracture and deformity if treatment is not carried out. These are the aims of physiotherapy: but perhaps the most important factor of all is the tremendous need for the boosting of morale. In

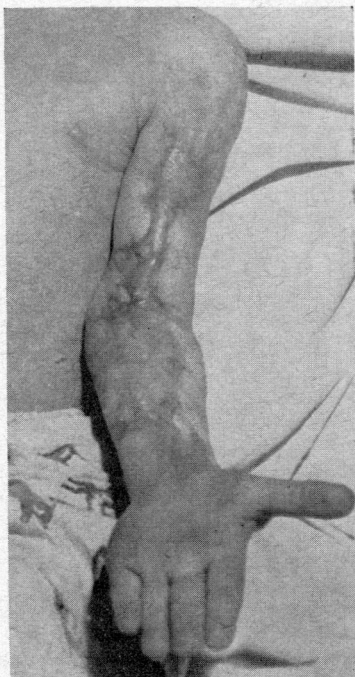

Fig. 45.—Scarring of arms resulting from burns. Note difference in colour and texture of scar tissue and skin on forearm. Keloid formation on arm and antecubital fossa. Note particularly the ridged effect of scar tissue with drag on surrounding skin and adherence to underlying structures.

dealing with patients who have suffered burns, the good physiotherapist is the one who has an intelligent appreciation of the overwhelming psychological effect the fear of disfigurement has on a patient. Much patience and encouragement is required of her.

METHODS OF TREATMENT.—

MOVEMENTS.—In the early stages treatment consists only of movements. These should be assisted active, and active, to begin with. *No passive movements should be given and no movement must ever be forced.* The patient should take the movement to the limit of his active range, with assistance if necessary. The physiotherapist then holds the position until such time as the patient can renew activity and gain a little in range. It is essential that all the movements of which a joint is capable are performed, but it should be stressed that *deformities, when they occur, are flexion deformities. Therefore accent is laid on extensor movements in order to overcome this danger.* Movements should be taught and performed slowly, smoothly, and co-ordinately. Treatment is given daily, ideally during immersion in the saline bath, to facilitate ease of movement and allay the patient's fears.

MASSAGE.—This is not given until the tissues can withstand it, i.e., when the burns are healed or almost healed except for some small areas. In ungrafted cases the skin will appear red, thin, and delicate; it will be easily broken, and *blister in response to slight injury or pressure.* (This is a point which must always be kept in mind when treating burns.) It will be stretched tightly over the finger-joints. Even if movements have begun, the joints will be stiff and the hand and fingers atrophied. The amount of disability varies according to the severity of the initial injury and the degree of sepsis, if any, which followed it. If the burn has been grafted, the graft will have taken by this stage, but will still be very delicate and liable to damage if roughly treated. A lanoline type of cream should be used in conjunction with massage to soften and lubricate the skin.

WAX BATHS.—These are invaluable in the later stages of the treatment of burns. Wax encircles the limb and assists the lubrication of the tissues and the restoration of function, particularly in cases where there has been arterial or venous impairment. It is very important to check the temperature, which should be 110° F., not only because of the patient's fear of heat, but also because their sensation will be abnormal.

ULTRA-VIOLET RADIATION.—At the Queen Victoria Hospital, East Grinstead, general irradiation is given for its tonic effect. Local treatments are not given, even in infected cases, as it is felt to lead to over-granulation.

BURNS OF THE HAND
(See Fig. 46)

PHYSICAL TREATMENT.—Bunnell has said, "Next to the brain, the hand is man's greatest asset", and as such the hand needs particular attention. It must be kept in a good functional position, i.e., with the wrist in dorsiflexion, the

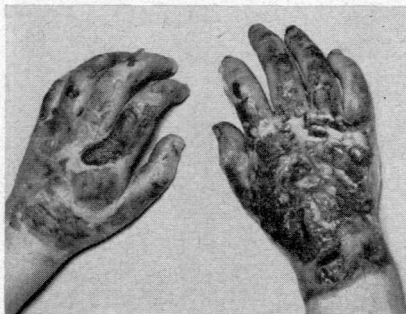

Fig. 46.—Severe second and third degree burns of hands with sepsis.

metacarpophalangeal joint in flexion, and the fingers extended. The thumb should be in slight flexion and opposition. This prevents the deformity of 'claw hand' which can easily arise in cases of palmar burns if care is not taken to prevent this. Although splinting of an adult hand is not ideal, since it leads to so much stiffening, it may none the less be necessary. A child does not suffer in the same way from splinting. It is possible to keep a child in a splint, night and day, for

6 months, and it will regain mobility in no time at all once the splint is discontinued. Webbing of the fingers is prevented by inter-digital dressings.

Another very important fact is that the hand should be supported the whole time, by the physiotherapist during treatment, and on a pillow when in bed. If necessary the arm should be elevated to prevent œdema.

It is essential that the physiotherapist should sit during treatment. By doing this she has a far greater contact and affinity with the patient, which assists the patient psychologically. She can watch the patient the whole time and her hand can support the patient's and can also act as a fulcrum during movement.

MOVEMENTS.—These begin as soon as possible and are given in saline when practicable. The joints of fingers and wrist should be stretched *very gently*. No force should ever be used. The movements should at first be assisted active movements. Too strong work may injure the joints and even a very moderate degree of pressure exerted on the newly formed skin, when giving massage or movements, may produce blisters. This distresses the patient, and holds up his treatment. More important still, *the patient must move his hand and fingers himself*. The patterns of movement and the precision and co-ordination of the hand *must* be regained. He may need a good deal of encouragement, as progress is naturally slow, and fits of depression are often an obstacle to recovery. If the thumb can be opposed to the fingers, a very small amount of increased movement in the latter will enable thumb and fingers to be brought together, and small objects can then be picked up. Various kinds of apparatus have been devised for exercising the fingers★ in the later stages, and an ingenious physiotherapist can invent new methods for herself. The other joints of the limb must be exercised, and the patient's posture should receive attention. A course of occupational therapy may, if necessary, conclude the treatment.

MASSAGE.—A lubricant, such as lanoline, or lanoline cream, should be used in the early stages, care being taken not to allow it to become contaminated, especially if there is any part of the wound unhealed. It should be washed off between treatments to prevent accumulation. The injured part—fingers, hand, or wrist—should be treated *very gently and carefully* with frictions or finger-kneadings. The rest of the limb above the site of the injury should receive light and stimulating massage, *but there should be no drag on the injured part*. Areas of healed skin-grafts must be kept supple.

OIL TREATMENT.—If the skin is very delicate, and cannot be touched at all without causing blisters, the patient should soak his hands in warm olive oil for 15–20 minutes, moving the joints gently while immersed. After this he practises active movements under supervision. Massage with oil or lanoline, and gentle stretchings, may be added later.

PARAFFIN WAX BATHS.—These should be given as soon as possible. The wax must not, of course, be applied over any unhealed area.

ELECTRICAL TREATMENT.—The muscles of the arm and forearm may sometimes be gently stimulated with the faradic current. This can be used in the later stages to strengthen the muscles or, at an earlier period, in place of movements if the skin shows a tendency to blister. Radiant heat or infra-red radiation may be used in conjunction with massage.

PRECAUTION.—In old cases, the massage can be deeper and the scar tissue can receive rather more vigorous treatment, *but no violent stretchings may ever be given to the finger-joints*.

Burns of the legs are treated on the same principle. It is, however, essential to give support to the leg following grafting, or the taking of a graft from the legs, to

---

★ *See*, for example, "An Elastic Exerciser for Injured Fingers", by P. Jobling, *J. chart. Soc. Massage med. Gymn.*, February, 1941.

prevent œdema. Firm crêpe bandages should be used and the patient gradually accustomed to dependent limbs. This is done by the patient sitting over the edge of the bed for 1–2 minutes per hour on the first day, gradual progression being made. When he walks again he must not stand for too long.

BURNS OF THE FACE

Treatment.—The treatment generally consists of careful frictions and finger-kneadings to loosen or soften scar tissue, and improve the circulation in the parts. It is sometimes given in preparation for plastic operations. Olive oil is used in preference to lanoline.

SKIN-GRAFTS

Skin-grafts may be used on any part of the body, in areas where there has been extensive destruction by burns, lacerated wounds, etc. Grafts may be autogenous or homogenous. For large grafts both autogenous and homogenous are required. For functional areas autogenous are used if possible. The two principal types of skin-grafts are:—

1. *Free Grafts* (*Fig.* 47).—These consist of slices of skin removed from one part of the body and grafted on to a raw surface in another part. They are of varying thicknesses, e.g., Thiersch or thin razor grafts consisting of the whole

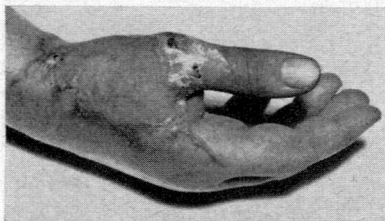

Fig. 47.—Free skin-graft over first metatarsal. Note smooth scar formation at junction of graft and skin. Small areas have yet to heal. Note keloid formation on ungrafted areas on thumb and first finger.

epidermis and part of the dermis; or Wolfe grafts, which consist of the full thickness of the skin. Grafts are fixed in place with dressings which are left undisturbed for 5 days whether or not saline baths are used. In about 14 days the graft begins to contract and harden, and cannot be moved freely over the tissues beneath it. Such grafts are treated very like the burns already described. The aim of treatment is *to soften and loosen the graft* and *improve its circulation*. Deep finger-kneading should be given from the margins of the graft to its centre. As in burns, olive oil or lanoline should be used. Sir Harold Gillies recommends the use of sterile paraffin for eyelid grafts, which must be treated very gently.★ He also says that fresh air benefits grafts, and that patients should be encouraged to keep them uncovered. Later, function must be regained in the affected parts. Paraffin wax baths (temperature 110° F.) are as useful for skin-grafts as for burns. They help the 'setting-in' process.

2. *Skin Flaps and Pedicle Grafts* (*Figs.* 48, 49) in which the skin to be transferred remains attached by one end to the part from which it is to be taken until it has grown securely on to its new site, the reason for this being that the blood-supply should remain intact in order to keep the skin alive during the transfer.

★ Olive F. Guthrie-Smith, *Rehabilitation, Re-education and Remedial Exercises*, Chapter XX (contributed by Sir Harold Gillies and Miss M. B. Penny).

These grafts consist of *whole skin thickness and subcutaneous tissues as well.* They may be applied direct to the area, the distal attachment being severed later, or they may be transferred via an intermediary, e.g. abdomen, arm, or chest, in two or three stages. In such cases three weeks elapse between each stage. Flaps sometimes become œdematous, because of the interference with the lymphatic circulation.

PHYSICAL TREATMENT.—The pedicle or flap will only have a tenuous hold on life in many cases, and physical treatment is seldom, if ever, required. Since, however, the raising of these flaps or pedicles often necessitates an abnormal posture, treatment may be ordered to relieve pain and discomfort from this—but no strain must be put on the flap or pedicle. Heat and massage may be given to the immobilized joints and static contractions should be given to the muscles of the immobile joints. *If heat is administered it must not impinge on the flap or pedicle or a grafted surface, as the heat causes too great a hyperæmia for these delicate tissues at this stage.* After immobilization full range must be regained. After grafting, treatment will be the same as for free grafts and burns. Besides being used to

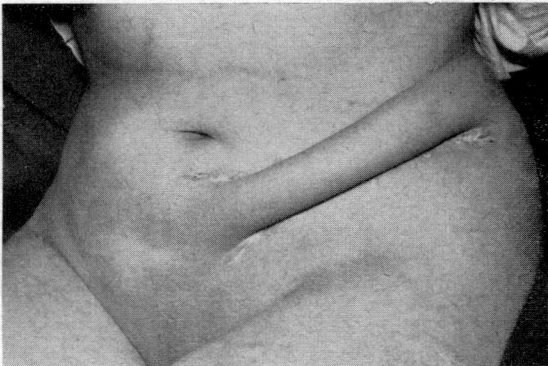

Fig. 48 A.—Pedicle graft, stage one: flap raised on abdomen.

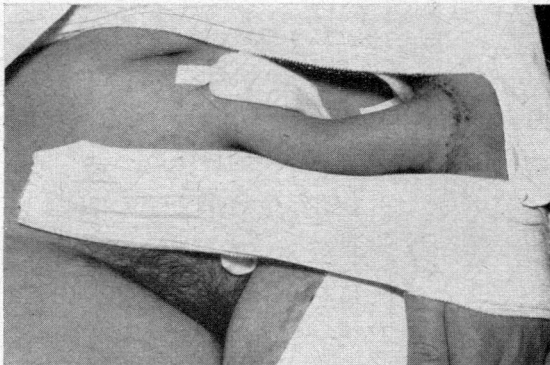

Fig. 48 B.—Second stage: flap joined to forearm. Distal portion will remain attached to abdomen until proximal attachment on forearm takes.

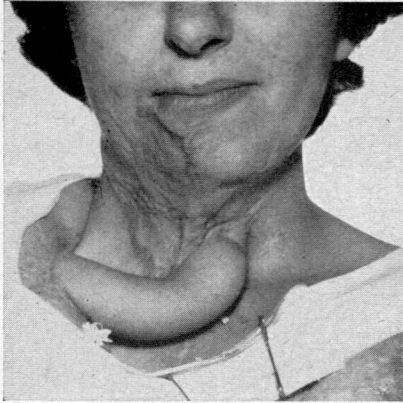

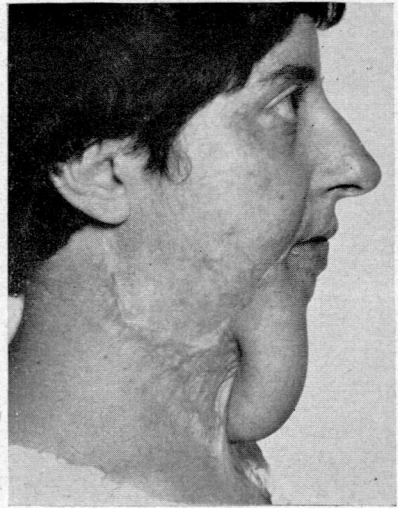

A

B

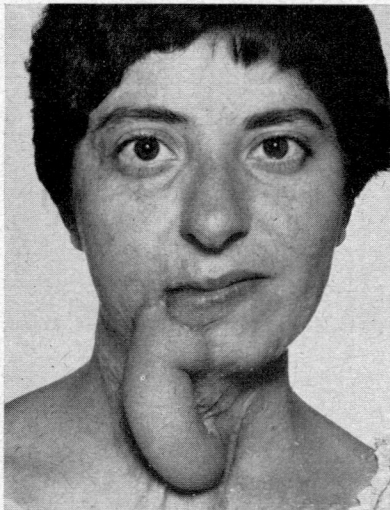

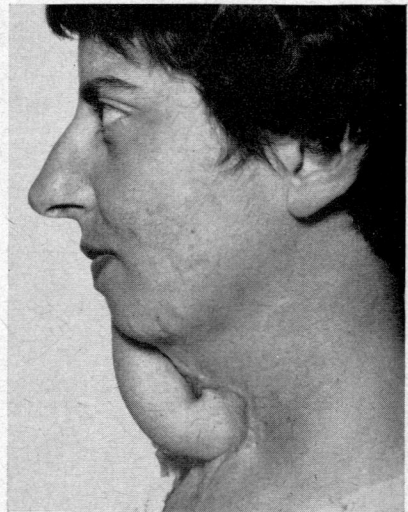

C

D

Fig. 49.—Third stage. A, Flap freed from abdomen and free end attached to neck. Forearm attachment will remain until graft takes on neck. Arm strapped into position to prevent movement meanwhile. When new graft takes final operation will be performed. Scar tissue will be excised, forearm attachment will be freed and applied to scarred area. B, C, D, Last but one stage of graft. It has now been detached from the arm and is in the final grafting position. Note the contraction of the scar and the hard ridged areas.

repair burns and wounds, such grafts are used in plastic surgery, in cases of post-burn contracture, or for cases of breakdown of a free graft.

IV. AMPUTATIONS

Amputation is performed when the state of a limb is such that its survival is incompatible with the health, but perhaps the life, of the patient. The four main reasons for amputation are:—

1. *Peripheral Vascular Disease* (arteriosclerosis) which, by diminishing the circulation, reduces the health and vitality of the tissues to such an extent that gangrene sets in.

2. *Trauma*, particularly the result of road, and industrial accidents.

3. *Malignancy*, in an attempt to arrest its spread.

4. *Diabetes Mellitus*, unhealed sores leading to gangrene.

The proportion of *lower limb* to *upper limb* amputations is 10 to 1, and of those performed on the lower limb, 80 per cent are due to vascular disease, whilst in the upper limb 60 per cent are due to trauma, of which 60 per cent are industrial.*

As in the case of burns, patients are, ideally, treated in a specialized unit, but whether or not this is so, pre- and post-operative care is in the hands of an expert team of which the physiotherapist is an important member, from the time a decision to amputate is taken until the final rehabilitation with the artificial limb (*prosthesis*), and certain basic principles apply to all forms of amputation.

Principles of Treatment.—

SURGICAL.—From the surgeon's point of view, and in the best interests of the future well-being of the patient, the stump must preserve as many joints as possible. This will ensure as good a lever as possible in order to obtain maximum muscle control. As has been stated in earlier chapters, an adequate circulation is essential for healthy tissue repair, and on the healing and health of the stump much depends. Unless the circulation is good, the wound will either fail to heal or, having healed at last, will be liable to repeated breakdown and ulceration—either of which can make the fitting of a prosthesis virtually impossible. In addition, the successful use of a prosthesis requires maximum control from the remaining muscles of the limb, so that the greater the muscle bulk which can be left, the higher the chances of a successful end-result.

PHYSICAL.—Physical treatment divides into two main stages: Pre-operative and post-operative, which sub-divide into early and late stages.

PRE-OPERATIVE TREATMENT.—The main aim is to prepare the patient for the operation and its after-effects. Ideally the patient enters hospital or attends the department two weeks before the operation. This allows sufficient time to become thoroughly acquainted with the post-operative routine. After-care of the stump should be fully explained, and it is helpful if he can meet patients who have had the operation, and watch part of their treatment. A start can be made on training specific muscle groups which will be of importance in the final rehabilitation, and if the amputation is to be a lower limb one, he should practise handling crutches, walking with them, and standing and balancing on one leg. As in the case of burns, the psychological effect of an amputation should not be overlooked. Most patients, particularly the young, will need much reassurance and help in overcoming the fear that they will no longer be useful, independent members of society.

---

* Recent statistics give the following percentage of causes:—
Lower Limb.—Disease, 81·4 per cent (80 per cent vascular); trauma, 17 per cent; congenital deformities, 1·6 per cent.
Upper Limb.—Trauma, 60 per cent; congenital deformities, 27 per cent; disease, 13 per cent (50 per cent malignancy).

EARLY POST-OPERATIVE TREATMENT.—At this stage there are three aims of vital importance.

1. *To Prevent Contracture.*—If these occur, the successful use of a prosthesis may be impossible and great difficulties arise, both for the patient and the limb-fitter.

2. *To Build up Muscle Control.*

3. *To Condition and Care for the Stump and Prevent Terminal Œdema.*

It should not, however, be forgotten that an amputation is a major operation, and that the risks attendant upon any major surgery are present in these cases. A general post-operative routine should therefore be included in the treatment, breathing exercises being given to avoid the possibility of chest complications, and foot and leg exercises to the sound limb, in order to avoid thrombosis.

Lower Limb Amputations

In the lower limb several factors have to be taken into account when considering the amputation site. As has been said, the surgeon aims at as long a stump as possible, with good circulation and muscle control, but both depend to a large extent on the condition for which amputation is undertaken.

Arteriosclerotic gangrene almost always necessitates amputation at, or above, the knee but the trend in modern amputation techniques is towards a *through-knee amputation* whenever possible. This allows a good circulation to the stump, through the superior genicular branches of the popliteal artery and the patellar anastomosis. It also retains the patella and allows knee joint control from the quadriceps. Another advantage of this method is that it provides what is known as an *end-weight-bearing stump*. Formerly the aim was to provide a conical stump, with the bone-ends covered by a thin layer of skin and fascia, the body-weight being transferred to the prosthesis by means of thigh or pelvic bands. The through-knee amputation allows a tapered stump, covered by muscle, soft tissue, and tough skin. It has been found that this gives a much better circulation and the stump heals more quickly. Because large muscles have not been divided, there is less tendency to hæmatoma, an all-too-frequent evil of the older methods, and, perhaps most important of all, the whole of the stump can transmit body-weight to the prosthesis. Thus the advantages of proprioceptive impulses can be fully used in the retraining of balance and leg control, which has proved of particular value in the treatment of the elderly.

In cases where an above-knee amputation has to be performed, the surgeon aims at achieving a stump 70 per cent of the length of the normal thigh. In cases of arteriosclerotic gangrene this is not always possible, however, and in cases of malignancy the whole limb may have to be disarticulated at the hip (hind-quarter amputation).

Above-knee Amputations

This will be taken as the standard amputation, the principles of treatment being the same for a through-knee or above-knee amputation.

PHYSICAL TREATMENT.—

PRE-OPERATIVE TREATMENT.—The patient will require strong shoulder-girdle and arm muscles, strong trunk muscles, and a strong sound leg, if he is to be retrained in balance and pelvic control. He will also need strong muscles and a mobile hip joint on the amputation side. Treatment should therefore include a general programme of exercises, as well as specific resisted exercises for the depressors of the shoulder-girdle and elbow extensors; the erector spinae and trunk rotators; and the muscles of the hip and knee (abductors and quadriceps in particular) on the sound limb. The exercises may have to be modified, depending on the age and general health of the patient, but the above should be the aim whenever possible. During this period he should also practise using crutches, crutch-walking (shadow-walking with the affected leg) and balancing on the sound limb.

EARLY POST-OPERATIVE TREATMENT.—Besides routine post-operative treatment, the three cardinal aims are prevention of contracture, the maintenance of strength and mobility, and care of the stump.

Prevention of Flexion Contracture of the Hip.—In an above-knee amputation, the great danger is a *flexion-abduction deformity.* It will be remembered that the abductors of the hip insert into the great trochanter, whereas the adductors insert into the femoral shaft or condyle. The adductors are, therefore, relatively weak, and, without sufficient training, cannot oppose the pull of the abductors. Similarly, the hip flexors remain intact, whilst the extensors, other than gluteus maximus, have lost their insertion. Added to this, the patient sits in bed for long periods which aggravates the tendency to flexor contracture.

In order to overcome this danger the mattress should be on fracture boards and the patient should lie perfectly flat in bed for an hour 2 or 3 times a day with the stump in extension and adduction. *A pillow should never be allowed to support the stump.* The patient may have two or three pillows for his head *but no others.* As soon as possible (within 2 or 3 days), he should lie prone in bed for the periods mentioned above, again with the stump in line with the sound limb.

Exercises start as soon as possible, the emphasis being on adduction and extension of the hip, but if a drain has been inserted these must be delayed until it is removed (2–3 days). Movements of the amputated limb are free to begin with and should include flexion, extension, abduction, adduction, and circumduction. Gentle resistance to the extensors and adductors can be added in a few days, and will gradually be progressed. To begin with the exercises are best done in side-lying.

Maintenance of Strength and Mobility.—Treatment for the prevention of contractures also maintains the strength and mobility of the stump, but, in addition, general exercises for the arms, trunk, and sound limb can begin the day after the operation. With the need for crutches in mind, the patient should be encouraged to move around in bed by pressing down on his hands and using his shoulder-girdle to move himself up and down the bed.

Care and Conditioning of the Stump.—The ideal stump is firm, healthy, well healed, and tapered or broadly conical in shape, so that it will fit comfortably into the socket of a prosthesis. The chief responsibility for this lies with the physiotherapist, and it is achieved by *pressure bandaging.* This does two things: It accustoms the stump to all-round pressure, such as the socket will supply, and it controls terminal œdema whilst holding the flabby tissues in a firm, tapered shape (*Fig.* 50 **A, B**). Bandaging begins as soon as the stitches are removed, and the bandage is applied three times a day. Aseptic precautions will be taken until the wound is healed, and if it shows signs of breaking down infra-red radiation or ultra-violet light may be ordered to check infection. As a further precaution against œdema, the foot of the bed is raised 40° for the first 7–14 days.

BANDAGING (*Fig.* 51).—Wide crêpe bandages (at least 6 in. in width) should be used. Usually three bandages are required. They should be smoothly sewn together and very tightly rolled, so that the bandage is put on the stretch and its elastic recoil can be made use of when the bandage is applied. The bandage is carried three times backwards and forward over the end of the stump so that it is completely covered, and the turns are continued *firmly* from above downwards, that is to say, a turn is taken from the lateral side up to the groin, round and down to the medial side of the stump again. This is repeated, lateral pressure being exerted to check the tendency to abduction. A few turns should be taken round the body towards the end of the bandage, both to fix the bandage and to check flexion. Great care must be taken to see that the bandage passes round the body from the *lateral* side of the stump across the abdomen, and is then brought across the back and down to the medial side of the stump. In this way the stump can be kept in extension, by means of a backward pull as the bandage is brought down

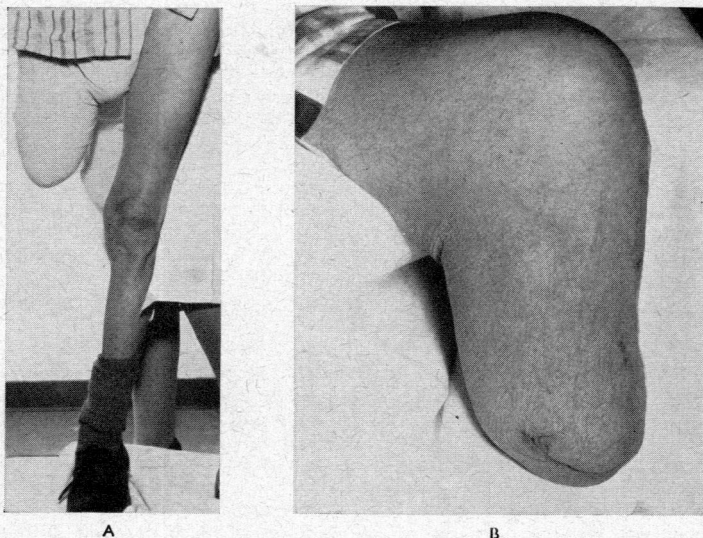

A   B

Fig. 50.—A, Above-knee amputation showing well-moulded stump. Patient has not yet learned to balance and take weight on one leg. Note gross inclination of pelvis as a result. B, Below-knee amputation (bandage removed): scar healing well; moulding progressing but slight œdema still present.

(*Fig.* 51 A–E). The pressure exerted by this bandage controls œdema, makes the stump firmer, and helps to produce the desired taper shape. The bandage is discarded once a limb has been fitted and is in use but the stump should again be firmly bandaged if the limb has to be left off. The patient must be taught to apply his own bandage at home, with the assistance of a relative or district nurse if necessary.

LATE POST-OPERATIVE TREATMENT.—At this stage (10 to 12 days after the operation) training for the prosthesis really begins. The principal aims are:—

1. *To strengthen the extensors and abductors*, by means of strong, resisted exercises.

2. *To retrain balance.*

3. *To teach crutch-walking*, making sure that the stump is used as an integral part of the movements. As the crutches are moved forwards, the hip must be brought into flexion, and then extended as the sound limb is carried through.

When the stump has fully healed, one of two things may happen. Either the patient is fitted with a pylon until prosthesis is ready (this is the ideal, since it ensures continuity of treatment, and accustoms the patient to the feel of the socket and management of an artificial limb), or the patient is discharged to await the arrival of the prosthesis. In this case it is vital to see that the strength and mobility of the stump are maintained, and the patient should attend for regular weekly checks. If pylons are used they are fitted as soon as possible and re-education in walking begins at once. To begin with the pylon is worn for 2 hours twice a day, the periods being increased until it is worn all day.

Re-education in Walking. This begins in parallel bars, with the feet 6 to 10 in. apart. Weight transference is practised from side to side, and forwards and back.

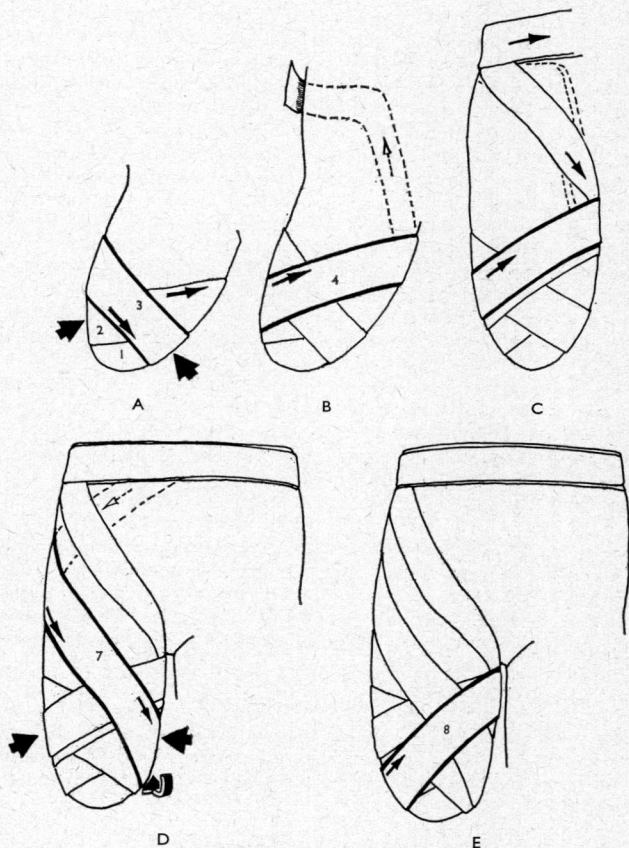

Fig. 51.—A, Tension applied from below upwards to apply pressure to the stump; B, Bandage taken high into groin to prevent overlap roll of flesh, then round waist from behind; C, Bandage taken round body (turn 4 repeated if necessary); D, Bandage brought down from waist, pressure being exerted in downward and backward direction to prevent flexion and abduction deformity; E, Bandage completed by repeating turn round waist and following with turn 8.

When this has been mastered, walking can begin, *emphasis being placed on taking even steps, and using the lateral flexors of the trunk to raise the pylon clear of the ground.* From work in the parallel bars, the patient progresses to four-point walking with crutches. Elderly patients may progress from crutches to sticks, but with young patients it is better to use sticks from the beginning, and to progress to walking unaided. Patients who have not been fitted with pylons must be taught crutch-walking, and it is important that they think of the stump as an integral part of themselves.

If pylons have been used, the transition to prosthesis is a relatively simple one. The main difference in the limb and the pylon is that with the limb, knee flexion and extension can be achieved. Whether pylons or crutches have been used, training in the use of the prosthesis is the same. To begin with the parallel bars are used, and the patient learns to swing the prosthesis forward with the knee in flexion. Placing the heel on the ground locks the limb in extension, and the stump must then be extended in order to stabilize the knee. The weight is thus over the prosthesis and the patient is ready to bring the sound leg through, but simple weight transference must be mastered before he is allowed to take steps. The first steps are again taken between the bars, the patient transferring his weight to the stump as described above, and carrying the sound leg right through. The stump is then flexed and the prosthesis swung through and locked in extension, in readiness for the next step. Two common faults must be controlled: the hip *must* be flexed and extended, *not* circumducted, and the steps must be *even*, the tendency being to take too long a step with the prosthesis.

Once the art of walking has been mastered, training continues towards full rehabilitation. Before the patient is discharged he must be able to do all the things a normal person can do*—walk forwards or backwards, side-step, turn, walk up and down stairs and slopes, get on and off buses, sit and rise from a chair, and lower and raise himself from the ground. This may not, of course, be possible with the elderly but it is an essential part of the rehabilitation of the young.

In the case of through-knee amputations the quadriceps are intact. They must, therefore, be strengthened to the full and fully used in walking. It has been noticed that these patients regain their balance far more quickly, presumably because of their increased kinesthetic sense.

Below-knee Amputations

Treatment.—In these cases treatment presents little problem, the chief factor being the acquiring of a good gait. The bandage is similar to that for an above-knee amputation but a 4 in. one is used. The first four turns cover the stump, and the fifth is continued behind the knee to the thigh. Two turns are then taken round the thigh and down, finishing with two turns round the stump (ten turns in all).

Upper Limb Amputations

Treatment.—The bandage in these cases is similar to that for below-knee amputation, with the fixing turns taken round the front of the shoulder and thorax. The important factor in physiotherapy is the maintenance of full shoulder and elbow mobility.

Hip and Hind-quarter Amputations

The important factor in these cases is the strength of the arms and trunk, which supply the motive power in walking.

PHANTOM PAIN

This is a phenomenon which sometimes occurs post-operatively, the patient complaining of pain in a part of the limb which has been amputated, e.g., the ankle or toes. It is wise to warn the patient that it may happen, and reassure him that it will disappear. There are many forms of treatment which can be

---

* This also applies to patients using pylons.

applied, either in the form of counter-irritation or analgesia. Quick, light percussion with a small hammer is often effective. It starts proximally, gradually extending to the painful area, where it is continued until the pain is numbed, a faradic brush can also be used. Infra-red radiation, or the application of crushed ice may be effective, and ultrasonic treatment is frequently used. Injections of novocain or hydrocortisone may be administered, and if the cause is thought to be a neuroma, it will be explored and excised if necessary.

PROSTHESES

The use of light-weight plastics in the manufacture of prostheses has led to a much wider variety of limbs, with greater freedom of movement and comfort, and a far more natural gait and appearance. It is not proposed to go into details of the various types. For further information the student should consult W. Humm, *Rehabilitation of the Lower Limb Amputee*, and *Physiotherapy*, Vol. 52, No. 6, June, 1966 (*Fig.* 52).

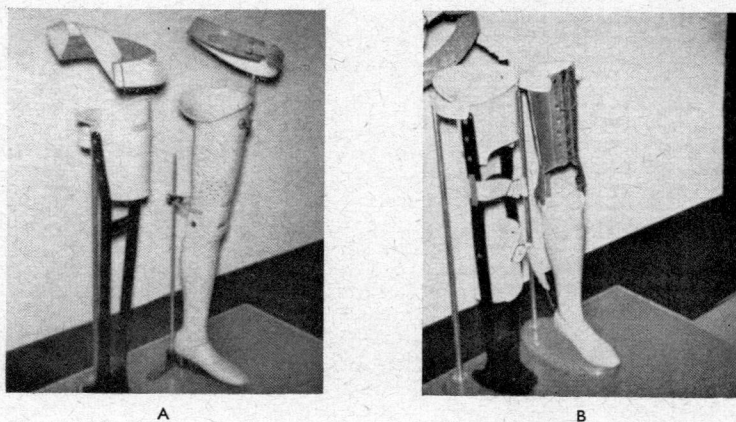

Fig. 52.—A, Above-knee primary pylon. Above-knee permanent prosthesis. B, Below-knee primary pylon. Below-knee metal permanent prosthesis. (*Reproduced by kind permission of Vessa Limited, Alton, Hants, from 'Rehabilitation of the Lower Limb Amputee' by W. Humm.*)

CHAPTER VI

TREATMENT OF THE AFTER-EFFECTS OF INJURY: STIFF JOINTS

Causes and principles of treatment—Stiff shoulder—Stiff elbow and superior radio-ulnar joint—Stiff wrist, hand, and finger—Stiff hip—Stiff knee—Stiff ankle, foot, and toes—Stiff spine—Specialized techniques and treatments.

DESPITE modern methods of treatment we are called upon, all too often, to treat the after-effects of injury—particularly those which have affected joint structures. There are two main symptoms with which we are faced. One is *stiffness and limitation of range*. The other is *pain*. Both can be due to a variety of causes and *before attempting treatment the physiotherapist must discover the cause in each individual case*.

CAUSES OF STIFFNESS.—

1. ADHESIONS, SCARRING, OR CONTRACTURES.—In cases where one of these factors is the chief reason for the disability, the tissues at fault must be stretched and their blood-supply stimulated before any increase in range can be achieved.

2. CHRONIC ŒDEMA.—The presence of fluid in the tissue spaces limits movement by causing pressure on the tissues. In addition, in post-traumatic œdema, organization may have occurred. This, by causing adhesions, still further limits range and activity. In order to achieve any increase in range the œdema must be dispersed as much as possible, and its recurrence controlled. Any resulting adhesions must be stretched.

3. DISUSE ATROPHY.—If a muscle is not fully used its power will diminish, and its range of movement decrease. Its strength must therefore be regained. Another way in which disuse can affect movement is by loss of a cortical pathway. If a muscle or group of muscles is not used the brain literally forgets the movement in which they are concerned. In such cases cortical re-education is required.

4. PAIN.—If movement is painful the muscles will go into protective spasm and the patient will not move beyond the limit of pain. If, therefore, protective spasm due to pain is the only limiting factor, relief of the pain leads to restoration of mobility.

CAUSES OF PAIN.—Adhesions, scarring, or contractures will give rise to pain when the affected structures are stretched. In the same way œdema can give rise to pain. In some cases nerve-endings may actually be involved in scar tissue. In such cases little can be done in the way of cure, but alleviation may be possible with analgesics.

It will be realized that in most cases of post-traumatic disability there may well be a combination of the above causes. However, there is usually one outstanding cause, to the relief of which the major part of treatment should be devoted.

PRINCIPLES OF PHYSIOTHERAPY.—The aims of treatment can be summarized as follows:—

To relieve pain when it is present.
To gain relaxation.
To stretch tightened structures.
To strengthen muscle power.
To increase mobility.

The physiotherapist has a wide choice of methods at her disposal. The routine treatments applicable to all forms of joint stiffness will be discussed first. More specialized techniques and treatments are considered at the end of the chapter.

HEAT.—Heat is invaluable in the treatment of post-traumatic stiffness. It relieves pain and improves circulation, thereby nourishing the tissues and assisting tissue fluid interchange. Because of the local hyperæmia which heat produces, the tissues tend to become more pliable and muscles are prepared for activity. Any form of heat can be used, but, since the joints are primarily affected, those forms of heat which enable the whole area to be treated, i.e., short-wave diathermy and wax baths, are perhaps the most efficacious.

MASSAGE.—The effects of massage are the same as those of heat, and in addition the tissues are moved. In cases of joint stiffness massage should be deep and vigorous, such manipulations as kneadings, frictions, and pétrissage being the most effective. When œdema or pain is present, slower, more soothing techniques should be used, the accent being on effleurage, stroking, and deep squeezing kneadings.

MOVEMENT.—Under this heading passive and active movements must be considered.

Passive Movements.—Here again *relaxed* passive movements and *forced* passive movements must be considered. In dealing with stiff joints it is the forced movements rather than the truly passive relaxed movements, which are of value, since force is required to stretch the tight structures. These forced movements include passive stretchings and manipulative techniques. *The term 'forced' does not, however, imply violence.* Where more than normal strength is required in order to break down adhesions, manipulation under anæsthetic will be performed by a surgeon. Following such treatment relaxed passive movements will be required to maintain the range achieved at the operation until the patient can do this by voluntary muscle control.

Active Movements.—These form the most valuable part of the treatment. Moreover, they have an advantage over forced movements in that *the patient does not contract the antagonists of the acting muscles as he would do, voluntarily or involuntarily, to resist a painful stretching carried out by another person.* Quick, swinging movements are used to increase the mobility of the joint itself, as the momentum acquired by the swinging limb carries it slightly beyond the existing range of movement. Such movements do not, however, increase power. To achieve this, *resistance* must be given. It may be manual or mechanical, whichever is most suitable. In the rehabilitation of stiff joints one must combine mobility and strength. In order to mobilize, free active movements can be used as described above, or assistance can be given by the use of pulleys, slings and springs, or water. These latter have the advantage that gravity is eliminated and all the energy is devoted to joint movement. In addition these media can be adapted to give resistance as well.

In order to strengthen muscles one must bring the greatest possible number of fibres into contraction. This not only increases the muscle bulk and power but also increases the range of movement. When considering muscle contraction, particularly in relation to stiff joints, the following principles should be borne in mind: (1) A greater contraction is achieved when a muscle starts to contract from a stretched position; (2) The greater the contraction, the greater is the subsequent relaxation; (3) The more fully the muscle relaxes the greater will be its subsequent contraction. Reciprocal relaxation occurs in the antagonists.

The movements of which the joints of the body are capable are considered below, and free and resisted exercises suitable for class-work, home exercises, or individual treatments are suggested in each case.

It must be clearly understood that most of the exercises listed are not suitable for cases in which there is any danger of recurrence of the original injury, or recrudescence of inflammation. Nor are *all* the exercises given for any particular joint appropriate to every individual case. The physiotherapist must consider her patient's requirements, as well as any complications that have been, or are, present before selecting the exercises. The starting positions of the exercises may, of course, be altered as required and two or more exercises may be combined in one. (*See also* Chapter XXIII, CLASS EXERCISES.)

STIFF SHOULDER

In the case of the shoulder-girdle, it is essential that exercises should be chosen which will restore *every movement of each of the three joints which it comprises*; no movement should be omitted from the table. The movements are as follows:—

Humeroscapular (Shoulder) Joint.—(1) Flexion and extension. (2) Abduction and adduction. (3) Internal and external rotation.

Sternoclavicular Articulation.—(1) Elevation of the clavicle and with it the scapula. (2) Depression of these bones. (3) Forward movement of the clavicle during which the scapula is drawn forward (abducted), on the chest wall. (4) Backward movement of both bones, the scapula being adducted, or carried back towards the vertebral column.

Acromioclavicular Articulation.—A movement of rotation of the scapula takes place in conjunction with abduction of the humerus and elevation of the clavicle. When the arm is lifted from the side, the inferior angle of the scapula is rotated outward, so that the acromion process is raised, allowing the deltoid to complete the abduction of the humerus. When the arm is lowered, the inferior angle is rotated inward towards the vertebral column.

All the above movements must find a place in the patient's table; elevation should be taken through flexion (Arm-raising forward and upward) and through abduction (Arm-raising sideways and upward).

FREE EXERCISES.—

1. Standing 2-Arm-swinging forward and upward, backward and downward.

2. Standing Alternate arm-swinging, as above.

3. Standing 2-Arm-swinging outward and upward to shoulder level, then across each other in front of body.

4. Standing- or (long-) sitting, 2-Arm-raising sideways and upward (quickly), clapping the hands over the head.

5. As 4, but bringing the backs of the hands together over the head instead of the palms.

6. Standing 2-Arm-swinging in circles.

7. Lying, or crook-lying, Alternate arm-swinging forward and upward over head.

8. As 7, but with the two arms together.

9. Standing (or sitting) Alternate arm-swinging forward and backward with elbow-flexion and -extension. This consists of loose alternate swinging of the arms, shoulder and elbow flexed together in the forward swing, and extended together in the backward swing. The arm is not raised above shoulder level. (*Fig. 53.*)

10. Standing 'Crawling up wall' (with one arm).

11. As 10, but with both arms together.

12. High reach-grasp standing. Trunk forward-bending. Chest-down-pressing. Exercise to stretch shoulder in elevation through flexion. The patient, with arms raised forward and upward grasps a wall-bar as high up as he can. He then bends forward until his body lies as horizontal as the stiffness of his

shoulders will allow. He then tries to press his chest down, thus forcing the arms upward and backward.

13. Standing, stride-sitting, or tailor-sitting 'Cabman's exercise'. This is well known to most people. The patient crosses his arms over his chest, and then swings them outward into extension and outward rotation. It should be done vigorously and in quick time.

14. Standing, or sitting, 2-Shoulder-shrugging.

15. Standing, or sitting, 2-Arm-bending and -stretching in all directions.

16. Forward-bend- (or neck-rest-) standing, or sitting, 2-Elbow-circling. The patient carries the elbows round in small circles, taking them back sharply and relaxing slightly as he brings them forward again.

17. Forward-bend-standing, or (ride-) sitting, 2-Elbow-backward-carrying. Performed much as 16, but the elbows are carried backwards in a series of jerks. Both these exercises are for the retractors of the scapula, and may be repeated about ten times; after a short rest a second series of ten may be given if desired.

18. Reach-standing 2-Arm-parting (quick or slow).

19. Bend-standing or (ride-) sitting 2-Arm-flinging.

20. Forward-bend-stride- or tailor-sitting Alternate arm-flinging.

21. As 20, with Alternate (head- and) trunk-rotation.

22. Standing, or sitting, 2-Arm-swimming.

23. Standing, or sitting, free (single) Arm-rotation with rod, poker, etc. The patient grasps the rod or poker near the centre. The elbow should be straight and the shoulder slightly flexed, abducted, or between flexion and abduction. He rotates the shoulder in and out. A dumb-bell may also be used. To make the exercise more difficult, the poker may be held progressively nearer and nearer the end, so lengthening the weight arm of the lever, and increasing the resistance

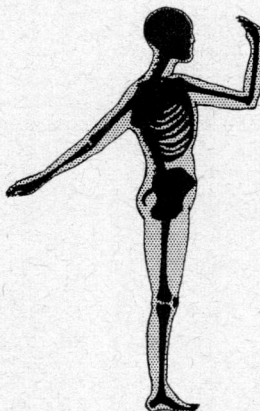

Fig. 53.—Standing Alternate arm-swinging forward and backward with elbow-flexion and -extension.

24. Standing, or sitting, Hand-placing behind neck (neck-rest position) and behind lumbar region. An exercise for inward and outward rotation of the shoulder. It should be done as quickly as possible, and the height to which the arm can reach from the lumbar region progressed.

25. Grasping partner's hand (elbow extended), Rotation in and out.

26. Standing, Sawing.

27. Prone-falling position and its variants. The patient stands with hands against the wall or some high piece of furniture, with arms only just below shoulder level. In this position he performs 2-Arm-bending and -stretching, allowing himself to fall close to the wall and pushing himself away. The support for the hands is gradually lowered, e.g., the patient will place his hands on (1) a table, (2) a high chair, (3) a low chair or stool, (4) the floor. Arm-bending and -stretching in the last position will only be possible for patients with very strong muscles, and forms a final strengthening exercise on recovery. *For many patients it is never possible with the hands lower than* (2), *either because the arms are not strong enough, or because of the strenuous work for abdominal muscles and quadriceps.*

28. For children: 'Cat washing its face' forms a variant of Arm-circling.

120 MASSAGE AND REMEDIAL EXERCISES

EXERCISES REQUIRING APPARATUS OR SKILLED RESISTANCE.—
1. Pulley exercises, double or single pulley. Exercises with spring resistance. (*See* Chapter XXIII.)

> Pulleys may often be extemporized in private houses. An ordinary roller towel on its rail is quite useful, the patient grasping both sides of it and pulling one side down thus drawing up his other arm. Or he may put a piece of cord or rope over a beam, hook on a door, etc., and holding the two ends use it as a pulley.

2. Stretch-half-lying 2-Arm-bending and -stretching. Mobility must be nearly complete before the arm can be brought up to, or near to, the stretch position.
3. Turning nautical wheel (elbow straight).
4. Turning handle of wrist machine with elbow straight.
5. Use of screw-driver.
6. Exercises with Indian clubs, dumb-bells, etc.

It will be noticed that some of the exercises given are directed especially towards the improvement of mobility, others towards the strengthening of muscles. Others, again, aim at attaining both these results at the same time.

Precaution.—A patient with limitation in both shoulders must not be allowed to compensate for his inability to raise his arms above his head by bending his trunk backwards; nor must one with one stiff shoulder be allowed to bend the trunk sideways when abducting or elevating the injured arm. Limited abduction in the humeroscapular joint must not be compensated for by shrugging the shoulder.

Specimen Table for a Shoulder Class, showing how each Movement can be included

EXERCISE	MOVEMENT
1. Standing Deep breathing	
2. Standing 2-Arm-swinging forward and upward, backward and downward	Elevation through flexion; depression and extension
3. Forward - bend - standing 2-Elbow-backward-carrying	Extension of shoulder: retraction of scapulæ
4. Long-sitting 2-Hand-clapping over head	Elevation through abduction
5. Sawing	Forward and backward movement of scapulæ, flexion and extension of shoulder, etc.
6. Standing 2-Shoulder-shrugging	Elevation
7. Tailor-sitting 'Cabman's exercise'	Flexion and extension in shoulder-joint
8. Standing 2-Hand-placing alternately behind neck and behind lumbar region	Internal and external Rotation in humeroscapular joint
9. Standing 2-Arm-swinging in circles	Circumduction
10. Standing (or crook-lying) Deep breathing	

STIFF ELBOW AND SUPERIOR RADIO-ULNAR JOINT

(For precautions in treating an injured elbow, *see* p. 24).
The movements possible are as follows:—
1. Flexion and extension of the elbow-joint.
2. Pronation and supination of the radio-ulnar joints.

Supination can be combined with flexion of the elbow, and pronation with extension. For mobilization of the inferior radio-ulnar articulation, *see* STIFF WRIST, p. 123.

FREE EXERCISES.—

1. Standing Alternate arm-swinging forward and backward with elbow-flexion and -extension (*see* No. 9, SHOULDER EXERCISES, and *Fig.* 53).

2. Standing 2-Arm-bending and -stretching in all directions (quickly).

3. Standing Alternate arm-bending and -stretching. The forearm is held between pronation and supination, and one elbow is flexed as the other is extended. Should be done quickly.

4. Standing (or sitting) 2-Arm-bending, touching shoulders. Both elbows are bent at the same time; the forearm is in supination. The movement may be quick or slow.

5. Standing 'Crawling up and down the wall'.

6. Standing with forearms resting on high plinth, Forward-bending. The exercises should be done with the forearms in supination and in pronation. (*Fig.* 54 A, B.) The same exercise may be done sitting at a low table.

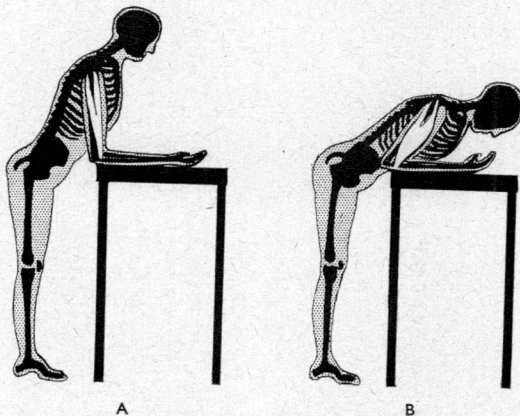

Fig. 54 A, B.—Standing with forearms resting on a high plinth, Forward-bending. (A table is used in this case.)

7. Climbing wall-bars, stretching elbows. The patient keeps hands and feet close together and stretches backward between each step.

8. Tug-of-war. The patient grasps his partner's or the operator's hand, and they pull against each other.

9. Forward-bend-standing (or tailor-sitting) 2-Arm-flinging.

10. Forward-bend-tailor-sitting Alternate arm-flinging with trunk-rotation.

11. (Stoop-) stride-standing Alternate arm-flinging with head-turning to same side ('sign-post').

12. Standing, Sawing.

13. Weight lifting and carrying.

14. Arm-swinging with weight.

15. Prone-falling position, with or without 2-Arm-bending and -stretching (*see* No. 27 SHOULDER EXERCISES).

16. Standing 2-Arm-swimming.

17. Standing (or sitting) Elbow-grasp Pronation and supination. The patient grasps his own elbow from behind with his other hand, to prevent rotation in the shoulder-joint. He quickly turns the palm of his hand upward and downward.

18. As 17, but grasping partner's hand; each resisting the other.

19. Elbow-grasp Pronation and supination with rod or poker. The grasp of the rod is as in No. 23 shoulder exercises. The position of the arm is as in No. 17.

20. Wringing a cloth.

21. Twisting a rod. The patient holds a short rod in front of him, hands pronated and about 3 inches apart. He twists the rod towards him (pronation) and away from him (supination) with his injured hand, resisting with his sound hand. (*Fig.* 55 A, B.)

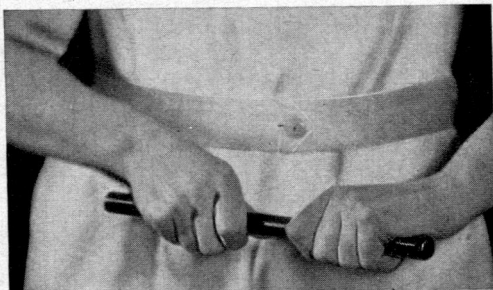

Fig. 55 A.—Twisting a rod. Complete pronation.

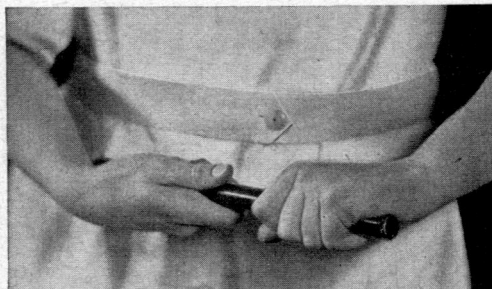

Fig. 55 B.—Twisting a rod. Complete supination. The patient is moving the right hand from one position to the other.

22. Turning door handle.

23. Use of small screwdriver, elbow kept flexed.

24. Hands palm to palm or clasped, finger-tips away from body. Turn finger-tips towards body, keeping palms together. This, of course, must include shoulder movement (flexion and rotation).

25. Hand-clapping (alternate pronation and supination). The elbows are kept close to the sides. The hands are clapped, each hand being placed alternately on top of the other.

APPARATUS AND RESISTANCE EXERCISES.—

1. Pulley exercises (*see* Chapter XXIII), or those with home-made substitutes.

2. Hitting the punch-ball, or a large ball suspended in the air.

3. Wrist machine Pronation and supination—elbow-grasp.

4. Stretch-half-lying 2-Arm-bending and -stretching.

STIFF WRIST, HAND, AND FINGER

The following movements are necessary:—

WRIST-JOINT.—Flexion, extension, abduction or radial deviation and adduction or ulnar deviation.

INFERIOR RADIO-ULNAR JOINT.—The radius moves round the ulna in pronation and supination.

CARPAL JOINTS.—Slight movements of flexion, extension and rotation between the carpal bones will take place in conjunction with those of the wrist and inferior radio-ulnar joints.

METACARPOPHALANGEAL JOINTS.—These are enarthrodial (ball-and-socket) joints and therefore are capable of: (1) Flexion and extension; (2) Abduction and adduction; (3) A very slight rotary movement is possible when passive movements are given. Since restoration of mobility in the hand is so important a little will be said here on the technique of passive movements. When moving the inferior radio-ulnar joint the forearm should be held in the mid-position. The radius should be grasped between the physiotherapist's index finger and thumb and should be moved backwards and forwards on the ulna, in addition to ordinary pronation and supination.

When moving the carpus, strong traction in the long axis of the forearm should be maintained.

1. Flexion and extension of metacarpophalangeal joints. Dr. Mennell has pointed out that there is a marked gliding element in the movements of this joint, as well as in that of the interphalangeal joints,* and that if the first phalanx is grasped well above the joint and forced forward, the posterior ligaments will be torn. Instead of this, the *head* of the metacarpal should be pressed back while the *base* of the first phalanx is moved forward over it, the pressure in both cases being exerted as close to the joint as possible.

2. Abduction and adduction. The first phalanx should be grasped firmly, and drawn out longitudinally. The finger should then be moved from side to side.

3. Rotation. The grasp is as above, but the joint is slightly flexed. Only very slight movement is possible.

INTERPHALANGEAL JOINTS.—These can be flexed and extended and passive movements are given in a similar manner to those for the metacarpophalangeal joints.

> The chapter in Dr. Mennell's book, referred to in footnote, is most valuable, and should be read by all who wish to make a success of this kind of work. It is written for surgeons, but many useful suggestions may be gathered by the experienced physiotherapist which should be of considerable assistance to her in her work. It is not, of course, intended for beginners.

FREE EXERCISES.—Cases to be treated in a *class* for hand injuries should be very carefully selected. Over-strenuous treatment may in many cases do irreparable damage and we have to remember how very serious hand disablement is for many patients. Cases in which sepsis has been present should be most carefully watched. Patients recovering from paralysis are not suitable for inclusion in classes until recovery is practically complete.

The following exercises are suitable for class-work or individual treatment.

1. Wrist-shaking, forward and backward.

2. Wrist-shaking, laterally. This combines abduction and adduction of the wrist with pronation and supination.

3. Standing, hand pronated on table, Trunk-falling-forward. For extension of the wrist.

4. Crawling on all fours (for children). For extension of the wrist.

---

* *Physical Treatment by Movement, Manipulation and Massage,* Chapter XVIII.

5. For pronation and supination, Exercises 17–25 in the list of elbow exercises (*see* pp. 121, 122).

6. Standing, hand on table, Wrist- and finger-flexion (*Fig.* 56).

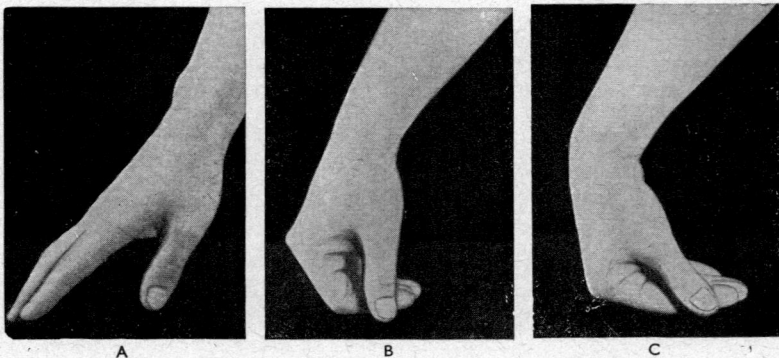

Fig. 56.—Standing, hand on table, Wrist- and finger-flexion. **A,** Starting position. **B,** Flexion of metacarpophalangeal and first interphalangeal joints. **C,** Flexion of wrist.

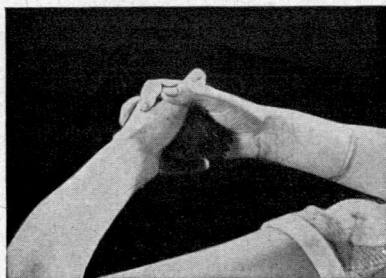

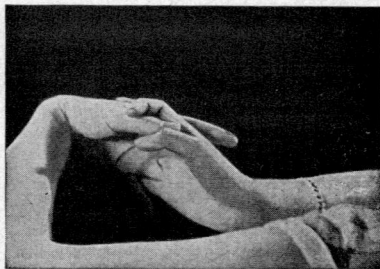

Fig. 57.—Exercise No. 13, for flexion and extension of wrist. For the purpose of showing wrist movement, the model's arms are raised to shoulder level and carried to the left. In the exercise as described, the hands are placed in front of the thorax just above the waist level.

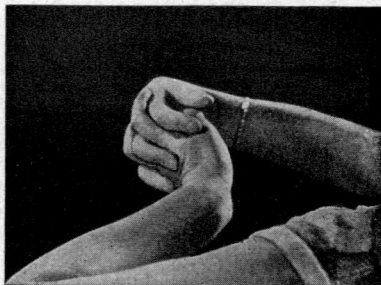

7. Hand-opening and -closing, with abduction and adduction of fingers.

8. As No. 7 plus flexion and extension of wrist. Closing of the hand accompanies extension of the wrist, opening accompanies flexion.

9. Hand-opening and -closing plus 2-Arm-bending and -stretching.

10. Squeezing a rubber ball.

11. Grasping rods of different sizes.

12. Palms together, arms stretched in front of body; draw hands in towards body, carrying elbows outwards, the palms being kept together. For extension of the wrist.

13. Hands clasped in front of thorax, elbows at side. Each forearm is brought alternately against the thorax, producing flexion of one wrist and extension of the other. A strong exercise if done quickly and vigorously. (*Fig. 57.*)

14. Finger-tips together, finger-tips pointing away from body, elbows at sides. Bring elbows out from sides, pressing palmar aspects of all fingers together, keeping palms of hands apart. For extension of fingers and thumb.

15. Touch each finger-tip in turn with the tip of the thumb. For opposition of the thumb.

See also exercises for MEDIAN and ULNAR PARALYSIS, Chapter XII. These are useful for strengthening the small muscles of the hand.

The beginner who finds massage difficult will find these exercises of assistance in helping to mobilize and stretch the hands, so that they become more flexible.

APPARATUS EXERCISES.—

Wrist Machine.—Begin by grasping the smallest bar. Turn: (1) Away from self for wrist flexion; (2) Towards self for extension. Progress to larger bars, and add resistance gradually. For pronation and supination, use as for elbow exercises.

For home exercises a rolling-pin held by an assistant answers quite well.

Sand-tray Exercises.—Patient picks up the dry sand, and tries to hold it in his closed hand. Beans, lentils, etc., can also be used.

STIFF HIP

The following movements are possible.

1. Rotation of the hip.

2. Flexion and extension of the hip. This may be combined with knee flexion and extension.

3. Abduction and adduction.

4. Circumduction.

Special attention must be paid to *abduction* and *inward rotation after all old injuries to the femoral neck*, and indeed in most cases of 'stiff hip' from whatever cause.

FREE EXERCISES.—

1. Half-yard-standing (or free standing) Leg-swinging forward and backward.

2. Cock-step marching, or marching with knee-raising.

3. Standing Alternate knee-raising, with knee-clasping. The patient raises each knee alternately, clasping it with both hands and drawing it into as full flexion as possible.

4. Knee-sitting position, or the endeavour to assume it.

5. Going up and down steps.

6. Reach-grasp-standing Leg-side-swinging.

7. Crook-lying 2-Knee-abduction and -adduction (free).

8. Reach-grasp-standing Leg-carrying (or -swinging) in circles.

9. Long-sitting (if possible) Forward-bending.

10. Stride-sitting Forward-bending.

11. Sitting Forward-bending and backward-falling to half-lying position. If in a gymnasium, the patient sits on the short end of a low plinth, the long end being raised. He alternately bends forward and falls back into half-lying position.

12. Stretch-standing Forward- and downward-bending and raising.

13. Standing, Hewing.

14. Wing- or reach-grasp-standing Heel-raising and knee-bending.

15. Heave-grasp-close-standing (in doorway) Alternate pelvic-rotation (free).

16. Crook-lying Pelvic-raising and -rotation.

17. Yard-close-standing Alternate trunk-rotation; or any trunk-rotation in which the pelvis is not fixed.

18. Crook-lying Pelvic-rotation. The patient swings both knees together, first to one side then to the other.

19. Prone-lying Leg-raising backward.

20. Any exercise in the list of knee exercises which involves movement in the hip also.

APPARATUS OR RESISTANCE EXERCISES.—

1. Pulley exercises (single pulley) (*see* Chapter XXIII).

2. Leg-forward-lying Trunk-forward-bending. The patient is in leg-forward-lying on a low plinth, or a high plinth with a stool in front. The feet are strapped, or supported by the physiotherapist. He places his hands on the floor, or stool, and gradually lowers his body over the end of the plinth by bending his arms.

3. Heave-grasp-lying, 2-Knee-updrawing and -down-pressing.

4. Crook-half-lying 2-Knee- (or leg-) abduction and -adduction (resisted).

5. Resisted Trunk- and Pelvic-rotations.

6. Stationary bicycle.

7. Rowing machine.

8. Skipping exercises.

9. Exercise with a 'skate'.

STIFF KNEE

The movements possible are:—

1. Flexion and extension.

2. Internal and External Rotation with the knee in semi-flexion (this is often forgotten). External rotation should not be given to knock-kneed patients.

Lateral and upward and downward movement of the patella should be given passively in all cases of stiff knee.

FREE EXERCISES.—

1. High-sitting free Leg-swinging. Later, a weight may be attached to the foot—first 1 lb., then 2 lb. etc.

2. Sitting Knee-bending and -stretching.

3. Wing-standing, or half-yard-grasp-standing Leg-swinging (knee swinging loosely).

4. Reach-grasp-standing Heel-raising and knee-bending (quickly and slowly).

5. Crook-sitting position, the patient drawing up the stiff knee towards his body with his own hands.

6. Wing-knee-standing, trying to assume knee-sitting position. This should only be given if the knee can already be flexed to a little beyond a right angle. Otherwise the patient assumes a position of lordosis, hollowing his back in order to keep the line of gravity within the base.

7. Half-kneeling Forward-bending. The patient kneels on the sound knee (*Fig.* 58 A). He then bends forward over the front knee (*Fig.* 58 B), so forcing it into flexion; a series of small movements backward and forward may be made when the limit of movement is reached. In order to obtain a further stretching he may bend the trunk as far forward as possible, stretching out the arm on the side of the injured knee and trying to touch the ground as far in front of him as possible.

8. **Prone-kneeling Backward-pushing.** The patient, on hands and knees, pushes his body backward with his hands till knees and hips are fully flexed, or as much flexed as possible.

9. Running on the spot with knee-raising.

10. Lunge position.

11. 'Frog-march'.

12. Lying, half-lying, or standing, quadriceps contractions.

13. Nos. 2, 3 and 5, in list of hip exercises.

14. Stride-sitting Knee-rotation in and out.

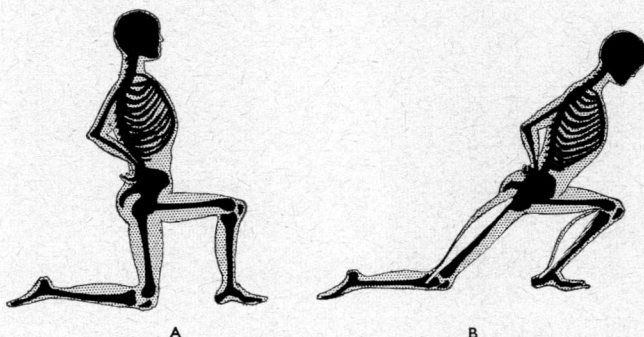

Fig. 58.—Half kneeling forward-bending. The knee can be still further flexed if the heel is raised from the ground; but this must not be allowed if the purpose of the exercise is to obtain full dorsiflection of the ankle.

APPARATUS OR RESISTANCE EXERCISES.—

1. Rowing machine (or rowing in boat with sliding seat).

2. Pulley exercises (*see* Chapter XXIII).

3. Kicking a football.

4. Progressive weight-resistance.

5. 'Bunny-jumping' over a form.

STIFF ANKLE, FOOT, AND TOES

Those movements which can occur actively are:—

1. Flexion and extension of the ankle.

2. Inversion and adduction, eversion and abduction, movement occurring in the talocalcaneal and mid-tarsal (transverse tarsal) joints.

3. Circumduction.

4. Flexion and extension of the toes.

It should be remembered that passive movements of the ankle, foot, and toe joints should be given on the same principles as those of the wrist, hand, and fingers (*see* p. 123).

FREE EXERCISES.—

1. (Wing) standing Single heel-raising and -lowering. (*See Fig.* 57.)

2. Standing 2-Heel-raising and -lowering.

3. Standing 2-Knee-bending (to curtsey-standing position).

4. Wing-standing Heel-raising and knee-bending.

5. Walking on the toes, and running.

6. Knee-sitting Trunk-raising and -lowering. Given for plantar-flexion of the ankle.

7. Stamp-and-toe-marching. Four steps on tip-toe, then four steps stamped.

8. Other fancy marches, in which the patient uses the feet quickly and actively.

9. Reach-grasp- (or wing-) standing Alternate heel- and toe-raising.

10. Half-kneeling Forward-bending. No. 7 knee exercises (*see also Fig.* 56 A, B). The exercise produces strong dorsiflexion of the foot of the leg in front.

11. Heel-support-standing Forward-bending.

12. Heel-support-standing Heel-raising and knee-bending. Both these exercises stretch the calf muscles as well as the hamstrings.

13. Standing Toe-flexion and -extension. (*Fig.* 59 A, B.)

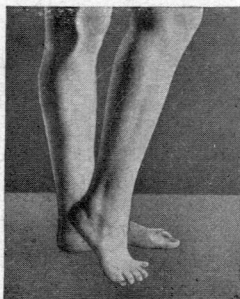 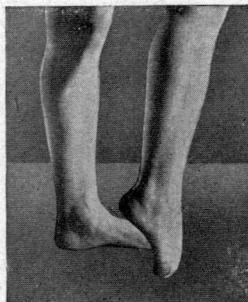

A   B

Fig. 59.—Standing Toe-flexion and -extension. A also represents the position taken in *heel-raising* in Exercise 1, Wing-standing Single heel-raising and -lowering.

14. Standing at edge of plinth, toes over the edge, Flexion and extension of toes of both feet.

15. Picking up objects with the toes—pencil, marble, golf-ball, etc.

16. Sitting (or half-lying) Toe-separating (if possible).

17. Standing Foot-shortening, re-forming arch (*see* Exercises for FLAT-FOOT, Chapter XV).

18. Sitting 2-Foot-inversion ('clawing').

19. Standing 2-Foot-inversion.

20. Standing on outer borders of feet. This exercise is much recommended by some but it produces a great strain on the outer side of the foot and should not be given to heavy patients, nor if there has been any damage to, or weakness of, the external lateral ligament of the ankle.

21. Sitting (on stool) with knees crossed, Active foot-rolling.

22. All dancing steps; jumping and skipping exercises.

23. Exercises for re-education in walking.

24. Walking and running with short steps.

27. 'Frog-march' and 'Snake-hop' for children. The latter is simply 'frog-march' in line, each child placing his hands on the shoulders of the one in front of him.

N.B.—If the Achilles tendon is shortened, no tip-toe exercises should be given.

APPARATUS AND RESISTANCE EXERCISES.—

1. Pulley exercises (*see* Chapter XXIII).

2. Half-lying Foot-bending and -stretching, Inversion and eversion, Toe-bending and -stretching (resisted).

3. Foot-stretching in apparatus.

An apparatus invented by Mrs. Guthrie-Smith stretches the tendo Achillis and produces full dorsiflexion of the ankle.

The patient's foot is fixed to a foot-piece by straps; it may also be inverted if desired by means of a wedge under the inner border. The end of the foot-piece is fastened by straps to a broad piece of webbing which passes behind the patient's body, so that by leaning back he puts tension on the calf muscles and tendo Achillis. This is a useful and easily constructed apparatus.

4. Rowing machine.
5. Stationary bicycle.
6. Walking on inclined board. The board is so constructed that it is highest in the centre and slopes down on both sides towards the edge, which is guarded by a rim. The patient's feet are thus kept in inversion as he walks.

STIFF SPINE
Cervical Region

The movements possible are flexion, extension, side-flexion, rotation and circumduction.

When giving passive movements, traction must be maintained throughout. This is very important.

FREE EXERCISES.—
1. Lying (or stride-sitting) Head-side-carrying. The patient may place his hands against the sides of his face at the level of the cheek bones, and press alternately against each. The head must not be *tilted* sideways.
2. Low-grasp-sitting Head-side-bending.
3. Reach-grasp-sitting Head-forward and -backward-bending.
4. (Reach-grasp) stride-sitting, or tailor-sitting Head-rotation.
5. Reach-grasp-sitting Chin-indrawing and forward-pushing. No head-flexion must take place.
6. Standing (or tailor-sitting) Head-nodding to centre, left, and right, three times each way.

APPARATUS AND RESISTANCE EXERCISES.—
1. Exercises 2–4 (*above*) resisted by operator.
2. The same movements in suspension apparatus.
3. Pulley exercises.
4. Spring resistance exercises.

Thoracic and Lumbar Region

The movements possible are the same as in the cervical region but the student will remember that *rotation does not occur* in the thoracic region.

FREE EXERCISES.—
1. Stride-sitting Back-raising Vertebra by Vertebra.
2. Back-support-standing Forward-bending and -raising.
3. Stretch-stride-standing Forward-bending, trying to touch heels. This may be done in a series of small rhythmic movements.
4. Long-sitting Forward-bending, trying to touch toes (as 3).
5. Walk-standing, Wing-knee-standing, or holding partner's hands Trunk-backward-bending.
6. Stride-standing Hewing.
7. 'Donkey' (abdominal and lumbar contractions).
8. (Heave-grasp-) lying 2-Knee-raising and lowering.
9. Lying Head- and shoulder-raising and 2-Knee-raising (clasping knees).
10. Stride-sitting Alternate side-bending. (This may be localized to thoracic or lumbar region.)
11. Stride-standing, or -sitting, quick Alternate side-bending.
12. Stoop-stride-sitting Alternate trunk-rotation and Alternate arm-flinging. The patient places his hands on the inner sides of his knees. He swings the right

5

arm and trunk to the right, helping the trunk-turning movement by pressing with the left hand against the knee. He then turns forward, replaces the right hand on inner side of knee, and repeats the movement to the left.

13. Stride-standing Sawing.
14. Half-yard-grasp standing Leg-swinging forwards and backwards.
15. Crook-lying Pelvic-rotation (*see* Exercise 18 for STIFF HIP).
16. Crawling exercises (Clayton).

See also ABDOMINAL EXERCISES, p. 459, and those for SACRO-ILIAC STRAIN, p. 69.

APPARATUS AND RESISTANCE EXERCISES.—

1. Heave-grasp-lying 2-Knee- (or 2-Leg-) updrawing and downpressing.
2. Wing-close-sitting or Wing-high-ride-sitting Trunk-rotation.
3. Pulley Exercises.
4. Spring-resistance Exercises.
5. Medicine ball Exercises.

These exercises are intended only as a guide. The student should learn to adapt them for any particular requirements, e.g., modifications and progressions should be worked out, and plans made for adapting them for inclusion in activities of daily living. Manipulations requiring special skill, and very strong exercises suitable only for men patients returning to heavy work after injury, are not included here. The former may be found in works by Dr. Mennell and Dr. Cyriax: the latter in the books by Mrs. Guthrie-Smith, Mr. Colson, Böhler, and others.

SPECIALIZED TECHNIQUES AND TREATMENTS

Before closing this chapter some consideration should be given to the Kabat method of treatment, and various forms of electrotherapy which can be used to advantage in the treatment of stiff and painful joints.

The Kabat Method of Treatment.—This is a highly specialized method of treatment which requires a thorough knowledge and understanding of the technique employed before it can be used effectively. It is, however, a method of treatment based on physiological principles and these can be applied when giving any exercises designed to assist joint mobility and muscle power. An outline of these principles is given here and in the chapter dealing with ANTERIOR POLIOMYELITIS, pp. 208–10.

The treatment is based on *normal physiological patterns of movement.** Whilst these movements are being performed, the physiotherapist assists muscle contraction by applying proprioceptive stimuli: (1) Pressure is applied on the surface in the direction of movement, e.g., if the knee is to be extended the hands are placed on the quadriceps and on the extensor aspect of the leg or foot. (2) The muscles are stretched over *all* the joints on which they work in order to initiate the stretch reflex and increase the contraction, e.g. if the ankle is to move into dorsiflexion and inversion, the movement starts from full plantar flexion and eversion. (3) Slight traction or, in some cases, compression, is given to stimulate the proprioceptive nerve-endings in the joint and increase the contraction. (4) Resistance is applied during muscle contraction. The term 'maximal resistance' is used in connexion with the Kabat technique. This means that the greatest amount of resistance is given, compatible with smooth controlled activity, *throughout the whole range of movement.* It may be very light or very heavy, depending on the state of the muscles concerned. It must never cause pain.

Two kinds of contraction are recognized: (*a*) *Isotonic contraction*, which is active shortening of the fibres. This occurs during voluntary muscle work. (*b*) *Isometric contraction*, which is a static muscle contraction. *During Isotonic or Isometric contraction the antagonistic muscle groups will lengthen eccentrically.*

---

* More details of these are given in Chapter IX.

In treating stiff and painful joints in which there is muscle spasm, the tight muscles must be relaxed before the range can be increased. Because of this spasm the antagonistic muscles will be weak from disuse *and for the same reason the tight muscles will also be weak*. Power must therefore be built up in both groups.

The principles of three simple Kabat techniques of use in such cases are given below.*

1. An *isometric (static) contraction* is given to the tight group followed by relaxation. *No movement is allowed to take place*. The tight muscles, having gone into strong contraction, relax more fully. This allows the passive range to be increased slightly. Taking limited elevation of the shoulder due to tight flexors as an example, the technique is as follows. The physiotherapist takes the arm into elevation as far as the limit of the pain-free range. She then asks the patient to resist her attempts to take the arm further into elevation. When she feels a strong contraction in the muscle she asks the patient to relax and, when relaxation is complete she takes the arm into the range it is now possible to achieve. The process is repeated in the new range and in this way progress is made. This technique is known as 'Hold Relax', and is of special use in the early stages to gain initial relaxation during the period when active movement causes pain.

2. An *isometric contraction* is given to both the tight group of muscles *and* their antagonists. Again, no movement occurs in the joint. Relaxation is gained, as in the above technique, through contraction of the tight muscles and is augmented by eccentric lengthening of these muscles brought about by the isometric contraction of their antagonists. At the same time power is beginning to be built up in both groups of muscles. Taking the same example as above, the arm is taken by the physiotherapist to the limit of the pain-free range of elevation. She then asks the patient to resist her attempts to take it further. As soon as she feels a good contraction in the tight muscles she changes her hands to the antagonistic surface (to give proprioception) and asks the patient to resist her attempts to take the arm down. Several alternating contractions are given in this manner, and after a final contraction in the antagonistic group the patient is allowed to relax. *No relaxation must be allowed before this*. This is useful when the pain and stiffness are less acute. It is known as 'Rhythmical Stabilization'.

3. An *isotonic contraction* followed by an *isometric contraction and relaxation* are given to the tight group of muscles followed immediately by an *isotonic contraction* of their antagonists. *Only a very small range of movement is allowed in the tight muscle group but a full range of movement with maximal resistance is given to their antagonists*. In this way relaxation of the tight muscles is achieved as in the technique described above. In addition, power is built up in the antagonistic group which is the essential factor in increasing active joint range. In order to gain elevation of the shoulder when the flexors are tight, the arm is taken to the pain-free limit of elevation. The commands are "Pull down and in; hold and relax". During the contractions maximal resistance is given. When relaxation is complete the physiotherapist changes the position of her hands and gives the command "Push up and out". This technique is known as 'Slow reversal, hold, relax', and is used in the later stages of treatment.

At this stage, techniques designed specifically for strengthening and mobilizing can be included in the treatment. These are given in the chapter dealing with ANTERIOR POLIOMYELITIS, *see* pp. 208–10.

---

* For a detailed description students should read the article "Proprioceptive Neuromuscular Facilitation in relation to Stiff Joints", S. Riddell, *Physiotherapy, Lond.*, November, 1958. Also "The Practical Application of Proprioceptive Neuromuscular Facilitation", by H. Kabat, M. McLeod, and C. Holt, *Physiotherapy, Lond.*, April, 1959, and "Proprioceptive Neuromuscular Facilitation", *Physiotherapy*, London, January, 1967.

Electrotherapy Treatments.*—Relief of pain, an increase in circulation, relief of œdema, softening of fibrous tissue, and strengthening of muscles can all be achieved by electrotherapy. A brief outline of the principles of the various techniques is given below.

RELIEF OF PAIN.—This can be achieved in three ways: (1) By the use of anodal galvanism, in which its analgesic properties are made use of; (2) By the introduction of analgesic drugs by ionization, e.g., calcium, aconitine, cocaine, or novocain; (3) By counter-irritation, superficial painful stimuli being applied to break through the painful pattern established by the deeper pain nerve-endings. For this cathodal galvanism, histamine or renotin ionization and local erythema doses of ultra-violet light can be used.

INCREASE IN CIRCULATION.—This is best achieved by: (1) The production of an artificial inflammatory reaction, either by histamine or renotin ionizations, or strong local erythema doses of ultra-violet light. These all produce an active hyperæmia and an inflammatory reaction; (2) Direct current can also be used, a better hyperæmia being produced under the cathode than under the anode, because of the increased sensory stimulus which leads to superficial vasodilatation.

RELIEF OF ŒDEMA.—This can be achieved by giving faradism under pressure, fluid being forced towards the drainage centres by pressure from the muscles contracting against restricting bandages.

SOFTENING OF FIBROUS TISSUE.—Certain drugs such as iodine and chlorine have a fibrolytic effect on scar tissue and adhesions. Another form of treatment which is often beneficial is ultrasonic treatment.

STRENGTHENING OF MUSCLES.—This is achieved by means of the faradic current. *The stimuli must be sufficient to cause a good contraction and should be augmented by voluntary muscle action.* The principle of eccentric relaxation used in the Kabat techniques can be achieved by reciprocal faradism in which opposing muscle groups are brought into contraction alternately.

Treatment of Œdema in Later Stages of Fractures.—The *massage manipulations* used are similar to those described on p. 96. The limb should be elevated on pillows or suspended in a sling for 20–30 minutes before treatment is begun. *Slow deep effleurage* should be given to assist the venous and lymphatic flow, beginning at the upper part of the limb so as to empty the lymphatics in that area. The part immediately below this should next be treated, to press on the fluid into the vessels which have already been cleared, after which a return should be made to the upper region. The physiotherapist should continue on this principle over the length of the limb, ending with long strokes from the fingers or toes, towards the lymph-glands in the axilla or groin. *Hand kneading*, also slow and deep, should next be given, with *finger-kneading* round joints or over small muscles; also *frictions* to stretch adhesions. The manipulations are followed by *active movements* of all joints of the limb, with circling movements of hip or shoulder, to promote venous and lymphatic circulation by muscle pressure. These may, if necessary, be assisted by the physiotherapist, or may be performed with the limb in suspension. The patient should also practise *deep breathing*.

Bandaging the limb with rubber or crêpe bandages may also help to reduce œdema, and *faradism* (graduated contractions) applied to the muscles with the bandages in place has also been recommended (Mennell). This not only causes the muscles to press more strongly on the vessels, but, since resistance to the contractions is provided by the bandages, the muscles themselves are strengthened.

N.B.—Any precautions necessary in special circumstances, e.g., thrombosis (pp. 434–6), scars, wounds, nerve involvement, etc., must, of course, be carefully observed.

---

* Heat treatments are not included here.

Buerger's Exercises (*see* p. 431), or *Contrast Baths* (*see* p. 93) may be suitable in certain cases.

MANIPULATIVE METHODS.—These are made use of by the surgeon: (1) *To replace the bones in their correct position*, i.e., to set the fracture; (2) *To mobilize a stiff joint, or joints*, when adhesions have formed to such an extent that full movement cannot be regained by active exercise alone. In such circumstances the patient is anæsthetized and the surgeon moves the joint forcibly, breaking down the adhesions which impede its free movement. This may be done in one operation, or the manipulation may be carried out in several stages. The reason for this is that if the joint is suddenly completely mobilized, the large amount of damage to the surrounding tissues may set up intense inflammation, which results in the formation of new adhesions. Also the severe pain suffered by the patient may make him unwilling to attempt to move the limb at all.

AFTER-TREATMENT.—The physiotherapist should, if possible, be present at the manipulation, so that she may see exactly what range of movement was obtained. If not present, this should be clearly explained to her by the surgeon. It is essential that this degree of restored movement should not be lost.

Massage.—Gentle kneading and effleurage may be given as in cases of recent injury, avoiding any specially painful point. Careful frictions round the joint may be added later.

Movements.—Passive movements should only be given *within the limit of pain*. The patient *must* move the limb actively in spite of the pain, or the joint will speedily stiffen up again. Rhythmic swinging movements are best, and the patient may be placed with the limb in a suspension sling. In this way, gravity being eliminated and friction reduced to a minimum, he will be able to move it more freely and with less discomfort. (*See* Chapter XXIII.) Appropriate exercises will be chosen, in suitable starting positions, e.g., lying with an arm in suspension sling for abduction movements; side-lying with leg in slings for flexion and extension of the hip. The patient is far more likely to relax in this position than he would do with an unsupported limb. Feeling the movement to be under his own control, he will ultimately come to relax his muscles instead of tensing them, voluntarily or involuntarily, to resist the force of gravity or even the 'assistance' of the operator. It is important, however, that whatever apparatus or assistance is used the starting position should be correct, and remain so throughout the movement; e.g., the thorax must be fixed and the shoulder girdle controlled for abduction in the humeroscapular joint, otherwise he may perform some trick movement such as shoulder shrugging or lateral flexion of the spine to the sound side, and may thus establish a habit. Later, in some cases, the single pulley may be used (*see* p. 485, *Figs.* 191, 192), so that the sound limb may at first *assist* and then *resist* the injured one. Free exercises, e.g., Arm-or leg-swinging forward and backward, or in circles, may be added as the patient improves. Muscle power may be worked up by gradually increased resistance, given by means of springs, weights and pulleys, the patient's own body-weight, or manual resistance by the physiotherapist. If any further treatment is required, a course of occupational or recreational therapy may be indicated. General and postural exercises should accompany the special movements.

Electrical Treatment.—Radiant heat, ionization, the whirlpool bath, or short-wave diathermy, are all used in the early stages to relieve pain and prepare the way for exercises. The last-named is often extremely effective.

CHAPTER VII

DISEASES OF JOINTS, SYNOVIAL MEMBRANES, AND BONES

I. Diseases of joints: Traumatic synovitis or arthritis—Bacterial synovitis or arthritis—Infective arthritis—'Rheumatoid' arthritis—Still's disease—Osteo-arthritis—Spondylitis—Tuberculous joints. II. Diseases of synovial sheaths, bursæ, etc.: Tenosynovitis—Bursitis—Ganglion. III. Diseases of bone: Osteomyelitis, Periostitis—Tuberculosis: Pott's Disease.

I. DISEASES OF JOINTS: SYNOVITIS AND ARTHRITIS

Synovitis means inflammation of the lining membrane of a joint; if the inflammation spreads to, or begins in, other structures of the joint, the condition is known as *arthritis*. The synovial membrane is a delicate structure, which is easily injured, and it also falls an easy victim to bacteria; hence disease often starts here and may, or may not, spread further.* Certain lesions, however, may begin in the cartilage, as does osteo-arthritis, or in the bone-ends, as does tuberculosis.

Synovitis and arthritis may be divided into two definite varieties, *traumatic* and *bacterial*. Certain forms—osteo-arthritis, gout, and chronic rheumatism—come into neither class, but appear to be due to defective circulation or metabolism. The last two will be dealt with among constitutional diseases.

TRAUMATIC SYNOVITIS OR ARTHRITIS

This condition arises as the result of injuries to joints (dislocations, sprains, fractures into or near joints, blows, and bruises); from continual overstrain; or from the habitual holding of a joint of the lower limb in a position incorrect for weight-bearing. For instance, in cases of genu valgum, or flat-foot, the joints are subjected to undue stress and synovitis or arthritis eventually occur. We may probably also include in the same class certain conditions of varied and uncertain origin, such as 'water on the knee' occurring from no ascertainable cause. All these types of synovitis may be *acute* or *chronic*.

Acute Synovitis

PATHOLOGY.—The changes in the *synovial membrane* are those of acute inflammation. There is a greatly increased exudation of clear serous synovial fluid, and the joint cavity becomes much distended. In severe injuries, blood may escape from torn vessels into the joint. The inflammation may, as mentioned above, spread to other structures and constitute an *arthritis*.

SYMPTOMS.—These, again, are the general symptoms of joint inflammation. *The joint may feel hot*, and the skin is sometimes *reddened* but this is not always so, as the inflammation, if deeply seated, may not extend to the skin.

Swelling is marked, owing to the exudation into the joint. *Fluctuation* may generally be detected by placing the fingers of one hand on one side of the affected joint and by giving gentle digital pressure and relaxation on the other side. The movements of the fluid can then be felt against the fingers of the stationary hand.

---

* The distinction between the two conditions is largely theoretical. Few infections or traumas would involve nothing but the synovial membrane.

Pain is a marked feature, dull and aching in character when the joint is at rest, but increased on movement, whether active or passive.

The patient holds the joint in such a position as to relax the ligaments: This is generally a position midway between two extremes of movement, e.g., semi-flexion at elbow or knee.

Atrophy of the muscles working on the joint occurs very quickly from disuse. In addition to these general symptoms there will probably, in the traumatic variety, be a tender spot at the site of the actual injury. There may be signs of fracture, dislocation, or other derangement of the joint.

Treatment.—The principles are the same for all joints. They are:—

1. To prevent the spread of inflammation by resting the joint until the inflammatory reaction subsides.

2. To relieve pain.

3. To relieve swelling, thereby assisting tissue-fluid absorption and thus preventing adhesions.

4. To prevent disuse atrophy and to regain joint range and function.

We will take the knee as an example, since it is so frequently the seat of synovitis of this type.

SUPPORT.—The limb may be raised and is usually rested on a splint in a semi-flexed position. Sometimes it is supported by pillows and sand-bags, but in severe cases a splint is more comfortable, since it procures complete immobilization, *and in these cases the least movement is intensely painful.*

RELIEF OF INFLAMMATION.—

IN THE EARLY STAGES.—During the first 24 hours or so, *ice-bags or cold applications* give great relief. For the latter, a piece of lint or flannel, or a small towel, should be wrung out in cold water and applied to the part. It should not be covered by a bandage or other dressings, since these would prevent evaporation. It should be replaced as soon as it gets warm.

Evaporating lotions (lead lotion, lead and opium lotion) are sometimes used. They are applied on lint and left uncovered in the same way. The heat, in the case of these lotions and in that of the cold dressing, is carried off by evaporation, the blood-vessels are constricted and the inflammation is reduced. If cold applications or evaporating lotions are to be used, the leg should be fixed by two bandages, one including the foot and leg to just below the knee, and the other loosely applied above the knee.

LATER.—If absorption of the fluid is slow, a *compression bandage* may be put on—that is, the joint is bandaged firmly over several thicknesses of wool. The latter, being elastic, prevents the exertion of too much pressure on the blood-vessels or nerves in the vicinity. Nowadays this method of treatment is often applied from the beginning, cold compresses or evaporating lotions being dispensed with.

PHYSICAL TREATMENT.—

POSITION OF PATIENT.—Half-lying. The leg may be unbandaged for treatment from the beginning, but should be left resting on the splint for a few days, until it can be moved without pain.

FIRST FEW DAYS.—

Heat.—Infra-red radiation, radiant heat, or very mild short-wave diathermy can be given to relieve pain and swelling.

Massage.—Many surgeons do not like massage given in the early stages, since they believe it increases the inflammatory reaction. If it is allowed, effleurage only should be given to begin with. It should begin above the knee and gradually approach the joint. If the synovitis is too acute for the patient to bear even this manipulation, gentle squeezing movements in an upward direction, placing one hand on each side of the limb, can be substituted and effleurage added later.

The effleurage is gradually brought lower and carried over the knee itself, until finally the whole leg is treated, *but a return should constantly be made to the thigh, in order to keep the lymphatic vessels clear in that region.*

As soon as the patient can tolerate them gentle finger-kneadings should be given round the knee, to reduce the swelling around the synovial cavity and prevent the formation of adhesions. Palmar kneadings on either side of the joint can be added a little later.

Meanwhile, any parts of the thigh that can be reached without moving the knee should be massaged fairly vigorously and the lower leg and foot should be included in the treatment in order to maintain the circulation in the limb.

Movements.—These should be given as soon as possible—either by the *relaxed passive method* first, *active contraction* following later, or as *assisted active movements* from the beginning. *In either case they must be painless and keep within the limits of pain.* Voluntary muscle contractions should begin as soon as possible to prevent disuse atrophy.

LATER.—When the inflammation has subsided and pain has gone, more vigorous massage can be given, particularly deep frictions round the knee to reduce the risk of adhesions. If short-wave diathermy is being given the degree of heat can also be increased.

Exercises should now be included, at first without the patient bearing weight on the leg, e.g., Sitting Alternate leg-swinging, and Knee-bending and -stretching with resistance. The patient may practise on the rowing machine and stationary bicycle, if these are available; finally, he is allowed to walk. Once he is allowed to take weight, treatment should include general leg exercises and any lost mobility or power must be restored. Forced passive movements,* strong resisted exercises and mobilizing techniques, will be used as required.

ELECTRICAL TREATMENT.—Faradism under pressure is sometimes given as soon as it can be borne, for the purpose of reducing œdema. The contracting muscles exert pressure on the lymphatics and hasten the flow in these vessels. Faradism and various forms of ionization can be used in the later stages.

SURGICAL TREATMENT.—This consists of treatment of the cause, if necessary; e.g., reduction of the dislocation or fracture; replacement of a slipped cartilage. Such conditions may necessitate modified treatments.

Chronic Synovitis

CAUSES.—Chronic synovitis may be the result of: (1) One or more acute attacks; (2) Repeated injuries or strains; (3) Loose bodies in the joint, or internal derangement of any kind.

PATHOLOGY.—Because of long-standing inflammation the synovial membrane becomes *thickened, vascular, and roughened* by organized fibrinous deposits. It also becomes *fringed*, and portions of these fringes may break off and form loose bodies in the joint. The exudation in the joint may continue indefinitely.

SYMPTOMS.—*Chronic swelling* may persist. The *ligaments become lax and the muscles atrophy*, hence the joint becomes unstable and tends to 'give way'. The *pain is of a dull aching kind.* There may be some *stiffness* in the joint due to disuse atrophy and the formation of adhesions.

Treatment, e.g., of the knee.—

SURGICAL TREATMENT is sometimes required for the removal of loose bodies in the joint, or to remedy other derangements.

SUPPORT.—A supporting bandage is sometimes applied.

* Provided the surgeon agrees and there is no likelihood of flaring up of the synovitis.

PHYSICAL TREATMENT.—Our primary aim will be to strengthen the atrophied muscles and thus restore the stability of the joint. In addition it may be necessary to soften or break down any adhesions and thickenings which have formed. It is also important to improve the circulation and so improve the nutrition of the joint structures.

HEAT.—Any form of heat, including wax baths, can be given to the joint.

MASSAGE.—Kneading and deep frictions should be given to the joint itself.

PASSIVE MOVEMENTS.—These are not often required. If they are, forced movements will be necessary.

ACTIVE EXERCISES.—These are essential, both for the restoration of mobility, and for the purpose of strengthening the muscles. A scheme of home exercises must be given, for example:—

1. Quadriceps contractions.
2. High-sitting Knee-swinging; free, and with self-resistance.
3. Heel-raising and knee-bending (quickly). (In reach-grasp or wing-standing.)
4. Half-yard-grasp-high-standing. Leg-swinging (knee being allowed to swing loosely).
5. Running on the spot, with knee-raising.

ELECTRICAL TREATMENT.—*See* p. 143. In the chronic stage fibrolytic drugs may be used. Ultrasonics and treatments designed to produce an artificial inflammatory reaction can also be used.

BACTERIAL SYNOVITIS OR ARTHRITIS

A large variety of types of joint conditions is included under the above heading. Some arise from the introduction of organisms by way of open wounds, or through direct infection from other local lesions in the vicinity, such as the bursting of a bone abscess into a joint. Others are due to such general conditions as rheumatoid arthritis, or arthritis arising in connexion with gonorrhœa, scarlet fever, enteric fever, or other diseases.

We have therefore to consider types of arthritis due to bacteria of known or unknown origin, and other types apparently due to defects of circulation or metabolism. In this section we shall deal with: (1) Infective arthritis, (2) 'Rheumatoid' arthritis, (3) Still's disease, (4) Osteo-arthritis, (5) Spondylitis ankylopoietica, (6) Tuberculosis of joints.

1. INFECTIVE ARTHRITIS

Under this heading are included arthritis due to gonorrhœa, scarlet fever, enteric fever, or other general diseases; or to infection with various bacteria whether from without, or from a focus elsewhere within the body.

PATHOLOGICAL CHANGES.—These vary in severity from those of a slight synovitis to those of an intense arthritis which destroys the whole joint ; with purulent exudation filling the synovial cavity, caries (wasting or necrosis) of bone, and involvement of all structures round or near the joint.

ACUTE FORM.—The changes are at first similar to those of the acute traumatic variety, but in some cases of virulent infection may be of a much graver nature. The serous exudate may become *serofibrinous* or *fibrinous* (i.e., containing little or much fibrin), *seropurulent* or *purulent* (i.e., containing a high or low degree of pus).

CHRONIC FORM.—This may be the final stage of the acute form, or the infection may be chronic from the beginning. If the chronic form is the final stage of the acute form an intermediary *sub-acute stage* will have occurred. In the sub-acute stage the acute inflammatory reaction is dying down *but there is a grave risk of flare up if the joint is subjected to strain or injury.* In the chronic stage, whether primary or secondary, the fibrin exuded becomes organized, i.e., turned into connective tissue in and around the joint. Blood-vessels grow into this newly formed tissue, bringing increased nutrition to it, and fibroblasts lay down fibrous tissue in it. This leads to *fibrous ankylosis*, that is, *fixation of the joint by fibrous tissue*. If other parts of the joint—bone, cartilage, or ligaments—are involved, the damage is still greater. The bones may become necrosed at the ends and knit together, producing a *true or bony ankylosis*.

SYMPTOMS.—These vary correspondingly in severity. They may resemble those of traumatic arthritis; or they may be those of intense inflammation, with *agonizing pain, muscle spasm,* and *loss of mobility,* ending in complete *ankylosis,* fibrous or bony. *Dislocations* can occur. In severe purulent cases, *constitutional symptoms* arise—rigors, fever, etc. Occasionally, even in mild cases, there is a slight rise of temperature. In some purulent cases the pus may track to the surface forming deep, discharging sinuses.

Principles of Treatment in the Acute and Sub-acute Forms.—The general principles are the same as those already described *but it is essential to control the infection and arrest its spread.* If pus is present drainage must be established, and later healing must be promoted.

SUPPORT.—The limb is kept at rest on a splint; if there is any tendency to deformity, or if the muscles are in spasm, traction is applied as for a tuberculous joint (*see* p. 155).

MEDICAL TREATMENT.—Hot or cold applications or anodynes may be applied to reduce the pain and swelling. Penicillin or other antibiotic injections are generally given, usually into the arm or buttock. If the exudation is only serous a pressure bandage can be applied.

SURGICAL TREATMENT.—The fluid is sometimes drawn off with a syringe. If the exudate is purulent, the joint is opened and the pus evacuated. Rubber tubes are inserted for a time to secure free drainage. If the disease is of such a serious nature that ankylosis is inevitable, the joint is put up in the position in which it will later be most useful to the patient. (*See* p. 155.)

PHYSICAL TREATMENT.—*The sub-acute stage must be reached before this begins.* After the pus has been evacuated, and when the wounds are healing well, careful massage and gentle relaxed, or active assisted, movements can be started.

Massage, if ordered, should be very gentle at first. The area of the joint must be given a wide berth till healing is complete.

No movement should ever be forced at this stage. Only *relaxed* or *assisted active movements* are permissible. They should be increased in range slowly and carefully and *the risk of a flare-up should always be borne in mind.* It will be indicated by a rise in temperature (local or general), swelling, and pain in the joint.

ELECTRICAL TREATMENT.—Local irradiation with ultra-violet light, or zinc ionization may be ordered if there are open wounds.

Treatment of the Chronic Form.—When the wounds are firmly healed and the infective processes are over, the principles of treatment are those of any chronic joint conditions.

Heat (in particular *radiant heat*) and *whirlpool baths*, if obtainable, give good results.

Massage should be vigorous and deep.

Active movements and strong passive stretchings will have to be continued for weeks or months, but should be given with discretion. Any joints which will be put to greater use, and therefore may become strained, must be strengthened to minimize this risk. If contractures have formed a series of splints may be required for day and night use to help stretch the contracted tissues.

In the slighter types of infective arthritis, in which pus has not been formed, the progression in treatment may be more rapid but, even in these cases, caution is imperative. Sometimes, if stiffness in the joint remains after recovery and the stiffness will not yield to passive movement and active exercises, the joint is *manipulated under an anœsthetic*. This is only done when all symptoms of infection have disappeared. The treatment will then be similar to that already described for such cases (p. 133).

2. 'RHEUMATOID' ARTHRITIS
(*Atrophic Arthritis*)

'Rheumatoid' arthritis and osteo-arthritis (considered below) are frequently confused with each other. The so-called '*rheumatoid*' *arthritis* is thought to be a toxic or bacterial condition, or one due to faulty metabolism, although its nature is not fully understood. It generally occurs in young people, though a chronic and less severe form of it appears also in middle age; whereas, broadly speaking, *osteo-arthritis* is a disease of old age, or later middle life, probably due to the strains to which the joints have been subjected in the course of life.

AETIOLOGY.—

SEX.—'Rheumatoid' arthritis, which must not be confused with the diseases generally known as *acute* or *chronic* rheumatism* (*see* Chapter XX), is more common in women than in men.

TYPES.—There seem to be two distinct types: *an acute form*, involving many joints, which usually affects young women between the ages of 15 and 30, though it may occur also in men or in children; and a *chronic form* from which middle-aged women, at or after the menopause, are the most frequent sufferers.

CAUSES.—The *actual cause* is not known; the disease may be bacterial in origin, though there is no evidence that organisms actually invade the joints (Davidson) and no virus or bacteria have yet been found to substantiate the theory. The most modern theory is that it is a manifestation of *auto-immunization*. It has been found that serum from experimental rheumatoid cases contains a protein (called 'rheumatoid factor') which has the characteristics of an antibody. It is therefore postulated that it is the reaction of this 'rheumatoid factor' with an unknown antigen which results in the inflammatory lesions of rheumatoid arthritis. It is also thought that genetic factors may contribute to the condition.†
It may be precipitated, or exacerbated, by emotional disturbances. (*See also* p. 146, on effects of Cortisone.) Both the joints and the body generally are affected.

Predisposing causes appear to be debility, overstrain, worry, or exhausting diseases. The poor are more often affected than the rich, and exposure, damp, or cold may favour the development of the disease. Malnutrition, or deficiency of vitamins in the food, especially of vitamin D, may also contribute to it.

PATHOLOGY.—The disease begins in the *synovial membrane*, which becomes hyperæmic and thickened, bone or cartilage forming in its substance. The *ligaments* are involved next. Fibrous adhesions are formed in them, or within the joint itself. The *cartilage* becomes soft through lack of blood-supply, degenerates, ulcerates, and is ultimately absorbed. Finally the *bone* atrophies and *softens*, the compact tissue being worn away by friction—hence the name 'atrophic arthritis'. Later, the cancellous tissue of the adjoining bone-ends knits together, and a true bony ankylosis occurs.

The *structures round the joint* all become fibrous and thickened. The muscles become markedly atrophied, much more so than in osteo-arthritis, and they often degenerate, forming contractures and deformities.

SYMPTOMS.—The *onset* may be *sudden* or *insidious*. On the other hand, the disease may run a *chronic course* with *intermittent acute attacks*. As in infective

---

* The connexion between the various forms of rheumatic disease is, however, still somewhat confused.

† *See Physiotherapy, Lond.*, March, 1964.

arthritis the condition manifests itself in three stages—acute, sub-acute, and chronic. The *acute polyarticular form* which attacks young people is far the most serious and the patient may, in a very short time, be entirely crippled with stiff and deformed joints. The heart may also be affected.* If the disease does not appear till the patient is middle-aged, it is not of such a virulent character and is much more amenable to treatment. The attacks are intermittent, and generally take place when the patient is run down. In particular the small joints of the hand and feet are subjected to repeated attacks of acute inflammation.

In the acute forms, the patient manifests *general as well as local symptoms*. She is thin, weak, and anæmic, and suffers from loss of appetite, languor, a feeling of cold, and functional nervous symptoms. Pulse and temperature are raised in the early stages, the blood sedimentation-rate is always raised, and blood-pressure is usually low.

LOCAL SYMPTOMS.—*Many joints are attacked, usually symmetrically* on both sides of the body; the smaller joints suffer first, generally the *interphalangeal articulations* of the hands. The deformity of the latter is typical, the enlargement of the joints being *fusiform* (*Fig.* 60). Wrists, elbows, shoulders, ankles,

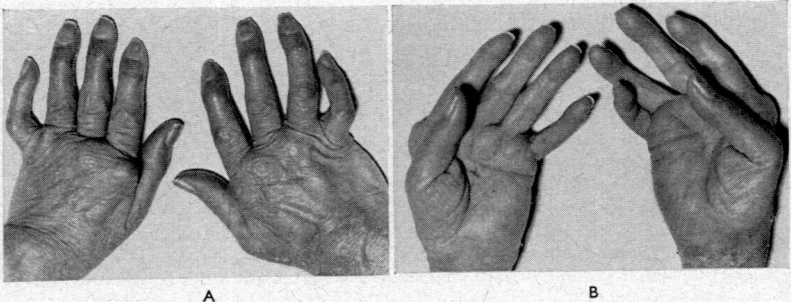

A   B

Fig. 60.—Rheumatoid arthritis of the hands. A, Note fusiform swelling of the joints and lateral deviation of the fingers. The skin is shiny and there are trophic changes in the nails. B, Flexion deformity of metacarpophalangeal joints with considerable wasting of muscles, particularly of the thenar eminence.

and knees may suffer later; the hips are rarely involved. During the acute phase, *the joints* are often hot, and the skin over them may be red. There is neuralgic pain in the joints, often worst while in bed at night. The *muscles* go into spasm, thus fixing the joints, and become very much wasted. *Deformities are marked*, particularly in the hands. As a rule, *the metacarpophalangeal joints are flexed, the first interphalangeal joint hyperextended, and the second interphalangeal joint flexed. The fingers are drawn over to the ulnar side of the hand*, partly by the influence of gravity, and partly by the manner in which a patient whose legs are affected grasps the sticks she uses when walking. Patients confined to bed may have *radial deviation. Trophic changes* are most marked in the skin, which becomes pink and glossy. The sweat-glands do not function normally and there is often a peculiar, characteristic, sour odour from the skin. *Creaking* in the joints is also a feature.

Principles of Treatment.—

GENERAL AND MEDICAL TREATMENT.—There is, as yet, no cure for this disease. Treatment is designed to alleviate the condition. This consists of

---

* *See* Chapter XVIII.

a search for any focus of infection that may be present in the body and its elimination by medical or surgical means. The patient may be treated by appropriate drugs (especially aspirin), vaccines, or gold injections and a diet is prescribed by the doctor. If she is thin and anæmic, as in the acute type described above, the diet is full and nourishing and rich in fats. If she is over-weight, as sometimes happens when the attack occurs in connexion with the menopause, the diet aims at reduction, since extra weight strains the already damaged joints. A sufficient supply of vitamins A and D is also essential. Vitamin A increases the resistance of the epithelial structures to infection, while vitamin D improves the assimilation of calcium, this being important in view of the softening of the bone-ends at the affected joints.* (As regards Cortisone, see p. 146.) Rest is essential at first. Patients with fever or anaemia, and those who are very weak, are kept in bed for varying periods.

Warm clothing should be worn and sufficient, but not excessive, exercise taken. If possible, the patient should live in a warm climate but, unfortunately, this is not often practicable !

PHYSICAL TREATMENT.—

ACUTE AND EARLY SUB-ACUTE STAGES.—The aims of treatment in the early stages are *to prevent contractures and deformity* and *to maintain joint range* as far as possible. *During the period of bed-rest the patient's posture calls for careful attention.* She should be on a firm mattress, with appropriate support during the day—a bed-rest, or carefully arranged pillows to maintain the head, shoulders and spine in correct position—and should lie flat at night, with only one pillow. The feet should be supported in *dorsiflexion*, with a cradle over them. It is a good thing for the patient to lie flat for an hour during the day, with a small pillow under the lumbar spine and, if she can manage it, she may turn into the prone position for a short time with a pillow under the abdomen. *It is most important that she should not develop flexion contractures of the knees. Pillows should never be placed under the knees.* The possibility of hip contractures should not be overlooked. These can easily occur if the hips are allowed to remain constantly flexed, even though the joints themselves may not be affected by the arthritis.

For patients not confined to bed, hydrotherapy is of great value in the treatment. This may be given at suitable spas—Buxton, Bath, etc. Failing this, ordinary local or general baths, hot packs, or the whirlpool bath if obtainable, are useful for relieving pain, stimulating the circulation so that the products of inflammation in the affected parts are carried away, and increasing the action of the skin and kidneys. This promotes the elimination of toxins, whether produced by the action of bacteria, or by some defect of metabolism. *Contrast baths* may be given for hands or feet, and paraffin-wax baths or packs for all joints of the extremities.

Radiant heat, short-wave diathermy, and *ionization* with salicyl, chlorine, or citrate are also of benefit.

Movements.—These are not begun until the B.S.R. (blood sedimentation-rate) is down, i.e., until the sub-acute stage has been reached. *Massage* should not be given because of the danger of flaring up the inflammatory reaction, but at this stage *each joint should be moved passively once a day* to prevent deformity. As the pain and spasm in the limb may be considerable, and because even the slightest activity may cause the condition to flare up, the movements must be given very slowly, only gradual progression being made. A careful watch must be kept for any untoward symptoms, e.g., rise in temperature (local or general), exacerbation of pain, or a rise in B.S.R. Any instructions given by the doctor must be carefully carried out. It must be remembered, however, that all the

---

* C. W. Buckley, *Arthritis, Fibrositis and Gout,* Chapter VI.

patient's joints may not be in the same condition. For instance, those of the hands may be in a state of acute inflammation, while the feet or knees are in the chronic stage, or vice versa. In such a case each must be appropriately treated according to its condition. The patient's general state of health must also be taken into consideration. Breathing exercises should be started as early as possible and general exercises given according to the patient's capacity, *but the rate of progression depends entirely on the B.S.R.*

Hot and painful joints should be comfortably supported in a good position by light splints or plaster.

> N.B.—It should be noted that certain doctors prefer the joints to be kept at *complete rest* in plaster for 7 to 14 days during the stage of acute inflammation. They consider that the symptoms of inflammation subside more quickly if treated in this way, especially in the case of weight-bearing joints, and that the danger of ankylosis has been over-emphasized (*see* p. 146). When the pain and swelling have subsided, the splints may be removed for active movements without weight.

LATER, SUB-ACUTE, AND CHRONIC STAGES.—Our aims are: (1) *To relieve pain, and to prevent extreme atrophy of muscles*; (2) *To maintain the mobility of the joints as far as possible*, but not to attempt to restore lost mobility by violent stretching of the tissues, unless expressly ordered to do so by the doctor; (3) *To strengthen weakened muscles* and those which will be called upon to take extra strain as a result of the disease; (4) *To improve the patient's general condition*, having particular regard to respiration and posture; (5) *To assist in the elimination of toxins* from the system.

The following is an outline of suitable treatments.

Supports.—Splints or plaster may be used to correct deformities, or to support weak joints. Light plasters which improve the position of fingers and hands may be worn at night. During the day these are usually exchanged for shorter splints which allow of more movement of the fingers. Plasters, or a succession of graduated plasters, are often required for the knees, both for correction of flexion deformities and for support when walking. If there is considerable flexion deformity of hips or knees traction may be applied by means of a Thomas splint with weight and pulley, or similar apparatus. Arch supports should be supplied for the feet when necessary and the patient should be advised to wear suitable shoes.

Massage.—General massage can be given to improve the condition of the patient's body as a whole. *Limb massage* should consist of brisk but gentle effleurage and kneading. Careful frictions may be given round the joints to reduce the thickening in the periarticular tissues, *but these manipulations should never be painful, and their effect must be carefully watched*. The treatment must not last too long.

Movements.—Passive (*relaxed*) movements can be administered to the joints to preserve mobility but *forced* movements would only increase pain and inflammation, and should never be used. *Assisted, free, and resisted active movements* are given to strengthen the muscles and increase joint range. The patient must be encouraged to work hard at the exercises, which should be performed many times daily. Where no movement is possible in a joint, *static contractions* of muscles should be taught. *Suspension exercises* in the Guthrie-Smith apparatus are most valuable, a simpler version of which may be arranged in the patient's home. *Pool therapy* is also invaluable. The warmth of the water increases the circulation and aids metabolism, whilst the buoyancy of the water assists movement and allows a greater range of movement. Later, the buoyancy can be made use of to resist movement and thus strengthen the muscles. *Breathing exercises*, diaphragmatic and costal, are necessary to maintain mobility and full expansion of the thorax. Everything possible should be done to encourage and cheer these patients, many of whom really come as much for psychological as for physical help. Any improvement, however slight, should be pointed out, and the physiotherapist must never lose patience, or, worse, let the patient think that she has given up hope, and that no further progress is possible.

Posture.—On getting up a patient may suffer from pain in the neck or back muscles, especially if postural training has not received proper attention in the early stages of the illness. A patient who has been neglected or inadequately treated tends to poke the chin forwards and extend the head at the atlanto-occipital joint. The shoulders are raised by the upper trapezius, and carried forward by the pectoralis major. The thoracic region is rounded, the scapulæ lying wide apart, the sternum is depressed, the ribs are oblique and the costal angle narrowed. The over-strain of the semispinalis capitis and the upper trapezius causes pain in the cervical region, while in the thoracic region the weak and stretched back muscles (longitudinal and transverse) cause pain and fatigue in this area. Because of weakened anti-gravity muscles there is the possibility of a flexion deformity developing in the spine. It is very important to see that when the patient first gets up, and indeed throughout subsequent treatments, the hips and knees are *extended* as much as is possible. Hip extension can be assisted either by gentle pressure over the hip-joint anteriorly, or just below the tuber ischii. The breathing may be shallow and the diaphragm moves minimally. Of course, none of this should have happened if the patient has been correctly treated throughout, but such cases do come to us and we must be prepared to deal with them. Moreover, even in a properly treated case, *what has been gained must be maintained.* The resumption of the erect position will present difficulties, and the physiotherapist must be ready to help the patient with these.

Walking.—A patient in the chronic stage who has lost the power of walking should be helped to regain it, provided that her deformity is not so severe as to render this impossible. She should start in a 'walking machine', then begin to use crutches,* and later sticks. If wearing knee-splints, she will probably find it easier to begin by walking in these. Later on the splints can be removed and the knees firmly bandaged. She should be taught to walk as correctly as is possible in the circumstances and attention should be paid to her posture throughout. *A careful look-out must be kept for crutch paralysis,* which is very likely to develop, since the patient's hands are often partially disabled and she is therefore unable to take much weight on them. With a heavy patient especially, damage to the radial nerve may occur as the result of pressure maintained for not more than a minute or so. No complaint of pain or pressure in the axilla should ever be disregarded.

Ultra-violet Irradiation (third-degree erythema dose with a Kromayer lamp) is sometimes prescribed for an individual joint, generally the knee, both for counter-irritation and to produce a local hyperæmia. The metacarpophalangeal and interphalangeal joints are sometimes treated by cautery.

Other Forms of Electrotherapy.—Various forms of ionization can be given. The following drugs may be made use of: *Histamine* for counter-irritation and local hyperæmic effects; *Choline* is sometimes used to induce vasodilatation and to increase the activity of the sweat-glands, thereby assisting excretion of the toxic products; *Aconitine, cocaine, or novocain* for their analgesic properties; *Iodine and chlorine* for their fibrolytic effects, or *Citrate*, which is particularly useful for treating the hands and feet. According to a modern theory the pattern of exacerbation in these joints is due to *anaphylaxis* (the response of the body tissues to the reaction of an antigen with its antibody). As a result of this reaction, platelets and leucocytes form a *thrombus* (clot) which breaks down

---

* *See* notes on crutch walking (pp. 47–8).

leading to H-substance liberation and an inflammatory reaction in the joint. Citrate prevents the thrombus formation. It is rapidly absorbed by the tissues and a deposit is formed which is slowly absorbed into the system.

Some cases respond well to direct current treatments.

HOME TREATMENT.—Many patients are unable to have constant treatment in hospital or by a private physiotherapist on account of distance, difficulty of transport, or the expense entailed. They should therefore—if intelligent and responsible—be encouraged to carry out simple treatment at home by themselves or with the help of their relatives. Radiant heat, paraffin-wax baths or packs, and contrast baths for hands or feet can all be used *after instruction by the physiotherapist*. The patient should be particularly warned against having either the water or the wax too hot, and the danger of burn or scald should be explained. A simple scheme of suitable exercises should be practised. A simple suspension apparatus can often be arranged, especially for movements of the larger joints, while hand movements can be carried out on a smooth surface or in a bowl of water. The physiotherapist should discover the principal difficulties of home care and daily living which face the patient and his relatives. Much help can be given by treatment designed to overcome these, and by simple adaptations in the home, such as handrails on the stairs and in the lavatory. Gadgets and mechanical aids can be devised to assist in dressing and personal care.★ (*Figs.* 61–63.)

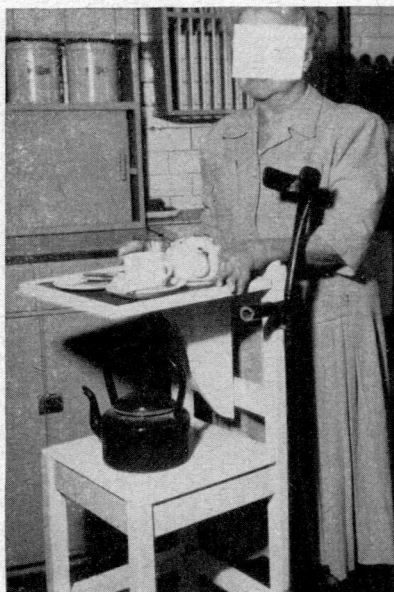 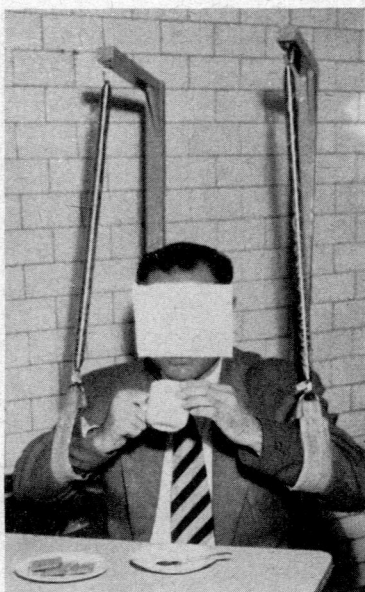

A   B

Fig. 61.—Aids for the use of handicapped patients. A, Table–trolley–chair, here used by patient badly crippled with rheumatoid arthritis. Note gross deformity of hand. B, Slings and springs attached to chair to help patient with stiff shoulders and elbows.

★ *See* articles "Physiotherapy in Medical-Social Rehabilitation" and "Through Activity to Rehabilitation", *Physiotherapy, Lond.*, March, 1960.

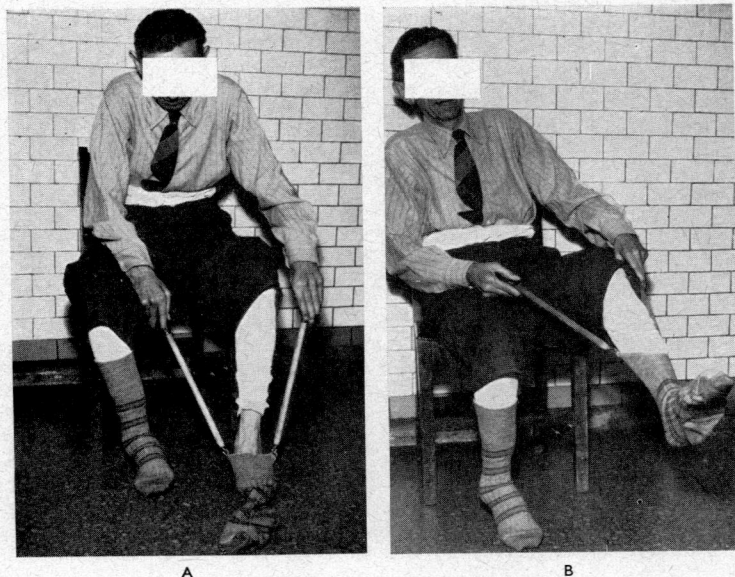

Fig. 62.—A, B, Dressing aids.

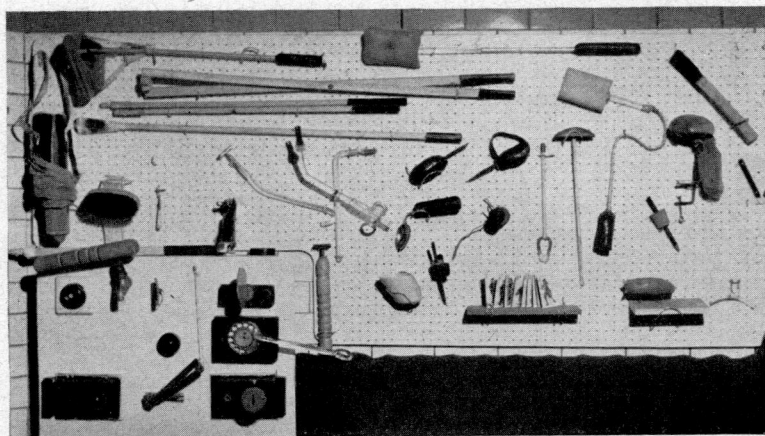

Fig. 63.—Wall board showing tools and household objects adapted for use by handicapped patients. Chief aids lie in length and breadth of handles; straps, hooks, or wires for holding or fitting into or on to hands; and slots and spikes for holding objects.

OCCUPATIONAL THERAPY.—Because of the crippling nature of rheumatoid arthritis and the mental depression which it induces, occupational therapy is invaluable, both for the benefits it gives to muscle and joint control, and for the stimulus it can give the patient. In some cases occupational training may be required, since some patients can no longer pursue their former occupation.

MODERN DEVELOPMENTS IN EARLY PHYSICAL TREATMENT*

During the past few years, experimental work carried out in connexion with the treatment of rheumatoid arthritis has led to the evolution of an entirely new regimen during the *active* stages of the disease. For the first 3 weeks, the patient is on complete bed-rest and splintage, his case being entirely in the hands of the nursing staff. Unpadded plaster-of-Paris splints are used—the arms being supported from axillæ to finger-tips, with the elbows in the position of rest (25° short of full flexion). The legs are supported from the gluteal fold to the toes, with the knees and feet in mid-position. During this period of splintage it is found that local symptoms rapidly abate and there is also a reduction in systemic activity. Also, far from an increase in bony ankylosis, which might be expected, there is actually an increase in joint range following the initial post-immobilization stiffness. At the end of 3 weeks the splints are discarded and the patient is allowed to move freely in bed, though no physiotherapy is given. At the end of the fourth week physical treatment commences and at the end of the fifth week the patient is allowed to sit out of bed for increasing periods, progressing to getting up for toilet purposes, and finally to walking and weight-bearing. The period in hospital lasts from 8–10 weeks and the patient attends the physiotherapy department for the last 2 weeks or so. *No passive movements are ever given*, it being held that this leads to protective muscle spasm and effusion, thus undoing the benefits of complete rest. The only form of movement used are *free* and *resisted* active exercise. In more chronic cases, joints in which there are signs of active flare-up are immobilized and the above routine carried out, whilst quiescent joints are treated along more conventional lines.

SURGICAL TREATMENT.—When the active stage of the disease is past, the surgeon sometimes decides to mobilize the joints by manipulation or by open operation.† This is only done if he is satisfied that (1) the focal sepsis has been eliminated, or (2) the metabolic defect has ceased to exist. On the other hand, he may perform an arthrodesis (*see* p. 151), fixing the joint, or joints, in the most favourable position for use (*see* p. 155), or an arthroplasty (*see* p. 149). Another form of surgical treatment, performed increasingly on wrist, hands, ankles, and feet, is the excision of granulation tissue from the soft tissues. This leads to relief of pain, greatly improved joint function, and appears to reduce the tendency to later involvement of tendons.

CORTISONE AND ACTH THERAPY.—A few years ago, there was no patient with rheumatoid arthritis—or, unfortunately, with any other form of arthritis—who had not heard about cortisone, and who was not eager for information on the subject. This was a pity, as the remedy had not been fully tried out, and a great deal more research was needed before it could—*if* it could —be used for the effective treatment of this kind of disease. A good deal of disappointment was inevitably caused, when the wonderful new substance proved not to be the almost miraculous cure that had been expected.

Cortisone is one of the many secretions of the cortex of the adrenal gland. Its action in rheumatoid arthritis is not easy to understand. It neither kills micro-organisms nor removes irritants, but seems to protect susceptible tissues from inflammation. As a result, the pain and general stiffness are relieved, the joints recover their mobility, and the nodules surrounding them may disappear. The anæmia associated with the disease clears up, the patient sleeps better, recovers an appetite and puts on weight. Moreover, a marked sense of well-being and optimism (euphoria) develops. Unfortunately, the patients almost always relapse when the administration of cortisone is discontinued and some may

---

even become worse than they were before. Cortisone, in fact, does not *cure*; it merely suppresses symptoms. Moreover, in a large number of patients, its continued administration produces very undesirable side-effects—e.g., nervousness, depression, glycosuria, obesity, increased growth of hair, acne, etc. Sometimes even more serious disorders arise.

Cortisone was originally derived from purified ox bile, but the quantity obtained from each animal was so minute that about 40 cattle were needed to provide the daily dose for one patient. The substance is now made synthetically, and may be given in injection, or orally in the form of tablets.

ACTH (adrenocorticotrophic hormone), which is the extract of the anterior pituitary gland, has exactly the same effects as cortisone, because it stimulates the adrenal cortex to produce this substance, but symptoms are relieved more rapidly. It is interesting to note in this connexion that sufferers from rheumatoid arthritis become remarkably free of symptoms during pregnancy, presumably because of the increased activity of the pituitary gland. ACTH is extracted from the glands of pigs and cattle and has not yet been made synthetically. It is given by means of injections. Unfortunately, it has the same undesirable side-effects as cortisone.

Because of these two disadvantages—the patient's relapse when administration of the hormones is discontinued, and the unfortunate side-effects entailed by their use—these substances have proved disappointing as a means of dealing with rheumatoid arthritis, though it is possible that research may reveal some other way of administration, or some combination with other substances which may make it a valuable form of treatment for this and other diseases.

N.B.—It must be recognized that some cases are too advanced for cortisone to bring about even much temporary alleviation. It cannot, for instance, do away with bony ankylosis. Few cases, however, would be incapable of some slight *improvement*. There is no likelihood of cortisone being of any benefit to sufferers from osteo-arthritis or fibrositis, which are aetiologically different diseases, but it has marked effects on rheumatic fever and ankylosing spondylitis.

3. STILL'S DISEASE

This is a form of arthritis occurring in children under eight years of age. It is so similar in its general symptoms to the rheumatoid arthritis of adults that it need not be described in detail here. In addition to the joint changes, the spleen and lymphatic glands are enlarged. The disease probably has a toxic origin. It is not fatal, but the child may be badly crippled and his development arrested.

Treatment.—This is generally given in the chronic stage, and is similar to that for rheumatoid arthritis.

4. OSTEO-ARTHRITIS
(Hypertrophic Arthritis)

AETIOLOGY.—There are two types: (1) A form which attacks one joint, generally a large joint such as the hip or shoulder. This is a disease of old age, and may follow repeated attacks of rheumatism, or other forms of arthritis. It attacks both men and women. The exciting cause is probably an injury. And (2) A form beginning in late middle age in the hands, and spreading to other joints. It probably attacks the hands because these joints have been so much used in the course of life. This type is commoner in women than in men and often begins at the menopause. Both forms are due to some fault of metabolism, and not to bacterial infection. There may be a hereditary defect in the articular cartilage.

PATHOLOGY.—In this type of arthritis, unlike the 'rheumatoid' form, the *cartilage* is first attacked; it becomes hyperæmic and fibrous and is worn away at the points of greatest pressure, allowing the bones to rub together. It lies in irregular masses round the edges of the articular surfaces. The *bone*, owing to the continuous friction, becomes polished and very hard, like ivory. This process is known as 'eburnation'. Moreover, at the articular margins, where the friction does not take place, osteophytes are thrown out and new processes of bone are formed. These interfere with the movements of the joint but *bony ankylosis does not occur.*

The *soft structures round the joint* next become involved, ischæmic degeneration taking place in the ligaments. The action of the muscle tendons inserted in the neighbourhood is hampered, and the muscles atrophy to some extent, though not so markedly as in the 'rheumatoid' form. Later, the *synovial membrane* becomes inflamed, thickened and fringed. Sometimes parts of these fringes break off, forming loose bodies in the joint.

SYMPTOMS.—In the first type the disease comes on gradually, one of the large joints, hip, knee or shoulder being generally the first to suffer, though other joints may be implicated later. The local symptoms are those of a *chronic inflammation*, the skin over the joint neither being red or hot nor very painful when touched. *Swelling* appears, and later the joint may become much enlarged owing to the formation of osteophytes. *Pain and aching* are felt in the affected joint, worse when the limb is kept constantly at rest, or, in the case of the hip,

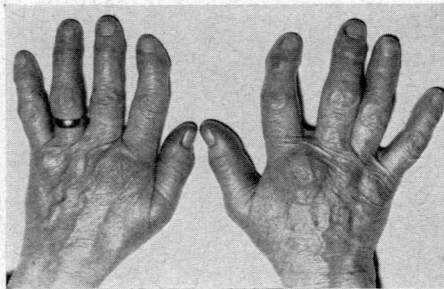

Fig. 64.—Osteo-arthritis of the hands showing deformity and Heberden's nodes on second interphalangeal joints.

when weight is put on the joint. *Stiffness* is present from the early stages and later there is *ankylosis* of the joint—not a true ankylosis, but one caused by the blocking of the movements by the bony outgrowths. *Creaking* in the joint is always present. *The muscles waste*, and *deformity* may develop owing to contractures.

In the polyarticular form, the small joints of the hands are first attacked, beginning with the second interphalangeal joints, which become enlarged (Heberden's nodes) (*Fig.* 64). The other phalanges are implicated later, and the hands become quite stiff and distorted. Later, the disease may spread to other joints. It is not *acutely* painful.

Treatment.—The principles of treatment are similar to those of rheumatoid arthritis, but in these cases there is no acute inflammatory reaction or active infection present. This obviates the need for prolonged bed-rest, and there are no acute or subacute stages. It is sometimes possible to attempt to restore mobility by strong *forced* passive movement. The doctor's advice should, however, be sought before doing so. Pulley exercises are useful and the active exercises can be stronger and more vigorous than in rheumatoid arthritis. *It is extremely* *important to prevent strain in joints which may be indirectly affected, and to strengthen the muscles to meet this contingency.* In both rheumatoid and osteo-arthritis, Kabat techniques can be used with advantage. Deep massage can be given and any accompanying fibrositis should be treated.

Heat and Electrical Treatment.—Dr. C. W. Buckley, in discussing the treatment of osteo-arthritis, writes: "Heat is of great service in improving the circulation in and around the joints. . . . For deep-seated joints like the hip or spine, diathermy or short-wave treatment will probably give the best results, but presents no advantage in the more superficial joints, where the ordinary form of radiant heat is as useful as any. Paraffin-wax baths are also very useful. . . ."*

The doctor will treat the case with analgesics, and sometimes injections into the painful joint are given. Deep X-ray therapy is sometimes advantageous.

SUPPORT.—The joints of the lower extremity, especially the hip-joint, may need support, or some form of apparatus to relieve the strain upon them (bandages, calipers, plasters, etc.). The patient may be obliged to give up some of his accustomed activities, if too strenuous, and periods of rest for the joint may be advisable during the day. Obese patients should take measures to reduce their weight, especially if the hips or knees are affected, as excess weight throws further strain on the joints. Arthritis of the cervical spine may be supported by a collar, or treated by traction followed by a collar support.†

SURGICAL TREATMENT.—When the quiescent stage of the disease is reached, these cases are sometimes treated by manipulation or by open operations.

MANIPULATION is undertaken to stretch the shortened ligaments, and to break down adhesions.

Post-operative Treatment.—The joint is treated in much the same way as any stiff joint after manipulation. In the case of joints of the lower extremity, the exercises are first given in lying or sitting.

OPEN OPERATIONS.—Occasionally the joint is opened and osteophytes and loose bodies are removed, or a synovectomy performed but the most usual operations performed today are *arthroplasty* and *arthrodesis*.

Arthroplasty is designed to produce a new joint (particularly in the case of the hip, which will be taken as our example). Several types of operation are in use today:—

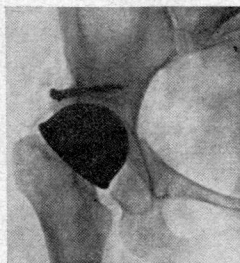

Fig. 65.—X-ray showing vitallium cup arthroplasty. (*Reproduced by kind permission from 'Essentials of Orthopaedics' by P. Wiles.*)

1. *Robert-Jones* in which the head of the femur is excised and the acetabulum trimmed.

2. *Smith Petersen* in which a vitallium cup is fitted over the head of the femur. It is free to move both on the head and in the acetabulum. (*Fig. 65.*)

3. *Judet's* in which the femoral head is replaced by a plastic prosthesis (*Fig. 66 A*).

4. *Austin-Moor* in which both the head and neck of the femur are replaced by a metal prosthesis (*Fig. 66 B*).

---

* C. W. Buckley, *Arthritis, Fibrositis and Gout,* Chapter XI. For a somewhat unusual view concerning the order in which massage and infra-red treatment should be given, *see* W. Beaumont, *Infra-red Radiation,* Chapter IV.

† *See* article by John G. Kuhns on "Osteo-arthritis of the Cervical Spine", *Brit. J. phys. Med.,* 1957, **20**, No. 6.

5. *The Fluon Arthroplasty* in which a small stainless-steel replacement of the femoral head and neck is fitted into a fluon plastic socket, this representing a completely new prosthetic hip-joint.

Post-operative Treatment after any operation designed to secure a *movable joint* is on the same lines as that following manipulations, the interval which must elapse between the operation and the beginning of active exercise depending on

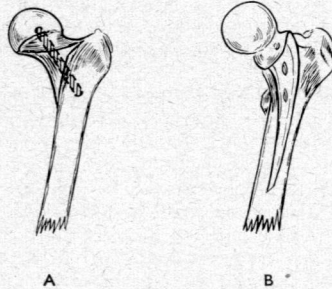

A   B

Fig. 66.—A, Judet's arthroplasty. The head of the femur is replaced by a plastic pros-thesis. B, Austin-Moor replacement. Both the head and neck of the femur are replaced by a metal prosthesis.

the nature of the operation, and on which joint is involved. After cup arthro-plasty of the hip (Smith-Petersen), the limb is put up on traction or on a splint resembling one of the Hodgen type (*see* p. 33). Foot and toe movements and quadriceps and gluteal contractions begin at once. In 3–4 days hip and knee movements can be given. Suspension exercises start in 3–4 weeks and resistance is added in 4–6 weeks. The patient then begins to take weight, progressing from crutches to sticks and finally to walking unaided. After Austin-Moor replace-ment the limb is either placed in abduction on traction on a Balkan frame, or in abduction in an anti-rotation plaster extending below the knee.* Treatment is lengthy and final results are often disappointing, with a return of pain and disability.†

Following fluon arthroplasty the patient wears a crêpe hip spica and a mattress is placed between the legs to maintain *abduction*. Active foot movements begin the same day and specific leg exercises (gluteal and quadriceps contractions and hip and knee flexion) on the 2nd day. Abduction and straight-leg-raising start in 2 weeks, and in 3 weeks the patient is allowed up, finally weight-bearing, using elbow crutches. The patient is normally discharged in 5 weeks and requires no further physiotherapy.

But whether treatment is long or short and progress slow or rapid, the basic aims remain the same. Namely *to increase strength and stability; to maintain or increase range and mobility* ; and *to achieve maximum independence*. As in cases of amputation the patient must not only be re-educated in walking, but must be able to change from standing to sitting, climb stairs and slopes, get on and off buses, etc., before he can again take his place as an independent member of society.

---

* Treatment following Austin-Moor replacement is based on that following cup arthroplasty, but hip and knee movements are delayed until the 7th day. Partial weight-bearing is allowed in 4 weeks and the patient is usually discharged at the end of the 7th week.

† N.B.—Short-wave diathermy must never be given to an area in which a metal prosthesis has been inserted.

Arthrodesis is designed to fix the joint, and, thereafter, no movement is allowed in it. Treatment is directed towards strengthening the unaffected muscles and joints, particularly the postural and weight-bearing ones, to compensate for the 'loss' of the arthrodesed joint; and to re-education in walking and daily living.

5. SPONDYLITIS ANKYLOPOIETICA
(*Spondylose Rhizomélique; Ankylosing Spondylitis*)

The condition known as spondylitis may be divided into two forms: (1) Spondylitis osteo-arthritis, which, as the name implies, is simply osteo-arthritis of the spine; and (2) Spondylitis ankylopoietica, which, once thought to be merely rheumatoid arthritis of the vertebral column, is now considered to be a separate entity.

Spondylitis ankylopoietica is characterized, as the name implies, by its tendency to ankylosis of the joints of the vertebral column and those adjoining them.

AETIOLOGY.—

AGE.—The disease is commonest between the ages of twenty and thirty years, although the onset may be earlier, i.e., from the late teens to twenty-five years of age.

SEX.—Unlike rheumatoid arthritis, it is much commoner in men than in women.

CAUSES.—The exact nature of this disease is not understood. No specific organism has ever been found and the cause is unknown.

Predisposing causes may be injury or strain or former attacks of rheumatism, and in some cases gonorrhœa.

TYPES.—Two types are recognized:—

1. THE MARIE-STRÜMPELL TYPE.—Beginning in the lumbar region, it spreads upwards. It involves the sacro-iliac, hip, and shoulder-joints, and sometimes some of the smaller articulations as well. The muscles are more wasted than in the other type and there may or may not be neurological symptoms. This is the more common form.

2. THE BECHTEREW TYPE.—Beginning in the cervical region it spreads downwards, but the joints of the extremities are never involved. The disease begins in the meninges of the spinal cord and sets up an irritation of the nerve-roots.

PATHOLOGY.—Two principal changes take place.

OSTEOPOROSIS.—This is a softening and rarefying of bone. The bodies of the vertebræ, and generally the sacrum and ilia, are affected.

OSSIFICATION.—This affects the articular processes with their capsules, the interspinous ligaments, the ligamenta subflava, the anterior common ligament, especially in the cervical region, and the outer part of the intervertebral disks. The bodies become constricted in the middle and broad at the margins, producing what has been called the 'bamboo-like' appearance (*Fig.* 67). The result of this ossification is that *the spine becomes entirely rigid in the affected area.* There is pain on pressure over the ossified joints.

SIGNS AND SYMPTOMS.—

LUMBAR REGION.—There is *pain* in the back, and often in one or both sciatic nerves. Because of rigidity and the fact that the patient lies down as much as possible, the lumbar spine is generally *flattened*.

THORACIC REGION.—*Kyphosis* appears early because of rigidity, but is never very marked; the *ribs* become joined to the vertebræ by ossification of the costo-vertebral joints, hence breathing becomes entirely abdominal. The patient is particularly prone to respiratory infection or disease because of the rigidity of the thorax. There is often *pain* along the course of the intercostal nerves.

LOWER CERVICAL REGION.—Here a *very marked kyphosis* may be present, because the weight of the head compresses the vertebral bodies and bends the spine forward; the head itself is hyper-extended to restore the line of vision. If the atlanto-axial joint escapes, as it commonly does, the patient is able to rotate his head.

OTHER JOINTS.—First the *sacro-iliac* and then the *hip-joints* may become fixed, if the disease begins in the lumbar spine. The knees and shoulders are rarely affected.

The blood sedimentation-rate is often raised.

The cases vary a good deal in severity. The position of ankylosis depends on the patient's habitual position—e.g., the hips may be flexed or extended, and

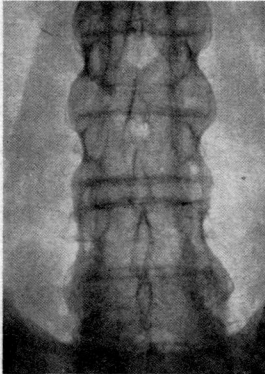

Fig. 67.—Ankylosing spondylitis with extensive ossification of the lateral longitudinal ligaments ('bamboo spine'). (*Reproduced by kind permission from 'Essentials of Orthopaedics' by P. Wiles.*)

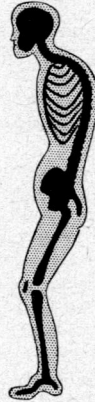

Fig. 68.—To show 'question mark' deformity in spondylitis ankylopoietica. There is also a flexion deformity at the hip and slight compensatory flexion at the knee.

the curves of the spine may vary slightly. On the whole, the spine assumes the shape of a question mark. The knees tend to fall into slight flexion to compensate for the position of the pelvis and hips (*Fig.* 68).

COURSE OF DISEASE.—The onset may be sudden or insidious, the progress rapid or slow. It may be arrested at an early stage, or continue till every joint from the head to the knees is ankylosed, in which case flexion deformities are severe.

The initial symptoms are often not severe, and there may be remissions in the early stages of the disease.

Treatment.—Dr. Buckley, in an article on this disease, says: "It would seem as though bony ankylosis occurred only where immobilization was secured by any means, and that treatment should be directed to preventing this." He also remarks: "It would seem a reasonable hypothesis that the softening of the vertebral bodies and the consequent danger to the vital structures in the spinal canal lead to rapid ossification of the ligaments to neutralize this risk." Our *aims* will therefore be *to preserve mobility in the joints, to strengthen weak muscles,* and *to stretch tight ones.* Special attention must be paid to the thorax; and both abdominal and, as far as possible, costal breathing must be encouraged. *No attempt should ever be made to forcibly mobilize joints which have already ankylosed.*

SUPPORTS.—In many cases, the patient needs some type of spinal support during the day; in others he is fitted with a plaster case in which he lies at night.

In some cases both may be necessary. The patient should get used to the night support gradually, and need not be expected to spend the whole night in it at first. Sedatives are often given until he does become accustomed to it, otherwise his general health may suffer from loss of sleep.

MASSAGE.—This may be given to the back and to the limbs, if required for the relief of pain, and should be sedative in nature.

EXERCISES.—These form the major part of treatment and the most important of all are *breathing exercises*, especially costal breathing. They should be given first in lying or half-lying with the patient on a plinth. One cannot give hard and fast rules for starting positions. They should be chosen with regard to the comfort of the patient, while still allowing as much freedom of movement as possible. If kyphosis is extreme, and the neck bent forward, the head should be supported by one or more cushions. Such exercises as the following should be given:—

1. Crook-lying Costal breathing, hands on sides of chest. The patient should be encouraged to grasp the ribs at the costal margin with both hands, pulling them outward on inspiration, on expiration he puts his hands on his lower ribs and exerts pressure on them. This will assist thoracic mobility and ventilation.

2. Crook-lying diaphragmatic breathing.

Other breathing exercises should be added, being chosen to get as full a range of movement as possible in all parts of the thorax. Later, the exercises may be done in sitting.

Arm Exercises.—Free and resisted exercises suited to the patient's condition should be chosen and respiratory exercises incorporated with some of them.

Leg Exercises.—Most *unilateral* exercises can be given: e.g., the patient, in lying, may bend up one knee over the chest, straighten the knee, and lower the leg slowly; or in the case of a weaker patient, bend up each knee in turn and lower it. *Most bilateral exercises are too strong, and, moreover, impede respiration.* Later, such exercises as Half-yard-grasp-standing, Leg-swinging forward and backward, or Reach-grasp-standing, Alternate knee-upbending, etc., may be added. Exercises for the *glutei* and *adductors and abductors of the hip* will be required.

General Exercises.—General spinal mobility exercises should be given whenever practicable. Back extension exercises are important in counteracting the tendency to flexion deformity. Abdominal exercises should also be practised. Some surgeons or physicians do not allow trunk flexion, but others allow it for general mobility purposes.

Head Exercises.—All head movements should be practised.

Suspension Exercises are most important in this condition, particular use being made of *total suspension*. The patient lies on his back, the head, trunk, arms, and legs being well supported in slings. Spring resistance is given to the head, arms, and legs. To begin with the patient moves head and limbs individually. Eventually, all are moved together and breathing is combined with the exercises.

The treatment, in fact, is not unlike that for Pott's disease (*see* pp. 166–7) but, as a greater extent of the spine is likely to be implicated, fewer exercises are suitable.

HEAT AND RADIOTHERAPY.—*Radiant heat or infra-red radiation* may relieve pain or aching in the joints. *Deep X-ray treatment* is given for the same reason and is very effective, especially in early cases and is regarded as the treatment of choice. It may, however, have very marked side-effects, headache, nausea, and depression.

SURGICAL TREATMENT.—In cases with marked deformity, spinal osteotomy may improve the patient's posture. If the hips are badly affected, arthroplasty (*see* p. 149) may be performed.

As regards cortisone treatment, *see* p. 146.

It is advisable to take a tracing of the patient's spine from time to time, and also to take and record the chest measurements on expiration and inspiration, not only as a guide to progress but also as an incentive to the patient.

6. TUBERCULOUS JOINTS

Patients with tuberculous joints are only referred for physical treatment when the infective process has subsided. Too much time need not be spent, therefore, in considering the symptoms, etc., in detail. Phthisis is dealt with in the chapter on lung disease. Children, adolescents, and old people are most often attacked, children and adolescents being particularly vulnerable. The poor are more often affected than the rich.

CAUSES.—

PREDISPOSING.—General weakness and debility; unhygienic surroundings and in some cases, heredity.

EXCITING.—Injury to a joint, which is then invaded by the tubercle bacillus.

PATHOLOGY.—The first structures affected are either the bone-ends, or the synovial membrane, which becomes thickened, soft, and spongy. Tuberculous foci form in it and some of them become *caseated* (*see* TUBERCULOSIS, Chapter XVII), and break into the joint. Sometimes there is pus formation. Caries occurs in the bones close to the cartilage, which at a later stage becomes eroded; the ligaments may ultimately be destroyed.

RESULTS.—The disease may terminate in *recovery, fibrous ankylosis, bony ankylosis,* or *dislocation.*

RECOVERY.—This may take place in slight cases, where no structure other than bone is attacked, or if the infection of the synovial membrane is checked at a very early stage.

FIBROUS ANKYLOSIS.—The synovial membrane and cartilage are replaced by fibrous tissue. The bacilli, if still living, are shut in and encapsulated by adhesions. Since these are living bacilli in the joint there is always a danger of recurrence of the activity.

BONY ANKYLOSIS.—The cartilage being destroyed, the bone-ends knit, forming a true ankylosis. In some cases the fibrous tissue surrounding the joint may become ossified.

DISLOCATION.—This is due partly to destruction of the ligaments and partly to neglect. The parts then become fixed in the incorrect position by fibrous tissue.

SYMPTOMS.—Generally *only one joint* is involved, but this is not invariably so, the *order of frequency* being the spine, the hip, the knee and ankle, and the elbow. Finger-joints may also be affected but this is less common.

In the early stages the well-known '*tumour albus*' or 'white swelling' is found —the skin over the joint being white and the swelling hard; *active or passive movement is painful,* and *the muscles waste rapidly.* These symptoms are due to disease of the synovial membrane. If the bone-ends are affected, any movement which tends to rub the joint surfaces together, or jar them, is intensely painful. Later, *pain increases* (ligaments and cartilages being involved) and *all voluntary movement ceases.* The muscles go into spasm, and ultimately produce *fixed deformity.*

Finally, to the above symptoms may be added *shortening of the limb, dislocation of the joint,* and *suppuration.*

Principles of Treatment.—Since there is an active infective inflammatory reaction the principles of treatment are similar to those of infective arthritis. *It is essential to control the infection or,* if this is not possible, *to render it comparatively harmless through encapsulation.*

REST AND PREVENTION OF DEFORMITY.—The patient remains in bed for a time, the affected part being immobilized during the period of inflammation, and for some time after the infective process is apparently quiescent. The limb is put up in the best possible position, muscle spasm being overcome by traction in some cases. If the joint is bound to become ankylosed, it is maintained in the most favourable position. The ankle is fixed in dorsiflexion to a right angle; the knee in extension; the hip in abduction to 20° or 30°; the wrist in dorsiflexion; the elbow in flexion at or near a right angle, so that the hand can be carried to the mouth (if both elbows are affected, one is rather more flexed than the other); the shoulder in abduction to 45°, and in inward rotation.

MEDICAL TREATMENT.—Local applications, injections, or counter-irritation are used for the joint condition. The patient often receives vaccine treatment.

SURGICAL TREATMENT.—This may consist of:—

1. OPENING OF ABSCESSES, when necessary.

2. EXCISION OF THE JOINT.—Only undertaken nowadays when general treatment has been of no avail, or if it is considered practicable, to remedy fixation or deformity.

3. AMPUTATION.—Only performed when all else (including excision) has failed and if the affected limb will otherwise be useless, or if the patient's general health is seriously threatened by the continued presence of the infected joint.

PHYSICAL TREATMENT.—As has been said this is only required when the disease is quiescent, and many patients are never referred for treatment. If it is required, *aims* of treatment are *to improve the patient's general health; to regain joint mobility and strength where possible or to maintain the existing range; to strengthen other joints to share the work of the affected joint.*

LIGHT TREATMENT.—The patient may be given general treatment, preferably with a carbon arc lamp, but *general irradiation must never be given if there is any suspicion of phthisis.* Appropriate local treatment may also be given to the affected joint.

ACTIVE MOVEMENTS can be given to the joint affected, *but no attempt should ever be made to mobilize it, or to break down adhesions, lest bacilli encapsulated by fibrous tissue be set free and the disease flare up again.* If the surgeon believes the lesion to be entirely healed, decides to mobilize the joint and wishes such movements to be given, he will issue orders to that effect. *Unless he does so, neither 'forced' movements given by the physiotherapist, nor active movements in which the weight of the patient's body or limb is used to produce a similar effect of mobilization, are permissible.*

The other joints of the limb must be kept mobile and their muscle power increased by passive (relaxed) movements and careful resisted exercises.

II. DISEASES OF SYNOVIAL SHEATHS, BURSÆ, ETC.

TENOSYNOVITIS

Inflammation in the synovial sheath of a muscle generally occurs at the wrist or ankle. Like synovitis of a joint, the condition may be traumatic or bacterial.

1. Traumatic Tenosynovitis and Tenovaginitis
(*Acute non-suppurative tenosynovitis*)

CAUSES.—(1) Overwork of a muscle. (2) Stretching or wrenching of the tendon; e.g., in sprained or dislocated ankle or wrist; or a blow on the tendon itself. (3) Spread of inflammation from surrounding tissues—skin, fascia, muscles, etc. (4) There is sometimes no ascertainable cause.

PATHOLOGICAL CHANGES.—The changes are those typical of inflammation. The fluid exuded by the membrane is *serous* or *serofibrinous*. When the inflammation subsides and the exudate is absorbed, the surfaces of both tendon and sheath remain rough, so that the movement of these surfaces on each other causes pain. In *tenovaginitis* the primary lesion is in the sheath itself.

SYMPTOMS.—There is *swelling in the line of the affected sheath or sheaths*, with *tenderness* and *pain* on movement. *Crepitus* can usually be detected, due to the friction between the roughened walls of the sheath and the tendon. This is absent in tenovaginitis.

TREATMENT

Tenosynovitis.—There are two methods of treating this lesion—by *operation* or by *massage*. The principle of treatment is the same wherever the trouble is situated, namely to smooth out the roughened surfaces, or to free the tissues from adhesions.

SURGICAL TREATMENT.—

OPERATION.—This consists of splitting the tendon sheath: it effects an immediate cure, since it abolishes friction between the tendon and its sheath. Active movements are begun the next day.

PHYSICAL TREATMENT.—

REST AND SUPPORT.—The limb may be splinted or strapped to prevent movement and thereby relieve the pain. In some cases rest, alone, leads to recovery in about 3 weeks, but since the pathological changes have not been affected relapses are frequent.

MASSAGE.—This consists of *deep transverse frictions across the affected tendon*. In this way, the sheath is moved repeatedly across the tendon, and the roughness, which causes pain on movement, is smoothed. *The tendon should be fully stretched during the massage in order to treat it to the fullest extent*. This method avoids the inconvenience of wearing a splint, as well as the disadvantage of a scar after operation, which may be noticeable at the wrist or in the hand. In chronic untreated cases, a longer course of treatment will be required before a cure is effected. While under treatment, the patient should not use the limb more than he can help. When the condition is cured, active exercises may be needed to strengthen the limb. In the case of the foot it may be necessary to correct a faulty gait which has arisen owing to pain.

Short-wave diathermy is sometimes given in the early acute stage, to relieve pain.

In *tenosynovitis of the Achilles tendon*, the foot may be strapped in plantar flexion and the heel of the shoe raised. Alternatively, and more usually nowadays, the condition is treated by deep frictions.

Tenovaginitis.—The treatment is similar to that for tenosynovitis—operation, or deep massage. Rest alone is of little use. In tenosynovitis *diagnosis of the exact position of the lesion is essential*, and should be conveyed to the physiotherapist by the doctor.

Tenovaginitis of the Extensors of the Thumb (Stenosing Tenosynovitis: Hoffman's Disease).—This consists of a fusiform thickening of the common sheath of the abductor longus pollicis and the extensor brevis pollicis, over the outer side of the lower extremity of the radius. It is 1½ to 3 inches in length.

AETIOLOGY.—The cause is unknown. It is more common in women than in men. It may be caused by trauma, but in many cases there is no history of injury.

SYMPTOMS.—There is *pain at the outer side of the wrist*, radiating down to the thumb and up the forearm. As a rule, it comes on gradually, and may increase until it causes great disability. There may be a visible *swelling* on the outer side of the wrist, *tenderness on pressure, and pain* on resisted, or even on active, extension and abduction of the thumb. There is no crepitus.

The condition is treated by *operation* (*see above*, p. 156) or failing that by *massage*. Immobilization is almost useless. As in tenosynovitis, *massage* consists of deep frictions across the tendon and is given if operation is not immediately possible, or the patient refuses it. Dr. Cyriax* says the massage treatment must be continued for 3 months, but hardly ever fails. He points out, however, that the tendons may be involved at more than one place—at the level of the carpus, at the insertion of abductor longus pollicis to the base of the first metacarpal, or where the tendons in their common sheath lie in the groove at the lower extremity of the radius, *and that it is essential to know at which of these points the trouble exists.* He recommends half an hour's friction twice weekly.† This treatment is very painful, but will fail to cure unless given deeply. Exercises are not given after treatment and the patient must not use the hand unnecessarily.

2. Bacterial (Suppurative) Tenosynovitis

CAUSES.—The causes of this type of tenosynovitis are injuries which break the skin and allow bacteria to gain access to the tissues. If the initial sepsis is in the thumb or little finger the infection may spread up the synovial sheaths of the flexor tendons from fingers to wrist. The flexor longus pollicis tendon has one continuous sheath from two inches above the wrist to its insertion, while the flexor sheath of the little finger is continuous with the common synovial sheath of the flexores profundus and sublimis digitorum. This does not occur in the three middle fingers, which have distal sheaths unconnected with the common sheath.

PATHOLOGICAL CHANGES.—The changes are those of typical bacterial inflammation, with pus formation. The pus may break through the sheath, spreading infection in the surrounding tissues, or the tendon itself may be attacked and destroyed.

The late results are *dense adhesions, extensive scarring*, and *limitation of movements* in the neighbouring joint or joints.

SYMPTOMS.—In the early stages these are typical of bacterial inflammation. The toxins formed locally enter the blood-stream and produce *general symptoms*, the patient's temperature rising to a variable extent.

After the infection is overcome, there may be *scarring, contractures*, or *deformity* of the limb. If the process was confined to the tendon-sheaths there is simply *loss or limitation of mobility* in the joints.

Treatment.—

EARLY ACUTE STAGES.—As long as the infective process is active, medical and surgical treatment are required. Incisions are made to liberate the pus, and drainage is maintained by means of rubber tubes or of gauze packing. Appropriate dressings or baths are used. The part is rested on a splint.

ELECTRICAL TREATMENT.—This will follow the lines of treatment described for infected wounds. Very mild doses of short-wave diathermy can be given twice daily for short periods of time, to assist drainage and promote repair. Sectional ultra-violet irradiation of the body can also be given to raise the general resistance. Penicillin irrigations are also used, and antibiotic dressings applied. *Movements must not be given in the very early stages.*

LATER SUB-ACUTE AND CHRONIC STAGES.—

SUB-ACUTE STAGE.—When the wounds are *clean and almost closed*, treatment is required to stimulate healing. Electrotherapy should be continued. Short-wave diathermy is increased in intensity; local ultra-violet irradiation of second

---

* *Text-book of Orthopædic Medicine*, Vol. I.
† *Ibid.*, Vol. II.

MASSAGE AND REMEDIAL EXERCISES

158   MASSAGE AND REMEDIAL EXERCISES
or fourth degrees intensity can be given, depending on the state of the tissues, or zinc ionization may be used instead of irradiation. Sectional ultra-violet irradiation should be replaced by general irradiation. Very gentle movements can now begin. Massage is often not allowed until the wounds have healed firmly.

CHRONIC STAGE.—When the wounds are *firmly healed and the inflammation has completely died down*, more vigorous treatment can be applied. This is similar to the late treatment for infective arthritis, but it should be remembered that the adhesions and contractures are in the tendon-sheaths and in the soft tissues over them, *not* in the joint itself, unless the infection has spread. The joint may, however, be stiff from 'passive inflammation'—stagnation of blood in the part— or from long immobilization. There may also be stiffness in joints higher up the limb, especially if the case has received no physical treatment before this period. *Deep effleurage, finger kneadings*, and *strong frictions* should be given to loosen adhesions and adherent scars; *passive* (forced) *movements* are required to mobilize joints and stretch adhesions, and *active* and *resisted exercises* are necessary to restore the strength of the limb. Olive oil is sometimes used to soften the superficial tissues.

Radiant heat, ionization, short-wave therapy, and *whirlpool baths* are often useful.

Much the same treatment is required for the *after-results of an acute cellulitis* or other septic conditions of the soft tissues. Great patience and perseverance are required on the part of both patient and physiotherapist. The progress is very slow and the result often disappointing, though in some cases a very marked improvement takes place, and an almost crippled hand or foot again becomes useful. If a nerve is involved, the outlook is, of course, much less hopeful.

BURSITIS

Inflammation of a bursa, generally of a superficial one.

ANATOMY.—Bursæ are small membranous sacs, lined with endothelial cells, which may or may not be in communication with joints. *Their purpose is to prevent friction between any two structures* (i.e., tendon and tendon, or tendon and bone), or to protect prominent bony points—the patella or olecranon process, for example. A *true bursa* is one normally present at some particular point; a *false bursa* is one which is not normally present, but which has formed over some bony point that has become unduly prominent through disease. Such is the bursa found over the metatarsophalangeal joint in hallux valgus (*see* Chapter XV).

Examples of inflammation of a true bursa are prepatellar bursitis, subdeltoid bursitis, 'miner's elbow' (inflammation of the olecranon bursa), and achillodynia (inflammation of one of the bursæ situated round the tendo Achillis).

Bursitis may be acute, subacute, or chronic.

CAUSES.—(1) *Trauma*. A severe injury causes acute bursitis, repeated lesser injuries cause the subacute or chronic variety. (2) *Rheumatism, gout*, or other metabolic diseases or infections.

PATHOLOGICAL CHANGES.—These are similar to those of synovitis.

SYMPTOMS.—In the acute form there is *pain, stiffness* of the joint near which the bursa is situated, with *swelling and fluctuation limited to the bursa itself*. This is most noticeable when it is a superficial one. The pain, also, is limited to the bursa, and increased in those positions of the joint which cause pressure to be exerted on it. There is no pain in the joint itself.

We shall here consider two typical examples of bursitis—the prepatellar and subdeltoid varieties.

Prepatellar Bursitis
('*Housemaid's Knee*')

'Housemaid's knee' may be a true prepatellar bursitis—that is, an inflammation of the bursa situated over the patella and beneath the skin; or it may be an affection of the bursa placed between the ligamentum patellæ and the upper part of the tubercle of the tibia.

CAUSES.—(1) A blow, or fall, on the knee. (2) Much kneeling. The frequency of its incidence in housemaids, charwomen, etc., gave this condition its name.

SYMPTOMS.—(1) *Pain* in the region of the bursa. (2) *Swelling*. If the prepatellar bursa itself is the seat of the trouble, the swelling is a large rounded one over the knee-cap; if that under the ligament is the one affected, the swelling is seen on either side of that structure. (3) *Stiffness* of the knee, but *no pain in the joint itself*.

In the chronic form there is little pain, though the swelling may be marked.

Treatment.—If causing little inconvenience, the bursa is sometimes left alone, only a bandage or pressure bandage being applied. Otherwise operative treatment is the rule.

SURGICAL TREATMENT.—This consists of removal of the bursa. It is carried out through a lateral incision, in order to avoid a tender scar at the front of the knee, which would be pressed upon in kneeling.

PHYSICAL TREATMENT.—

POST-OPERATIVE.—*Radiant heat*, or some other form of heat, can be used if there is pain.

WHEN THE WOUND IS HEALED.—*Massage* is given to all the muscles of the thigh with *frictions* to the knee-joint and round the patella. *Lateral movement of the patella should be given to regain its mobility. Active and resisted exercises* are required for the knee, gradually increasing in range. Quadriceps contractions must begin at an early stage.

> *Redness* and *heat* in the region of the bursa indicate a *septic* or *infective bursitis*. This can be treated by penicillin but if the infection recurs, the bursa is excised. Post-operative treatment is as above, but the surgeon will decide when it may begin.

Subdeltoid Bursitis

The subdeltoid bursa is a large sac situated, as its name implies, between the deltoid and the capsule of the shoulder. It does not communicate with the joint.

CAUSES.—(1) Trauma—a fall or blow on the shoulder; or injury to the muscles in that region. It may complicate a fracture of the great tuberosity. (2) Rheumatism or infection.

The name 'subdeltoid bursitis' probably covers a variety of conditions which give rise to similar symptoms. According to different authorities, these symptoms may be due to: (*a*) a tearing of the periosteum at the insertion of the tendon of the supraspinatus, or an injury to the tendon itself; (*b*) calcareous nodules in this tendon; (*c*) a tearing away of the subscapularis from the capsule of the shoulder (*see* p. 77); or (*d*) inflammation of the subdeltoid bursa, sometimes with calcification (a deposit of lime salts) in the bursa itself.

SYMPTOMS (Acute Bursitis).*—(1) These are similar to those of an acute synovitis, but are *localized*, there being one particular painful spot. (2) The pain is worst *if the arm is abducted*, the acromion process then pressing on the inflamed bursa. Owing to the pain, active abduction is always limited to some extent. (3) The patient sometimes has *fever* and *general symptoms*. In

---

* Owing to the variety of conditions included under the term 'bursitis' and the difference of opinion among doctors concerning its treatment, it is almost impossible to give a list of symptoms applicable to all cases, or a description of treatment suitable for all patients.

some cases the onset is sudden, in others gradual. The pain and limitation of movement vary from case to case according to the actual nature of the lesion.

Principles of Treatment.—Treatment is designed *to relieve pain* and later *to restore mobility and power* in the joint.

ACUTE STAGE.—For the first few days the condition is treated by: (1) *Rest*, the arm being supported in a sling; (2) *Heat*. Any other injury such as fracture or dislocation will receive appropriate treatment.

PHYSICAL TREATMENT.—After a few days physical treatment can begin.

POSITION OF PATIENT.—The patient should sit with the arm close to the side. It should be supported by a table or pillow.

MASSAGE.—The chest and upper part of the back should first be treated with effleurage and kneading; then the shoulder and upper arm are carefully approached, using gentle effleurage followed by kneading. At first the painful area is avoided but it should be gradually included as the pain subsides. Gentle frictions are added later. This treatment needs great care and skill.

MOVEMENTS are given within the limit of pain *but abduction is not allowed*.

SUBACUTE OR CHRONIC STAGE.—When the pain has subsided, treatment can be given as follows:—

MOVEMENTS.—Careful re-education of the deltoid and supraspinatus must be undertaken as soon as this can be done without undue pain.* The patient should begin in the lying position, the movements being given in the same way as for paralysed muscles (*see* Chapters IX, XII). The back of the plinth can be raised day by day until the patient is sitting upright. Resistance will be added as soon as possible to increase power, and the course of treatment will conclude with general arm exercises, pulley exercises, etc. The pain will probably not be completely relieved until the full range of movement in the shoulder has been recovered.

ELECTRICAL TREATMENT.—Dr. Mennell recommended radiant heat in the early stages and, if the injury is to the supraspinatus or subscapularis, graduated faradic contractions. Short-wave diathermy and various forms of ionization may, or may not, help.

OTHER METHODS OF TREATMENT.—*Radiotherapy* is sometimes given, and relieves some patients. *Cortisone* or *ACTH* may be injected. Sometimes the only treatment given is injections of analgesics such as novocain. In the late stages the shoulder may be *manipulated under anæsthetic* to break down adhesions. This is sometimes done in several stages. Physical treatment is then given in the usual way.

SURGICAL TREATMENT.—If other measures fail, the following operations may be considered—division of adhesions, removal of calcified deposits, or excision of the bursa. In more severe cases, the surgeon may resort to excision of the acromion process, or even arthrodesis of the glenohumeral joint.

POST-OPERATIVE TREATMENT.—After manipulation, exercises are given to maintain the range of movement obtained; after removal of calcified deposits, or excision of the bursa, massage may be given to the shoulder. Movements are given in small range until the stitches are removed and then gradually increased; after *arthrodesis*, massage and active movement may be given to all other joints of the shoulder-girdle and arm.

Inflammation in other bursæ is treated on the same lines.

GANGLION

A ganglion is a cyst of synovial membrane, generally found on the dorsal surface of the wrist, but it may appear in other places also—in the palm of the

---

* Some authorities advocate passive movements as well as active, to maintain the range of movement as far as possible.

hand, on the dorsum of the foot, or on the outer side of the knee. In appearance, the ganglion is a rounded swelling, which, as a rule, develops gradually. It may be quite small, or as large as a walnut. Some ganglia disappear spontaneously and most give no trouble unless situated in a part which is subject to pressure, e.g., the wrist.

SYMPTOMS.—In ganglion of the wrist there is weakness of that joint, and sometimes pain when doing laborious work—for instance, in lifting heavy weights. The symptoms may, however, be very slight.

PATHOLOGY.—Ganglia are fibrous sacs containing a viscid material. Their origin is uncertain. They may be small pouches which have become separated from tendon-sheaths or the synovial membranes of joints during foetal life and which for some reason—irritation or strain of the parts—become distended with fluid and form swellings.

Treatment.—If the ganglion has a thin wall, it can sometimes be burst by digital pressure. Then the fluid is dispersed into the surrounding tissues. Failing that it can be punctured in one or more places by a needle and the fluid expressed. The ganglion not infrequently recurs, in which case it is excised. Even then, it occasionally reappears. Post-operative treatment, if required at all, consists of massage of the arm and hand, with proper precautions as regards the scar, and careful movements of wrist and fingers to regain mobility. Another method of treatment is to aspirate the ganglion and inject sclerosing fluid into it.

Success in the treatment of ganglia has also been claimed for radiotherapy.

III. DISEASES OF BONE: OSTEOMYELITIS, PERIOSTITIS, AND TUBERCULOSIS: POTT'S DISEASE

OSTEOMYELITIS

As an example of bone infections we may take *osteomyelitis*, the late results of which we sometimes encounter in the course of our work. All infective processes in joints and bones need rather similar treatment. It is, however, necessary to have some understanding of the nature of these conditions, in order to appreciate the dangers which confront us when dealing with them.

AETIOLOGY.—

AGE.—The disease is commonest in children and in young people at puberty (10–14 years). This is because of the active bone growth taking place at this time of life, as well as the frequency of injuries at this age.

SEX.—Males are much more often affected than females.

CAUSE.—Infection (direct or indirect) of the bone tissue by micro-organisms.

PATHOLOGICAL CHANGES.—The bones most often affected are, in order of frequency: (1) The upper end of the tibia (hence the frequent involvement of the knee-joint); (2) The lower end of the femur; (3) The upper end of the humerus; (4) The ulna; (5) The fibula; (6) The radius; (7) The metacarpals and metatarsals.

The inflammation generally begins close to the epiphysial cartilage where growth is proceeding, the soft new tissue being a favourable situation for the growth of the bacteria. An abscess is formed and from thence the infection spreads to the medullary cavity of the diaphysis or shaft, and also outwards along the epiphysial disk to beneath the periosteum. The inflammation is intense, pus forms, and parts of the bone die. The pus, unless evacuated by surgical means, ultimately forces its way to the surface of the body and escapes. Surrounding tissues—muscles, ligaments, or fascia—may become involved, and infection may also be carried by the blood to other parts of the body.

REPAIR.—Bone has a wonderful capacity for recovery and as soon as the pus is evacuated it begins to grow again, the periosteum and bone-marrow laying

6

down new bone round the dead parts. The latter ultimately become detached from the new tissue and have to be removed by operation. In some cases, however, the condition may become chronic and in such cases the patient suffers periods of acute exacerbation. Discharging sinuses may persist.

SYMPTOMS.—

GENERAL SYMPTOMS.—Fever and other general symptoms arise in most cases. These may be serious, or even fatal.

LOCAL SYMPTOMS.—*Great pain* in the affected bone. *Swelling*, appearing as a marked and early symptom if a superficial bone is affected, but at a later stage in the case of a deep bone. *Fluctuation* may be apparent. *Changes in the skin over the affected bone*; it is first white, then red and angry-looking. If the pus is not surgically liberated, the abscess bursts.

COMPLICATIONS.—Involvement of joints; spontaneous fractures; displacement of epiphyses. Involvement of organs (the liver, spleen, kidneys, or heart may become diseased).

LATE RESULTS.—(1) *Shortening* of the limb, as the result of a displaced epiphysis; or *lengthening*, due to overgrowth caused by hyperæmia. In either case *deformity* results, especially where one of two parallel bones is affected, e.g., talipes valgus or varus, or club-hand (*see* Chapter XV). (2) *Ankylosis, deformity*, or *dislocation* of joints.

PROGNOSIS.—This used to be bad, but the discovery and use of antibiotics (penicillin, etc.) has revolutionized the treatment. The infection can now generally be controlled, and the late results avoided. The mortality has been reduced from 20 per cent to less than 1 per cent. The fatal cases are those in which general symptoms predominate—the *fulminating type*.

Principles of Treatment.—The aims of treatment are to control the infection. Rest is essential.

ACUTE STAGE.—

MEDICAL TREATMENT.—Administration of penicillin, or, if this is ineffective, some other antibiotic. It should begin as early as possible and continue for some time.

SURGICAL TREATMENT.—Incisions are made to evacuate the pus, and to remove as much dead bone as is necessary.

LATER STAGES.—

SURGICAL TREATMENT.—Operations of various kinds may be required; for example:—

Sequestrotomy, or removal of the dead pieces of bone (these are known as *sequestra*).

Bone-grafting.—If the bone has been extensively destroyed, bone-grafts are inserted into the gap; e.g., the patient's own fibula may be used to replace parts of the tibia, humerus, or femur; or chips of cancellous bone are inserted into the gap.

PHYSICAL TREATMENT.—We generally meet these cases at one of two periods: (1) When the wounds are just healed, or almost healed; and (2) When the wounds are firmly healed. These are old cases. The nearest joint may be partially or completely fixed by a bony or fibrous ankylosis. The muscles are probably much wasted. In either case the aims are the same, namely to strengthen muscles and to regain mobility.

1. *Cases with Unhealed or Recently Healed Wounds.*—It is essential to begin treatment very gently and carefully. The patient is often weak, nervous, and apprehensive and the physiotherapist must reassure him, making it quite clear that he is not going to be hurt. If the wounds are not quite healed, the bandages should be left in position for a day or so, or a clean (i.e., sterile) piece of gauze put over the wound.

If the physiotherapist touches the dressings or the skin near the wound, she must take proper precautions with regard to asepsis. In any case, she should be very careful as to the cleansing and disinfection of her hands. Any skin lesion should be protected by a gauze and collodion dressing.

Massage: If given, this will be much the same as for infective arthritis. The physiotherapist should begin by treating a part well away from any of the wounds, and she should not approach them closely for some days.

Active movements: These should be encouraged from the beginning. They may be assisted by the operator but *no force should ever be used until all risk of flaring up the infection is at an end.* In the case of a lower extremity lesion, the date for weight-bearing is for the surgeon to decide. Re-education in walking may then be necessary.

Electrical treatment: Zinc ionization, using soaked ribbon gauze packed into the wound, may be ordered for unhealed wounds. This is, however, acutely painful and should therefore be used with discretion in treating children. Local ultra-violet irradiation is perhaps a better method of obtaining healing.

2. *Old Cases, with Wounds Long Healed.*—In these cases we shall need to restore the power of the muscles. With regard to movements, we must be guided by the condition of the nearest joint. It may or may not be ankylosed; if it is, the ankylosis may be bony or fibrous. The physiotherapist should have seen a radiograph of this joint, or should have been informed by the surgeon of its actual condition.

If there is bony ankylosis, it is obviously useless to attempt movement. A patient with an ankylosed knee, for instance, will have to be taught to walk as correctly as possible with a stiff knee; or if, unfortunately, the knee is fixed in a more or less flexed position, with whatever apparatus is prescribed for him. If the ankylosis is fibrous—that is, due to adhesions within the joint and to contractures in the soft tissues surrounding it—an attempt may be made to mobilize it; forced movements may be given *but only in cases where all infection is over and no danger of its recurrence exists.*

In either case, we may endeavour to loosen adherent scars by frictions and vibrations though, if soft tissues have become adherent to *bone,* our efforts are not likely to meet with much success. Olive oil can be tried. The whirlpool bath, if available, is useful in these late cases. Ultrasonics, chlorine or iodine ionization is sometimes given.

Precaution.—A watch must always be kept for signs of inflammation in or near the wounds or scars. A recrudescence of inflammation with a small amount of discharge in a previously healed area probably means that another small fragment of dead bone has come loose and is setting up irritation. Anything of this kind should be reported at once.

Cases in which the condition has subsided without operation need no physical treatment, except, possibly, active exercises.

ACUTE TRAUMATIC PERIOSTITIS

This is a condition which arises as the result of a blow on the bone—generally the shin bone, which is subcutaneous and thus especially exposed to injury.

PATHOLOGICAL CHANGES.—The changes are those of simple inflammation. Suppuration rarely occurs. The bone does not die, but is merely a little thickened at the site of the injury.

SYMPTOMS.—These consist of *swelling*—not excessive—*pain*, and *tenderness*.

Treatment.—

MEDICAL AND SURGICAL TREATMENT.—The condition is treated by rest, suitable lotions, and sometimes counter-irritants. Occasionally the fluid is drawn off with a syringe.

PHYSICAL TREATMENT.—As for acute traumatic synovitis, but as the condition does not affect a joint, and therefore movement is less painful, progression may be quicker. Sometimes accompanying muscular strain may call for treatment; or, for instance, in periostitis of a rib or ribs, movements of the shoulder girdle may cause pain, owing to the pull of the serratus anterior on the injured area. In such cases, the physiotherapist must see that the patient does not lose mobility in these joints. Many cases do not require physical treatment at all.

TUBERCULOSIS (POTT'S DISEASE)

Tuberculosis is similar, from the point of view of the physiotherapist, to that of tuberculous joints, and the aims and treatment are alike. As our example we will take Pott's disease which is a tuberculous affection of the spine. It generally attacks the vertebral bodies, producing an angular deformity. The infection spreads from some other focus, and affects the lower thoracic region particularly.

AETIOLOGY.—Like all tuberculous diseases, spinal caries (Latin, caries= decay) is seen more often amongst the poor than the rich, though it is far less common today than formerly. It is probably not hereditary and is usually seen in children under 10 years old. The majority of cases occur under the age of 5 years, though adults may be attacked.

PATHOLOGICAL CHANGES.—The tuberculous process generally starts in the *metaphyses of the upper and lower surfaces of the vertebral body* in children, and in *the front of the vertebral body* in adults. From thence it spreads to neighbouring vertebræ. It destroys the bone substance and finally forms a large cavity, so that the vertebra collapses under the body-weight transmitted through the bones above (*Fig.* 69). The whole spine bends forwards and downwards at this point. One or more spinous processes project noticeably, forming the 'lump' or break in the normal contour of the back. This is known as a *gibbus*. Repair is by fibrous replacement of the destroyed tissue. In course of time this tissue may be converted into bone.

COMMON SITES OF THE LESION.—The *lower thoracic region* is most frequently attacked, then the *upper lumbar*. Caries of the upper thoracic region is much less common, and cervical caries is rare.

SYMPTOMS.—*Pain* is felt at the site of the lesion, and in the form of 'referred' pain when it radiates round to the front and sides of the body in a girdle-like manner. Any jarring of the spine causes sharp pain, as does palpation over the spinous processes. *Rigidity* is due to spasm of the back muscles. The patient uses these muscles, voluntarily and involuntarily, to immobilize the spine and so avoid pain. Moreover, he will not attempt to bend his back and, if asked to pick up an object from the floor, does so by flexing his hips and knees, keeping the spine rigid.

POSTURE AND GAIT.—The attitude is characteristic, always being one which will procure support for the affected part of the spine, thus relieving pressure on the diseased vertebræ and decreasing pain. In advanced cases, the child either will not stand at all, or else he holds on to objects round him and will not walk unless he can obtain such support. A limp is common in lumbar disease.

DEFORMITY.—There is *an angular deformity in the normal contour of the curves of the spine*, best seen when the child bends forward. It is usually anteroposterior and, although very slight in early cases, may develop to an extreme degree if untreated—the patient becoming a 'hunch-back'. *Lateral angulation*, leading to scoliosis, is sometimes seen if the *side* of the body of a vertebra is diseased and collapses, but it is rare.

COMPLICATIONS.—

PRESSURE.—In bad cases of thoracic caries, there may be serious pressure on the *heart and lungs*, and grave interference with their functions.

ABSCESS FORMATION.—Abscesses commonly form, either at the site of the lesion, or elsewhere, due to tracking of pus along fascial planes and sheaths.

COMPRESSION PARAPLEGIA.—This is generally spastic, and is caused by compression of the spinal cord, the neural canal being narrowed by the collapse of the vertebræ and the bending of the spine.

We need not further discuss the disease in its early stages, as we are not much concerned with its treatment until a later period.

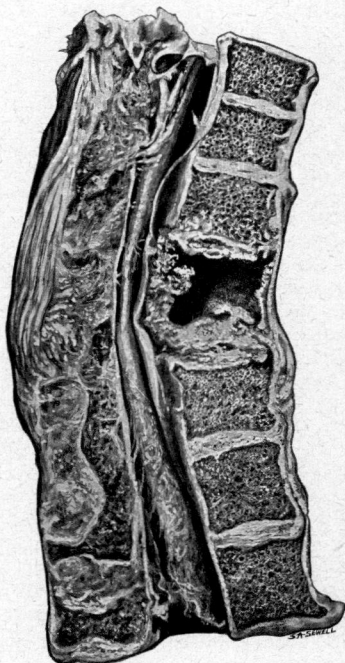

Fig. 69.—Tuberculous disease of the body of a vertebra.

Principles of Treatment.—

GENERAL TREATMENT.—In all cases of tuberculous infection of bone, rest, good food, hygiene, fresh air and sunlight are essential. That the sun is our best ally in such cases has been abundantly proved at Leysin in Dr. Rollier's clinics for the treatment of surgical tuberculosis. Similar treatment, as far as is possible in our climate, is carried on at the Treloar Home at Alton, and at many other homes and hospitals, where it has been wonderfully successful. During the summer, the patients, wearing a minimum of clothing, spend all their days in the sun—having been, of course, accustomed to this by gradual exposure—their heads being protected by a shade. Artificial sunlight is also used when necessary, *providing there is no phthisis.*

LOCAL TREATMENT.—Immobilization is necessary until the disease is quiescent, i.e., there is no radiological evidence of further decalcification, and the pulse-rate, blood-sedimentation rate, and temperature have remained normal for 2 or 3 months. In cases of Pott's disease the patient is placed in the recumbent position, with *the spine in hyperextension*. This attitude diminishes the pressure on the diseased vertebral body, or bodies, and thus relieves pain, prevents flexion deformity, and gives the spine a chance to heal. This is brought about by partial replacement of the destroyed bodies by new bone, and by ankylosis of the joints between the affected vertebræ. *The position also reduces the risk of para-plegia.* The type of support used for the immobilization depends on the preference of the surgeon in charge of the case. It may consist of some form of frame, e.g., a *Whitman frame*★—a rectangular frame made of steel tubing, about 6 in. longer than the patient and about three-quarters of his width, the two side bars being connected by stout canvas. The patient lies on his back, rubber squares being laid under the buttocks, and felt padding so arranged as to protect the diseased vertebræ, or the gibbus, if one exists. The frames are angled in such a way as to produce hyperextension of the spine in the affected area. *Plaster beds are also in common use today.* The patient will lie prone or supine for the majority of the time, depending on the surgeon's views, but in either case the spine will be hyper-extended. The *prone* position has the advantage that when the head is raised the spine is kept in hyperextension, whereas in the *supine* position it causes flexion of the spine.

When the disease is quiescent, the patient is gradually allowed to sit up, to stand, and finally to walk. He must, however, continue with some form of support, either a plaster jacket or a spinal brace, until the repair is consolidated. This may well take 12–18 months, and the duration of the treatment is long. It may continue for three or four years in thoracic caries, rather less if the disease is in the cervical or lumbar regions. Supervision is necessary for a considerable time in order to obviate all danger of relapse.

PHYSICAL TREATMENT.—

DURING THE PERIOD OF RECUMBENCY AND SUPPORT.—As in any case requiring lengthy immobilization physical treatment is directed towards *the prevention or minimization of complications attendant on enforced recumbency*, such as *stiffness*, *atrophy*, and *pressure sores*. In adults there may also be a risk of respiratory infections or thrombosis. Treatment, therefore, follows the same lines as that given for fractures requiring prolonged immobilization. *Massage* may be given to maintain circulation and nutrition of the tissues, and gentle *passive* and *active movements* should be given to prevent stiffness and disuse atrophy. Breathing exercises should also be included. If *compression paraplegia* is present treatment as for SPASTIC PARAPLEGIA may be required but this condition generally disappears in the course of the general and mechanical treatment of the disease.†

WHEN HEALING HAS TAKEN PLACE.—The spine is consolidated at the seat of the lesion and the main aim of treatment is *to strengthen all the patient's muscles* and, if necessary, to *increase mobility in any joint in which it is impaired, except those in the area attacked by the disease*. Since it is difficult to confine movement entirely to one region of the spine, this means, in practice, that no *forcible stretching or mobilization* of the spine is to be attempted.

MASSAGE.—This is rarely used today. It can be given to the limbs but the back should be approached with caution and the diseased area must be given a wide berth.

EXERCISES.—These are essential *provided that no attempt is made to increase the range of movement in that part of the vertebral column which has been the seat of the disease*. No overstretch or overpressure should be given in any trunk

---

★ For descriptions of other spinal frames, the student should consult one of the standard text-books on orthopædics.

† If recovery does not take place, an operation may be undertaken for its relief, after which treatment may proceed as before, but it must be very gentle and careful, as these operations are very severe ones, and not always successful.

exercise. The thorax needs mobilizing, *but this has to be done with care*, and *no movement should be undertaken which could put any strain on the spine*. Special care is necessary with regard to any movement which takes place most freely in the affected region, e.g., specific trunk-turnings (or, indeed, any exercise including rotation of the trunk in the lower thoracic region) and forward flexion, particularly if the disease has involved the cervical or lumbar regions of the spine. The best trunk exercises are free movements done in rather slow time. They should include back exercises, abdominal exercises, and side-flexions. *Breathing exercises* are most important in order to mobilize the thorax and improve respiration. The patients should be instructed in costal, diaphragmatic, and apical breathing so that they use the whole of the thorax and fully expand the lungs. Most free movements may be given to the arms and legs and simple resistance may be added, but there must be *no overstretching when the arms are raised above the head*, and leg exercises in which the abdominal muscles work concentrically and eccentrically are not suitable. Any form of hanging is, of course, contra-indicated, since the stretching of the spine by the drag of latissimus dorsi (attached to the spinous processes from the seventh thoracic vertebra downwards) may cause the repaired tissue to break down and the disease to become active again. In thoracic or lumbar cases, head movements can be performed in the ordinary way but in *cervical* cases they must be given with great care. There must be no overstretch and they should be performed slowly with little or no resistance. Probably few exercises of ordinary strength would be harmful to these patients, provided that all forced movements were avoided, but spinal caries is too serious a disease to justify the taking of any risks, and it is better to err on the safe side. The following are, however, definitely contra-indicated: strong mobility exercises (e.g., Trunk-rolling); pressures of any kind; exercises with overstretch or over-pressure; movements with strong resistance by the force of gravity, or by the physiotherapist; free exercises in very quick time, producing a jerk at the end of each movement (e.g., Hewing, Yard-standing (quick) Alternate trunk-rotation). Obviously the exercises selected must be carefully graduated.

CHAPTER VIII

DISEASES OF THE NERVOUS SYSTEM: GENERAL CONSIDERATIONS

Aetiology of nervous diseases—Pathology—General symptoms—Classification—Principles of treatment.

AETIOLOGY OF NERVOUS DISEASES

LESIONS of the nervous system, whether of the brain, of the spinal cord, or of the peripheral nerves, may be due to *injury* or to *disease*. The principal causes are as follows:—

INJURIES.—Fractures of the skull, vertebral column, or limbs; dislocations, or any application of force to the tissues sufficiently strong to sever, lacerate, bruise or otherwise injure a nerve. In the case of fractures, the nerve may be damaged at the time of the accident, or may be compressed afterwards by displaced bone or by callus.

DISEASE.—Under this heading we may include: (1) *Infection by micro-organisms*, as in 'infantile' paralysis, tabes dorsalis, or post-diphtheritic neuritis. These micro-organisms generally have a *selective affinity* for some particular part of the nervous system—that is, they attack that part and no other, e.g., the virus of acute anterior poliomyelitis attacks only the anterior horn cells of the cord, or the corresponding cells of the cranial nerves. Bacterial inflammation may also, of course, spread to nervous structures from the surrounding tissues. (2) *Poisoning*, e.g., by lead, arsenic, alcohol, etc. This generally affects the peripheral nerves. (3) *Tumours or congenital malformations*, producing pressure on some part of the nervous system. (4) *Vascular lesions*, hæmorrhage, thrombosis, embolism, etc. (5) *Rheumatism*, the products of which bring about compression of nerves, as in some forms of facial paralysis, or irritation of nervous structures, as in chorea. (6) *Any other conditions causing compression* of these structures, e.g., Pott's disease. The origin of certain nervous diseases is at present unknown or uncertain, e.g., progressive muscular atrophy and disseminated sclerosis.

The symptoms vary according to the cause and site of the lesion.

PATHOLOGY

A nervous disease may consist of (1) *acute inflammation* or (2) *chronic degeneration* of some part of the nervous system.

ACUTE INFLAMMATION.—The usual changes are present. The blood-vessels are distended, and there is *swelling and destruction of cells*, as well as *pain due to pressure on sensory neurons* if such are in the neighbourhood. The inflammation may clear up, often leaving behind it more or less permanent damage (*in the case of the central nervous system some degree of permanent damage is inevitable*); it may progress to a fatal issue or it may be succeeded by a *chronic* process of degeneration.

DEGENERATION means the transformation of a highly specialized tissue into one of a lower order—for example, of nervous or muscular structures into fibrous connective tissue. In the case of nerves, the cells or fibres are destroyed and their place is taken by *neuroglia*.

DEGENERATION OF FIBRES.—If a nerve-fibre is cut off from its trophic centre that is, from its cell of origin, it dies. The *cells of origin of the motor neurons are situated in the cerebral cortex (upper motor neuron)*, or in the *anterior horns* of the spinal cord *(lower motor neuron)*. Their axons pass *downwards*. Therefore that part of the fibre *below* the lesion degenerates. If the cell itself is destroyed, the whole axon dies; this is known as *descending degeneration (Fig. 70). The cells of origin of the sensory neurons are situated peripherally*. Those of the lowest neurons are in the ganglia on the posterior roots of the spinal nerves, and their axons pass *upwards* in the cord. Therefore, if the cell or fibre is injured, the part *above* the lesion dies, that is, there is an *ascending degeneration (Fig. 71)*. (The fibre passing into the ganglion from the skin or other areas is, physiologically, a *dendron*, and will die, too, if separated from its cell.) The same rule applies to the high sensory neurons, which have their trophic centres in the medulla, thalamus, etc.

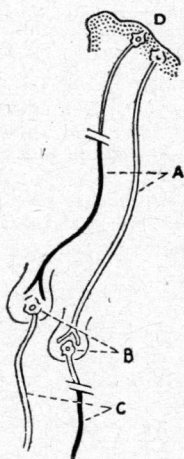

Fig. 70.—Descending degeneration of efferent (motor) neurons. A, Upper motor neuron; B, Anterior horn cells; C, Lower motor neuron; D, Cerebral cortex. In *Figs*. 70 and 71 the site of the lesion is shown by two parallel cross lines, the degenerated part by a solid black line.

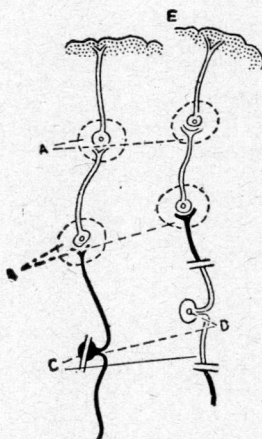

Fig. 71.—Ascending degeneration of afferent (sensory) neurons. A, Thalamus; B, Nucleus cuneatus; C, Lowest sensory neuron; D, Posterior root ganglion cells; E, Cerebral cortex.

Changes of Degeneration in Fibres.—(1) The medullary sheath degenerates first, breaking up into fatty globules which are ultimately absorbed. (2) The axon is later broken up and disappears. (3) The neurilemma sheath remains, and its nuclei increase in number. It is filled at first by a soft protoplasmic substance; later, this becomes fibrous tissue.

Regeneration of Fibres.—Peripheral nerve-fibres *outside* the cord are capable of regeneration in favourable circumstances, but *not fibres within the brain* or *cord*. The process begins in the central end. New axis-cylinders are laid down by the cells of the neurilemma and grow down into the peripheral portion, i.e., into the sheaths of the dead axons, or the spaces between them. It is essential that the ends of the severed nerve should not be too widely separated, and that its outer sheath should be intact. The medullary sheath is reproduced later. The new nerve grows downwards at the rate of about 1 millimetre a day. At the point where the axons have been newly laid down, a gentle tapping over the nerve will produce a tingling sensation in the limb. This is known as *Tinel's test*, and by it we can discover exactly how far the regeneration of the nerve has proceeded. The sign may be elicited before there is any indication of returning sensation or motor power.

DEGENERATION OF CELLS.—A cell may be destroyed by injury, compression, the action of bacteria, etc. It atrophies and dies, and its place is taken by the neuroglia, which increases in quantity. *The death of the cell involves the destruction of the whole neuron*, all the process degenerating with it. The blood-vessels in the part become thickened, and many of them disappear altogether. This condition is also known as *sclerosis* (Greek, *skleros*=hard). *No nerve-cell is capable of regeneration, nor can any existing cell, after birth, produce another by division*. The higher tissues have paid for their specialization with the loss of their reproductive power.

A cell which has been deprived of its axon undergoes certain changes, *but it is capable of recovery so long as its nucleus remains intact*.

GENERAL SYMPTOMS

The symptoms appearing in any particular condition depend, of course, on the position of the lesion in the nervous system—that is, on exactly what cells or fibres are involved (*see* CLASSIFICATION, p. 177). We shall therefore consider briefly the chief effects of the various lesions as regards the movements, sensation, and trophic conditions of the parts affected.

MENTAL SYMPTOMS.—These occur either when there is injury or disease of the frontal lobes of the brain (*Fig.* 72), or when some important 'association area' is affected, that is, when the communication between the various parts of the brain is cut off or disorganized.

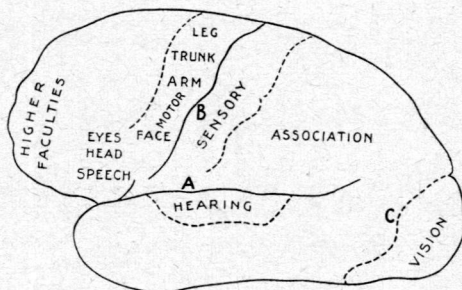

Fig. 72.—Localization of function in the brain. **A**, Sulcus lateralis (fissure of Sylvius); **B**, Sulcus centralis (fissure of Rolando); **C**, Parieto-occipital sulcus.

MOTOR SYMPTOMS, EFFECTS ON MUSCLES AND MOVEMENTS.— When considering the effects of defects in the central nervous system on muscles and movements *it is important to remember that throughout the central nervous system facilitatory and inhibitory mechanisms exist*, as it were, side by side. The *facilitatory mechanisms* lead to *muscle contraction* and the *inhibitory mechanisms determine the degree of contraction and the way in which the movement is performed*. Under normal conditions the inhibitory mechanisms prevent over-activity, and lead to smooth co-ordinated performance. The patient may suffer from: (1) *Flaccidity* of muscles, with *complete loss of power* and *true atrophy*; (2) *Spasticity* of muscles; (3) Involuntary movements of various kinds; (4) *Atonia* (loss of tone), or *hypotonia* (decrease of tone) of muscles, *without loss of power*.

1. FLACCID PARALYSIS WITH TRUE ATROPHY.—This condition is characteristic of the *lower motor neuron lesion*, i.e., injury of the anterior horn cells of the spinal cord, or of their axons (*see Fig. 73*). The muscles are at first pale and flabby; later, they become much wasted, and the limb is cold and blue. This is because the motor nerve-supply to the muscles is entirely cut off. No messages come through to them, therefore all power of contraction is lost. No movement at all can take

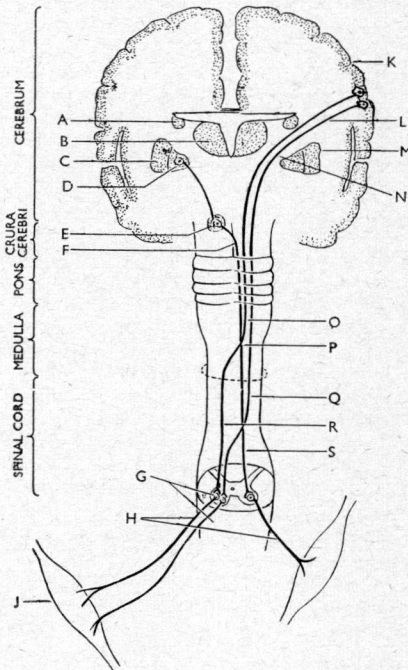

Fig. 73.—The motor path (descending tract). A, Caudate nucleus; B, Thalamus; C, Putamen; D, Globus pallidus; E, Red nucleus; F, Ventral segmented decussation; G, Anterior horn; H, Final common pathway (motor nerve); J, Muscle; K, Motor cortex; L, Corona radiata; M, Lentiform nucleus; N, Internal capsule; O, Pyramid; P, Decussation of pyramids; Q, Anterior cerebrospinal (direct pyramidal) tract; R, Lateral cerebrospinal (crossed pyramidal) tract; S, Rubrospinal tract.

place, and even the normal tone of muscles at rest cannot be maintained. Moreover, the anterior horn cells appear in some way to control the nutrition of the muscles, since, if these cells are destroyed, the muscles atrophy more than is compatible with mere disuse. The circulation of the whole limb is disorganized, and if bone growth is not complete, it may be gravely impaired.

If a nerve is severed, or its cells of origin destroyed by an accident, the resulting paralysis appears immediately. If an acute inflammation arises in the neurons, it comes on in a few days or hours but if a degenerative process sets in, the development of the paralysis may extend over months or years.

2. SPASTICITY OF MUSCLES.—This is *characteristic of the upper motor neuron lesion*. The inhibiting power of the suppressor zones of the cerebrum and of the reticular formation is lost, so that the lower motor neuron is uncontrolled, all sensory stimuli producing exaggerated responses. Moreover, impulses coming down from the cerebellum and the semicircular canals of the inner ear are destined to *increase* the tone of the muscles. Since these are no longer balanced by the inhibiting impulses, the muscle tone becomes abnormally great in the affected parts of the body, and we have the development of the *spastic state*. This results in the peculiarities of gait and posture which are to be seen in upper motor neuron lesions. These are described in detail later (*see* HEMIPLEGIA, pp. 181, 189).

3. INVOLUNTARY MOVEMENTS.—These are of many different kinds, and may be due to:—

Injury of the Basal Ganglia, i.e., the caudate and lenticular nuclei (*see Fig.* 73).—This may produce: (1) *Athetosis*, a strange twisting, squirming movement, generally of the fingers or toes, but sometimes seen in the head, wrist, elbow, or shoulder. It occasionally accompanies hemiplegia or diplegia in children (*see* pp. 189–90); (2) *Tremors*, of the kind seen in paralysis agitans (*see* p. 223). These consist of fine shaking movements, continuing when the limb is at rest, but less evident when the patient performs purposive, i.e., *willed*, movements. Both athetosis and tremors of this kind are due to the loss of the controlling actions of the above-mentioned ganglia (in particular the caudate nucleus) over various other groups of cells in the brain (e.g., the red nucleus in the midbrain), which, unchecked, produce these disordered movements. Purposive movements are less affected, because the cerebral cortex then becomes more active. The diffuse rigidity of paralysis agitans (*see* p. 223) is also thought to be due to the failure of this inhibition, since those parts of the brain which produce overtone of muscle are not sufficiently balanced.

Injury to the Cerebellum.—This produces *tremor during the performance* of *purposive movements*, i.e., *intention tremor, nystagmus*, etc. (*see* pp. 226, 228). The cerebellum controls, or partly controls, co-ordination during movement. It is responsible for *the synergic action of muscles* and *the timing and force of individual muscle contraction*, as well as the maintenance of posture, balance, and equilibrium. Hence injury to this part of the brain, or to the tracts passing to or from it, brings about a kind of jerky incoordination.

Irritation of Motor Nerves in any Part of the Nervous System.—This is *the result of pressure of inflammatory products on the nerves*. The upper neurons may be affected, as in chorea, or the lower neurons as in various conditions of cramp, and possibly in spasmodic torticollis. The spasm in such cases may be *tonic* or *clonic*. In the tonic variety, the muscles go into a condition of fixed over-contraction or tetanus, as in the well-known cramp of the calf-muscles. Clonic spasm consists of a series of twitches or jerks, as in chorea or spasmodic torticollis.

4. ATONIA OR HYPOTONIA.—The former means *loss* of tone in the muscles, the latter *diminution* of their tone below normal. If present *without loss of power of contraction*, it would be more correctly classed as a sensory symptom, being generally due to a lesion of the afferent tracts, for example, the fasciculi gracilis and cuneatus (columns of Goll and Burdach) in tabes dorsalis (*see* p. 215).

DISTRIBUTION OF PARALYSIS.—This depends on the site of the lesion. It may be unilateral or bilateral, according to whether one or both sides of the brain or cord are involved. It may be on the opposite side of the body from the lesion, or on the same side, according to whether the lesion occurs above or below the crossing of the fibres of the neurons concerned (*see Fig.* 73). It may affect many or few movements or muscles. Broadly speaking, a lower motor neuron lesion produces a paralysis of *muscles*—a group or part of a group, one single muscle, or even only part of that muscle—because the cells for each muscle lie together in the anterior horns. In upper motor neuron lesions there is a paralysis of *movement* rather than of *muscles* themselves. This is because the cells in the motor area of the cerebral cortex are arranged according to movements, not according to muscles.

REFLEXES.—The nature of a reflex is well known to all students. It depends on the integrity of the reflex arc. *If this is broken in any part, the reflex is lost.* For instance, in tabes dorsalis, the *afferent (sensory) impulse* is prevented from reaching the cord by the destruction of the posterior nerve-roots and ganglia; in 'infantile' paralysis, the *motor response* to the stimulus cannot take place, because the anterior horn cell—*the discharging station*—is lost; in peripheral nerve lesions, the *efferent fibre* is out of action. Therefore, in diseases or injuries of *the lower motor neuron* or of the lowest sensory neuron, *the reflex is lost* (*Fig.* 74). In *upper motor neuron* lesions—for example, in hemiplegia or primary spastic paraplegia—the *reflex response is increased*, because the arc is intact but *the controlling power of the cortical cells is lost.*

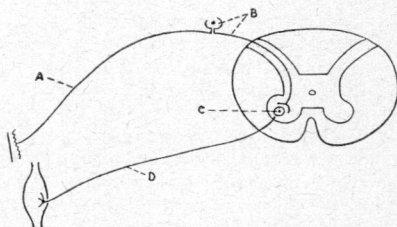

Fig. 74.—Showing the different situations in the reflex arc where a lesion may occur, resulting in loss of the reflex. A, Sensory nerve—e.g., by severance; B, Posterior nerve-root and ganglion—e.g., in tabes dorsalis; C, Anterior horn—e.g., in anterior polio-myelitis; D, Motor nerve—e.g., by severance, neuritis.

If a lesion involves both grey and white matter in the cord at some particular level, the reflexes are *lost* in the parts of the body supplied by the cells in that area. They are, however, *increased below* the site of the lesion because the upper motor neuron fibres of the pyramidal tracts are interrupted on their way to the anterior horn cells lower down in the cord. They are, of course, *normal above* it. There is often a hypersensitive area corresponding to the upper edge of the lesion, the degenerate or inflamed part acting as a foreign body and irritating the living tissues above (*see* TRANSVERSE MYELITIS, p. 236, and TABES DORSALES, p. 215). The reflexes are little affected in extrapyramidal or cerebellar lesions.

The reflexes which are best known and most easily obtainable in healthy persons, and therefore most valuable as a diagnostic test in disease, are, among deep reflexes, the knee- and ankle-jerks and, among superficial or skin reflexes, the abdominal and plantar.

THE KNEE-JERK (patellar reflex) is obtained by means of a sharp tap on the common tendon of the quadriceps, the patient sitting on a chair with one leg crossed over the other, or on a bed with the legs hanging over the side. It consists of a single sharp contraction of the quadriceps. It is a test of the integrity of the reflex arc at the level of the second, third, and fourth lumbar nerves (that is, roughly, of the *lumbar plexus*).

THE ANKLE-JERK (Achilles tendon reflex) is elicited by tapping that tendon, with the foot hanging free in dorsiflexion, i.e., the patient kneels on a chair with his foot over the edge. It consists of a contraction of the calf-muscles, and corresponds to the fifth lumbar, and the first and second sacral segments (that is, roughly, to the *sacral plexus*).

The reflexes in the arm, e.g., the biceps, triceps, and supinator jerks, are more difficult to elicit, and are often absent even in healthy people.

THE ABDOMINAL REFLEXES are three in number. The *upper one*, corresponding to the *sixth and seventh thoracic segments*, is obtained by tickling the skin over the epigastric region; the *middle one* (Thoracic 8 and 9) by stimulation of the skin above the umbilicus, and *the lower* (Thoracic 10, 11, 12) by stimulation of the skin below it. They all result in contractions of various parts of the abdominal muscles.

THE PLANTAR REFLEX (Lumbar 5, Sacral 1 and 2) is produced by drawing some sharp object along the inner side of the sole of the foot. It normally causes *flexion* of the big toe, except in infants who have not yet begun to walk, when *extension* is the normal response.

Abnormal responses to stimuli, known as *pathological reflexes*, occur in upper motor neuron lesions. These are ankle-clonus, knee-clonus, and Babinski's sign.

ANKLE-CLONUS.—To elicit this, the knee should be flexed, and the ankle dorsi-flexed by putting pressure on the ball of the foot. A series of quick contractions of the calf muscles takes place. The normal reflex response to pressure on the ball of the foot in walking is extension of the ankle, but in these cases it takes place in an uncontrolled and incoordinate manner, owing to lack of cerebral inhibition.

KNEE-CLONUS.—This is less often seen. The patella is drawn down, and a tap is given to its upper margin. A similar tremor results.

BABINSKI'S SIGN is, in adults, the pathological form of the plantar reflex. Extension of the big toe follows the stimulus instead of flexion. It is a return to the infantile type, the acquired reflex brought about by the necessity of pressing the toes on the ground when walking, being lost.

N.B.—For the STRETCH REFLEX, *see* p. 130.

Certain other special reflexes, or reflex patterns, are seen in infants. These may persist throughout life, or disappear, in normal babies, during infancy or childhood, as the child's movements come under voluntary control. They are valuable in diagnosis, because in patients with brain or cord lesions they may be absent or exaggerated, or may persist beyond the normal period. They can sometimes be made use of in treatment. Examples★ of such reflexes are:—

THE GRASP REFLEX.—Everyone knows how a baby will grasp a finger placed in his hand. This reflex diminishes between the second and third month, when he begins to grasp voluntarily.

THE TONIC NECK REFLEX.—If a baby's head is turned to one side, he contracts the arm and leg of the opposite side. The reflex begins to die away at the end of the fourth month, and disappears at some time before the end of the third year.

THE LABYRINTHINE RIGHTING REFLEX.—By this the child keeps his head upright, in correct relationship with his body, however he is turned or tilted. The eyes must be covered to prevent righting by means of sight. This reflex appears at two months and continues throughout life.

THE EXTENSOR THRUST.—The lower limb is extended when pressure is applied on the sole of the foot. In athetoid cases extension may be produced in the affected part of the body (often the spine) without apparent stimulus, if startled or excited, or on attempting movement.

TROPHIC CHANGES.—

MUSCLE ATROPHY has already been discussed; *it is characteristic of lower motor neuron lesions only* and does not appear in other types of nervous disease, except as the result of disuse of the part.

★ For description of other such reflexes, *see* Viola Cardwell, *Cerebral Palsy*, p. 100.

CHANGES IN THE SKIN, NAILS, BONES, OR JOINTS may also take place in *lower motor neuron lesions, or in those of the sensory nerves.* The skin becomes glossy and sometimes thickened and hard, the nails longitudinally streaked, and abnormally curved from side to side. The sweat-glands may over-secrete or under-secrete in the affected area. Any injury to the skin heals slowly and with difficulty, and ulcers may appear. The bones may become brittle, and fractures occur as the result of trivial violence; in children, bone growth is arrested. Arthritic changes may take place in the joints, or they may become the seat of intense effusion (Charcot's joints).

SENSORY SYMPTOMS.—The most important of these are *pain, anæsthesia or paræsthesia,* and *hyperæsthesia.*

PAIN.—This is due to pressure on sensory nerve-fibres, exerted by inflammatory products within or without their sheath, by displaced bone, by formation of callus, scar tissue, etc.

ANÆSTHESIA (Greek, *an*=not, *aisthesis*=sensation).—This means loss of sensation, due to interruption of sensory nerves or tracts.

Anæsthesia due to Injury of Peripheral Nerves.—The student will remember that there are two kinds of sensibility, superficial and deep. *Superficial,* or *cutaneous, sensibility* may be divided into *protopathic* and *epicritic,* each type of sensation being carried by special fibres. The *protopathic* type of sensation

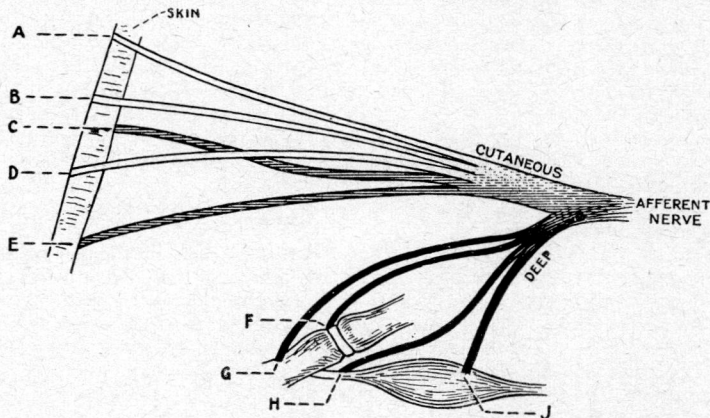

Fig. 75.—Types of sensation and their distribution. A, Light touch (discriminative sensibility); B, Localization; C, Pain; D, Finer differences of temperature; E, Extremes of temperature; F, Joint sense; G, Bone sense; H, Tendon (muscle sense); J, Muscle (deep sensation).

includes the perception of painful stimuli, of pressure, and of extremes of temperature; the *epicritic* type, the perception of light touches, of finer shades of temperature, and of cutaneous localization (i.e., of knowledge of what area of skin is touched, whether it is touched in one or two places at the same time, etc.). *Deep sensibility* is that of the muscles, tendons, joints, and bones, and the impulses arising in these organs are those of 'muscle sense' and 'joint sense'; or, as regards the bones, the sense of vibration. Put shortly, *muscle sense* keeps our brain informed as to the state of contraction or relaxation of our muscles, *joint sense* as to the position of our joints. Both are necessary if we are to co-ordinate our movements correctly. Pain, and a sensation of pressure, may also be felt in these deep structures (*Fig. 75*).

If a single peripheral nerve is injured, there may be little or no impairment of deep sensation, and the loss of epicritic sensation is always more extensive than that of protopathic. *Epicritic sensation* is tested by touching the part supplied by the nerve, with cotton-wool; *protopathic sensation* by means of pin-pricks, or the application of the faradic current. *Deep sensation* may be tested by strong pressure on the part; *muscle sense* by active movements, and *joint sense* by passive movements. All these tests should be carried out with the patient's eyes shut.

Anæsthesia due to Injury of Tracts in the Cord.—The fibres carrying all the above types of sensation enter the spinal cord by way of the posterior nerve-roots, and are then distributed to the various ascending tracts. Roughly speaking, there are three main tracts going upwards to the brain: (1) *The fasciculi gracilis and cuneatus* (posterior columns). These carry impulses of muscle and joint sense, and tactile discrimination (i.e., the finer shades of touch). (2) *The anterior and lateral spinothalamic (Gower's) tracts*, carrying sensations of pain and temperature, and of crude touch and pressure. (3) *The posterior spinocerebellar (Flechsig's) tract*, carrying impulses connected with the maintenance of co-ordination and equilibrium (e.g., certain types of muscle sense) (*Figs.* 76, 77).

If all these tracts are destroyed, there is *complete anæsthesia below the level of the lesion. Dissociated anæsthesia* means loss of some particular form of sensation, while other kinds remain intact—for example, in syringomyelia (*see* p. 222), there is loss of pain and temperature sense, but not that of touch, muscle contraction, etc., because the spinothalmic tracts only are affected.

PARÆSTHESIA (Greek, *para*=beyond).—This means *abnormal or perverted sensation*, the afferent nerves carrying up false impressions, such as the feeling of walking on cotton-wool in tabes, 'pins and needles', etc. It is due to *partial* lesions of the nerves or tracts. The latter may also cause *diminished or delay sensation*—the patient may not feel the touch until several seconds after it has actually taken place.

HYPERÆSTHESIA.—This is a condition of *over-acute sensibility* to stimuli *owing to irritation of nerves.*

ATAXIA.—This has been defined as *pathological incoordination.* Although it is manifested by *disordered movements*, it is a defect of the *afferent* tracts. It is mainly the result of loss of muscle and joint sense through lesions of the posterior columns, or spinocerebellar tracts. The cerebrum or cerebellum are not kept informed of the state of contraction of the muscles or of the position of the joints, so that they are unable to co-ordinate the movements of the body. For a description of the two types of ataxic gait, *see* TABES DORSALIS and CEREBELLAR ATAXIA (pp. 215, 226).

ELECTRICAL CHANGES.—In *upper motor neuron disease* the electrical reactions are normal. In *lower motor neuron affections* we find the condition known as *reaction of degeneration* (R.D.). The characteristics of this reaction are, in the first place, increased excitability to both interrupted direct current and a faradic, or faradic type of current. After a short time there is a decreased response to the faradic current (because the dying nerve is less and less able to carry the stimulus to the muscle), but an increased response to the galvanic (which can stimulate the muscle tissue directly if there is no nerve conductivity). Finally there is no reaction to a faradic current but the galvanic response will persist unless, or until, the muscle itself degenerates.

DEFORMITIES.—These often occur in nervous diseases and are due to *contractures.* In lower motor neuron lesions contractures are caused by the unopposed pull of healthy antagonists, sometimes assisted by the action of gravity. In upper motor neuron disease their cause is the action of spastic muscles, which maintain the limbs in abnormal positions.

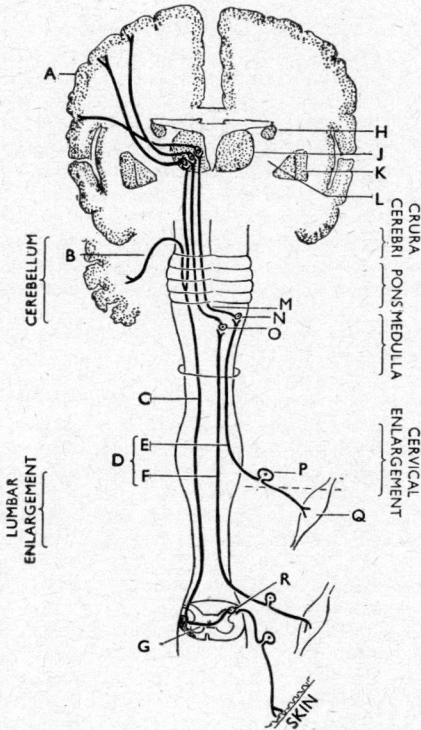

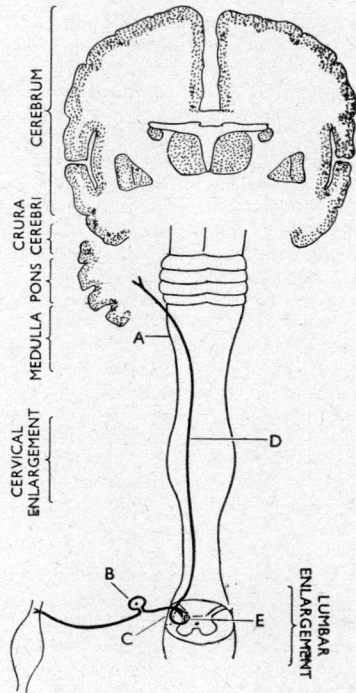

Fig. 76.—The sensory path—the fasciculi gracilis and cuneatus (columns of Goll and Burdach) and the anterior and lateral spinothalamic (Gower's) tracts. A, Sensory cortex; B, Superior peduncle; C, Lateral spinothalamic tract; D, Posterior columns; E, Fasciculus cuneatus; F, Fasciculus gracilis; G, Grey commissure; H, Claudate nucleus; J, Thalamus; K, Lentiform nucleus; L, Internal capsule; M, Sensory decussation; N, Nucleus cuneatus; O, Nucleus gracilis; P, Posterior root ganglion cell; Q, Muscle; R, Cell of posterior horn.

Fig. 77.—The posterior spinocerebellar (direct cerebellar) tract; A, Inferior cerebellar peduncle; B, Posterior root-ganglion cell; C, Posterior horn; D, Posterior spinocerebellar (direct cerebellar) tract; E, Cell of thoracic nucleus (Clarke's column). The posterior spinocerebellar (direct cerebellar) tract ends by passing through the inferior peduncle into the cerebellum.

CLASSIFICATION

Nervous diseases may be divided into *diseases of the brain, diseases of the spinal cord,* and *diseases of the peripheral nerves.* It will, however, be more convenient here to take together those which have similar groups of symptoms according to which neuron, or neurons, are affected. We shall therefore consider in order:—

I. Lesions of Brain and Cord.—

(1) The upper motor neuron. (2) The lower motor neuron. (3) The sensory tracts. (4) Other lesions.

II. Lesions of Peripheral Nerves.—

Injury or disease of individual nerve-roots or -trunks. Neuritis, neuralgia, and cramp.

PRINCIPLES OF TREATMENT OF NERVOUS DISEASES

So far we have been concerned with conditions and lesions which respond well to physical treatment. They have been relatively simple cases of muscular weakness and joint immobility, caused by factors which can be altered by the application of certain forms of treatment. In dealing with lesions of the brain and spinal cord we are faced with pathological changes which can in no way be altered by any form of treatment, *the damage done is permanent and irreversible as far as the substance of the tissues is concerned.* Such lesions, however, give rise to *symptoms* which add their crippling effect to the disabilities produced by the lesions itself. *It is with the symptoms that the physiotherapist is concerned, since their effects can be considerably alleviated by treatment.* Certain principles of treatment are common to all forms of nervous disease, although specific aims and methods will vary with each case.

The primary aim of treatment is *to restore the maximal functional ability* to the patient in order that he may be independent of others for his personal care. Broadly speaking this means: (1) *Relieving incapacitating symptoms,* e.g., spasticity; (2) *Training faculties left to the patient* to compensate for those which are lost, e.g., using sight and sound to take the place of muscle and joint sense; (3) *Preventing contracture and deformity;* (4) *Maintaining and improving joint mobility;* (5) *Teaching the patient to live with his disability,* both from the physical and mental point of view.

In order to treat any patient suffering from a lesion of the central nervous system intelligently, and with the maximum benefit, the physiotherapist should consider the following points:—

1. *What state is the patient in?* Is he bed-ridden? Is he confined to life in a wheel-chair? Is he comparatively mobile and self-sufficient?

2. *What appears to be the principal disability?* Is the primary *neurological symptom* flaccidity, spasticity, or incoordination? In order to assess this, watch the patient in bed, in his chair, or as he walks into the department: test passive and active movements, and ask questions of him and his relatives if possible.

3. *What can he do?* How much voluntary movement has he? How much, if at all, has he compensated for what he has lost?

4. *What can he not do?*

5. *What must he be able to do in order to become functionally independent, and what matters most to himself and to his family?* This last factor is of paramount importance. Valuable time can be wasted teaching him to manage stairs when he lives in a bungalow, but if he could open a door unaided his life would be altered! These last three questions can best be answered by asking him to perform simple tasks essential to normal living, and by questioning him and his relatives about his disabilities and the problems which face them.

6. *Why can he not do certain things?* This is *the most important factor of all.* Are his disabilities mainly due to: (*a*) *Loss of motor unit activity?* If so, is it a *cortical lesion?* This will be manifested by spasticity and grossly abnormal patterns of movement, e.g., dorsiflexion of the foot may only be possible if the hip and knee flex as well. Or is the lesion one of the *anterior horn cells?* This is manifest in flaccid, wasted muscles and loss of, or greatly diminished, power. (*b*) *Loss of sensory perception?* Particularly that of muscle and joint sense. A simple test for this is to ask the patient to close his eyes. While the eyes are closed a joint, preferably a small one such as a finger or the big toe, is flexed or extended and the patient is asked to give the position of the joint. (*c*) *To incoordination?* If so, is it *sensory*—demonstrated by the above test—or *cerebellar?* (*d*) *Spasticity?* If spasticity is not obviously demonstrated by the position of the

limb, its presence can be detected by testing tendon reflexes and by eliciting ankle-clonus. When considering spasticity it is important to realize that *spastic muscles for all their apparent strength are, in fact, weak muscles.* (*e*) *Muscle weakness?* If so, is the weakness due to spasticity, to disuse (in cases of spasticity disuse weakness will appear in the antagonistic muscles), or to a lesion of the anterior horn cells? (*f*) *Muscle imbalance?* This will occur, as stated above, in spastic cases in which the pull of the spastic muscles is so strong as to inhibit movement in their antagonists; or, in the case of anterior horn cell lesions, where the weakened muscles cannot overcome the tone of the unaffected group. The last three factors can all lead to deformity. This *must* be prevented. (*g*) *Lack of will?* The patient's powers of co-operation will depend on many things. His intelligence, his environment, and the effect his disability has had on him psychologically, will all determine his desire to recover. In assessing the amount of recuperation possible these factors must be taken into account, because without the patient's co-operation, physical treatment can do little: with it, it can achieve much.

Having made a first assessment of the principal disabilities (reviews will be necessary from time to time) how can we deal with them?

LOSS OF CORTICAL MOTOR UNIT ACTIVITY.—Briefly, we have two problems— that of *spasticity*, and of *deranged movement patterns.* We must, then, reduce spasticity and re-educate more normal control. Spasticity can be reduced by heat or by cold; by deep rhythmical sedative massage; by prolonged, stretching, passive movements; by positioning; by active contraction of both the antagonistic *and* the spastic group of muscles. Having reduced spasticity, re-education of normal movement must then begin.

LOSS OF ANTERIOR HORN CELL ACTIVITY.—By bringing as many sensory stimuli as possible to bear on the anterior horn cells, activity can be induced in cells which have been damaged, but not completely destroyed. Methods of proprioceptive facilitation already mentioned should be used fully in all re-education of the anterior horn cells.

SENSORY PERCEPTION.—Where possible, proprioceptive and exteroceptive stimuli should be used; where this is not recoverable the eyes and ears must be trained to give the necessary information. By training one or other of these mechanisms the effects of incoordination can be considerably alleviated.

MUSCLE WEAKNESS.—This must be overcome by the use of resisted muscle work. By so doing, muscle imbalance, joint stiffness, and the possibility of deformity will be considerably reduced.

LACK OF WILL.—*The patient's co-operation must be encouraged in every way.* The physiotherapist's manner and approach are of great importance, and everything possible must be done to stimulate the patient's interest. A high standard must be set, but it must not be out of reach; praise should be given when praise is due; but above all, the *rate of progress must never be too fast for the patient's capabilities.*

It is hoped that this rather formidable list of information required for the adequate treatment of patients with nervous diseases will not prove too forbidding to the student. Expert knowledge can only come with experience, but if she genuinely tries to put these principles into practice, the student will find that what may at first sight appear a hopeless task becomes not only very worth while, but of absorbing interest as well.

CHAPTER IX

DISEASES OF THE MOTOR NEURONS

I. Lesions of the upper motor neuron: Hemiplegia—Cerebral paralyses of infancy—Primary spastic paraplegia—Spastic paralysis due to injuries of the spinal cord. II. Lesions of the lower motor neuron: Acute anterior poliomyelitis—Progressive muscular atrophy—Amyotrophic lateral sclerosis.

I. LESIONS OF THE UPPER MOTOR NEURON

HEMIPLEGIA

By this is meant a spastic paralysis of the arm, the leg, and sometimes of the face, on the opposite side to that of the brain lesion. The trunk muscles and the diaphragm are not severely affected as a rule, since these are bilaterally innervated—that is, they receive nerve impulses from both sides of the brain. Thus, if one side is injured, the centre on the other side supplies the deficiency.

AETIOLOGY.—The principal *causes* of hemiplegia are: (1) *Hæmorrhage* into the brain substance; *embolism*; or *thrombosis* of one of the arteries in the brain. (2) *Tumours* of various kinds, or *inflammatory conditions* of the brain. (3) *Traumas*, such as fractures of the skull.

CEREBRAL HÆMORRHAGE.—

Predisposing Causes.—(1) *Arteriosclerosis* is the commonest predisposing cause. It is a condition in which the arterial walls become hard and brittle. It is either a physiological change of old age—hence the greater frequency of 'apoplexy' in old people—or the result of various diseases—heart or kidney disease, syphilis, lead-poisoning, etc. (2) Cases are often found among men engaged in occupations entailing *continual hard physical work* (dock-labourers, etc.), because the constant exertion keeps the blood-pressure high and so irritates the artery walls, bringing about degenerative changes. It is also frequently seen among those in whom a large intake of nitrogenous food or alcohol produces similar effects. (3) Hæmorrhage tends to occur in men of a *certain physical type*—plethoric individuals of heavy build with short thick necks. (4) *Blood diseases*, e.g., pernicious anæmia. (5) *Aneurysm.*

Exciting Causes.—Anything which causes a sudden rise of blood-pressure may bring about a hæmorrhage in one predisposed—sudden violent exertion, e.g., running to catch a train, lifting a heavy weight, an attack of coughing, or even violent emotion.

Pathological Changes.—It is always an *artery* that is ruptured, *never a vein*, since the pressure in the veins is low. The hæmorrhage lacerates the brain tissue in the area where it occurs. The common sites of hæmorrhage are *the internal capsule, the corpus striatum,* and *the thalamus.* The blood then clots, the serum being gradually absorbed. The clot itself may in some cases be absorbed also, leaving only a small scar. This happens most often in young people, and the result is, to all intents and purposes, complete recovery. More usually the clot becomes organized. Inflammation is produced in the surrounding tissues by the presence of the clot, leading to an increase of connective tissue, which forms a fibrous capsule round it. This is more common in elderly people, and in this case recovery does not take place, though there may be slight improvement as the inflammation subsides.

EMBOLISM AND THROMBOSIS.—

A *thrombus* is a clot formed on the wall of a blood-vessel. An *embolus* is the whole or part of a clot formed elsewhere in the body, which has been broken off. It then circulates in the blood-stream, until finally it lodges in some artery or vein—generally an artery, since these vessels are of smaller calibre than the veins. Fragments detached from vegetations on the valves of the heart may also form emboli. Thrombosis in the brain is usually due to arteriosclerosis or syphilitic disease of the artery walls; embolism is often a complication of disease of the mitral valve. In *thrombosis* the onset is *gradual*, in *embolism, sudden*.

Pathological Changes.—The result of either embolism or thrombosis is *softening and degeneration of the brain* in the area thus deprived of its blood-supply. If, for instance, the branches of the middle cerebral artery which supply the internal capsule are blocked, the fibres in that part degenerate, and the ultimate result is much the same as would have taken place had there been a hæmorrhage (*see below*).

TUMOURS.—

In the case of tumours, the progress of the disease is very slow—spread over many months. Headache, giddiness, or coma appear gradually, as do the 'localizing symptoms', the nature of which depend on the situation of the new growth. Hemiplegia occurs if the tumour is in the motor or precentral (Rolandic) area.

It must be remembered that there is such a thing as 'functional hemiplegia', appearing in hysterical patients.

SYMPTOMS ARISING AS THE RESULT OF THE ABOVE-MENTIONED LESIONS.—There is not the space here to consider the characteristic symptoms of lesions at all the various levels of the upper motor neuron. The student who knows her anatomy can easily work them out for herself. We must confine ourselves to enumerating those found as the result of the commonest type of lesion—a hæmorrhage from a branch of the middle cerebral artery into the internal capsules. A brief note is added later as to two other types of lesions.

SYMPTOMS OF A TYPICAL CASE OF HEMIPLEGIA DUE TO A LESION IN THE INTERNAL CAPSULE (*Fig.* 78 B).—Symptoms really fall into three stages: (1) those of *the acute stage of the attack and the initial stages*; (2) those of *the period of recovery*; and (3) those of *the period of residual spasticity*.

THE ACUTE STAGE OF THE ATTACK AND THE INITIAL STAGES.—The occurrence of a large hæmorrhage is manifested by a sudden loss of consciousness known as an *apoplectic fit*. The outflow of blood raises the pressure in the cranium, *disorganizing the whole brain*, not only that part in which the bleeding takes place. The attack may be ushered in by headache or dizziness, or it may occur without warning. *The patient's face becomes flushed*, in contradistinction to the pallor of syncope; *breathing is stertorous*, because impeded by the paralysed tongue and palate; *the pupils* of the eyes are *dilated*, sometimes one more than the other, from paralysis of the iris, and *the eyes are turned towards the side of the lesion in the brain*, because of the paralysis of the rectus lateralis (external rectus) on the contralateral side; *the head is turned towards the same side. The pulse* is *strong, full, and slow. The limbs are completely paralysed and flaccid, and all reflexes are lost.* For the time, the whole nervous system is out of gear. However, there is slightly more tone in the muscle of the sound side, so that an expert observer can determine on which side the paralysis will appear.

The 'fits' vary in their details, according to the extent of the hæmorrhage and its site in the brain. In some cases they begin with convulsions; in others, the hæmorrhage is small, consciousness is lost more gradually, or never entirely lost. The case may end fatally, or the patient may regain consciousness in the course of hours or days. Sometimes *trophic changes* develop. The hand and/or foot may become œdematous, and blisters or bed-sores may form.

THE PERIOD OF RECOVERY.—When *reaction* sets in the pulse quickens, the temperature rises, and the patient becomes restless, excited, or even delirious. *The reflexes return gradually*, those on the sound side first. Sometimes the flaccid muscles become spastic, constituting what is known as *early spasticity*. This sometimes passes off till *late spasticity* sets in, usually some weeks afterwards. More usually the muscles remain flaccid on the affected side for a period varying from a few days to 2–3 weeks. It is thus that the physiotherapist usually sees the patient. There is *spasticity* and *weakness* throughout one side of the body, but the arm is the most seriously affected, particularly the fingers and hand, all

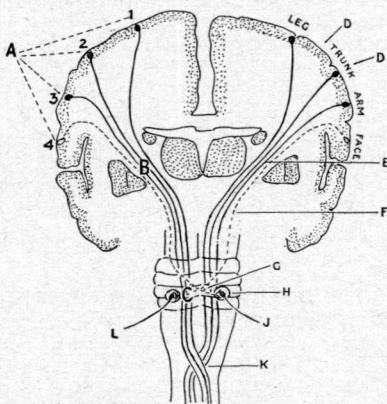

Fig. 78.—Positions of lesions of upper motor neuron (hemiplegia). A, Motor cortex: B, Internal capsule; C, Pons. The remaining letters indicate structures. D, Cerebral cortex; E, Internal capsule; F, Upper neuron fibres for face; G, Decussation of facial fibres; H, Facial nucleus; J, L, Facial nerves; K, Decussation of pyramids (fibres for limbs).

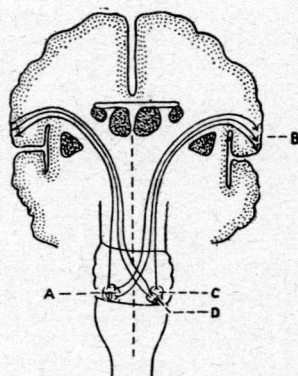

Fig. 79.—Connexions of facial nucleus with cerebrum. A, Facial nucleus; B, Pyramidal cells; C, Upper part of nucleus; D, Lower part of nucleus.

skilled movements being completely lost. The position of the head will have returned to normal but there may still be some affection of the eyes for a week or so. The trunk and abdominal muscles will be weak and because of this the patient will take his weight on the unaffected side, whether he is lying or sitting up.

THE PERIOD OF RESIDUAL SPASTICITY.—

THE MUSCLES AND REFLEXES.—The reflexes now return on the affected side but are exaggerated; ankle-clonus and Babinski's sign (*see* p. 174) can both be elicited.

CONDITIONS OF LIMBS AND FACE (*see Fig. 81*).—(1) *The arm* continues to be more seriously affected than the leg or face. It is usually held close to the side in a position of *adduction*; the *elbow* is *semi-flexed*, the *forearm pronated*, the *wrist* and *fingers flexed*.★ Whatever degree of recovery takes place, the arm is always the last to be restored, and since, in both limbs, the coarse movements return before the fine ones, the small movements of hand and fingers are the last to be re-established. (2) *The leg* is held stiffly with the *knee* in *extension and external rotation* with the *foot strongly plantar-flexed*. (3) *The face* is the least affected, and recovers first. The paralysis is most marked in the lower part. This is because the upper part of the facial nucleus receives fibres from both

---

★ The student may meet atypical cases in the course of her career, but since the principles of treatment remain the same, they will not be dealt with here.

sides of the cortex, the lower part from the opposite side alone (*Fig.* 79). *The tongue*, when put out, inclines towards the paralysed side, being drawn across by the spasm of its intrinsic muscle supplied by the hypoglossal nerve. *The muscles of mastication* are unaffected, since the fibres for these, and for the extrinsic muscles of the eyes, are the farthest forward in the internal capsule, and so escape. The patient, however, finds that, though he has no difficulty in chewing his food, it collects between his teeth and his cheek on the affected side. This is due to paralysis of the buccinator, which maintains the tone of the cheek. For the same reason he is unable to whistle.

DISTRIBUTION OF WEIGHT.—From a feeling of instability and the fear of falling the patient continues to take weight on *the unaffected side*.

GAIT.—The patient leans towards the sound side and swings the paralysed leg forward in a half-circle. Both these movements are for the purpose of bringing his dropped foot clear of the ground, since he has lost the ability to flex the hip and knee.

THE SPHINCTERS are unaffected, as is usual in unilateral lesions.

SENSATION is often found to be altered to a varying degree. In particular, *postural* and *kinesthetic* sense is lacking.

THE HIGHER FACULTIES are rarely impaired.

APHASIA, or loss of the power of speech, is sometimes found if the lesion is on the *left* side of the brain, that is, in a *right-sided* hemiplegia. This is not due to paralysis of the muscles of articulation, but to inability to co-ordinate and combine the various nervous impulses by which speech is produced—*the fibres from the speech centre being cut off in the internal capsule*. Later, the patient may be able to say a few simple words, such as 'Yes' and 'No'. We do not know whether this is done by means of a few remaining fibres from the centre on the left, or by means of the rudimentary centre on the right. Frequently the patient has difficulty with speech, although he does not actually suffer from aphasia. In *left-sided hemiplegia*, which is rare, there is no interference with speech, except in left-handed persons whose speech centre is in the *right* hemisphere.

LATE SYMPTOMS.—In addition to the above symptoms *involuntary movements* and *trophic changes* may be seen in long-standing cases.

Tremors may appear in the paralysed limbs (damage to the lentiform nucleus?); also *athetosis* (*see* p. 189), due to involvement of the caudate and lenticular nuclei, or a kind of *chorea*, the last two symptoms being more common in children.

Trophic changes are sometimes seen in the skin. Muscular atrophy may occur in the hand, and arthritis may also develop, making movement painful. In these cases it would appear that the anterior horn cells must have become affected.

SYMPTOMS IN ATYPICAL CASES.—

LESION IN THE MOTOR CORTEX (*Fig.* 78 A).—This produces a *monoplegia* (paralysis of a single limb), in whatever part of the body is controlled by the injured area, i.e., in the arm or leg on the opposite side to that of the lesion. The extent of the paralysis varies according to the size of the lesion; for instance, an injury at A.1 in the diagram may cause a spastic paralysis of the whole leg, or may affect one movement only, e.g., extension of the ankle. A *hemiplegia* in a cortical case could only arise from a lesion so extensive as to make it very improbable that the patient would survive.*

LESION IN THE PONS (*Fig.* 78 C).—As a rule this produces a *hemiplegia* of the arm and leg on the *opposite* side to that of the lesion, and of the face on the *same* side, the fibres for the face being injured *after* they have crossed the middle line, the pyramidal fibres *before* their decussation. This constitutes what is known

---

* But as regards *infantile* hemiplegia, *see* p. 188.

as *crossed paralysis*. If the facial nucleus itself is injured, the paralysis in the face is of the lower motor neuron type. Sometimes the fibres which have crossed over to go to the nucleus of the sixth cranial nerve (abducens oculi) are also involved.

Treatment of the Apoplectic Fit.—

FIRST AID.—The patient should not be moved more than is absolutely necessary. If the fit occurs indoors, he should not be taken from the room where he fell, but should be placed on a couch, or even on the floor, until the doctor arrives. All tight clothing should be loosened, and the head should be raised. He should be placed in a position which facilitates breathing, and a free circulation of air allowed in the room. If the fit comes on out-of-doors, an ambulance should be summoned, and the patient should not be moved until it arrives, unless he is in a position of danger, e.g., in the road amongst the traffic. Hot-water bags or bottles, with a cover or wrapped in a blanket, may be placed at the feet, and ice, if obtainable, applied to the head. Nothing should be given by the mouth, and no further steps should be taken until the doctor arrives. The patient's recovery depends on the severity of the initial damage and recuperative power. If the clot is absorbed and little damage has been done to the surrounding structures, the patient will recover; if it is not absorbed, he will remain disabled to a certain extent.

Treatment of the Hemiplegic Patient.—

TREATMENT DURING THE FLACCID STAGE.—During this stage treatment is of supreme importance, since *much can be done by early treatment to minimize the residual disability*. Should recovery take place it will be some time before the limb is functioning normally, and during this period joints may stiffen, and deformities arise which hinder the return of function. In many cases which result in spasticity, early treatment can actually minimize the degree of residual spasticity. It is probable that if the patient is allowed to lie like a log in the flaccid stage, the complete inertia, together with some degree of sensory involvement, add to the resultant disability. In order to overcome this and to assist the restoration of functional independence we may be said to have the following aims of treatment during this stage:—

1. To prevent joint stiffness and deformity from muscle contracture.
2. To re-educate sensory perception.
3. To re-educate movement patterns.
4. To restore functional independence.

THE PREVENTION OF JOINT STIFFNESS AND DEFORMITY.—All the affected joints should be put through a full range of passive movements daily, particular attention being paid to the shoulder-joint which is the most vulnerable. A simple pulley circuit, or sling suspension apparatus, can be rigged over the bed to allow the patient to give himself passive exercise. *Positioning of the limbs is very important.* Since the spastic pattern in the arm is flexion, adduction, and internal rotation with the forearm in pronation, the arm should be kept out to the side by means of pillows, in such a way as to maintain *the opposite pattern to the spastic one.* The head and trunk should be straight and the leg should be prevented from externally rotating by means of a sand-bag. The knee should be slightly flexed and the position of dorsiflexion should be maintained at the ankle. Splints are not recommended because of the danger of pressure sores. A bed cradle should be used to prevent pressure of the bedclothes forcing the foot into plantar-flexion.

RE-EDUCATION OF SENSORY PERCEPTION.—During passive movements the patient should 'think into the limb' and try to do the movements with the physiotherapist. To help this he may be asked to do the movement with the unaffected limb as the physiotherapist moves the other one. In addition skin sensation should be stimulated by stroking, light slapping, and brushing with a soft brush or the back of the hand. *By far the most important factor is the re-introduction of weight-bearing on the affected side.* It is noteworthy that the arm is usually far more spastic than the leg and this is thought to be due to the fact that the leg is a weight-bearing limb. The patient should be made to lie, and as soon as possible sit, on the affected side and be moved from one to the other to initiate a 'feeling' of difference. The arm and leg should be held in positions in which weight can be taken on the hand or foot until such time as the patient can do this for himself, e.g., the patient should sit over the side of the bed with the leg on a stool and the arm at the side or behind him (*Fig.* 80). In this position simple balance reactions may be given. It is equally important to get the patient to stand and take weight on the affected limb as early as possible. The knee should be adequately supported to prevent the patient from falling. *It is important to see that no fall or loss of balance occurs during treatment, as this can adversely affect the patient's confidence in himself and his physiotherapist.*

RE-EDUCATION OF MOVEMENT PATTERNS. —By asking the patient to 'think into'

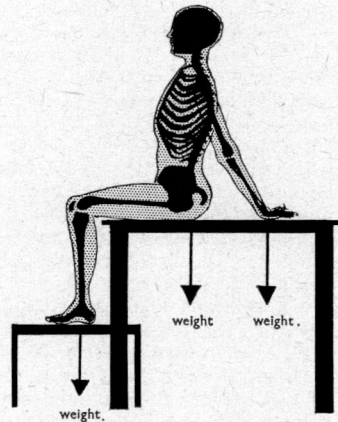

Fig. 80.—To show sitting position for weight-bearing in hemiplegia. Hip and knee at 90°. Foot dorsiflexed. Arm in extension and external rotation.

passive movements and attempt to do the with them physiotherapist, this form of re-education is begun. The limb *as a whole* should be taken through complete flexion or extension movements along natural lines, thus continuing a *pattern* of movement rather than an individual joint or muscle action. For this a knowledge of the Kabat patterns is extremely useful. As soon as any sign of functional activity appears in the limb it must be encouraged.

RESTORATION OF FUNCTIONAL INDEPENDENCE.— Whilst the patient is in bed he must be taught how to turn over, to move up and down the bed, to sit and reach for what he wants unaided. Much assistance can be given to the paralysed side by means of the unaffected limbs, and he must be taught how to do this as soon as possible. By making the patient use his sound side to help the affected side the strength of the unaffected muscles should be maintained, but specific exercises must be given if required.

TREATMENT DURING THE SPASTIC STAGE (*Fig.* 81).—Whether the patient has received treatment in the flaccid stage, or whether he first comes for treatment in the later stages of the condition, the problems are the same. We are confronted with a patient whose limbs are held in abnormal positions, and whose attempts at movement induce a flood of impulses into the spastic group of muscles *throughout*

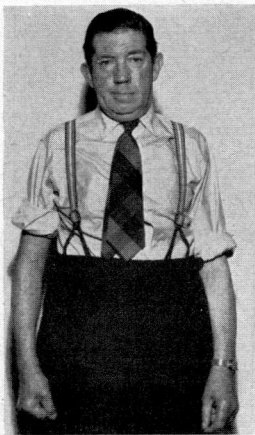

Fig. 81.—Patient with right-sided hemiplegia. The patient has responded well to treatment. Asymmetry of face still marked. There is considerable residual spasticity in hand and fingers and the elbow is still slightly flexed.

the limb, or limbs, thus enhancing the abnormalities. The aims of treatment now are as follows:—

1. To reduce spasticity.
2. To re-educate movement.
3. To strengthen weakened muscles.
4. To re-educate functional activities.

REDUCTION OF SPASTICITY.—This is too vast a subject to be discussed in detail here. An outline only will be given of various methods which may be used.

Massage.—This should be of a soothing and rhythmic character, slow and fairly deep. It should consist of effleurage, kneading, and stroking. *No stimulating movements should be used, as they enhance spasticity.* In some cases stroking induces spasticity, in which case it must not be given.

Passive Movements.—These should be given smoothly and slowly, but strongly enough to ensure the stretching of the spastic muscles to their full extent. The shoulder and the hand need special care and attention. When spasticity has set in, the beginning of the passive movement is difficult. For instance, in extending the elbow, the spastic flexors resist strongly at first, but as the stretching continues, their resistance weakens and the end of the movement is easy. This is known as '*clasp-knife rigidity*'. Care must be taken not to jerk the limb at this stage, or spasm will again be excited (stretch reflex).

The beginner is often worried by the occurrence of ankle-clonus when she attempts to dorsiflex the ankle. Pressure under the balls of the toes sets up a reflex producing plantar-flexion of the ankle—this happens normally in walking (*see* p. 174). In the hemiplegic patient the reflex cannot be inhibited, but takes the pathological form of clonus. Clonus is also elicited by initiation of the stretch reflex during passive movement. It can sometimes be avoided by keeping the knee in extension while the ankle is dorsiflexed. If the ankle can be taken beyond the point which stimulates the stretch reflex it will stop. In some unfortunate cases clonus presents a serious obstacle to walking.

Reflex Inhibiting Postures.—A very brief outline only can be given here of this valuable method of treatment devised by Madame Bobath.* Broadly speaking *the patient's limbs are taken out of their abnormal postures into positions which block the flood of impulses leading to these abnormal postures, and which allow more normal patterns of posture to be superimposed on them.* To put the limb into *the completely opposite patterns only induces greater spasticity.* The abnormal patterns are therefore broken up, *one or two components of the abnormal pattern being kept* (*Fig.* 82 A, B). Gradually, as spasticity decreases, further break-up of the abnormal pattern may be possible. To begin with the new positions must be passively held by the physiotherapist, until the patient learns control of these positions and can assume them himself. Finally he learns to move from these positions. At first into a 'normal pattern', later, if possible, into one which tends to evoke spasticity.

Kabat Techniques.—Various techniques of treatment may be used which involve isometric and isotonic contractions of the spastic muscles, and isotonic contraction of their antagonistic muscles. The technique described for treatment of stiff joints may be used to gain relaxation in spastic muscles (isometric contraction), followed by relaxation, followed immediately by an active (isotonic) contraction of the spastic muscles.†

---

* B. Bobath, "Some Observations on Adult Hemiplegia and Suggestions for Treatment", *Physiotherapy, Lond.*, December, 1959, January, 1960.

† H. Kabat, M. McLead, and C. Holt, "Neuromuscular Dysfunction and Treatment of Corticospinal Lesions", *Physiotherapy, Lond.*, November, 1959, and R. Barroclough, "Re-education of the Hemiplegic Patient", *Physiotherapy, Lond.*, September, 1958.

RE-EDUCATION OF MOVEMENT.—As spasticity is controlled, activity can commence, whether or not reflex inhibiting postures or Kabat techniques are used. *Early active movements should be as simple as possible* and should take place in only one joint at a time, so that the patient may give all his attention to the control of that joint. Later he learns to hold one joint corrected while exercising another, e.g., he may extend the elbow while holding the forearm supinated, or extend the wrist with the elbow straight. He thus learns to control two joints at a time. Gradually he is taught to control the whole limb. *Active movements should begin in the proximal joints and gradually extend distally.* The small fine movements of the hand and fingers will be the last to return and, indeed, may never do so. During active movements of a limb the other limb

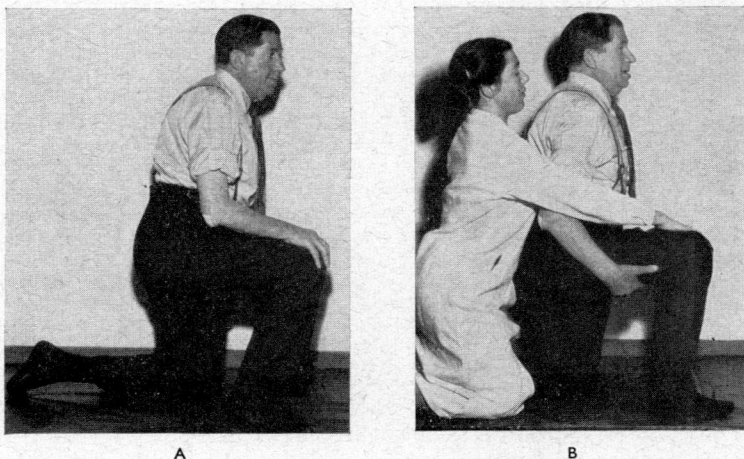

A   B

Fig. 82.—Balance and weight-bearing positions for hemiplegia. A, Half-kneeling position adopted by patient. The fingers are straightened over the knee. Note adduction of knee and thigh with foot in eversion. Weight taken on left leg. B, Corrected position. Thigh and knee will be held in corrected position until patient can hold it corrected himself. Lower leg and foot are straight. Patient's weight being pulled over towards the right.

should be placed in an inhibiting posture if possible, e.g., during arm movements the leg may be fixed in *extension* and *abduction of the hip* with the *knee in flexion* and the *foot in dorsiflexion*.

Suspension and Pulley Exercises.—These are invaluable in re-educating movement when the spasticity is reduced. They may also help its reduction. Both can be adapted to give resistance to movement in the later stages. Mrs. Guthrie-Smith has treated hemiplegics successfully by relaxation exercises in suspension. (Cf. Chapter XXIII.) Ball games and occupational therapy are of value in the later stage, to assist movement and co-ordination.

STRENGTHENING WEAKENED MUSCLES.—As spasticity is decreased and activity is made easier, power can return to the muscles. Resistance may be given, providing that it does not re-introduce spasticity in the limb. If the Kabat techniques are employed, relaxation and strength are achieved together. With other methods resistance should not be given until the muscles are ready for it.* *It must be*

---

* *See* B. Bobath, "Some Observations on Adult Hemiplegia and Suggestions for Treatment", *Physiotherapy, Lond.*, December, 1959.

remembered that the spastic muscles and their antagonists will be weakened from disuse and in the case of the spastic muscles considerable sensory stimuli may be required to facilitate muscular activity following reduction of spasticity. *It must also be remembered that the unaffected side of the body may bear considerable strain as a result of the hemiplegia,* and exercises should be given to strengthen specific muscle groups, in particular the *hip extensors* and *abductors*.

RE-EDUCATION OF FUNCTIONAL ACTIVITIES.—This should not be neglected. As movement is restored steps should be taken to see that it can be put to functional use. Activities required for the ordinary business of feeding, dressing, etc., should be practised, and help and advice given regarding gadgets and aids. Not least of functional activities which the patient requires is *the ability to walk.* We have to teach the patient to *flex* his *hip* and *knee,* and *dorsiflex* his *foot* if possible, in order to avoid the abduction of the hip, and the exaggerated tipping of the pelvis as the leg is carried forward. He has also to be taught to walk up and down stairs, to sit down and get up. All these complex movements may at first be broken up into their component parts, as in the case of a tabetic patient (*see* pp. 218–20). Correct weight-bearing must be practised, and to assist this various kneeling positions (4-foot kneeling; $\frac{1}{2}$-kneeling; and full kneeling) are valuable. (*Fig.* 82 **A, B.**) They also serve as reflex inhibiting postures and, as such, assist reduction of spasticity and re-education of postural sense. In severe cases, however, *the only way in which the patient can stand is through evocation of spasticity in the extensor pattern in the leg. One should therefore always be wary of too much reduction of spasticity in the leg.*

Needless to say, despite all efforts on the part of physiotherapist and patient, some patients recover very little, others make great progress. Each case must be judged on its own merits and treated accordingly. Neither in hemiplegia, nor in any other kind of nervous disease, is it of the least use to attempt to hurry progress, or push the patient on too quickly. To do so is to defeat one's own object, and no physiotherapist who is not prepared to have patience should undertake the treatment of such cases.

CEREBRAL PARALYSES OF INFANCY

CAUSES.—These affections are due to disease or injury of the brain before birth, during birth, or in infancy or early childhood. (1) *Before birth*, the trouble is due to injury or disease of the mother affecting the fœtus. (2) *During birth*, injuries may occur in the course of a difficult labour. (3) *After birth*, the chief causes of trouble are the infectious diseases of childhood which may lead to meningitis or encephalitis.

EXTENT AND AREA OF PARALYSES.—These consist of: (1) *Hemiplegia*, affecting the upper and lower extremities on one side of the body only. (2) *Paraplegia*, paralysis of both lower, or both upper, extremities. The legs are much more often affected than the arms. Occasionally the paralysis is confined to one limb and is then known as *Monoplegia*. (3) *Diplegia* or *Quadriplegia*, a paralysis of all four limbs, though sometimes in varying degrees.

Hemiplegia usually arises in infancy as the result of some infectious disease. Paraplegia and diplegia are more often caused by an injury at birth, or by a pre-natal infection. They are sometimes known as 'Little's disease'.

TYPES AND SYMPTOMS OF CEREBRAL LESIONS.—The symptoms vary according to the area of the brain which is affected. We may distinguish three main types—the *spastic*, the *athetoid*, and the *ataxic*.

1. THE SPASTIC TYPE.—This results from a *release phenomenon* similar to that described in adult hemiplegia. The suppressor mechanisms do not function normally, so that there is *hypertonia* in the muscles and attempts at activity result in a flood of impulses which increase the spasticity and hinder movement.

In these children *voluntary movement*, though it may be possible, is *jerky, slow*, and *uncontrolled*. *The stretch reflex is exaggerated*, so that excessive movement takes place, especially if the muscles concerned are quickly or jerkily stretched. The muscles themselves may at first appear normal but in time secondary changes take place—wasting, contractures, etc. The hemiplegic child shows symptoms very similar to those of an adult hemiplegic patient, and the aims of treatment are the same. In diplegia and paraplegia, the problem is rather different. The child's development is retarded, and he remains at a more primitive level than does a normal child. Several reflexes which are normally discarded during babyhood or infancy remain with the child through life, and

higher reflexes which succeed the more primitive ones are not attained. The '*scissor-gait*' is often a most marked symptom. Pressure on the soles of the feet, which in a normal individual gives rise to postural tone, produces a *crossed extensor reflex* in these children. The legs are strongly *adducted* and *extended*, which causes the child to cross his legs as he walks (*see Fig.* 83), the knees being held stiffly in extension. Moreover, he cannot bring his heels to the ground because of spasticity of the calf muscles. Before the child begins to walk this reflex appears if the spine is extended, often in conjunction with flexion of the arms. The child is slow in developing, and does not sit up until long after the usual time, nor does he attempt to walk until very late, the above-mentioned spasticity making it almost, or quite, impossible for him to maintain his balance. *Aphasia* may be present, but more often the speech is very indistinct owing to spasticity of

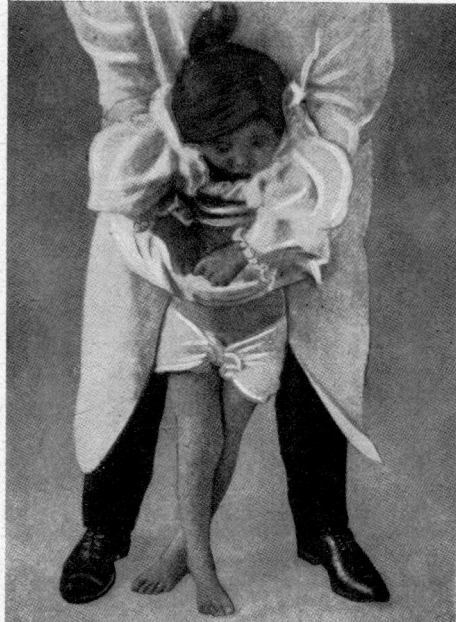

Fig. 83.—Congenital cerebral diplegia. Cross-legged progression.

the muscles of articulation (*aphoria*). *Deformities*, especially talipes equinus, are liable to occur as a result of the spasticity.

2. THE ATHETOID TYPE.—Athetosis is due to injury to the corpus striatum (basal ganglia, *see* p. 172). Involuntary movements (*see* p. 172) are the most striking symptom—strange writhing movements of the hands and arms or other parts—and the patient may assume very strange positions if startled or excited.★ The movements are absent or slight when the limb is at rest, but increase with voluntary motion. Reflexes are normal and the muscles are able to contract, but

★ These are caused by disturbance of normal reflexes, or persistence of infantile ones. The subject is too complex to be dealt with here. The student may consult *Cerebral Palsy* by Viola Cardwell, or other similar works.

the movement produced is abnormal and unduly slow. This is due to *rigidity* (*not* spasticity) of muscles. The symptoms, posture, and gait vary from patient to patient, but the latter is generally of a stumbling, lurching type. If arms and legs are affected, the arms are generally the worst. The forearm is usually held pronated, the fingers spread out, and the arm drawn back. The feet may be inverted and the toes hyperextended. The head may be drawn back, the mouth held open with the tongue protruding, or the patient may grimace in a way that suggests a mental deficiency which is not, in fact, present. The muscles of speech and mastication may be involved.

3. THE ATAXIC TYPE.—Ataxia is less common and is of a mild type which tends to improve. It is of the *cerebellar type*, balance and equilibrium being disturbed. The muscles are *hypotonic*. There may be nystagmus and staccato speech. (*See* p. 230.)

In any of these cases there may be *mental* deficiency. It is most common in *diplegic* children, less so in the athetoid type, such children being usually of average, or above-average, intelligence.

THE OUTLOOK.—In these cases, we have to recognize the fact that the patients cannot be entirely cured; they can, in fact, never be physically quite as other children, or, later, as other men or women. The actual damage to the brain is done, and cannot be undone. What we have to do is to teach the children so to adapt themselves to their disability as to be able to take their places in society as happy, useful, and efficient men or women. Of late years, an enormous amount of excellent work has been done on these cases. The importance of dealing not only with a child's spastic muscles, but with *all* his needs, mental and emotional, as well as physical, has been increasingly realized; and the necessity of *team-work* in carrying out his rehabilitation has been emphasized. Ideally, this should be undertaken by specialists in many fields—neurologists and psychologists, nurses, physiotherapists, occupational and speech therapists, social workers and educational and vocational specialists. Indisputable in theory, this is very difficult to obtain in practice, but something of the kind is necessary if the child is to attain the full development possible for him. In this team-work the physiotherapist should willingly and loyally co-operate. The importance of obtaining the co-operation of the child's parents, and of the child himself when old enough, cannot be stressed too much.

There are, of course, many different degrees of disability.

1. THERE IS THE MENTALLY DEFICIENT CHILD WITH DIPLEGIA OR PARAPLEGIA.—Here we can do little. Mercifully, this child will not realize what he has lost. If possible he should be placed in an institution, where he will generally be happier than he would be at home. *We have to remember, however, that many of these children are not really mentally deficient, but merely backward because they are deprived of the normal child's opportunities of acquiring information, especially if their speech be affected.* This type of child needs training by those skilled in this kind of work, so that they are able, after receiving physical treatment and careful educational preparation (preferably at a special school) to take their place with, and be accepted by, normal children.

2. THERE IS THE DIPLEGIC, HEMIPLEGIC, OR PARAPLEGIC CHILD WHOSE SPEECH IS UNAFFECTED AND WHOSE MIND IS NORMAL.—If the arms are not involved, this child has a future before him, since he may undertake (and often excels in) any sedentary occupation. If the arms are seriously affected, the handicap is much greater. Fortunately, this is rarely the case. The victim of a right-sided hemiplegia is possibly at a greater disadvantage than the paraplegic child, though some slight cases do so well that little disability is apparent. Fortunately, however, in all these patients much improvement can often be produced. Many have had extremely successful, and sometimes brilliant, careers.

3. THE CHILD WHOSE ARMS, LEGS, AND SPEECH HAVE ALL SUFFERED, BUT WHOSE MIND IS NORMAL.—This is the most pathetic case of all. The aphasic child often suffers from some degree of mental impairment, but it is quite possible for the speech to be extremely indistinct (from spasticity or incoordination of the muscles of articulation) and yet for the patient to have a normal, or even supernormal, mentality. He will sooner or later realize the extent of his deprivation, and very sympathetic treatment is necessary in the training of such a child, to counteract the effects of frustration and enable him to take his place in society. Efficient speech-training may effect a marked improvement, and even in such circumstances it is possible for him—like the even more tragically handicapped blind, deaf-mute—to lead a reasonably happy and purposeful life.

Inexhaustible patience is required in treating these cases. Sympathy, tact, love of children, the spirit of play, the power of stimulation and encouragement are all needed. But it is infinitely worthwhile.

Treatment.—

GENERAL.—*Instructions to Parents.*—Parents need to be taught how to care for a child with cerebral injury—physically and psychologically. Care of the skin in infants and small children, balanced feeding, correct application of splints or braces, protection from injuries and infections are in their hands, and must be carried out conscientiously, or the child will suffer. Also, he must be made to feel himself a loved and valued member of his family. It is often difficult for some parents to overcome a sense of guilt, shame, or in some cases revulsion. Sometimes they feel a stigma attached to themselves or the child. Nor is it easy to adjust the child's requirements to those of normal brothers or sisters. Many parents need wise and sympathetic advice from someone well qualified to give it. If a frustrated and antagonistic attitude is produced, either in the child himself, because he feels resented or unwanted, or in the normal children, who think that their interests are being sacrificed to his, an atmosphere is engendered which is very unfavourable to the spastic child's habilitation and development. On the physical side, the mother should be taught how to prevent bad postures, and encourage the child in useful activities: when and how to assist him—and when *not* to assist him, but allow him to act independently: what toys to choose for him, and how to teach him to play and amuse himself, alone or with other children. The physiotherapist should show the parents simple exercises to be practised at home between treatments.

PRINCIPLES OF PHYSICAL TREATMENT.—

1. THE SPASTIC TYPE.—The principles are similar to those given for Adult Hemiplegia, but it is essential to realize that whereas an adult patient has *lost* the power to move normally and to control his movements, *the cerebral palsied child has never had such power.* So that whereas the adult patient must be re-educated along old, familiar lines, the spastic child must be taught to develop. Our aims are *to prevent contractures* due to the disproportionate pull and secondary shortening of the spastic muscles, or to correct such contractures if they have already occurred; *to obtain*, as far as possible, *relaxation and reduction of spasticity; to gain control over exaggerated reflexes*; and *to train the child in the activities required in ordinary life.*

Splints, calipers or braces are used as required. They should be as light as possible, and must be carefully adapted to the child's growth. If contractures have become established before treatment is started, they will have to be corrected by progressive splinting, passive movements, and appropriate active movements. It is extremely important to see that a scoliosis does not develop. If the deformities are too severe for passive correction, surgical methods may be employed (*see* pp. 193 and 211).

Passive movements are essential not only to preserve or regain the mobility of the joints, but also to assist reduction of spasticity and to teach the patient to inhibit the stretch reflex—or, as it has been put, 'to push back the point at which the stretch reflex occurs' (Cardwell).* These movements must be given *rhythmically* and *slowly* at first, but the pace may be quickened as improvement takes place. No joints should be neglected.

General Relaxation.—This was once considered a primary necessity in this type of patient and it remains so in *athetoid* cases. It has, however, been pointed out that a spastic child can be taught (by prolonged training) to relax on command, but is no better able to perform some purposeful activity than he was before. He has learned to relax, 'but the minute he tries some purposive activity the tenseness, spasticity, and incoordination return'. (Hipps.)† Certainly, it is well that these children, often nervous, excitable and easily fatigued, should be able to relax as much as possible in order to rest, but their education, or re-education, in simple movements, patterns of movement, and everyday activities are more important still.

Active Exercises.—Simple active movements of the weak antagonists of the spastic muscles and of the spastic muscles themselves must be practised. They should be given on the same lines as for the adult patient (*see* pp. 186–8) and with the same aims in view. The movements may be given in single joints to begin with, the movement later taking place in several joints together, or activity may begin at once with patterns of movement.

Daily Activities.—These must be taught following the lines of a child's normal development, with which the physiotherapist should be familiar. If the child cannot sit up at the appropriate time, efforts must be made to teach him to do so. He must first be taught *to hold up his head and balance it.* Next he must learn to *maintain the sitting position,* at first with support and then unaided. Then *to take the position himself from the supine position,* by flexion of neck, spine, and hips. He must also be able to turn from the prone-lying to the supine position. At the same time, he begins to learn to use his arms and hands, to grasp and release, and make other simple movements. Gradually, he is taught to use his legs in reciprocal (alternate) movement, and to crawl. In this way he learns to control his muscles and acquire balance. Having achieved control on all fours, he must *next learn to stand and finally to walk.*

One by one, he learns the skills necessary for daily life, feeding and dressing himself, attention to his own toilet, speech, writing. One activity should be taught at a time. It must be carefully demonstrated, and then practised until it is as perfect as is possible. The child should not be required to learn several skills at the same time. Constant practice is necessary, and the parents should be required to co-operate. Sometimes various appliances are helpful, e.g., special spoons or forks to facilitate eating. As soon as he is old enough, the patient's own co-operation is all-important and the physiotherapist should endeavour to gain it by praise and encouragement, as well as by explanation of the reason *why* he should attempt to do certain things.

Games can have an important place during this stage, both from an educational and from a recreational point of view. We should try to get the child to keep his legs apart by riding astride rocking-horses, wheeled horses, or toy tricycles, and to play at ball games, nine-pins, etc. We need not be too particular as to how

---

* Viola Cardwell, *Cerebral Palsy: Advances in Understanding and Care.*
† Hipps, G., *Brit. J. phys. Med.*, 1957, **20**, 2.

such movements as these are performed, so long as we are preparing the child to get about and help himself.*

As regards *walking*, the suitability of aids, such as various kinds of crutches, must be considered. The patient may begin with walking frames or rails and later walk between parallel bars. From there he proceeds successively to axillary crutches, elbow crutches, and sticks. Some patients may ultimately be able to walk unaided. The advisability of training a child in the use of a wheelchair (in addition to tuition in walking, not *instead of* it) has also to be considered, as this may be necessary for him later when, in the course of his career, *speed* of progression from one place to another may be required of him.

SURGICAL TREATMENT.—Operations are sometimes performed for the relief of spasticity of the calf muscles, adductors, etc. These consist of severance or crushing of the nerves, or parts of the nerves, to these muscles, e.g., the obturator nerve, or the branches from the medial popliteal nerve to the gastrocnemius; of tenotomies, e.g., of the tendo calcaneus (tendo Achillis), which is divided or lengthened, of the hamstrings to correct knee flexion, of the adductors of the hip; or bone and joint operations, such as fixation of the wrist in extension, triple arthrodesis of the foot for varus deformity (*see* p. 330), or osteotomy of the femur to correct rotation of the hip. These operations are rarely performed on young children, because of the shock and emotional disturbance which may be caused. Special apparatus is used afterwards to retain the limbs in the correct position and, as soon as walking is allowed, re-education is continued. Careful after-treatment is essential.

2. The Athetoid Type.—Here our principal aim is *to teach control of useless movements*, and *to reduce the general rigidity of the patient's muscles*. To this end, we must try to teach him to relax consciously, and to carry out movements from the relaxed position. *It is extremely important to teach control of the head* since the unwanted head movements seem to govern those in other parts of the body.

Relaxation.—The patient should be treated in a quiet place, apart from other children, as he finds it very difficult to concentrate. We may attempt to obtain relaxation by means of warmth, soothing massage, and slow, rhythmic, passive movements. Later, actual teaching of conscious relaxation is added. He should be taught to relax the muscles, controlling one joint at a time, beginning with the head and the least affected proximal joints, and going on to the more seriously affected distal joints. We must try to get him to acquire the *feeling* of relaxation, either by contracting the muscles and then relaxing them, or by relaxing them in the position they are already occupying. He must then try to remain relaxed for increasing periods. At first the relaxation exercises should be given in the lying position; later, the child must be taught to relax in half-lying, sitting, and as far as possible in other positions. Breathing exercises are useful in assisting relaxation.

Active Movements.—As control is gained rhythmic active movements are added, the relaxed position of the body being maintained. They should be performed slowly at first and should be confined to simple movements of one joint. Gradually the rate and number of joints involved is increased.

Daily Activities must be taught as to spastic children.

3. The Ataxic Type.—This type is less common, and the defect is not generally recognized until the child tries to walk. Most cases are comparatively mild in

---

* Some patients with very slight hemiplegia or monoplegia may join with other children in an exercise class, provided the gymnast keeps an eye on them and allows for their disabilities. It is far better for them not to regard themselves as quite different from other children, and joining with others in class may obviate this. Such treatment is, of course, only suitable for those with very slight disability.

7

type, and the prognosis is better than in the other forms of cerebral lesion. The symptoms are of the cerebellar type, and are similar to those of adults. (*See* p. 228.) In principle the treatment resembles that for cerebellar ataxia (*see* p. 229) and tabes dorsalis (pp. 217–21).

THE USE OF MUSIC IN TREATMENT.*—Music is considered by many authorities to be a most useful adjunct in treating these patients. It has been found specially useful: (1) With mentally maladjusted children in breaking down inhibitions and providing release for pent-up emotions. Cerebral cases may well be maladjusted owing to unwise or unsympathetic treatment of their disability. (2) With the frustrated type of aphasic child, who can express himself in this way, and to whom music may appeal strongly from an emotional and imaginative point of view. (3) With all types of 'cerebral palsy' children, particularly athetoid cases, since it helps to improve rhythm in their movements. As well as co-ordination and control, it gives pleasure and satisfaction to most, and stimulates them to attempt more activities than they would otherwise have done. It is also claimed that certain bodily movements can be associated with certain tunes or songs, so setting up 'conditioned reflexes' and thus facilitating these movements.

THE PATIENT'S APPEARANCE.—Stress is laid on the necessity of spastic, and athetoid patients in particular, achieving as normal an appearance as possible. As well as receiving training in gait, posture, and the avoidance or control of abnormal movements (especially of *hand* movements which are particularly noticeable in the daily activities of life), the patient should be taught to avoid grimacing, and to acquire control of lips and tongue. This is necessary to prevent the dribbling which is sometimes a distressing symptom in such cases (special dental treatment may sometimes be necessary). The patient should be encouraged to take a pride in his—or her—appearance. 'On this (normality of appearance) depends the favourable or unfavourable first impression which the individual makes on people he meets, and which may mean the difference between being considered employable or unemployable'. (Cardwell.)† Also, from a psychological point of view, the elimination of abnormalities of personal appearance assists the child's own emotional development, or at least removes obstacles to it.

MENTAL AND SPEECH TRAINING.—Such training of dull, or backward children, who are also cerebrally injured, is a matter for experts. Nevertheless, while treating the physical condition, we must try to arouse the child's interest in his surroundings—to make him notice the objects with which he plays; to count his nine-pins, balls, or beads, or to tell us the colour of them. We may show him pictures in books and ask him what they represent. If the speech is affected, we may try to get him to say single words, followed by short sentences. For instance, he may be taken to the window and asked what he sees, as well as other simple questions, requiring at first only one word as an answer. Some of these children are best treated away from other patients for a time, in a room alone, or in a screened-off corner, in order to secure their attention—a difficult matter among distracting influences.

SPECIAL METHODS OF TREATMENT.—There are many special approaches to physical treatment of 'cerebral' patients in this country and elsewhere. Space unfortunately forbids more than a brief mention of these, but workers in this branch of physiotherapy will be wise to study these methods for themselves, so that even if they do not adopt any one of them in its fullness, they will be able

---

* It must be realized, of course, that not all physiotherapists are suited by natural endowment, or by training, to carry out skilled 'music therapy'. To put a record on the gramophone is not enough!
† Viola Cardwell, *Cerebral Palsy: Advances in Understanding and Care*, p. 192.

to gain many valuable suggestions to assist them in their treatment of these patients. The best known of these methods in this country are:—

1. THE PHELPS METHOD.—This includes many elements commonly used in other methods of treatment. Phelps used 15 special techniques, or 'modalities', and the workers in this system choose, or combine them, according to the type of patient to be treated. They are massage, passive movement, assisted active movement, free active movement, resisted movement, conditioned movement, automatic or confused movement, rest, relaxation, movement from a relaxed position, reach and grasp, and skills. The basis of Phelps' treatment is *individual muscle re-education*, founded on an accurate estimation of the condition of each muscle, progressing gradually to skills, walking, etc. The *athetoid patient* is taught to relax and perform movements from the relaxed position, as has already been described. Specific exercises are given for muscles which require strengthening. Since the athetoid child's movement needs to be slowed down, the establishment of a suitable rhythm for each is important. Much use is made of the conditioned reflex, induced through music. The *spastic patient* starts with *slow* passive movements, their speed gradually being increased. Later, active movements are given. Movements are practised first in single joints, and later in two or more simultaneously. Automatic movement (confusion technique) is used for 'cerebral flaccid' muscles, that is to say if a muscle cannot contract voluntarily because of a *cerebral* lesion, resisted movement of some other muscle may bring about a contraction, e.g., if a hemiplegic cannot voluntarily dorsiflex his ankle, he may be able to do so when hip and knee are flexed at the same time, and may be taught to produce the required action in this way. Most of Phelps' other 'modalities' are used in the 'orthodox' types of treatment. He considers treatment every other day the ideal.

2. THE TEMPLE FAY METHOD.—Temple Fay based his treatment on the teaching of *evolutionary patterns of movement*. Certain primitive movements have not been destroyed by the injury to the cerebrum, since they depend on the medulla, midbrain and spinal cord. The individual, like the race, goes through certain stages of development as regards movement. The young normal infant, Fay says, when placed prone on the ground is *amphibian* in his movements. He does not raise himself from the ground and he moves the arm and leg on the same side, turning his head to the opposite side. The movements then become *reptilian*, as he raises himself on hands and knees, and later still they become *mammalian*, with alternate limb movements, as in crawling. Fay considered that simple progressive exercises based on these primitive movements make it easier at a later stage to train the child in the human activities of standing and walking. The exercises should be practised for an hour, twice daily, and results should be apparent in from six weeks to three months. These special exercises should be in addition to, and not instead of, other forms of treatment.

3. THE BOBATH METHOD (Use of Reflex Inhibition).—This, certainly one of the most important methods, is also one of the most difficult to describe in a few words. *Madame Bobath considers that dominance of the postural reflex system, upsetting the rhythm of both voluntary and involuntary movement, is the main cause of the disorders of movements in these patients.* Therefore, treatment must be directed to the development of inhibitory control over the exaggerated postural reflexes. Perhaps the best short summary of the method is one contained in an article by Madame Bobath herself: 'The primary object of treatment is to teach control of primitive reflex reactions, and is attained by a special technique of performing passive movements without allowing any reflex contraction. The patient must be taught neither to assist nor to resist these passive movements. With increasing degrees of relaxation and improved control, he gradually becomes

aware of normal sensations while under treatment. He must then learn how to recapture these new sensations, which are the foundation on which normal movement patterns can be built.'*

This method can be used in treating children with spasticity, athetosis, ataxia, or any other type of cerebral lesion.

4. A word must also be said on the treatment practised at St. Mary's Hospital, Carshalton, by Mrs. Collis. Mrs. Collis points out that the cerebrally injured baby lacks the power of the normal infant to develop the ability to deal with forces outside himself, including that of gravity. 'The spastic type of infantile cerebral palsy is early recognizable by the expert as a generalized motor immaturity.' Mrs. Collis believes that, if possible, the training of the baby should begin at 4 months. He is then responsive to treatment, and he acquires the components of ordinary movement by the use of those postural responses, which follow deliberately organized postural variation. The patients will perform certain movements when they get into the appropriate posture for doing so. Hence the frequent, planned, alterations of posture which are a feature of this system. In the various postures, 'the fundamentals of movement are learnt— by the repetition of the simplest motor components, for example, arm bending and stretching, and other simple joint movements'.† Appliances for support or correction are rarely used at Carshalton.

5. THE KABAT METHOD.—The Kabat Technique of Proprioceptive Neuromuscular Facilitation may also be used in the treatment of cerebral palsy, especially of the spastic type, particular use being made of *Reversal Techniques*.

SPASTIC PARALYSIS DUE TO INJURIES OF THE SPINAL CORD
(*Secondary Spastic Paraplegia or Quadriplegia*)

AETIOLOGY.—This may be due to *trauma*, the injury causing compression, or section, of the cord at various levels—*tumours*, or *myelitis* (*see* p. 234). The majority of the lesions are due to accidents of a more or less violent nature. If the lesion is in the *cervical region* a *quadriplegia* ensues. If *below the cervical region* a *paraplegia* will occur, with *trunk involvement* if the lesion is in the *thoracic region*. The extent of this involvement will depend on the level at which interference occurs.

The resultant paralysis is of the *spastic* type. There are two clinical forms of paraplegia: (1) paraplegia in flexion; (2) paraplegia in extension.

PARAPLEGIA IN FLEXION.—This form always results from *compression injuries* or *section of the cord*, and follows the period of spinal shock during which there is complete flaccid paralysis of the whole body. Apart from the tendency to *contracture in the flexed position*, which can result in fixation of the legs in a fully flexed position if no relief is given, this form of paraplegia is characterized by *involuntary flexor spasms* which cause the patient much distress and discomfort. In addition to the involuntary spasms, any form of sensory stimulus applied to the limbs evokes a violent flexor response.

PARAPLEGIA IN EXTENSION.—This is the first stage in cases of *tumour* or *disease*. The onset is gradual and is first seen by *weakness of the dorsiflexors*, so that the foot drags. Weakness next appears throughout the flexor muscle groups and the *gait becomes shuffling*. At this stage the *tendon reflexes will be exaggerated*. Finally

---

* Berta Bobath, "The Importance of the Reduction of Muscle Tone and the Control of Mass Reflex Action in the Treatment of Spasticity", *Occup. Ther.*, 1948, **27**, 371, 383. (Quoted by Viola Cardwell in *Cerebral Palsy: Advances in Understanding and Care*.) The student may also consult the article by K. and B. Bobath, "Spastic Paralysis: Treatment by the Use of Reflex Inhibition", *Brit. J. phys. Med.*, **13**, 121–7.

† Eirene Collis, "Infantile Cerebral Palsy; III. The Basis of Treatment", *Physiotherapy, Lond.*, 1949, **35**, No. 9, 146.

the limbs become *spastic in extension and adduction.* In these cases there may be *extensor spasms* and *clonus* in response to sensory stimuli. If the lesion is confined to the pyramidal tracts, the paraplegia in extension will remain. If other tracts become involved, the paraplegia in extension is succeeded by paraplegia in flexion.

In either type general symptoms consist of *anaesthesia* in the area corresponding to the paralysis, with *trophic changes,* from which *bed or pressure sores* are very liable to develop. The legs tend to become *œdematous* owing to lack of supporting muscle tone. Both *bladder and bowel are affected.* At first there will be *retention of urine,* but later the patient becomes *incontinent* and cystitis is often a complication. If a tumour is the cause of the lesion, *pain* may be a prominent symptom.

Principles of Treatment.—

MEDICAL AND SURGICAL.—Appropriate treatment will be given for the cause. In cases of tumour, deep X-ray therapy or surgery may be used. In cases of trauma any displacement or subluxation will be reduced, to assist any regeneration which may be possible. If necessary, internal fixation will be employed to maintain reduction. Although the injury sustained by the cord results in permanent damage, these measures may make the difference between the patient's being completely bedridden, or able to lead a reasonably active life with the aid of a wheel-chair, calipers, and crutches. Catheterization will be needed at first to overcome retention. Later, the patient will have to wear some form of appliance.

GENERAL TREATMENT AND NURSING.—The following points are important from the point of view of physiotherapy as well as nursing:—

1. *Recumbency must be avoided.* Although it may be necessary for him to remain in bed for some time, the patient should be encouraged to make what movements he can, as soon as possible after the injury.

2. *Prevention of contracture and deformity.* There should be no actual fixation of the limbs, but they should be supported in as correct a position as possible. *It is particularly important to avoid flexion deformities at the hips, since their occurrence will prevent the patient being able to use calipers.* Sensory stimuli, particularly pressure on the feet or toes must be avoided, and the bedclothes kept clear of both.

3. *Care of the skin.* Bed-sores, or pressure-sores of any kind, must be prevented, since they will be indolent, and readily become infected. They will not only cause pain and discomfort to the patient, but they may endanger his life from septic absorption. His position must be changed at frequent intervals, and pressure on prominent bony points must be relieved by rings, pillows, special mattresses, etc.

4. *Nutrition.* This must receive careful attention, especially in patients suffering from sores or bladder trouble. A special diet is required, and blood transfusions may be necessary.

5. *The care of bladder and bowels* is most important. Infection of the former is a frequent and dangerous complication. The patient *must* drink plenty of water.

PSYCHOLOGICAL TREATMENT.—This is of tremendous importance in all neurological disorders, but particularly so when dealing with traumatic paraplegic cases. They are often young and their whole life has been shattered. They suffer severe mental and physical shock, and often become depressed, resentful, and despairing. It is vital that they overcome these feelings and that their morale is restored. Cheerfulness, encouragement, and enthusiasm are necessary to obtain the patient's co-operation, without which little can be done.

PHYSICAL TREATMENT.—Since paraplegia in extension is dealt with in other neurological diseases (pp. 228–30), we will consider here a *traumatic paraplegia in flexion.* The aims of treatment are: (1) *To reduce spasticity* in order to *prevent the establishment of contractures*; (2) *To strengthen the normal muscles so that they may compensate for those paralysed*; (3) *To re-educate the patient in walking*, and *self-care*; and to *re-establish him in some form of occupation*.

PREVENTION OF CONTRACTURES.—The patient's *position* should be carefully regulated. The paralysed limbs must not be allowed to become fixed in any position. Pillows under the knees are inadvisable because they produce flexion contractures. If the upper limb is affected, flexion contractures at the elbow must also be guarded against.

Passive movements should be carried out several times a day, to prevent or remedy contractures. They also assist the circulation.

Massage, if given, should be deep, rhythmical, and soothing. It is sometimes useful in connexion with passive movements, particularly for *œdema*, for which *a controlling bandage may also be used*. Great care must be taken not to stimulate a flexor spasm.

TREATMENT OF INTRACTABLE SPASM.—From the point of view of the physiotherapist, this part of the treatment is linked with that of the prevention of contractures, because 'the irritation of sensory organs in contracted joints and tendons increases spasm' (Guttmann), and the spasm, if neglected, leads to contractures. The flexor and adductor spasm, especially, causes great discomfort and distress to the patient. *Passive movements*, given smoothly and slowly, are our great resource. Sir Ludwig Guttmann has devised a form of stationary bicycle, or pedal exerciser, to produce passive movements of the joints of the lower limbs. This is fixed on a couch in such a manner that the patient can work the pedals with his hands, his feet being strapped to the pedals. The long-continued passive movements produce a fatigue effect, which tires out and relieves the spasm, so that sometimes, the patient can proceed at once to walking or other active exercises.

It has also been shown that *posture* influences the *tone* of muscle groups. In the upright position the tone of the *extensors* of the hips and knees is increased, while in lying, the tone of the *flexors* predominates. Flexor spasm is therefore less marked when the patient is exercising on parallel bars, than when he lies in bed.

RE-EDUCATION.—Following passive movements for the spastic limbs, *strong resisted exercises are given to the normal parts of the body*, in order to hypertrophy the muscles and enable them to compensate for the paralysed muscles. For instance, in a patient with paraplegia, the *trunk*, *abdominal*, and *back muscles* (especially the erector spinæ, quadratus lumborum, and latissimus dorsi) must be over-developed, because their action will increase the mobility of the spine, improve balance, and help the patient to regain his powers of locomotion. They tilt and rotate the pelvis, and swing the trunk, thus partly compensating for the lost, or impaired, leg movements. (The strengthening of the abdominal muscles also facilitates the restoration of bladder and bowel control.) In a patient whose *abdominal muscles* are affected, e.g., in one with a lesion in the mid-thoracic region or above, the *pectoral*, *shoulder*, and *arm* muscles must be trained and developed. This enables the patient to use crutches, to take his entire body-weight on his arms, and to swing his body forward when doing so. In this respect, the *latissimus dorsi* is of very great importance. He must also learn to move in bed; to move from bed to a chair and back; and finally to stand from a sitting position. Calipers, or some form of support, will be required in most cases to enable the patient to stand.

Suspension Exercises are of great value. The patient's head and shoulders rest on the plinth, and the rest of his body is supported in slings. The patient, grasping the vertical bars at the head of the suspension apparatus in order to fix the shoulders, swings his lower limb and trunk from side to side, and practises starting and stopping to command, thus strengthening the trunk and shoulder muscles as described above. These exercises have also been found to assist the patient's circulatory mechanism, so that he does not feel faint or giddy when assuming the upright position.* Pulleys and weights, or springs, can be used as resistances at a later stage, or to train individual muscles. After this, exercises between horizontal bars are practised, the patient learning to swing himself in that position in which the spasm is less troublesome than when lying (*see above*). If calipers are not used, the physiotherapist sometimes needs to help him by keeping his knees straight.

If the lesion is high up in the spine, causing paralysis of most of the trunk muscles, the patient's balance will be disturbed, and this must be restored by means of *balance exercises*. These must begin as early as possible, first in lying, then in half-lying and sitting. He then practises arm-raising in different directions, forwards, outwards, and upwards, until he can keep his body upright with the arms in any position. Later, he will learn to do this between horizontal bars, raising one arm at a time from the support.

As soon as possible, the patient is encouraged to become independent. He learns to dress himself in an increasingly short time, and then to walk by means of pelvic tilting movements, forward swinging, etc., first between the horizontal bars, or in a walking machine, and then with arm or elbow crutches. Any *supports* (calipers, etc.) should be as light as possible, and should not include the pelvic area or trunk unless this is absolutely necessary for support.

Games, Occupational Therapy, and Re-training.—It is most important from a psychological, as well as from a physical point of view, that suitable occupations should be found for these patients. Many games can be played at a very early stage—ball games, darts, etc., and many others can be adapted to their disabilities. Occupational therapy is of great value, both from a mental and physical point of view. Finally, training in a trade or profession which will make them fully independent should be given. Any necessary adjustments such as the installation of rails and ramps, and the adaptation of toilet fittings and furniture, should be made in the home.

SURGICAL TREATMENT.—In cases of *intractable spasticity*, Dr. Guttmann injects alcohol into the spinal theca. This temporarily transforms the spastic paralysis into one of the flaccid type, relieving the patient from the intense discomfort and distress caused by the reflex spasm. The effect is said to last 6 months or more.

Primary Spastic Paraplegia

Occasionally the symptoms are first manifest in both legs. This was at one time thought to be due to disease of the pyrimidal tracts but it is now believed to be a form of amyotrophic lateral sclerosis (*see* p. 213).

II. LESIONS OF THE LOWER MOTOR NEURON

ACUTE ANTERIOR POLIOMYELITIS
(*Infantile Paralysis*)

This is an acute inflammation of the anterior horns of the spinal grey matter (*Fig.* 84), giving rise to flaccid paralysis.

AETIOLOGY.—The disease is due to a virus, specific in its action, which primarily attacks and destroys the anterior horn cells, though it may also attack the grey matter of the brain-stem and the motor cells of the cerebral cortex. Recent researches have revealed that several different viruses may cause poliomyelitis.

---

* For a full explanation of this *see* O. F. Guthrie Smith, *Rehabilitation, Re-education and Remedial Exercises*, 2nd edition, p. 445.

Susceptibility is increased following removal of adenoids or tonsils, dental extractions, and during pregnancy and lactation. Excessive exertion after infection has taken place is followed by severe and extensive paralysis.

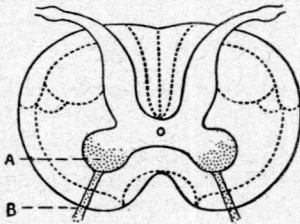

Fig. 84.—Acute anterior poliomyelitis. A, Anterior horn; B, Anterior nerve-root.

The disease may be *epidemic* or *sporadic*, both forms generally appearing in late summer or autumn. The epidemic form attacks both children and adults, and is often fatal. Serious outbreaks occur from time to time in America, Norway, Sweden, etc., but are less frequent in this country, though the incidence has increased since the 1947 epidemic which assumed quite formidable proportions. The sporadic form, though its after-effects are often lamentable, is very rarely fatal. In the epidemic form, the diaphragm and intercostal muscles may be affected, and the patient may die from respiratory paralysis. Children between the ages of 1 and 4 years are most often attacked, though no age is immune. It is to be hoped that with the increasingly widespread use of anti-poliomyelitis vaccines this disease will soon be controlled.

The disease is *contagious* and it can be spread by 'carriers' as well as by those who are in the incubation period, or early stages of the disease. It may be spread by droplet infection from the nasopharynx, or via the fæces, the latter now being thought to be the principal mode of conveyance. It may therefore be transmitted by ingestion or inhalation, the virus entering by way of the gastro-intestinal tract, or the nose and throat. Swimming-baths, milk, and fruit have all been blamed for the spread of the disease. The *incubation period* is 7–14 days.

PATHOLOGICAL CHANGES.—The virus probably passes from the site of infection along the axons of the nerves whose endings are in the area, and thence reaches the spinal cord, where it attacks the anterior horns. The blood-vessels in this region become engorged and inflamed, and the membranes around the affected part become hyperæmic. At first the large motor cells of the anterior horns hypertrophy, and later they degenerate. This degeneration spreads to the anterior nerve-roots and to the nerve-trunks. *The nervous elements are thus destroyed, and the neuroglia, which is increased in amount, takes their place.*

As a result of the destruction of these

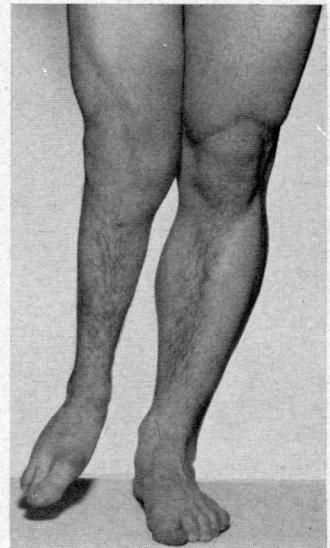

Fig. 85.—Muscle atrophy following anterior poliomyelitis affecting right leg, particularly anterior and posterior tibial groups and calf muscles.

neurons, the muscles, cut off from the trophic centres, also show signs of degeneration; they become *flaccid*, and *atrophy* sets in early (*Fig.* 85). If a whole muscle is thus destroyed, it ends by becoming merely a fibrous or fatty mass.

Polio-encephalitis or *bulbar form* is the result of the same virus, but in this case it is the *grey matter of the higher centres* that is attacked. The nuclei of the *cranial nerves* are generally involved, particularly the facial nerve and the abducens oculi. At the same time there may be a lesion in the cord. It is common following tonsillectomy.

SYMPTOMS.—

Not all patients who contract the disease suffer from paralysis. There is a *non-paralytic* or *abortive form*, in which the patient has a febrile attack, or may develop symptoms resembling meningitis, but these soon pass off leaving no disability. (Probably many people have acquired immunity through an unrecognized abortive attack.) In the *bulbar form* (polio-encephalitis), in which one or more of the nuclei of the cranial nerves are involved, the nerves of the larynx or pharynx are also affected and the patient is nursed in a respirator. Mortality is high in this type of case.

The *paralytic or spinal form* is that with which we, as physiotherapists, are chiefly concerned. The symptoms of this are as follows:—

THE ACUTE STAGE.—(1) Pre-paralytic; (2) Paralytic.

Pre-paralytic Stage.—*The onset* is often *acute*, and usually *febrile*, the fever reaching its height at about the third day. The febrile stage may or may not be preceded by a period of *malaise*—headache, sore throat—lasting from 4 to 7 days. In two or three days the paralysis appears, but before this there are signs of irritation of the meninges—*cervical* and *back rigidity, hyperæsthesia,* and *tenderness of the limbs*—with vomiting or even convulsions. The pain in the limbs persists for some weeks, and is increased by movement. The early rigidity is due to the meningitic inflammation which causes reflex contraction of the muscles to take place, in order to avoid pain from the movement which would cause stretching of the inflamed cord and meninges. With the onset of paralysis, *spasm* is to be found in the muscles deprived of their nerve-supply. *This must not be confused with the spasticity of upper motor neuron disease.* It is a protective reflex. Stretching movements would tear the newly-formed fibrous tissues in these muscles, thus causing pain, and any remaining fibres in the muscles go into protective contraction to prevent this.

Paralytic Stage.—*The paralysis* is often very extensive at first and may involve all four limbs and the trunk. This is because, during the acute stage, many cells not actually destroyed are compressed by the products of the inflammation, and thus temporarily put out of action. Others, though infected with the virus, are not so seriously damaged as to be incapable of recovery. Gradually signs of recovery appear. As the inflammation subsides, the compressed cells gradually resume their activities and the spasm and tenderness in the muscles diminish. This may take anything from 2 to 5 weeks, after which time the patient enters the *convalescent stage. The residual paralysis* varies greatly in extent. All four limbs may be involved in different degrees; only one muscle group; or even a single muscle. *The lower limbs are more frequently affected than the upper,* the *anterior tibial group* and *peronei* being most often paralysed. Next to these in frequency come the *quadriceps* and *glutei.* In the arm, the *deltoid* is often the chief sufferer. The paralysis may be symmetrical or asymmetrical. It is more often the latter, e.g., the anterior tibial group may be affected in one leg, and the quadriceps in the other. Complete recovery is very rare. Spinal or abdominal and respiratory muscles may also be affected. If the respiratory muscles are involved the patient will suffer from dyspnœa, and expiratory efforts such as coughing may be affected. One attack confers immunity against a virus of the same type.

CHRONIC STAGE.—

The flaccid muscles soon atrophy. The part looks fairly normal at first, but soon the wasting becomes apparent. If the whole limb is affected, defective circulation causes it to look cold and blue. *The reflexes* are lost in the affected parts. *Trophic changes* may take place in the skin and nails and the growth of bone may be arrested, causing shortening of the limb. *Reaction of degeneration* is present. *Deformities* tend to develop in the later stages. They are due to *muscle imbalance*, i.e., the unopposed pull of healthy antagonists of the paralysed groups, often assisted by the pull of gravity which leads to adaptive shortening. In some cases they are due to the *adaptive shortening* of the affected muscles themselves, which leads to reciprocal lengthening, and consequent loss of power, in their antagonists. For example, talipes equinus results from paralysis of the anterior tibial group alone, while the calf muscles are intact; or flexion deformity can occur at the elbow from paralysis of the biceps and brachialis, although the triceps may be healthy. Scoliosis appears either because one leg is shortened, or one arm is powerless, or else because of the unilateral paralysis of abdominal or back muscles, or of the psoas. The sphincters are usually unaffected, and sensation remains normal. In the epidemic form the lesions are more extensive, and the symptoms, therefore, more serious. Secondary changes may occur in the lungs or urinary tract.

Principles of Treatment.—For the purposes of describing the treatment, the course of the disease will be divided into three stages: the acute, the convalescent (i.e., stage of recovery), and the chronic (i.e., stage of permanent disability).

The Acute Stage

This includes the initial attack, and the period immediately succeeding it, and lasts from four to six weeks.* The most important part of the treatment at this time is *rest*, with appropriate medical measures and nursing. Proper precautions have to be taken against infection. If the respiration is seriously hampered, the patient may have to be placed in the 'iron lung', or some other form of apparatus for artificial respiration. So long as the limbs are tender and painful, physical treatment is chiefly directed towards *the relief of pain and spasm*, and *the prevention of deformities*. A start may be made even at this stage, however, in assisting recovery of muscles. Appropriate splints or supports may be applied as necessary, but these should be as light and simple as possible, and it is better to rely on *positioning* to prevent deformities. The optimum position is chosen as follows: the patient lies flat on his back with *hip* and *knee slightly flexed* by a very small pillow under the knee; the *foot* is in *dorsiflexion* to a right angle, neither inverted nor everted. The *arm*, if affected, should be in *abduction* to shoulder level, with *elbow semiflexed*, *wrist dorsiflexed*, *thumb in opposition*, and *fingers slightly flexed*. Hot packs may be used to relieve pain (Kenny treatment), moist heat being more effective than dry in the relief of spasm. At this stage treatment should also include passive movements to help in the prevention of contractures. *They must always be given within the limit of pain*, and this is particularly important when dealing with children. A child who has been hurt will become frightened of treatment, and much time may have to be spent in regaining his confidence before he will submit to further treatment. As the condition becomes less acute (that is, as soon as the tenderness of the limbs has disappeared), during what may be called the *transitional* period, between the acute and convalescent stage, more intensive treatment can begin. To begin with, the treatment sessions should be short and the patient treated twice if not thrice a day.

PHYSICAL TREATMENT.—

MASSAGE, if given, should consist only of very gentle *effleurage* and *kneading*, with, perhaps, light frictions round the joints. It is most important to maintain the circulation in paralysed muscles, which, cut off from their trophic centres,

---

* Trueta describes the acute stage as lasting from two to three weeks, followed by a transitional stage of from one to eight weeks, before the stage of recovery is reached. Its length depends mainly on the severity of the meningitic symptoms.

are unable to obtain a proper blood-supply. It cannot be over-emphasized, however, that in *any case of flaccid paralysis*, especially in the early stages, the *massage should only be of the gentlest kind*, great care being taken not to exert too much pressure on the delicate muscles, which might so easily be bruised or injured. We have also to remember, as Dr. Mennel points out, "how simple it is to overdo massage treatment in these cases Any excess leads to paralytic dilatation (of vessels), which means that the stagnation of the circulation—already present to some extent as the result of the paralysis—is increased by our manipulations, and thus the very evil which we are attempting to remedy is actually enhanced."*

PASSIVE MOVEMENTS.—These must begin as soon as possible, in order to obtain at least a useful range of movements in the joints. This is important in the early stages of the illness, because *it is at this time that degenerative changes are taking place in the muscles deprived of their nerve-supply*. Again they may either become shortened or lengthened, and it cannot be stressed enough that *these movements must be given very gently*. Stretching nerve-roots, or pressing on tender muscles will cause pain and increase spasm, and, in children, the joints themselves may be injured. Sister Kenny advocated hot packs to relieve pain and spasm in the muscles. These should cover the affected muscle groups entirely, and the treatment should be continued as long as pain and spasm persist. Not only do they give great relief and comfort to the patient, but they enable passive movement to be carried further, so that joint mobility is better maintained.

With regard to the 'transitional stage', it has been pointed out† that during this period, i.e., while any inflammation of the central nervous system or meninges persists—shown by lethargy, irritability, or feelings of fatigue—the patient must be allowed adequate rest. The question of fatigue is a moot point. At one stage it was a widely held belief that to work the paralysed muscles to the point of fatigue led to further damage to nerve-cells, and thus increased the residual disability. Nowadays, however, it is generally accepted that this does not occur and that the muscles should be worked to their maximum capacity if recovery is to take place. Such intensive re-education should not, however, begin for 4 to 6 weeks, by which time all meningeal symptoms should have disappeared.

RESPIRATORY COMPLICATIONS.—These may occur in *spinal* as well as *bulbar* cases. In the latter, because of paralysis of the muscles of the jaw, tongue, palate, pharynx, and larynx, the patient is unable to keep the passage of the lungs free from secretions of saliva, food, vomit, etc. In spinal cases the respiratory passages cannot be cleared owing to paralysis of the muscles of respiration. Sometimes both spinal and bulbar factors may be present. Such cases will require artificial respiration in an iron lung or respirator, and in some cases *tracheotomy* may also be necessary. In addition, postural drainage and percussion, with assistance in coughing, will be a necessary form of physiotherapy. This cannot be dealt with in detail here. Students should consult Trueta's *Handbook on Poliomyelitis*, or some other standard work on the subject.‡

The Convalescent Stage or Stage of Recovery

This lasts for about two years, though the patient sometimes shows definite improvement after this period. *It is the most important time from the point of view of physiotherapy*. It is the period of recovery, and this can not only be hastened, but made more complete, by careful and efficient physical treatment.

Physical Treatment by Movement, Manipulation, and Massage, Chapter XXIV.

† Joseph Trueta, A. B. Kinnier Wilson, and Margaret Agerholm, *Handbook on Poliomyelitis*, Chapter XI, p. 8.

‡ *See also* M. Agerholm, "Respiratory Paralysis in Poliomyelitis", *Physiotherapy, Lond.*, February, 1959, *and* A. M. Symmons, "Physiotherapy in the Management of Respiratory Poliomyelitis" *Physiotherapy, Lond.*, October, 1959.

Probably *true recovery*, i.e., that of damaged nerve-cells and muscles, takes place during the first six months. The improvement noted later is mainly due to increased mobility in the joints, the hypertrophy of healthy motor units in partially paralysed muscles which compensate for those lost, and the increasing ability of the patient to adapt himself to his disability. Our aims, briefly stated, are *to prevent the development of contractures and deformity, to check atrophy,* and as far as possible *to re-educate the patient in the use of the injured muscles*; or, in cases where these are damaged beyond recovery, *to teach him how best to use his other muscles to make up for their loss.* It is during this stage that the degree of damage can really be assessed. It will be found that the injured muscles will fall into 2 or 3 groups: (1) Those which have had their anterior horn cells completely destroyed and for which there is no likelihood of recovery; (2) Those of which the cells have been severely damaged, but in which there will be some degree of recovery; (3) Those of which the cells have been only slightly damaged and which should recover completely.

GENERAL TREATMENT AND SUPPORT OF THE LIMBS.—
APPROPRIATE SPLINTING OR SUPPORT is important for two reasons: firstly, to prevent the shortening of the healthy antagonists of the paralysed muscles, or in some cases, of the injured muscles themselves, and, secondly, to avoid too continuous stretching of these paralysed muscles—which may retard their recovery. If there is paralysis of back muscles, a *spinal jacket* may have to be worn. If the patient is a child he may require calipers or special boots when he is allowed to walk.

Splints should be made as light as possible, and are usually designed to keep the joints in an optimum position. Aluminium splints with appropriate straps are excellent, but expensive. Cheaper splints are made of alloys of aluminium or metals. These are not much heavier, and are certainly a great improvement on the cumbrous supports applied in the past. Light removable plaster splints may also be used. All splints should be well padded and special care is taken to protect bony points. Splint-sores develop very easily on these patients, and, once developed, may be difficult to heal. If a leg supports includes the knee, a small pad should be placed beneath the joint to prevent hyperextension.

INSTRUCTIONS TO PARENTS OF PARALYSED CHILDREN.—The patient is generally discharged from hospital at some time during the convalescent stage. If he is wearing splints or supports (other than walking apparatus), the parents should not remove them *unnecessarily.* Foot-splints, especially, are sometimes difficult to re-apply correctly. If the child is being treated by a physiotherapist every day, there will probably be little need for removal; but in the case of a baby, or very young child, wearing any form of leg-splints, the mother should be taught how to re-apply them if they have to be removed for purposes of cleanliness. Damp or soiled splints may cause much discomfort to the child and irritation to his skin, and such accidents may occur at week-ends when the child does not attend the hospital for treatment, or during any temporary absence due to childish ailments. The physiotherapist in charge of the case should not merely show the mother how to put on the splint, but see that she is able to do it, making her apply it several times under supervision if there is any difficulty. Any padding on the splints used for little children should be covered with some waterproof material which can be sponged if it becomes soiled, a thick layer of wool being placed between this and the patient's leg, which should be wrapped up warmly. Some extra wool and a spare bandage should be given to the mother, if the support is not fixed by straps. She should also have explained to her how she may assist the treatment by keeping the paralysed limb warm, a long straight knitted stocking, made like a bed-sock and large enough to go over the splint, being the best covering for arm or leg. Cleanliness is also most important. The skin should be washed with warm water, and carefully dried, a good powder being used, especially on the flexor aspects of joints. It should also be impressed upon the mother how much her child's recovery depends upon keeping the limb supported in the correct position when off the splint, e.g., in not allowing the foot to be plantar flexed by bedclothes.

With growing children it is extremely important to maintain the range of joint mobility achieved in the early days of treatment, during the two-year convalescent period. During certain periods of development, when growth is rapid, there is a tendency, particularly in muscle groups around which there is a lot of fibrous tissue (e.g., the lumbar region or foot) for tightness in these structures to enhance a tendency to deformity. The process can be insidious, but the late results are disastrous if it is unchecked. Since there is a very real danger of a child who is kept on treatment for too long becoming 'hospitalized', a certain responsibility for preventing deformity must rest on the parents. How much they will be able to do, or should be expected to do, must remain at the discretion of the physiotherapist in charge of the case, and will depend to a large extent on their intelligence. Whenever it is felt that treatment can profitably be continued at home, the parents should be instructed in the art of stretching tight structures, supervising and possibly assisting exercises, and correcting bad habits or faults. *Before leaving this to the parents, however, the physiotherapist must really teach them the necessary techniques and satisfy herself that the treatment will be conscientiously and responsibly carried out.** The patient should, of course, attend the physiotherapy department periodically for a check-up to see that all is well, and in order that the parents may be given any further help or advice which may be necessary.

PHYSICAL TREATMENT.—

POSITION OF PATIENT.—The limb must be adequately supported in the optimum position during treatment. *It is particularly important to see that a dropped foot is kept at a right angle.*

MASSAGE.—If massage is used it can now be more stimulating, but it should never at any stage be heavy or forcible. *Effleurage* and *kneading* are best for the affected muscles, but stretching manipulations—*picking up* or *frictions*—may be used as well on the antagonists.

PASSIVE MOVEMENTS.—These are continued as before, in order to prevent contractures and preserve the mobility of the joints. There is no need to move the joint more than once *provided the full range of movement in the required direction has been attained.* The muscles which are especially liable to need stretching are the *adductors of the shoulder*, the *hip muscles*, the *calf muscles*, the *back muscles*, and the *dorsiflexors of the ankle*.

In untreated cases, where contractures have already become firmly established, considerable force may be required to stretch them; but the movements should never be violent.

ACTIVE MOVEMENTS: RE-EDUCATION.—*This is the most important part of the treatment* and it is essential to obtain the patient's co-operation, even if he is only a small child.

Our *aims* are *to induce the partly paralysed muscles to resume work*, so that any healthy fibres in them may *hypertrophy* and in some measure compensate for those whose nerve-supply is lost; and also *to strengthen the unaffected muscles*, especially those of the same group as the damaged ones, or those which have a

---

* Too much emphasis cannot be laid on this. Indeed, many authorities still feel that because of the very serious damage which may result from unskilled treatment, no relative should be asked to give it. The author believes, however, that, provided sufficient precautions are taken, much benefit can be derived from home treatment.

similar action. Failing this, we have, as stated above, to teach the patient to do *the best he can in the circumstances*. It is in cases like this that any 'trick movements' which are useful should be deliberately encouraged. *But this should not be done until it is certain that recovery of the muscles concerned is impossible.*

We have to watch carefully for the least sign of returning power, and as soon as a flicker of movement can be discerned in a paralysed muscle, re-education should begin. This is, of course, easier in children who are old enough to understand what is required of them, but even in babies some progress can be made by one who can understand and amuse them.

In the re-education of muscles in poliomyelitis, or indeed in any form of flaccid paralysis, a certain *procedure* and certain *rules* must be observed.

1. *The actual condition of the muscles must be assessed.* A chart should be kept recording the power of each muscle. The usual way of grading the muscle is as follows. There are 6 grades:—

0 = no contraction.
1 = a flicker of contraction, not sufficient to move the joint.
2 = a contraction sufficient to move the joint with gravity eliminated.
3 = a contraction sufficient to move the joint against gravity.
4 = a contraction sufficient to move the joint against gravity and some resistance by the operator.
5 = full power of contraction.

Improvements in muscle power should be watched for and recorded. The weakest muscles (grades 0 and 1) should receive special attention (Trueta), particularly in the early stages of recovery but, since those with the higher grading have the highest chance of recovery, they must never be neglected.

2. *The patient's limbs should be warmed, before and during treatment*, by radiant heat, hot packs, whirlpool baths, or in the heated pool.

3. *Make sure that the patient knows what is required of him.* The physiotherapist should show him what movement she wishes him to try to make, by means of a passive movement. If there is a corresponding sound limb, he should make the movement with that first; if there is not, the physiotherapist demonstrates on her own limb, or on that of some other person. In babies, the exercises must take the form of play, e.g., the child may be persuaded to try to touch toys or brightly coloured objects, or the operator's finger.

4. *The muscles should be placed in the most favourable position for working.* In the earliest stages the patient's position should be chosen so that the pull of gravity *assists* the movement. A little later he is so placed that the pull of gravity is *eliminated*. Friction is reduced as much as possible by using a piece of smooth cardboard powdered with French chalk, on which the limb moves easily. A suspension apparatus may be used, the paralysed limb being supported in slings (*see* p. 485) suspended from a beam over the bed or couch. This eliminates gravity, practically abolishes friction, and gives the patient the advantage of the rhythmic swing of 'pendulum movement'.* A 'skate' may also be of assistance. Later, gravity may be used to *resist* the movement,† and further resistance may be added by means of weights and pulleys,‡ springs of varying strength, or manual resistance by the operator. It is often possible to fit up simple suspension apparatus with weights or springs in the patient's own home. This type of exercise is specially suitable for adolescents and adults. The angle of pull of the

---

* *See* Olive F. Guthrie-Smith, *Rehabilitation, Re-education, and Remedial Exercises*; Diana B. Kidd, *Physical Treatment of Anterior Poliomyelitis*; John Colson, *The Rehabilitation of the Injured*, Vol. II.
† For application of these principles, *see* Chapter XIII.
‡ *See*, as well as books previously quoted, Dr. Mennell, *Physical Treatment by Movement, Manipulation and Massage.*

working muscles and that of gravity must be considered in relation to the movement, and it should be remembered that a force is most effective when applied at right angles to a lever.*

5. *The weaker muscles should be exercised only statically, and at first only a few contractions can be expected.* If techniques of proprioceptive facilitation are practised this theory is discounted, and an active contraction is expected (*see* p. 208).

6. *The patient should be worked hard but should never be exhausted.* He should not be asked to contract a muscle too many times in succession without resting. As the muscle grows tired, its contraction will decrease in strength and, if continued, will finally cease altogether. If a short rest is given when the muscle shows definite signs of fatigue, it will often recuperate sufficiently to perform another series of contractions later. Massage and movement may therefore be given alternately, or short rests may be taken between the attempts at movement. A perceptible improvement cannot be expected every day, but when any definite improvement does take place the fact should be pointed out to the patient, if he is old enough to appreciate its significance, and to the parents in the case of a baby, or child.

General fatigue can be caused by too much practice of complicated movement such as walking. If he is allowed to continue the exercise when he shows signs of bad posture or gait, these may easily become habitual.

7. *Finally, the healthy muscles of the limb must not be neglected.* There is a danger that unaffected groups will undergo a certain amount of atrophy from disuse, and this must never be allowed to happen. It must also be remembered that the *antagonists* of any paralysed groups will need exercise. It is very important to maintain healthy *postural muscles*, and strengthen any muscle groups which can assist compensation. Healthy trunk, neck, hip, and arm muscles should always be included in the treatment. If the trunk muscles are affected balance exercises should be practised before a mirror.

It depends on the individual case, how long it is before a child is allowed to walk. Some doctors prefer to keep a child off its feet for eighteen months, some less. In any case, when walking is allowed, adequate supporting apparatus should be worn if any muscles remain paralysed, and the patient should never be allowed to walk without it. The child with paralysed anterior tibial muscles will wear a toe-spring; the one with powerless hip muscles will need a walking caliper. Careful re-education in walking must be undertaken. A very careful watch should be kept for *scoliosis* both during this stage, and in the chronic stage. Breathing exercises should be given if the diaphragm, intercostals, or abdominal muscles are involved.

THE WHIRLPOOL BATH, when it can be obtained, is excellent for improving the circulation. Ordinary warm baths are also useful.

POOL THERAPY.—Swimming-baths have been installed in many orthopædic and general hospitals for the purpose of giving exercises to these and other patients. The heated† pool is perhaps the most valuable adjunct to treatment and can be used as soon as the patient can be taken to it. Many exercises can be done in the water which would otherwise be impossible. The patient can begin with simple movements and advance to more complex ones. Moreover, all the muscles of the body can be exercised in the one medium. The warmth of the water improves the circulation and thus prepares the muscles for work; gravity is eliminated and the buoyancy of the water can at first be used to assist movement,

---

* *See* M. Dena Gardiner, *The Principles of Exercise Therapy*; Edith M. Prosser, *A Manual of Massage and Movements.*

† The temperature of the water is kept at 98° F., and it is chlorinated.

and later the starting positions can be adapted so that the water resists the movement. Rubber rings are provided for support. *Care must be taken to obtain true movement.* For instance, the pelvis must be held firmly by the physiotherapist when teaching hip movements. Re-education in walking can begin in the pool. At first the water should reach half-way up the patient's chest, so that he receives support from the water and his leg movements are given assistance. He gradually progresses to shallower water which will render the movements more difficult, as the shallow water tends to resist the movements. Pool therapy is enervating, and the patient should be dried and wrapped in warm blankets following treatment. He should then rest for 20 to 30 minutes at least.

THE KABAT SYSTEM.—This extremely valuable method of treatment of paralysis was originated by Dr. Kabat and Miss Margaret Knott in America. They *re-educate the neuromuscular system* not by using individual muscles, but *by physiological patterns* of movement, e.g., in re-educating the flexors of the hip, the mass movement may include, as well as *flexion, adduction,* and *lateral rotation of the hip, flexion of the knee and inversion* and *dorsiflexion of the foot*—in fact, the movement made by the forward-moving leg in walking. Flexion of the shoulder may be combined with abduction or adduction. Patterns of movement for the trunk consist of flexion or extension of the spine, combined with side flexion and rotation. All movements take place through a *diagonal plane and have a rotary component,* these last two factors being very important. The reason for using patterns of movement is that such movements are more natural, an individual muscle not normally being used alone. Also, particularly in re-education of weak muscles, the strong muscles can be used to facilitate movement in the weak muscles. Great emphasis is also laid on *proprioceptive and exteroceptive facilitation.*

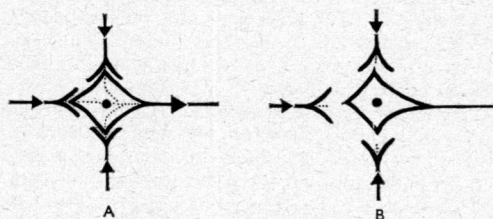

Fig. 86.—A, Normal cell synapse; B, Damaged cells; increased synaptic space.

In treating anterior poliomyelitis *every possible assistance must be given to encourage the firing of the anterior horn cells.* Those which have been completely destroyed will never function again, but those which have not been permanently damaged will respond, *provided there is a sufficient build-up of stimuli at the synapse.* The reason for this is that the damaged cells shrink, so that there is a greater space than normal at the synapse (*Fig.* 86 B) and there is therefore a greater 'resistance' to overcome. Besides making use of various sensory stimuli, an 'overflow' of impulses can be created by maintaining healthy muscles in a strong static (isometric) contraction. By preventing active contraction of the muscles, impulses directed towards producing such movement can be shunted into the weaker muscles and thus lead to a contraction in them (*Fig.* 87). For example, if the patient has weak rhomboids but strong extensors of the shoulder and arm, the arm is taken to its strongest point in its extensor range and the patient is then asked to hold the movement at that point whilst concentrating on retracting the scapula. *Maximum resistance is applied* to the extensors of the shoulder and arm throughout, by means of a hand placed on the ulnar border of the forearm. *Proprioception* is given to the scapula by placing the other hand on its lateral border.

A thorough knowledge of the patterns is essential in this work, in order to make the best possible use of their combinations. In treating anterior poliomyelitis cases, the distribution of paralysis will govern the choice and combination of patterns. For example, if the hip and knee flexors are weak, re-education may be given to the hip flexors as already described, but *extension* of the knee will replace flexion. Wherever possible the *proximal* muscles are used to give 'reinforcement' or 'overflow' but if the proximal muscles are not strong enough, *distal* ones can be used. Failing this the other limb, or even an opposite limb, can be used, i.e., if both legs are paralysed the arms may be used to give reinforcement.

The most useful techniques for the treatment of anterior poliomyelitis are those which *primarily strengthen*, but which *mobilize* as well. The simplest and most important of these is known as 'Repeated Contraction'. In this the patient carries a movement against maximal resistance, throughout its entire range, starting from a fully stretched position. The movement is punctuated at intervals by isometric holds, *but there must be no break in resistance and no relaxation until the end of the movement.* Other useful techniques are 'Reversals' and 'Rhythmical stabilizations', which have been described in Chapter VI. In giving reversal techniques the strong muscles are contracted first. *For both these techniques the antagonists must be strong.*

In all Kabat re-education of this kind the following rules must be rigidly applied:—

1. The hands must be placed on the surface in the direction in which the movement is to take place (*exteroception*).

2. The muscles must be fully stretched and slight traction, or sometimes apposition, given to the joint surfaces (*proprioception*).

3. Movement must be in a *diagonal* plane and must contain a *rotary component*. To ensure that this is maintained the physiotherapist's feet

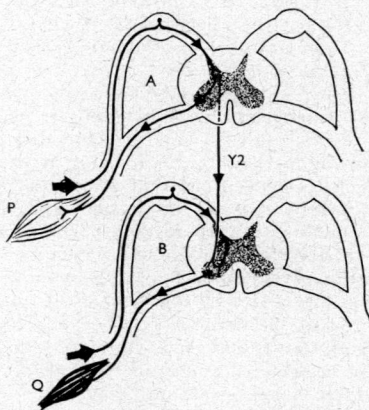

Fig. 87.—A, Section of grey matter of cord containing healthy anterior horn cells; B, Shows damaged cells; P, Healthy muscle; Q, Damaged muscle.
   Normal stimuli in A and B travel via post-ganglion cell to anterior horn cells, leading to contraction in P only. When contraction is blocked in P, impulses overflow via internuncial pathway Y2 to post-ganglion cell in section B. Normal impulses augmented and followed by contraction in Q.

be placed in the same diagonal. She can then apply even resistance, in the correct line, by turning her body on her feet.

4. Besides proprioceptive stimuli, exteroceptive stimuli are given via the skin (*see above*), eyes, and ears, the patient watching the movement and hearing the physiotherapist's commands.

Balance reactions are also used in the treatment of these patients, particularly when trunk muscles have been affected. The patient is pushed 'off balance', and taught to maintain equilibrium against these pushes. In this way various postural reflexes and balancing reflexes are brought into use. Weak muscles, as well as strong ones, will be brought into action to do this, and will thus be strengthened. This method is also used for cases of spasticity and ataxia.

This necessarily inadequate account of an important system should be supplemented by a study of the literature on the subject, as well as by practical experience. The student should consult the article by Miss Martin Jones in *The Principle of Exercise Therapy*, by M. Dena Gardiner, and the authorities quoted there.

ELECTRICAL TREATMENT may be useful with the older patients, faradism being used according to the needs of the case. We do not personally consider that it is at all suitable for small children.★ The constant current may sometimes be given by the bipolar method, the patient sitting or lying in a bath, suitably supported, the purpose of this being to improve the nutrition of the paralysed limbs. Dr. Cumberbatch recommends the use of the surging sinusoidal current. This may also be given in a bath. Short-wave diathermy has also been recommended, for the purpose of warming the deep structures of the paralysed limbs, a longitudinal field being used. This method would obviously not be possible in the case of infants or small children.

RADIANT HEAT OR INFRA-RED RADIATION is useful before exercise, particularly if the patient's limbs are very cold.

ULTRA-VIOLET RAYS AND ARTIFICIAL SUNLIGHT are sometimes given for a general tonic effect.

Much patience and conscientiousness are needed during the long course of this treatment, and much ingenuity is required to keep a child's interest and prevent boredom, but we have to remember that *the patient's fate is more or less decided during these two years,* and on the completeness and care with which the treatment is carried out that fate largely depends. A medical man, lecturing to the Chartered Society, once said that the hopeless cripples seen as the result of infantile paralysis are a reproach to our treatment. This seems a harsh judgement, but nevertheless there is truth in it. We have to see to it that the defective circulation is maintained as far as possible, so that growth of bone may continue, and the structures of the limb are kept in good condition. We must never allow preventable deformities to occur. *But above all we have to develop to the utmost, any power of movement that may be left.* If, through weariness or lack of interest, we neglect to do any of these things to the utmost of our power, we certainly assume a grave responsibility.

The Chronic Stage

This may be said to begin after two years, or even longer in cases that have received no physical treatment. Any recovery that is possible may now be presumed to have taken place. Muscles which are completely paralysed have become mere fibrous bands, with no response to any form of electric current. Our aims are *to restore what useful function we can,* and the principal methods of treatment at this stage include the provision of suitable apparatus for support; operations of various kinds; post-operative physical treatment, re-education in walking, occupational therapy, education and training for children, and re-habilitation, or perhaps re-training, for adults.

APPARATUS.—The forms of apparatus worn cannot be described in detail here. In serious cases, where many muscles round the hip are paralysed, the patient may need to wear some form of caliper with a special boot.† First he learns to walk between horizontal bars, then uses crutches, progressing to sticks, and, finally, dispenses with the latter if possible. Intensive training may be necessary in compensatory muscle groups; for example, if the *abductors of the hip* are quite powerless he is taught to use the *lateral flexors of the spine* to tip the pelvis.

★ They are generally frightened and upset by the treatment, and cannot bear enough current to do them any good. In any case, it causes them to associate pain and fear with their treatment, and this, it seems to us, is a fatal thing. The child should *enjoy* his visit to the hospital or the visit of his physiotherapist, and only if he does shall we be able to get the maximum of effort from him.

† Many surgeons prefer to dispense with calipers whenever possible because of their weight. Even the lightest instruments add considerable resistance to the patient's movements.

Each case has to be carefully studied and treated on its own merits. 'Trick movements' in arm or leg should now be encouraged if they increase the patient's general efficiency. Many useful gadgets have been invented to assist the patient with paralysis of arms, legs, or trunk in the activities of daily life.

SURGICAL TREATMENT.—The operations performed are of many different kinds. They may be briefly summarized: (1) *Operations on tendons*: tenotomy and tendon transference (muscle transplantation). (2) *Operations on bones and joints*: osteotomy, arthrodesis, and bone-grafting. (3) *Operations on nerves*: nerve anastomosis.

OPERATIONS ON TENDONS.—

Tenotomy is the severing of a tendon, generally by passing a knife beneath the skin, in order to overcome a contracture of the muscle attached to it or of the tendon itself: e.g., tenotomy of the Achilles tendon in talipes equinus. The tendon heals, but the contracture is abolished, the joint having been meanwhile held in the correct position post-operatively. *Myotomy* means division of a muscle for the same purpose: *fasciotomy* that of deep fascia.

Tendon transference consists of either cutting the tendon of a healthy muscle and attaching it to that of a paralysed one, or of removing a tendon from its attachment to the periosteum of a bone and inserting it into bone elsewhere. An example of the first method is one of the operations for dropped wrist. The flexores carpi radialis and ulnaris are transplanted into the extensors of the extensores (communis) digitorum, indicis, and minimi digiti, and the extensors of the thumb. The second method is used when, in the case of paralysed peronei, the tibialis anterior is transferred to the outer border of the foot to act as an evertor. Similarly, the peroneus brevis may be used to replace a lost tibialis anterior: or the biceps and semitendinosus may be inserted into the patella, or tibial tubercle, to act as extensors of the knee when the quadriceps are paralysed. These operations often succeed very well as far as voluntary (purposive) movements are concerned but they are not so satisfactory as regards automatic movements. Hence, they are generally more successful in the hands than in the legs and feet. A patient in whom for instance one of the peronei has been transferred to the inner side of the foot to replace the tibialis anterior, may be able to invert his foot quite strongly, even against resistance, but it does not follow that he will perform this action correctly when walking.

OPERATIONS ON BONES AND JOINTS.—

Osteotomy means cutting a wedge from a bone and then closing the incision, so as to alter the line of the bone (*see* p. 305).

Arthrodesis is used most often for joints of the lower extremity which have become unstable, so that the limb will not support the patient, e.g., in cases of flail knee or ankle, talipes valgus, etc. Stabilization of the joint allows the patient to dispense with apparatus and it is brought about by removing the articular cartilage, cutting thin slices from the bones, and fixing them in apposition so that they knit together. Examples of this operation are Whitman's operation and Robert Jones's operation (*see under* TALIPES).

Bone-grafting operations are sometimes performed to produce fixation of some part of the vertebral column in cases of paralysis of the spinal muscles.

OPERATIONS ON NERVES.—

Nerve anastomosis is a much less common operation than the above. It consists of joining the central end of a severed healthy nerve to the distal end of a cut nerve, the cells of origin of which have been destroyed and which is therefore degenerate: e.g., the spinal accessory nerve, or part of it, is sometimes grafted into the facial nerve in facial paralysis, causing regeneration of the latter.

PRE-OPERATIVE AND POST-OPERATIVE TREATMENT.—This is described in Chapter XV (TREATMENT OF PARALYTIC FORMS OF TALIPES), pp. 330–1.

PROGRESSIVE MUSCULAR ATROPHY

This disease is due to degeneration of the anterior horns of the spinal cord, and is therefore a typical lower motor neuron lesion. The disease is *progressive and incurable*, though it occasionally becomes arrested at a late stage. It may end by extension of the degenerative process to the medulla, involving the vital centres and giving rise to bulbar paralysis, or the patient may die of some intercurrent disease.

AETIOLOGY.—Men are more frequently attacked than women. The disease is one of middle life. The actual cause is as yet undiscovered. In some cases mental worry may be a predisposing factor.

PATHOLOGY.—The changes are those of sclerosis. The *cells of the anterior horns degenerate* one by one. The degenerative process may spread upwards into the pyramidal (lateral cerebrospinal) tracts (*Fig.* 88) and the muscles, cut off little by little from their nerve-supply, *atrophy*, become *flaccid*, and finally *degenerate*.

SYMPTOMS.—

The first symptom to appear is *atrophy and weakness of the small muscles of the hands* (the lumbricales, interossei, and those of the thenar and hypothenar eminences). The patient's hand later assumes a claw-like appearance. The atrophy spreads gradually to the forearm and shoulder muscles, and then to those of the back, missing out the upper part of the trapezius. Then, after an interval, often quite a long one, the legs become similarly affected, symptoms arising first in the muscles of the feet, the anterior tibial group, and the peronei.

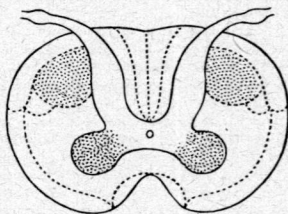

Occasionally the legs suffer first and the arms later. *Interference with respiration* owing to paralysis of the diaphragm and intercostal muscles may lead to a fatal issue. The degenerating muscles exhibit peculiar twitching movements—'*fibrillary twitchings*'. *The reflexes* are gradually lost. There is *partial reaction of degeneration*.

Besides the above, there is another variety of progressive muscular atrophy known as the *peroneal type*. This begins in childhood in the peronei and foot muscles, and extends from the lower leg to the thigh, of which it generally affects the lower third. Later it attacks the

Fig. 88.— Progressive muscular atrophy. The darker shading indicates the parts affected first, the lighter shading those affected later.

arms, the muscles becoming involved in the same order as in the adult type. The child may develop talipes equinovarus. This form is hereditary, or at least a familial type of affection.

COURSE OF THE DISEASE.—From 2 to 20 years; generally about 10 years.

Treatment.—No cure is to be expected in progressive muscular atrophy and although a slight improvement may take place in a hitherto untreated case, the patient is bound to go steadily downhill. The disease does sometimes become arrested, but this is very rare and not before much irreparable damage has been done. But undoubtedly its progress is considerably *retarded* by means of physical treatment, and the patient remains much happier if he feels something is being done for him. The principal aim is to maintain useful power in the muscles for as long as possible, and one cannot work for long among cases of progressive paralysis without realizing that *any* form of treatment which helps the patient to keep up his courage in the face of so terrible and incurable an illness, is abundantly worth while. He needs encouragement to fight every inch of the ground, even though he knows the battle to be a losing one. The physiotherapist should give all the encouragement and sympathy she can and whilst never holding out false hopes impossible of fulfilment, should be quick to point out any favourable sign. Treatment often affords a welcome break in the monotony of a bedridden patient's day, and should be as helpful and inspiring as possible.

SUPPORT.—The hands are not splinted as a rule, even at night. Provided the joints are kept supple by passive movements, the tendency to contracture of the muscles will disappear as the latter gradually become paralysed. The feet, however, should be supported in dorsiflexion when the patient is in bed, since the calf-muscles may retain some power long after the paralysis has spread to the muscles of the thigh, and a talipes equinus will prevent the patient from walking much earlier than would otherwise be the case.

PHYSICAL TREATMENT.—

MASSAGE.—This may be given to assist circulation and nutrition of the muscles. It should mainly consist of brisk but light effleurage, and kneading.

PASSIVE MOVEMENTS.—These are given in the usual way to prevent contractures and maintain joint mobility.

ACTIVE MOVEMENTS.—In the early stages, general exercises should be given; leg exercises should not be neglected even when the arms only are affected, nor arm movements, when the legs are first to be attacked. Dr. J. Goldthwait* points out the importance, in these and similar cases, of correcting the patient's posture as far as possible.

As regards the affected limbs, movements should be given according to the usual rules, except that, instead of being made stronger, they will have to be modified as time goes on. Resisted and free exercises may be possible at first; later, this work has to be assisted. We have to be careful not to produce fatigue and in this the Kabat method can be of much value. Hip movements, for instance, are a terrible effort to the patient when the muscles in this area are seriously weakened, even with gravity eliminated and with assistance from the operator. Suspension apparatus is valuable, particularly in the later stages, the slings being arranged so as to assist the movements.

The patient should not be allowed to become bedridden and should be kept on his feet for as long as possible.

AMYOTROPHIC LATERAL SCLEROSIS

This is really a variety of progressive muscular atrophy, but in this case the degeneration begins in the pyramidal tracts and spreads downwards to the anterior horns and nerve-roots. It begins, therefore, as an *upper motor neuron* disease, and ends as one of the *lower motor neuron* (*Fig.* 89).

AETIOLOGY.—The cause, like that of progressive muscular atrophy, is unknown. Both men and women are attacked, generally between the ages of 25 and 50. It is neither hereditary nor the result of syphilis.

PATHOLOGICAL CHANGES.—The same as in progressive muscular atrophy.

SYMPTOMS.—The disease begins as a *spastic paralysis* in the fingers and hands and spreads up the arms, the upper extremity assuming an appearance like that seen in hemiplegia. At the same time the muscles

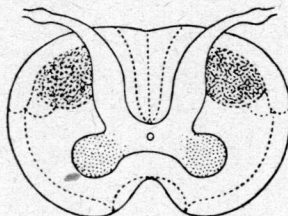

Fig. 89. — Amyotrophic lateral sclerosis. The darker shading indicates the parts affected first, the lighter shading those affected later.

of the limb *atrophy* very slowly, as the cells of the anterior horns degenerate one by one. *The reflexes* are increased at first, but gradually decrease and are finally lost. Ultimately, therefore, the *spasticity* disappears, and its place is taken by *flaccidity*, the symptoms due to the lesion of the lower motor neuron masking those caused by that of the upper motor neuron. *Sensory symptoms* are not marked; there may be tingling or numbness of the hands (paræsthesia) but not anæsthesia.

Later, the *legs* are attacked, spastic symptoms appearing first, as the whole of the crossed pyramidal tract becomes involved. The disease spreads into the anterior horn cells of the lumbar enlargement, and atrophy and paralysis follow in the same way as in the arms. The legs, therefore, may be in the spastic stage when weakness and atrophy are well advanced in the arms. *The reflexes* in the

---

* *Body Mechanics in the Study and Treatment of Disease.*

legs, as in the arms, are first exaggerated, ankle clonus and Babinski's sign being present, but these are finally lost. *The sphincters* are unaffected.

COURSE OF THE DISEASE.—This is shorter than that of progressive muscular atrophy, generally 1 to 3 years.

FINAL SYMPTOMS.—Death is due to *intercurrent disease*, often pneumonia or bulbar paralysis, the disease spreading up into the medulla. The respiratory or cardiac centres may be involved. In some cases swallowing becomes difficult and the patient may choke, this being due to paralysis of the tongue and soft palate. *Speech* becomes indistinct or impossible.

Treatment.—Little can be done in these cases. *During the spastic stage* massage may be of the same type as that used in hemiplegia. Passive and active movements should be given from the beginning and are most necessary in order to counteract the advancing atrophy as far as possible. *When the spastic phase is past,* the treatment is the same as that for progressive muscular atrophy. The onset of bulbar paralysis makes further treatment useless, unless massage and passive movements increase the comfort of the patient.

CHAPTER X

DISEASES OF THE SENSORY NEURONS

Tabes dorsalis—Syringomyelia.

TABES DORSALIS
(*Locomotor Ataxia*)

THIS disease involves a progressive degeneration of the posterior nerve-roots and ganglia, and the fasciculi gracilis and cuneatus (columns of Goll and Burdach) (*Fig.* 90).

CAUSES AND AETIOLOGY.—The disease is usually a late result of syphilis, and with the improved methods of early treatment it has become comparatively rare. Its incidence is commoner in men than in women and it manifests itself between the ages of 20 and 50. It is possible that, in a few cases, some other toxin is responsible.

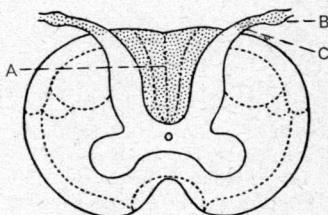

Fig. 90.—Tabes dorsalis. A, Posterior columns (fasciculi gracilis and cuneatus); B, Ganglion; C, Posterior nerve-root.

PATHOLOGICAL CHANGES.—The lesion consists of a chronic degeneration of the posterior nerve-roots and ganglia which spreads up the posterior columns. The nerve-fibres are destroyed and the neuroglia increases. In some cases, the sclerosis may extend to other afferent columns, such as the anterior and lateral spinothalamic (anterolateral), or posterior spinocerebellar (direct cerebellar) tracts. The optic nerve may be involved, and the motor nerves of the eyes also suffer.

COURSE OF THE DISEASE.—The onset is insidious, and the course very slowly progressive. It may be divided into three periods, each lasting roughly ten years. They merge into each other, and the progress of the disease varies in different patients, with certain special symptoms occurring sometimes in one stage, sometimes in another. The disease sometimes becomes arrested but this does not generally occur until a fairly advanced stage. The three stages are known as the *pre-ataxic*, the *ataxic*, and the *paralytic*.

SYMPTOMS.—

PRE-ATAXIC STAGE

As a rule, these are confined to *sensory symptoms* and *eye symptoms*.

SENSORY SYMPTOMS.—The chief of these are *lightning pains* (sharp, shooting pains at right-angles to the limb) and *girdle sensation* (feeling of a cord being drawn tightly round the body) due to irritation of sensory fibres in the posterior roots and ganglia and the intercostal nerves, and *parœsthesia* or *numbness* in the soles of the feet.

EYE SYMPTOMS.—The chief of these are *Argyll-Robertson Pupil*, loss of the pupillary reflex response to light (contraction) and *Diplopia* (double vision). There may also be *ptosis* (drooping of an upper eyelid); *squint*; *miosis* (abnormal contraction of the pupils) and *blindness* from atrophy of the optic nerve.

Both sets of symptoms may appear either in this stage or the next. If the patient becomes blind, the *ataxia* develops slowly and is rarely complete. Many of the eye symptoms may pass off later on.

ATAXIC STAGE

ATAXIA, or 'pathological incoordination', now develops owing to the degeneration of the posterior columns, causing loss of conscious muscle and joint sense. The patient is unable to tell the position of his joints, or to judge of the direction and extent of his movements without watching them. Loss of *joint sense* is tested by a *passive movement* while the eyes are shut. In this state he is quite unable to describe the state of the joint. The *effect of the sensory loss on muscle activity* can be demonstrated by asking the patient to perform an *active movement* with the eyes shut and with them open. In the former case he is unaware of whether or not he has moved. In the latter, unless he watches very carefully, the movement will be jerky and incoordinate, as he has no knowledge of the degree of correction required. The ataxia is specially manifested by two signs, Romberg's sign and his gait.

Romberg's Sign.—The patient cannot stand with his eyes closed and his feet together. He becomes unsteady and falls, since he can control his movements neither by muscle and joint sense, nor by sight.

Ataxic Gait.—The patient lifts the feet too high, throwing them forward with too much force, and stamping them down heavily, heels first. He keeps his feet apart to assist his balance by widening his base, and tends to fall if he places them too close together. He watches them all the time—often he cannot walk at all in the dark. There is great difficulty in turning round, or in avoiding obstacles. This is, of course, a picture of the typical gait in a *late* stage. If the ataxia is worse in one leg than in the other, if muscular hypotonia is extreme, or if there is ataxia of the *trunk* muscles as well as of those of the legs, the gait becomes even worse.

SENSORY CHANGES.—These increase and may be very marked. There is *hypotonia* or *atonia* due to loss of muscle and joint sense, *but there is no loss of power*. The limbs can be placed in all sorts of extraordinary positions, and this increased range of movement exposes the joints to the danger of strains, or even of dislocation. The atonia may also cause the patient to fall suddenly and injure himself. If the *parœsthesia* in the soles has already appeared, it now grows worse, the patient feeling as if he were walking on cotton-wool; finally, it may deepen into *anœsthesia* but even so, it is not so marked as the loss of muscle and joint sense. *Reflexes* are lost in the affected parts, the afferent part of the arc being broken in the posterior roots and ganglia.

TROPHIC CHANGES are present in skin, nails, bones, and joints. *Perforating ulcer of the foot* is common and, since it causes little pain, is liable to be neglected by the patient. The bones become brittle, and fractures occur as the result of trivial violence. *Charcot's joints* are a common complication. This consists of a painless swelling in one or more joints, which become distended with fluid. The articular surfaces are destroyed, new bony tissue forming in the structures round the joints. The ligaments becomes stretched and lax, with the result that abnormal mobility develops and the joint may become completely flail.

VISCERAL CRISES may occur; these constitute attacks of pain occurring in various organs. They may be *gastric*, with pain and vomiting, *laryngeal*, with paroxysmal cough and dyspnœa, *renal, vesical*, etc. *Bladder troubles* (retention of urine, imperfect sphincter control) are generally present.

PARALYTIC STAGE

The patient's symptoms increase to such an extent that he is unable to walk at all, and becomes completely bedridden. The bladder trouble increases, and may result in *cystitis* (inflammation of the bladder), or *kidney disease*. The patient usually dies of this or of some intercurrent disease, often pneumonia.

Principles of Treatment.—Apart from treating the cause, if necessary, treatment is chiefly directed towards preserving what kinesthetic pathways are left to the patient and training other sensory faculties to compensate for those which are lost.

MEDICAL.—If the Wassermann reaction (the blood-test for syphilis) is still positive, suitable treatment for the causative condition will be administered. This is effective in the early stages but once extensive degeneration of neurons has taken place, restoration of function is no longer possible.

PHYSICAL TREATMENT.—It is in the ataxic stage, if at all. that we see the patient and the primary aim is to treat the main symptom—*ataxia*. We must endeavour to re-educate what remains of the patient's muscle sense, or if this has almost ceased to exist, to train him to use the *sense of sight* and possibly *sound* as, in some measure, a substitute for it. At the same time we aim at a general improvement of the patient's health and bodily condition. He must not be allowed to take to his bed, but should be encouraged to continue his ordinary work as long as possible. It is important to remember that these patients should not be fatigued. They will not find the concentration required of them tiring and they do not know when they are tired. Consequently, frequent rests must be allowed during treatment.

MASSAGE.—This is far less valuable than exercises, but if required should be of the light stimulating variety.

EXERCISES.—The most usual form of treatment is by Frenkel's exercises, or by a combination of these with free, active movements. All exercises should be done slowly and rhythmically. In cases where the arms are unaffected, while the legs are ataxic, the remedial movements may be used for the former, the Frenkel's exercises for the latter. Breathing and trunk exercises should be included in the treatment. *Strong exercises* are not required, since there is no loss of muscle power. If the hypotonia of the muscles is extreme, some kind of support should be used to protect the joints of the lower limbs when the patient takes weight on them, especially the knees, where hyperextension may be very marked.

Frenkel's Exercises

These consist of a carefully planned series of exercises which aim at making the patient employ what is left to him of muscle sense in an attempt to prevent its further decrease, or even effect an improvement. Frenkel considered that, despite the damaged sensory path, a tabetic patient could learn to make the fullest use of what is left in the way of muscle sense by constant repetition— much as a normal person acquires complex skills. In fact this principle is illustrated in cases where optic atrophy has supervened early, for in these the ataxia develops slowly and incompletely, since the blind man is *obliged* to depend on his muscle and joint sense, and so uses it to the utmost of his capacity. If, however, the muscle sense is practically non-existent by the time a patient comes for treatment, the object of the exercises is to teach him to replace his lost sense by the sense of sight. Treatment should begin as soon as possible. If the patient is in the pre-ataxic stage, he should perform the most complex movements possible. In the later stages the exercises should begin with very simple movements and gradually advance to more complicated ones. Certain rules must be observed at whatever stage the patient may be.

RULES FOR GIVING FRENKEL'S EXERCISES.—

1. *Commands* should be given in an even, monotonous, sing-song voice; and the exercises should be done to counting.

2. Each exercise, or set of exercises, should have been mastered by the patient— that is, he should be able to do it accurately and smoothly—before he is allowed to proceed to a more difficult one. *Precision of performance must be attained*, but the exercises should be sufficiently varied to prevent boredom.

3. Exercises involving strong muscle work should not be given. Progression is by *complexity*, not strength.

4. Movements in *complete range* are easier than those in *small range*, therefore the former should be given before the latter, but no movement should be taken beyond its normal limit, because the hypotonia of muscles and laxity of ligaments render the patient vulnerable to dislocation or the onset of Charcot's joints.

5. The movements should first be given rather *quickly*, then *more slowly*, this being more difficult since it requires greater control.

6. The patient should practise movements first with his eyes open, and then with them shut.

7. Each patient should have individual attention, and should not be left unattended in case he should fall and injure himself.

8. *Rests* must be given between the exercises; after so many minutes' work, an equal number of minutes' rest should be taken.

9. It is necessary, when planning the treatment scheme, to take into consideration the patient's general health and mental attitude, the state of his muscles, and any complications such as Charcot's joints. A careful record should be kept of exactly what work the patient is doing from day to day.

The exercises themselves are given in *lying*, in *sitting*, or in *standing*.

EXERCISES IN LYING.—The patient lies on a bed, plinth, or couch with a smooth surface along which the feet can move easily. *His head must be sufficiently raised for him to be able to watch his feet*. The exercises in this group begin with simple movements, and gradually become more difficult and complicated.

The first set are as follows (One leg moved at a time; legs moved alternately):—

1. Flexion of one leg, at hip and knee, foot kept on plinth; extension.
2. Flexion as above; abduction, adduction; extension.
3. Flexion as above, but only half-way; extension.
4. Flexion as above (half-way); abduction; adduction; extension.
5. Flexion (voluntary halt made by patient during flexion); extension.
6. As 5, but halt at physiotherapist's command.

The exercises are done slowly three or four times, using each leg in turn. The foot should be kept dorsiflexed, so as not to stretch the hypotonic anterior tibial group. The physiotherapist should count four during each movement.

At a later stage both legs are moved together.

Examples of more difficult exercises in the lying series:—

1. Flexion of one leg at hip and knee, with the heel raised some inches from the plinth; extension.
2. Heel of one leg placed on patella of other leg; return.
3. As above, with voluntary halt.
4. As above, with halt to command.
5. Heel is placed on the middle of the other tibia, lifted off, and put by side of leg; extension.

6. Heel placed on other knee; down on bed at side; leg extended till heel reaches middle of tibia; placed on tibia, then again on bed at side; extended to level of ankle; placed on ankle, then on bed at side; complete extension.

7. Heel placed on knee; heel slides along tibia to ankle-joint; extension.

8. As above, but heel carried from ankle back to knee; extension.

9. Flexion and extension of both legs, with heels off bed.

10. As above, with halts.

11. One leg (e.g., left) flexed; left leg abducted and right leg flexed, simultaneously; left leg adducted and right leg extended; left leg extended. (Repeat with legs reversed.)

12. Left leg flexed, right leg abducted and flexed (all at the same time); right leg adducted; both legs extended, without heels touching bed till end of movement.

N.B.—These asymmetrical exercises are very difficult for the tabetic patient.

13. The physiotherapist places her finger on various places on the leg; the patient places his other heel on her finger.

14. As above; but as the patient reaches the finger, the physiotherapist moves it, and the patient tries to follow its course.

15. Right heel is placed on the knee of the other limb, which is in extension; with right heel in this position, the left leg is flexed and extended.

16. Right heel is placed on left knee, and slides down the tibia to the ankle; as it slides down, the left leg is flexed; as it is brought back to the knee, the left leg is extended.

These are only a few examples of the whole series of nearly 100 exercises. Anyone who has to treat cases of tabes should make a point of studying the lists in Frenkel's book.* Frenkel's exercises may *seem* 'old-fashioned', but they are still effective, and no one has yet improved on them. It is, of course, quite possible to invent other similar exercises if desired, and to adapt them to purposeful movements, e.g., to assist the patient to dress himself more easily.

EXERCISES IN SITTING.—These are not necessarily *progressions* on those in lying; they are considerably easier than some of the more advanced exercises in that series. Those given by Frenkel consist of rising from a stool or chair, and sitting down again. The patient has literally forgotten how to perform these 'stock' movements—he has lost his 'formula' for them. The rising movement, therefore, is divided into its component parts, the operator counting three. At *one*, the patient draws his knees under the stool. At *two*, he bends his trunk forward. At *three*, he rises extending hips and knees. He then sits down again, reversing the above process.

These movements may be done at first in the reach-grasp position, the patient sitting close to the wall-bars. Later, he rises unsupported. Later still, he attempts to do so with his eyes closed.

Other exercises may be given in sitting:—

1. The patient may be directed to raise his knees and place his foot on, say, the second rail from the bottom. This is done in three movements: (1) Flexion of hip; (2) Extension of knee; (3) Lowering of foot on to bar. He then replaces the foot on the ground.

2. He may be made to touch marked points on the floor with his foot. (Frenkel gives this type of exercise in lying; but it necessitates apparatus in that position.)

---

* *Tabetic Ataxia*, trans. Freyberger: Heinemann.

EXERCISES IN STANDING.—These are designed to give *re-education in walking*. They should be performed in as large a space as possible preferably where lines can be marked out as seen in *Figs.* 91, 92.

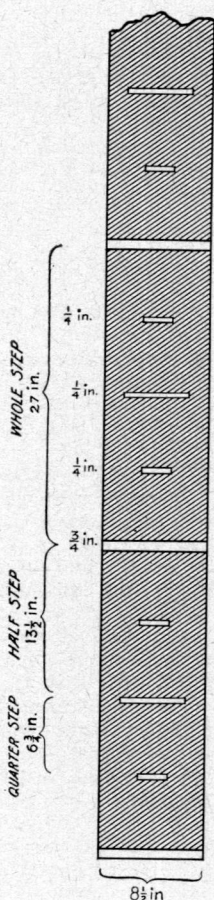

Fig. 92.—'Footsteps' for tabes treatment. (*After Frenkel.*)

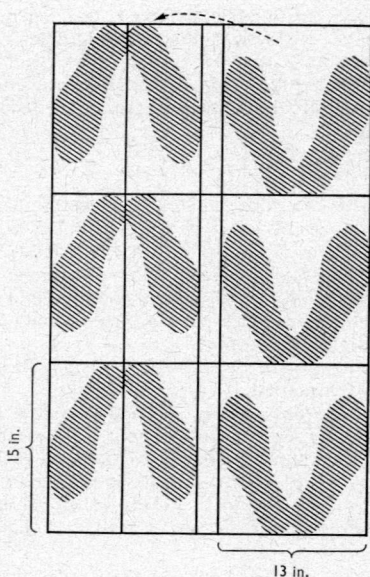

Fig. 91.—Diagram of 'steps' used in treating tabes. (*After Frenkel.*)

1. *Walking sideways*: The patient, accompanied by the physiotherapist—who must be prepared to support him if necessary—begins by walking sideways. Balance is easier in this way, because, except in the long step, he does not have to rise on the toes of one foot, thus decreasing his base.

He should begin by taking *half-steps*, which are easiest, alternately to left and to right, the physiotherapist counting three for each step, e.g., for half-step to right (1) he places the right foot on the ground half a step away, (2) he transfers his weight from the left to the right foot, (3) he brings the left foot up beside the right.

He then practises *quarter-steps*, then *long steps*, and finally combines all three lengths in one exercise, e.g.: (*a*) Three-quarter-step to right—one—two—three. (*b*) Quarter-step to left—one—two—three. (*c*) Half-step to right—one—two—three. (*d*) Whole step to left—one—two—three.

The long steps are more difficult because the toes have to be put on the ground first. The heel is raised and the patient's base is therefore smaller.

2. *Walking forwards*: Whole, half- and quarter-steps forwards, beginning with each foot alternately, counting three as before. Thus, in beginning with the right foot: (*a*) Place right foot forward, heel on the ground. (*b*) Transfer weight to this foot, raising heel of left foot. (*c*) Bring left foot up beside right foot.

3. *Walking backwards*, in a similar manner.

4. *Walking heel to toe.*

5. *Walking in footsteps* painted on the floor (*Fig.* 92).

6. *Turning round*, also in footmarks on the floor (*Fig.* 93), practised in three

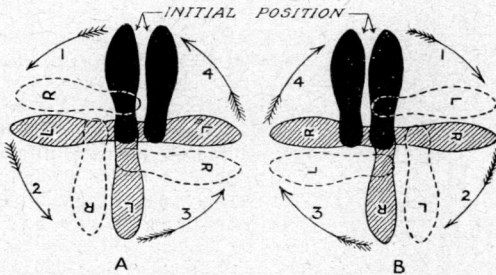

Fig. 93.—'Footmarks' for turning round, in treatment of tabes. A, Turning to the left; B, Turning to the right. (*After Frenkel.*)

movements; e.g., turning to right: (*a*) The patient turns on the right heel; (*b*) He raises the left heel and turns on the toes of this foot; (*c*) He brings the left foot up beside the right. This should be done four times, completing the full turn, and then repeated to the left.

7. *Walking up and down stairs or steps* : (*a*) The patient first goes up one step at a time. Later, he practises walking up the steps as a normal person would. (*b*) He walks up and down, with support to begin with, later without.

8. Finally, he is taught to walk while using his arms at the same time, carrying parcels, getting out of the way of obstacles, etc.

WHEN THE ARMS ARE AFFECTED, which is much more rarely the case, exercises of a similar nature are given, special attention being paid to the fine movements of hands and fingers, placing the fingers in holes in a board; inserting pegs or matches into holes; picking up small objects like marbles, and arranging them in piles or patterns. He should also practise going over diagrams with a pencil, writing, drawing, etc.

In the paralytic stage, only very simple movements can be given, but breathing exercises are important if treatment is ordered at this stage. Every effort must be made to avoid pressure sores, and treatment along the lines described in Chapter V may be required if these develop.

SYRINGOMYELIA

This is a rare condition, cases of which are occasionally referred for treatment; it consists of dissociated anæsthesia and paralysis.

AETIOLOGY.—The cause is not really understood, but it is thought to be due to a *congenital defect* of development in the spinal cord. The incidence is about the same in men and women. It generally appears in young people under 30, and may well be preceded by a *kyphoscoliosis* which develops in childhood or early adolescence.

PATHOLOGY.—The disease starts as a new growth of connective tissue round the central canal of the cord. Later this tissue breaks down and forms cavities, destroying the structures in the immediate neighbourhood of the canal, and exerting pressure on the regions beyond. The anterior grey commissure is first affected, and this entails destruction of some of the *pain and temperature fibres of the spinothalamic (anterolateral) tract* as they cross over to the opposite side, soon after entering the cord. Next, the pressure falls on the anterior horns.

Later, the sensory and motor tracts are affected and their fibres degenerate (*Fig.* 94).

The disease generally starts in the cervical or thoracic regions, and may spread upwards or downwards.

SYMPTOMS.—The earliest and most characteristic symptom is *dissociated anæsthesia*, i.e., loss of sensation of *pain and temperature*, but not of the sense of touch or muscle sense in the same areas. The latter sensations are at first unimpaired, because the posterior columns are not involved until considerably later. These patients tend to burn or otherwise injure their hands, where the loss of pain and temperature sense first occurs. Later, the anæsthesia spreads up the arms and to the trunk.

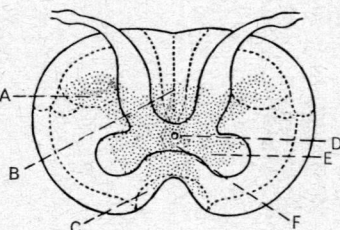

Fig. 94.—Syringomyelia. A, Lateral cerebrospinal (crossed pyramidal) tract; B, Posterior columns; C, Anterior cerebrospinal (direct pyramidal tract); D, Central canal; E, Anterior horn; F, Anterior grey commissure. The darker shading in the centre indicates the initial lesion, the lighter shading the parts affected later. The former should include a little more of the anterior grey commissure.

Muscular atrophy and paralysis appear as soon as the anterior horns are subjected to pressure. As in progressive muscular atrophy, they begin in the hands and spread up the arm, extending to the trunk in the same order as does the anæsthesia. Later, the feet may be similarly affected.

At a still more advanced stage, there may be *loss of sensation to touch*, with *ataxia* (posterior columns), or *spastic paraplegia* of the legs (crossed pyramidal tract). The disease may spread up to the medulla, producing bulbar paralysis.

Trophic changes—bone or joint changes, similar to those of tabes dorsalis, may appear. The patients often get painless whitlows on the fingers—painless since the sense of pain is lost.

COMPLICATIONS.—Scoliosis or kyphoscoliosis.

Principles of Treatment.—The aims and methods of treatment are similar to those in progressive muscular atrophy. Treatment may be requested for kyphoscoliosis in the child or adolescent, before the condition is actually diagnosed. Later, if ataxia develops, exercises of the Frenkel type may be tried. It is, in fact, as well to begin these before ataxia actually appears, starting with the more complex movements. If spastic paraplegia is the more marked, this must be appropriately treated (*see* HEMIPLEGIA, pp. 185-8, and SPASTIC PARAPLEGIA, pp. 197-9).

PRECAUTIONS similar to those required in tabes are necessary when giving movements to joints, great care being taken not to strain any joint or carry any movement beyond its normal limits.

CHAPTER XI

OTHER DISEASES OF THE BRAIN AND SPINAL CORD

Paralysis agitans—Encephalitis lethargica—Cerebellar ataxia—Disseminated sclerosis—Combined sclerosis—Friedreich's disease—Transverse myelitis—Chorea.

PARALYSIS AGITANS
(*Parkinson's Disease*—'*Shaking Palsy*')

AETIOLOGY.—This disease, which affects the basal ganglia, is commonest in advanced life, generally appearing after the age of 50 or 60 years. It attacks both sexes equally. The *cause* is unknown, but it may well be a form of senile degeneration. It is not hereditary, nor due to syphilis or any definite infection, though some patients have histories of encephalitis or Spanish 'flu, and in a very small proportion carbon-monoxide and drug or metal poisoning is responsible. Shock, worry, or an accident seem to excite it in some cases.

PATHOLOGICAL CHANGES.—Degenerative changes leading to the formation of minute perforations occur in the corpus striatum (particularly the *globus pallidum* of the *lentiform nucleus*) and the *substantia nigra* of the midbrain. This part of the nervous system presides over *automatic movements*, e.g., the swing of the arms in walking, and such movements are lost in paralysis agitans. It also controls normal muscle tone and activity, and synergic group action of muscles, so that *rigidity* and *tremor* are features of the disease.

SYMPTOMS.—These are often grouped together under the term *Parkinsonism*.

TREMOR.—This begins in one hand, and is very characteristic. The fingers are alternately flexed and extended, especially at the metacarpophalangeal joints, while the thumb rests against the index finger. This produces the so-called 'pill-rolling' movement. The tremor generally spreads to the arm and leg of the same side, and then to the other arm and leg. The head and trunk are rarely affected, the eyes never. This is not an 'intention' tremor; it is often absent during voluntary movement but continues when the limb is at rest, especially when unsupported. It is aggravated by emotional stresses or when the patient is conscious of scrutiny. It ceases during sleep.

CHANGES IN MUSCLES.—Because of the lack of control of muscle tone there is *hypertonus* in all muscle groups. This leads to a diffuse rigidity known as 'lead-pipe' rigidity, because, unlike that seen in upper motor neuron disease, *equal resistance to passive movement is maintained throughout the full range of movement*. This produces peculiarities of posture and gait, as well as a characteristic facial expression.

Posture.—The patient bends his body forward from the hips, and stands with hips and knees flexed. The head is also carried forward. The arms are slightly abducted, the elbows standing out from the sides and flexed to a right angle. The wrists are slightly extended, while the fingers are flexed at the metacarpophalangeal joints and extended at the interphalangeal joints.

Gait.—This is what is known as 'festinant' (hurrying). The patient walks with short steps, which tend to get faster and faster. If pushed forward, he will run in that direction; if pulled backward, he will run backward. The automatic swing of the arms is lost.

Facial Expression.—This consists of the 'Parkinsonian mask', rigidity causing the face to become immobile and expressionless. The blinking reflex occurs less often than usual, hence the patient appears to have a fixed stare. Because of the mask-like appearance it is easy to underrate the intelligence and mental capabilities of the patient. Since changes of facial expression are few and infrequent, the inexperienced tend to assume that the mind is equally 'vacant'. This is not so, the mental powers remaining normal throughout the disease, unless dissociated degeneration occurs elsewhere in the brain.

Speech.—This may be shrill and monotonous, or there may be hesitation, followed by rapid speech.

Muscular Weakness.—This is also a feature of the disease, not only because of rigidity but also because *the facilitatory pathways from the lentiform nucleus to the motor areas are interfered with.* Fine movements are most affected, e.g., those of the hands. There is also a lack of precision, caused by weakness and inability to co-ordinate. Because of the weakness and the rigidity in the antagonistic group, movements are slow and delayed, and fatigue sets in early.

REFLEXES.—Normal or sometimes increased.

SENSORY CHANGES.—The patient often suffers sensations of great heat, with sweating and rise of local temperature. He may suffer from cramps and aches, sometimes severe in the later stages of the disease.

Principles of Treatment.—Although the disease is slowly progressive and incurable, physical treatment may retard its course and relieve the symptoms, as well as having a psychological effect. Our *aims* will be *to lessen the rigidity of the muscles* and *obtain relaxation,* as far as possible; *to encourage rhythmical, active movement, to assist co-ordination,* and *to keep the patient on his feet* as long as we can.

PHYSICAL TREATMENT.—In order to reduce the rigidity, we may use massage, passive movements, and relaxation exercises. Radiant heat or other forms of heat can also be helpful. Active exercises will be used to assist co-ordination and muscle power. As in any case of nervous disease, an assessment of the patient's capabilities and disabilities should be made when he first attends the department, or at his first treatment, and a record should be kept of his progress.

MASSAGE.—General massage can be used to improve the circulation and obtain relaxation, but it is more usual for the limbs, alone, to be treated. The massage should, of course, be of the soothing type (effleurage, kneading, and stroking).

PASSIVE MOVEMENTS.—These should be slow, rhythmical, and in full range. They should be given to all joints to induce relaxation.

RELAXATION EXERCISES should also be given, particularly of the pendular, rhythmical variety. Use of the Guthrie-Smith apparatus may be found helpful. The Kabat techniques for gaining relaxation can be used to advantage, particularly those involving an isometric contraction followed by an isotonic contraction. The same group of muscles can be put through both types of contraction, or a reversal technique can be used.

ACTIVE EXERCISES.—These may be assisted, free, or resisted, according to the patient's capabilities. It will be noticed that when the patient is performing free rhythmical movements, the rhythm and range of movements tend to fade. To overcome this, music or counting is helpful in giving fresh impetus at flagging points. Voluntary, controlled movement must be encouraged, because the cerebral cortex now has to be responsible for movements which are normally automatically controlled by the basal ganglia. Success has been claimed by some for *Frenkel's exercises.* Re-education in walking and practice in ordinary occupations should form part of the treatment. Many patients do well in, and enjoy, class-work, the stimulus of other people acting as an incentive. Frequent rests should be given, and deep breathing and relaxation should form part of the work.

SURGICAL TREATMENT.—In recent years *stereotaxic surgery* has afforded relief to many patients by reducing rigidity and tremor. It consists of electro-coagulation of areas in the globus pallidum and thalamus. The former relieves rigidity, the latter tremor, but these symptoms cannot be totally abolished.

POST-OPERATIVE TREATMENT.—The patient remains in hospital for about 3 weeks. Physical treatment begins the day after the operation, with breathing exercises and gentle mobilizing of arms and legs. As soon as the patient is allowed up for an hour, usually the third day, he attends the physiotherapy department, and balance re-education and correction of posture begins. On about the fourth day he joins a class which consists of general mobility exercises (mobility of back and trunk being particularly important), co-ordination exercises, weight-transference, and re-education of walking. The patient should continue with home exercises for 6 months after the operation if he is to gain maximum benefit from the operation.

ENCEPHALITIS LETHARGICA

This terrible disease, much in evidence a few years ago and popularly known as 'sleepy sickness', occurred both in epidemic and sporadic form. It is now rarely seen, but nevertheless we may be called upon to treat its after-effects.

AETIOLOGY.—The actual cause is unknown, but is thought to be a virus.

PATHOLOGY.—It consists of an acute inflammation of the connective tissue of the brain, with degeneration of the nerve cells, especially those of the basal ganglia, the midbrain, and the cells of origin of the motor nerves of the eyes, which lie in the floor of the aqueduct of the midbrain.

SYMPTOMS.—The illness begins with an acute attack, the first symptoms of which are *fever* and *paralysis of eye muscles*. Then appear the *lethargy* and drowsiness which have given the disease its name. The patient often remains lethargic all day, but at night become restless, or even delirious. At no stage of the disease, however, is there any form of *motor* paralysis, other than that of the ocular muscles, neither is there anæsthesia nor are the reflexes affected.*

In fatal cases (about 25 per cent) the patient dies from respiratory failure, due to involvement of the vital centres in the medulla oblongata. In some slight cases in which there has been little or no destruction of nerve-cells, he may recover completely or almost completely. In 50 per cent of cases *a syndrome develops later, resembling that of paralysis agitans* (*Parkinsonism*) with tremor, athetosis, and the 'Parkinsonian mask', due to injury of the caudate and lentiform nuclei; more rarely one sees *spastic paralysis* or *cerebellar ataxia* (Purves-Stewart). In such cases the cerebrum or cerebellum has been injured.

LATE SYMPTOMS.—The after-effects of this disease are often tragic. Many patients remain mentally dull, and those who before their illness were quick, clever, and efficient are often quite unable to resume their former work, being no longer either physically or mentally equal to it. The patients are slow in all their movements and react slowly to commands, holding their limbs stiffly. Improvement may follow, but more often the reverse is the case, and even in the event of apparently complete recovery, a relapse is liable to take place during the three or four years after the illness. Pregnancy aggravates the sequelæ.

In children, symptoms such as *hemiplegia* or *diplegia, tremor, athetosis*, etc., may persist. Respiration may be affected, the child breathing through his mouth, which remains open, giving him an imbecile expression. Worst of all, there may be a *complete alteration in the child's character*.

Principles of Treatment.—The aims of treatment and methods used will depend on the symptoms. Where they are those of Parkinsonism the aims and methods

---

* At the same time, the symptoms tend to vary, and many cases are not typical.

are those described above; where there is cerebral or cerebellar involvement they will be similar to those described in the section dealing with CEREBRAL PARALYSIS OF INFANCY in Chapter IX.

CEREBELLAR ATAXIA

This constitutes a congenital or acquired deficiency, or disease, of the cerebellum, causing defective synergic control of the muscles. Cerebellar ataxia itself is a rare disease, though, of course, the cerebellum or its afferent or efferent tracts may be involved in multiple lesions such as disseminated sclerosis; in extensive degenerations, such as Friedreich's disease, or certain forms of infantile cerebral palsy.

SYMPTOMS.—The effects of a cerebellar lesion are *loss of the postural tone* of muscles (Chapter XVI), the patient being unable to stand steadily, and *asynergia*—lack of co-ordination and harmonious action of muscles in complex movements. These two defects of control are manifested by the following symptoms.

THE CEREBELLAR GAIT.—A reeling, lurching mode of progression which varies according to the actual site of the lesion in the cerebellum. The basic cause is lack of co-ordination of the movements of the limbs and trunk. In the most usual form, the trunk is held rigidly, while the legs appear to run away from it, because the trunk muscles cannot adapt themselves quickly enough to the changes in position of the body brought about by the movements of the limbs. The patient staggers and may fall to one side or the other, or even backwards. In other cases, the trunk is apparently the first part to move, and the legs are unable to respond in time, so that the trunk falls forwards, backwards, or to the side whenever the patient attempts to walk. He finds great difficulty in turning round. The reeling and staggering is often so marked that the unfortunate sufferer is not infrequently thought to be in a state of intoxication, which impression is confirmed by his indistinct or incoherent speech.

DISSOCIATION OF NORMALLY COMBINED MOVEMENTS.—Movements are broken up into their component parts, instead of being performed simultaneously; for instance, if told to raise his leg (in the lying or standing position) he will first flex the hip and then extend the knee, instead of holding the knee in extension while the hip is being flexed.

DYSMETRIA.—An incorrect estimation of how much a muscle should be contracted in order to perform any particular movement; for instance, if asked to drink a glass of water, the patient will probably over-contract the arm muscles and throw the water over his shoulder or into his own face. Symptoms of incoordination may appear in various special groups of muscles.

The 'heel-to-knee' test may be used in this condition as well as in lesions of the posterior columns. The patient being as unsuccessful in performing it as is the tabetic, though for a different reason—dysmetria being the reason here, and loss of kinesthetic sense being the cause in the tabetic patient.

INTENTION TREMOR occurs in the head, neck, and limbs, together with NYSTAGMUS, SCANNING (*staccato*), EXPLOSIVE, OR SLURRING SPEECH.—These three, which form the 'diagnostic symptoms' of disseminated sclerosis (*see* p. 228), are also present in cerebellar ataxia. In the former case they are probably due to some of the multiple lesions being situated in the cerebellum.

THE REFLEXES are normal, the reflex arc and the pyramidal pathway being intact; but the *knee-jerk* is peculiar, a swinging movement being produced in response to the stimulus ('pendular knee-jerk') instead of a single twitch.

THE MENTAL CONDITION is normal.

Similar symptoms would be produced by the destruction of tracts to and from the cerebellum.

Principles of Treatment.—Our aim is to try to teach the patient to co-ordinate his movements by means of voluntary control, through the higher centres in the cerebrum. For this purpose we may make use of Frenkel's exercises, though we shall not find sight such a valuable auxiliary as we do in the tabetic, since cerebellar ataxia is as bad with the eyes open as when they are shut. However, the same type of exercises is suitable, and the same rules should be observed. The patient should also be given exercises in which first two, and then more, joints have to be moved simultaneously, or one has to be moved and another held in some particular position—e.g., Lying or standing Leg-lifting (flexion of hip with static extension of knee); Reach-grasp-standing placing the knee on a stool in front (flexion of hip and knee); Bend-sitting (or half-lying) Arm-stretching upward (abduction of shoulder, extension of elbow, elevation of shoulder girdle, etc.—an advanced exercise).

The condition is a discouraging one to treat (*see, however*, p. 193, *regarding ataxia in children*), but occasionally a marked improvement can be noted, and the lesion is at least not progressive. (*See also* treatment of TABES DORSALIS, pp. 217–21.)

DISSEMINATED SCLEROSIS
(*Multiple Sclerosis*)

In disseminated sclerosis, as the name implies, the lesions are *multiple*; there are scattered patches of sclerosis found throughout the nervous system—in the spinal cord, in the brain, or in both. Grey and white matter may both be involved, though the latter is usually affected first.

AETIOLOGY.—The disease generally begins in young adults, during the third decade, though it may begin earlier or later in some cases. Both sexes are affected, but women much more often than men, in the proportion of 3 to 2. The patients are otherwise healthy.

CAUSE.—This is as yet unknown, but for some time it has been thought that it might be due to an unidentified enzyme or virus, which attacked the nervous tissue, or to some form of metabolic defect. Recent research has pointed to some form of vascular deficiency, probably in the capillaries, which, whilst not directly affecting the nervous tissue, leads to impairment of its vitality and subsequent degeneration. In some cases there appears to be a hereditary factor, and in many cases the initial attack follows a period of fatigue or emotional stress. Under *precipitating causes* we may list, therefore, a period of fatigue or emotional strain ; injury; shock; and sometimes a specific fever, such as typhoid, scarlet fever, etc. Pregnancy may also precipitate an attack, and symptoms are exacerbated in patients who already have the disease.

PATHOLOGICAL CHANGES.—The condition begins with small scattered patches of inflammation in various parts of the nervous system. The inflammation first appears in the spinal cord in many cases. The myelin sheaths of the nerve-fibres are affected, the axis cylinders remaining intact. Later, these inflamed patches degenerate and become sclerosed and necrotic (*plaque formation*). Almost any part of the nervous system may be affected—cerebrum, cerebellum, medulla, cord, etc., but the vital centres are not attacked.

THE COURSE OF THE DISEASE is long and slow, spread over many years. In most cases there are a series of attacks followed by a period of 'remission' during which the symptoms become less severe. To begin with the attacks are usually slight and the intervals between them are long, but they gradually become more frequent. Each attack is a little worse than the one before, and the patient becomes increasingly disabled. Only a very small percentage of patients grow steadily worse, without these remissions. Diagnosis is difficult at the beginning, because the symptoms are so transient, and the earliest attacks often seem to clear up completely, leaving such slight after-effects that they are unnoticed even by the patient.

SYMPTOMS.—

EARLY STAGE.—

Spinal symptoms are usually the first events which cause the patient to seek medical aid, the lower extremities being mainly affected. The patient suffers from weakness of the legs which, on examination, may also reveal spasticity. She complains of fatigue when walking, and also that one leg drags when she is tired. In some cases *one or both arms* also give trouble at this stage. They become clumsy and of little use, the finer movements of the fingers and hand being most affected.

Eye symptoms are an important diagnostic feature and are due to the disease having affected the nuclei of the optic nerve, or of the motor nerves of the eyes. There may be *blurred vision, diplopia* (double vision), or even *transitory blindness*. In many cases questioning reveals that such eye symptoms occurred fleetingly months, or years, previously. The condition then cleared up completely and was forgotten by the patient until a recurrence again brought it to her notice.

Sphincter trouble may cause a temporary loss of control of the bladder or rectum.

All these symptoms tend to pass off and the disease becomes quiescent until a second attack occurs.

LATER SYMPTOMS.—

At this stage appear what are known as the three diagnostic symptoms. (1) *Nystagmus*, which consists of an oscillation of the eyeballs when the patient looks sideways. It may be seen if she is asked to follow with her eyes the operator's finger, which is carried slowly to the right or to the left. (2) *Intention tremor*. When the patient starts to perform a definite movement a tremor begins, getting worse as the movement continues but there is no tremor when the limb is at rest. It is generally tested by asking the patient to touch her nose with her finger ('finger-to-nose test') but similar tests have been devised for the lower extremity. The tremor may be worse in one leg or arm than in the other. (3) *Scanning or staccato speech*. The patient pronounces every syllable of every word separately. These three symptoms are all probably due to lesions in the cerebellum, or in the tracts leading to or from it. They are manifestations of loss of co-ordination and control in the eye muscles, limb muscles, and muscles of articulation.

Definite spasticity develops, generally worse in one leg than in the other. The leg is held stiffly in *extension* as in a case of hemiplegia or paraplegia. In the very late stage of the disease, when the brain is practically cut off from the spinal cord, the reflex arc takes command entirely. The strongest reflex in the leg is that of the *flexors*, because this is the protective reflex by which the limb would be withdrawn from anything painful or dangerous; therefore in the later stage there is *paraplegia in flexion*, the patient having both legs flexed at hips and knees. *Contractures* form, the muscles degenerate, and the position becomes fixed.

Ataxia is often combined with spasticity, or it may be the more marked symptom of the two, depending on the areas of the nervous system which are most severely affected.

Sensory changes are usually slight or absent, though in many cases there is a *loss of kinesthetic sense*.

The gait therefore may be spastic, i.e., like that of hemiplegia, or more usually like the scissor gait of a cerebral paraplegia; or ataxic, i.e., unsteady and reeling, like that of tabes or cerebellar ataxia. Again, it may be a combination of both. Owing to the apparently haphazard distribution of the disease, a combination of spasticity and ataxia (sensory and/or cerebellar) is to be found in most patients.

It is not uncommon, for instance, to see a patient with marked spasticity of the legs who, at the same time, displays predominantly sensory symptoms in the arms, i.e., ataxia and incoordination. Again, the student may be disconcerted to find, on examining a patient who is obviously suffering from cerebellar ataxia, that the limbs exhibit a certain degree of spasticity. In some cases, of course, spasticity or ataxia predominates, but on the whole these are in the minority.

The reflexes are generally exaggerated, ankle clonus and Babinski's sign being present.

Loss of muscle power is present in all cases.

Mental or temperamental changes occur. There is no question of insanity, but in the later stages the patient becomes *euphoric*, that is to say she is prone to laugh and giggle, and is amused at trifles or at things that are not really amusing. *Loss of sphincter control* becomes more marked and the patient eventually becomes completely incontinent.

Trophic changes are not marked but the skin sometimes becomes dry. Bed-sores, or the tendency to them, may form a complication in the later stages.

Principles of Treatment.—For many years disseminated sclerosis has been treated by conventional means, depending on the stage it has reached and the primary symptoms exhibited. As a result of the research into the possible vascular cause of the disease, a revolutionary 'athletic regimen' was devised for use in treating these patients and results have been encouraging. Both methods will be considered here, but it is proposed to deal with the conventional treatment first.

CONVENTIONAL TREATMENT.—It is important that the student should realize the complexity of the symptoms which the patient may exhibit, for only by so doing can she apply treatment rationally and intelligently. Each case will require at least two, sometimes three, types of treatment. (1) *Palliative treatment* directed towards improving the affected parts. (2) *Compensatory treatment* directed towards training unaffected areas to take over or assist in the work of the affected areas. (3) *Preventive treatment* directed towards staving off possible consequences in areas as yet unaffected or only slightly affected. For example, a patient with markedly spastic legs will require palliative treatment to reduce spasticity and enable her to walk with the aid of sticks or crutches. In order to use these she will need to rely on her arms. Compensatory treatment should therefore consist of training the muscles of the arms. If they are already slightly ataxic, preventative treatment will be required to maintain, and if possible, improve co-ordination in order to keep the patient mobile for as long as possible and to stave off the inevitable reduction to life in a wheel-chair. It is essential, therefore, that the physiotherapist should be able to foresee possible difficulties and complications, and take them into account when planning treatment.

Depending on the condition of the patient when she first receives treatment the overall aims can be summed up as follows: either *to maintain the patient's functional independence for as long as possible and where possible to increase it*, or *to help her to regain some measure of that independence*. If, for instance, she is ambulant when she first receives treatment she must be kept on her feet for as long as possible; if she is in a wheel-chair we must aim at enabling her to walk again; if she is bedridden it may be possible to restore her to a wheel-chair life, and even, in some cases, to progress beyond that; in other cases it may only be possible to relieve the symptoms as much as we can and to make her reasonably independent in bed.

PHYSICAL TREATMENT.—Each patient must be thoroughly examined before treatment is undertaken. If possible the patient should first be watched while she is unaware of it. This will give a general impression of predominant signs and will provide a basis on which to conduct more detailed examination. She should next be examined when lying or half-lying, and all joints should be subjected to a full range of passive and active movement, not forgetting 'daily activities'. A thorough examination will take time, but it is time well spent. During the examination the following questions should be in the forefront of the physio-therapist's mind: *What can she do?*; *What can she not do?*; *Why can she not do it?*

The more specific aims and the methods used will depend on the actual symptoms present.

In cases where spasticity is present the main aims will be to reduce the spasticity; to prevent or stretch contractures; to regain mobility; and to increase muscle power. The methods which can be used to achieve this have been described in detail in Chapter IX. They may include heat, massage, passive movements and stretchings, the use of reflex-inhibiting postures, active exercise (assisted, resisted, and free), and mobilizing and strengthening Kabat techniques.

In cases where ataxia is present the aims will be to restore the power of co-ordination and balance. *It must first be discovered whether this is mainly sensory or cerebellar.* In cases of sensory ataxia much help can be given by using Frenkel type exercises and by making use of the principles of proprioceptive neuromuscular facilitation, but the results will not be so good in cerebellar lesions. Balance reactions, and simple balance exercises, should be included in the treatment scheme. Some patients may be suitable for class work.

In all cases re-education in walking should be given wherever possible, and this should be continued for as long as is practicable. Muscle power must also be built up and attention should be paid to facilitating the performance of everyday activities. This may include devising and training the patient in the use of appliances, mechanical aids and gadgets, and suggesting possible modifications in the home. Light plaster splints may be required for night wear in the case of spastic patients.

N.B. *Fatigue* is a big problem in all these patients, and allowances must be made for this when planning treatment schemes, either by the provision of specific resting periods, or by changing the nature and direction of treatment. Again, it cannot be over-stressed that the wise physiotherapist is the one who is alive to every change in the patient's condition, and who can therefore adapt the treatment to the changing circumstances.

In the case of bedridden patients in the very late stages of the disease it may only be possible to give massage and passive movements, but as long as the patient derives either physical or psychological benefit from treatment it is well worth while. If massage increases spasticity, it must not, of course, be given. At this stage the patient may have difficulty with respiration, and breathing exercises and percussion may be helpful.

ATHLETIC REGIMEN (*devised as a result of recent research*).—During the research into the possibility of vascular insufficiency as a possible cause of disseminated sclerosis, it was noted that no athlete at the height of his training and performance ever succumbed to the disease, although cases had been reported in athletes who had given up their activities. It was therefore concluded that the rigours of an athletic training kept the circulation, as a whole, at such a high pitch, that tissue health was also at a peak. Research was accordingly started into whether or not a comparable form of exercise programme could induce a similar type of circulation, *particularly with regard to the brain and spinal cord*, in patients suffering from disseminated sclerosis. This posed the question of whether or not 'fatigue' from such a programme would be detrimental. It was, however, considered that the fatigue following hard physical exercise was in a different category from that following emotional or physical strain, or from being 'on the go' all day, and treatment was undertaken experimentally, with the proviso that *adequate periods of rest* were given following exercise, and that hand in hand with exercises went the avoidance of 'overdoing' things.

Patients who co-operated in the experiment showed a dramatic improvement, particularly those in the early stages of the disease, and results have been sufficiently encouraging to hope that its use will be more widely adopted.

Basically the treatment consists of periods of physical activity, carried to the point of maximal effort, followed by definite periods of recumbency during the day, the main aim being *to improve the circulation to the brain and spinal cord*, as well as to the body as a whole, but *at the same time to avoid the danger of fatigue*.

Stimulation of the circulation to the brain and spinal cord is best achieved by *strong exercises* performed in prone or supine-lying, and all the basic exercises are done in these positions. All the exercises are simple ones which can easily be carried out at home, and they are done two to four times a day. The programme *must* be religiously carried out *and interspersed with regulated rest periods*. Each programme is worked out individually, and modifications and adaptations are made according to the patient's needs, the patient spending a short time in hospital, until a programme has been accurately assessed.

Exercises are of short duration, and a typical programme might be:—

1. Prone-lying; 10–12 press-ups.
2. Lying: Lifting a 7-lb. medicine ball from waist to above the head, ten to twenty times.
3. As above, lifting the ball from chest towards the ceiling.
4. As above, holding the ball in both hands and carrying it from the shoulder to the opposite hip.

These exercises have the double advantage of strengthening the shoulder-girdle and upper trunk muscles, as well as improving the circulation. Household objects of equivalent weight can be used to take the place of medicine balls at home.

Modifications may have to be made in the range of movement, and the number of times the exercises are performed. If the patient cannot get down to the floor a bed can be used.

Progressions are best made by *increasing weight rather than time*, and in the extent and range of the movement. *No patient should ever remain tired at the end of the day, and if this occurs the régime must be modified*. Swimming, skipping, running, cycling, and rowing can be used as additional activities, for such patients as can manage them.

Spasticity has been found to be little problem. Initially the most spastic areas are usually the legs and lower trunk, and in all test cases there was a marked decrease in spasticity following treatment.

Incoordination presents a greater problem, and has not yet been satisfactorily resolved. It has, however been found that holding a large object in both hands leads to greater stability, and that once the patient is strong enough to do press-ups, the incoordination can often be overcome.

COMBINED SCLEROSIS
(*Posterolateral Sclerosis. Ataxic Paraplegia*)

An affection of the posterior and lateral columns of the white matter of the spinal cord.

AETIOLOGY.—The disease is one of middle age, and is more common in men than in women. *The cause* is unknown: but it is sometimes connected with pernicious anæmia.

PATHOLOGY.—There is degeneration of the lateral columns, including the lateral cerebrospinal (crossed pyramidal) tract, the anterior and posterior spino-cerebellar, and anterior and lateral spinothalamic tracts. *Symptoms due to the lesion of the pyramidal tract predominate*. There is also sclerosis of the posterior columns, but the posterior nerve-roots are not affected, so that the reflex arc is not broken (*Fig.* 95).

SYMPTOMS.—These resemble the early symptoms of disseminated sclerosis. The *onset is insidious* and there is *weakness and spasticity* of the legs (due to the pyramidal lesion). There is also *ataxia*, from the involvement of the posterior columns and cerebellar tract. *Gait* is unsteady. *Reflexes* are exaggerated; ankle clonus and Babinski's sign are present, consistent with a lesion of the pyramidal tract. As in disseminated sclerosis, the spasticity becomes much more marked than the ataxia in the later stages. There is *no anæsthesia*.

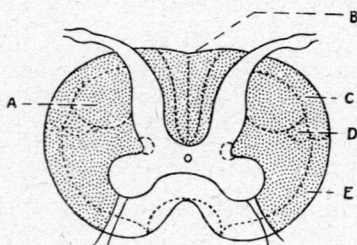

Fig. 95.—Combined sclerosis. A, Lateral cerebrospinal (crossed pyramidal) tract; B, Posterior columns; C, Posterior spinocerebellar tract; D, Rubrospinal tract; E, Lateral spinothalamic tract.

Treatment.—The disease is so similar in its main symptoms to cases of disseminated sclerosis, that a similar form of treatment can be given to combat the spasticity and ataxia.

FRIEDREICH'S DISEASE

AETIOLOGY.—A *familial* disease, affecting both males and females of the same family. The *cause* is unknown but it appears in many cases to be due to a genetic disturbance. It generally begins in childhood, but may not appear until early or late adolescence.

PATHOLOGY.—The changes are those of chronic degeneration, or sclerosis, involving both posterior and lateral columns of the cord. The fasciculi gracilis and cuneatus, the anterior and posterior spinocerebellar tract, the spinothalamic tracts, and part of the lateral cerebrospinal tract are implicated. Of the grey

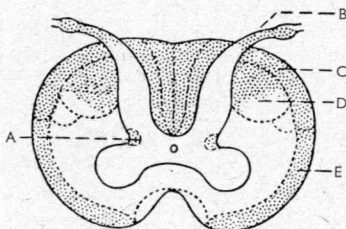

Fig. 96.—Friedreich's disease. A, Thoracic nucleus; B, Posterior nerve-root; C, Posterior spinocerebellar tract; D, Lateral cerebrospinal tract; E, Anterior and lateral spinothalamic tract.

matter, the thoracic nucleus and some of the cranial nuclei suffer. The posterior nerve-roots are also affected, though, as a rule, some of their fibres escape (*Fig.* 96).

SYMPTOMS.—It is difficult, in so extensive a lesion as this, to work out the exact symptoms likely to be present, but *those produced by the destruction of the pathways to the cerebellum seem to predominate*. We therefore find an ataxia of more or less cerebellar type but there are *skeletal* symptoms as well. The principal symptoms are:—

DISEASES OF THE BRAIN AND SPINAL CORD   233

NEUROLOGICAL SYMPTOMS.—

Ataxia and Muscular Weakness.—The first sign is often a slight unsteadiness, followed almost immediately by definite signs of muscular weakness. The incoordination spreads to the arms at a later stage. In an advanced case there is a *jerky kind of incoordination*, with a *reeling, staggering gait*, resembling that of cerebellar ataxia.

Intention Tremor develops in the arms, head, and neck, but usually remains slight.

Nystagmus is apparent at an early stage.

Speech is *hesitant* or *staccato*. It has been described as being of the 'hot-potato' type.

The above three symptoms are all probably due, in the main, to cerebellar defect.

Reflexes.—The knee-jerk is lost. The extensor form of the plantar reflex (Babinski's sign) is sometimes found.

Sensory Changes are slight as a rule. Sometimes there is paræsthesia, but rarely anæsthesia.

SKELETAL SYMPTOMS.—Deformities occur, especially scoliosis or kyphoscoliosis, talipes equinus or equinovarus, pes cavus, or a combination of the last two. In cases in which the neurological symptoms develop late in adolescence the skeletal signs have usually been present from an early date.

COURSE AND PROGNOSIS.—The disease is progressive and incurable, and usually runs a long, slow course. Occasionally, the symptoms undergo spontaneous arrest comparatively early in the disease. It is not fatal, and the patient dies of some intercurrent disease.

Principles of Treatment.—Treatment is unfortunately not very effective, since the disease is progressive, but a temporary improvement seems to take place in these patients, especially when they first start treatment. This may be psychological, but in all progressive diseases any alleviation is worth while.

As in all incurable nervous diseases, we are concerned with treating the symptoms, and with improving the patient's general condition. Our chief aims, therefore, are: (1) To deal with the ataxia as far as is possible by co-ordination exercises; (2) To take any possible measure to reduce the spinal or foot deformities*; (3) To increase the patient's comfort, and keep his general health at as high a level as possible.

PHYSICAL TREATMENT.—

This will mainly consist of treatment to improve co-ordination and power.

FRENKEL'S EXERCISES, or movements of a similar nature, can be tried to improve co-ordination and to maintain, or regain, some measure of control of muscle. Movements of the head and neck must not be forgotten. Again, Kabat techniques, particularly the balancing reactions, may be helpful.

PASSIVE MOVEMENTS, taken to the normal limit, but not beyond, can be given to prevent contractures, especially in the feet. They may also help to relieve spasticity.

RESISTED EXERCISES should be given whenever possible, in order to regain muscle power.

RHYTHMIC MOVEMENTS AND RELAXATION EXERCISES for trunk and limbs should be included, to counteract any skeletal rigidity that may be present. This would lead to loss of mobility, and fixation in a position of deformity. Free rhythmic trunk-rotations, trunk-rollings, alternate side-bendings of head

---

* These unfortunately tend to occur in spite of all precautions against them. The talipes is not as a rule treated by surgical methods, since the progressive nature of the disease renders any improvement so attained merely temporary.

and trunk are all suitable, with swinging arm movements, leg-swinging, etc. These exercises can be done in sitting, except for the last, for which the patient can stand between, and grasp, two parallel bars.

BREATHING EXERCISES should also be included, both to obtain relaxation and preserve the mobility of the thorax, and to promote metabolism by increasing the interchange of gases in the lungs.

TRANSVERSE MYELITIS

This disease consists of an acute inflammation of the spinal cord, involving either the grey matter alone, or both grey and white matter.

AETIOLOGY.—It is commoner in men than in women. People of any age may be attacked. *Causes* are many and varied. It is a bacterial or toxic condition, following various acute infections. Syphilis is often a factor. Injury of the spine, or severe chill, may be the exciting cause.

PATHOLOGY.—The changes in the cord are those of acute inflammation.

SYMPTOMS.—*The onset is generally sudden*, the patient's temperature rising very high. This is soon followed by the development of *paralysis and anæsthesia*. The exact symptoms depend on the level of the lesion of the cord. *The lower part of the thoracic region* is generally the seat of the trouble.

The table below shows the chief typical symptoms due to lesions in the cervical, lower thoracic, or lumbar regions, if the whole cord has been involved at one of these levels. It should be realized that if the lesion involves both grey and white matter in the cervical enlargement, the paralysis of the arms will be *flaccid*, that is, of the lower motor neuron type, because the anterior horn cells, the fibres of which are destined for the brachial plexus, have been destroyed; while that of the

TABLE TO SHOW THE CHIEF TYPICAL SYMPTOMS IN TRANSVERSE MYELITIS

	CERVICAL ENLARGEMENT	LOWER THORACIC REGION	LUMBAR ENLARGEMENT
Arms	1. Flaccid paralysis of arms 2. Atrophy and other trophic changes 3. Reflexes lost 4. Complete anæsthesia	Normal	Normal
Trunk	Possible involvement of phrenic nerve; if so, fatal result	1. Probably girdle sensation corresponding to upper limit of lesion 2. Otherwise normal, or little affected	Normal
Legs	1. Spastic paraplegia, with contractures 2. Trophic changes due to sensory loss. Bed-sores 3. Reflexes exaggerated; clonus and Babinski's sign 4. Complete anæsthesia	As in cervical lesion	1. Flaccid paralysis 2. Atrophy of muscles, and other trophic changes. Bed-sores 3. Reflexes lost 4. Complete anæsthesia
Sphincters	1. Bladder: Retention, due to spasticity; later incontinence 2. Rectum: Constipation, later incontinence	As in cervical lesion	Bladder and rectum: Complete incontinence due to involvement of their centres in cord

legs will be *spastic*, because the pyramidal tracts are interrupted, though the anterior horn cells of the lumbar and sacral plexuses are intact.

PROGNOSIS.—Lesions in the cervical region generally prove fatal, because the involvement of the phrenic nerves causes paralysis of the diaphragm. Cystitis (inflammation of the bladder) and nephritis may complicate the case, and ultimately cause death. Recovery, if it occurs, is seldom complete. The anæsthesia clears up first, followed by the paralysis to a greater or less degree.

Principles of Treatment.—These will be according to the kind of paralysis present. It is important to prevent contractures and deformity by positioning the patient correctly, and if necessary by the use of splints. Bed-sores must also be prevented. The problem is either one resembling anterior poliomyelitis, or one resembling spastic paraplegia due to injuries of the cord (*see* Chapter IX).

PHYSICAL TREATMENT.—Physical treatment is not usually undertaken until the acute stage is past and the patient is convalescent.

Flaccid cases need treatment suitable for anterior poliomyelitis. *The Re-education* will also proceed on a similar plan (*see* pp. 205–10). Passive movements will be required for all joints of the affected limbs, and splints or other suitable supports must be used to prevent contractures due to the pull of gravity, or to the shortening of denervated muscles, e.g., foot-drop. Other muscular contractures are unlikely to occur in complete lesions, as there are no healthy muscles in these cases. Re-education of muscles will follow similar lines to that given for poliomyelitis.

Spastic cases, commoner than the flaccid ones because the disease so often attacks the cord in the lower thoracic region, are more difficult to treat because of the intense spasm which is sometimes brought on by the merest touch. They are dealt with in the same way as the cases of spastic paraplegia already described. (*See* pp. 196–9.)

Incomplete lesions have to be treated according to the symptoms they produce.

SURGICAL TREATMENT.—*See* injection treatment in spastic paraplegia, p. 199.

CHOREA
(*St. Vitus's Dance*)

This is the result of an irritation of the cerebrum, the most characteristic symptom being that of involuntary spasmodic movements.

AETIOLOGY.—Chorea occurs most often in children between the ages of 5 and 10 years, though occasionally cases are seen among adolescents. The patients are often debilitated and undernourished. It is much commoner in girls than in boys, and is liable to recur. The disease also occurs in very young women during pregnancy and it is usually severe.

CAUSES.—Chorea is caused by a toxin of rheumatic origin, and there is often a history of other rheumatic symptoms—vague aches and pains, sore throats, etc.

PATHOLOGICAL CHANGES.—There is an irritation, or diffuse inflammation, of the cerebral hemispheres due to inflammatory changes in the meninges. Endocarditis due to the rheumatic toxin may also be present, though this is not often apparent in an initial attack but follows after subsequent ones. This may lead to valvular disease of the heart, generally of the mitral valve.

SYMPTOMS.—

INABILITY TO CONCENTRATE.—An attack often begins by the child's showing an inability to concentrate on her school-work. She is fidgety, irritable, and difficult.

LOSS OF CO-ORDINATION.—The patient becomes clumsy and awkward in performing fine movements. The gait may be unsteady if the incoordination extends to the trunk or leg muscles. Respiration may be affected, through failure of co-ordination among the respiratory muscles. There may be loss of the swing of the arms in walking as in paralysis agitans.

INVOLUNTARY MOVEMENTS.—These are jerky, purposeless, and irregular. They may affect one or both sides of the body, or be more marked on one side than on the other. Most frequent in the arms and the face, they may also appear in the legs and trunk, and sometimes affect the tongue and soft palate as well. They increase when the child is excited or nervous; when she is conscious of being watched; or when she attempts to perform specialized movements. They cease during sleep.

MUSCULAR WEAKNESS, WITH HYPOTONIA.—This occurs shortly after the condition is first noticed. The extent of the weakness varies in each case, and in some cases is more marked than the choreiform movements.

HEART SYMPTOMS.—The pulse is quick and irregular, and there may be other symptoms of valvular disease.

Since there is no destruction of nervous tissue, sensation and reflexes remain normal.

COURSE AND PROGNOSIS.—The patient recovers gradually in a few weeks or months. The prognosis is good, but the condition may recur.

Principles of Treatment.—

GENERAL TREATMENT.—Rest is required to allow the inflammation to die down and the cerebral irritability to subside. The length of the resting period will depend on the severity of the condition. The patient is kept in bed in the early stages, away from other patients or children. Nourishing food, avoidance of all excitement, and adequate sleep are all-important.

MEDICAL TREATMENT.—Suitable mild drugs are given to produce sleep.

PHYSICAL TREATMENT.—It is unlikely that the student or qualified practitioner will be required to treat many of these cases. Those for whom treatment is requested should be treated as cases of rheumatic fever (*see* Chapter XIX). *Exercises* will not be given until authorized by the physicians in charge of the case. The pulse-rate must be taken before and after treatment and if the rate is abnormally increased or remains raised for too long, modifications must be made. Before planning an exercise table, the condition of the heart should be ascertained. The table should include free relaxed movements, movements requiring co-ordination and control, and balancing exercises. Since the patients are children the tables should be short, varied, and interesting, and games should be interspersed with the exercises. When giving active exercises the larger movements should be given first, as these require less co-ordination and control. Progression is made to the finer movements. The child should practise keeping still—for a short time at first—that is, a few seconds only. Later, the length of time may be increased; but it must be borne in mind that it is not natural for any small child to remain motionless for long! General ultra-violet irradiation may be requested during convalescence for its tonic effect.

CLASS-WORK.—Before being discharged the patient may be sent to the gymnasium for an individual scheme of exercises, or for class-work.

TABLE TO SHOW ESSENTIAL DIFFERENCES IN NERVOUS DISEASES

The following table has been compiled to show at a glance the chief differences between the symptoms, and principles of treatment, of diseases of the upper and lower motor neurons, afferent neurons, and basal ganglia. The reasons for these are explained in the sections dealing with the conditions themselves.

CHIEF SYMPTOMS AND PRINCIPLES OF TREATMENT IN LESIONS OF MOTOR AND SENSORY NEURONS AND PARALYSIS AGITANS

	LOWER MOTOR NEURON	UPPER MOTOR NEURON	AFFERENT NEURON (POSTERIOR COLUMNS)	PARALYSIS AGITANS
Sites of lesion	1. Anterior horn cells of spinal cord 2. Anterior nerve-roots 3. Peripheral motor nerves	1. Cerebral cortex 2. Pyramidal tracts	Fasciculi gracilis and cuneati	Basal ganglia
Mental changes	None	1. Mental deficiency often occurs in diplegic children 2. Occasionally present in hemiplegic children or adults	None	None
Condition of muscles	1. Flaccidity 2. Atonia 3. Atrophy	1. Spasticity 2. Hypertonia 3. In cases of irritation, tonic or clonic spasm	Hypotonia or atonia	Diffuse rigidity
Function of muscles	Loss of power of movement	Loss of control of movement	Ataxia	Weakness. No paralysis
Involuntary movements	None	1. Clonic spasm 2. Athetosis 3. Tremor } In some cases (The last two are due to involvement of the basal ganglia)	None	1. Tremor, especially during rest; most marked in limbs. Head rarely affected; eyes never affected; loss of certain automatic movements
Distribution of paralysis, weakness, etc.	1. According to lesion; commonest in legs 2. May be unilateral or bilateral, symmetrical or asymmetrical 3. A paralysis of special muscles, or parts of muscles	According to lesion may be:— 1. Hemiplegia 2. Paraplegia 3. Diplegia A paralysis of certain movements rather than of muscles	Commonest in legs	1. Affecting all skeletal muscles 2. Involuntary muscles unaffected
Speech	Normal, unless laryngeal muscles affected	1. Aphasia, due to lesion affecting the speech centre; or 2. Aphonia, from spasticity of laryngeal muscles	Normal	May be shrill and monotonous; hesitation followed by rapid speech

CHIEF SYMPTOMS AND PRINCIPLES OF TREATMENT IN LESIONS OF MOTOR AND SENSORY NEURONS AND PARALYSIS AGITANS

	LOWER MOTOR NEURON	UPPER MOTOR NEURON	AFFERENT NEURON (POSTERIOR COLUMNS)	PARALYSIS AGITANS
Reflexes	Lost in affected region	1. Exaggerated reflexes; 2. Pathological reflexes: clonus or Babinski's sign	Lost	Normal or sometimes increased
Posture and gait	According to muscles affected	Spastic gait (in paraplegia, 'scissor-gait')	Ataxic gait	1. Characteristic posture (joints flexed, head forward, etc.) 2. Parkinsonian mask 3. Festinant gait
Sensory changes	None	None	1. Lightning and girdle pains 2. Muscle and joint sense impaired or lost 3. Cutaneous sensation dulled 4. Paraesthesia 5. Complete anaesthesia rare, but sense of pain may be much decreased or even lost in affected parts	1. Sensations of great heat; sweating; rise of local temperature 2. Cramps and aches, sometimes severe in late stages
Trophic changes	1. Marked changes in skin, nails, etc. 2. Atrophy of muscles 3. Arrest of bone growth in children	None, except disuse atrophy, and sometimes arthritis in old people	1. Marked, especially in bones and joints 2. Liability to perforating ulcer of foot	None
PRINCIPLES OF TREATMENT	1. Maintenance of nutrition in affected parts 2. Prevention of deformities 3. Re-education of patient in use of affected muscles 4. General re-education of patient in walking, etc. 5. Provision of suitable supports, etc., if necessary	1. Attainment of relaxation, and rhythm of movement 2. Prevention of deformity 3. Gradual re-education of patient in control of movements 4. Re-education in walking, stock movements, etc., with restoration of patient's 'formula' of movement 5. Re-education in finer movements if possible	1. Maintenance of nutrition in affected limbs 2. Prevention of injury or overstrain to joints 3. Re-education in co-ordination of movement by means of sense of sight 4. Re-education in walking, etc. 5. Provision of suitable supports in cases of extreme atonia	1. Attainment of a certain measure of general relaxation 2. Improvement of general circulation 3. Re-education, as far as possible, in freedom of movement, posture and gait 4. Maintenance of patient's general health and spirits

CHAPTER XII

LESIONS OF THE PERIPHERAL NERVES

General considerations; Principles of treatment. I. Nerve lesions of the upper extremity: Ulnar paralysis—Median paralysis—Musculospiral paralysis—Paralysis due to injury of the circumflex nerve—Erb's paralysis—Klumpke's paralysis. II. Lesions of the lower extremity: Anterior crural paralysis—External popliteal paralysis. III. Winged scapular. IV. Facial paralysis. V. Operation on nerves.

PERIPHERAL nerves may be affected by *disease, trauma,* or an *inflammatory reaction* in their structure. The former (anterior poliomyelitis, progressive muscular atrophy, and syringomyelia) have been dealt with in Chapters IX and X. The latter will be dealt with in Chapter XIII. Here we are concerned with injuries of the peripheral nerves themselves. Such injuries include *compression, contusion,* and *severance,* which may be partial or complete. A nerve-root, a nerve-trunk, or even a whole plexus may be involved. The possibility of recovery in these lesions depends primarily on the *nature and degree of the initial injury.*

DEGREES OF TRAUMA.—There are three degrees of trauma. The mildest form consists of *an obstruction to the conduction of nerve-impulses,* with little or no actual structural damage, so that once the obstruction has been removed the nerve recovers. Such a state is known as *neurapraxia.* If, however, the pressure is prolonged, *the axoplasm may become compressed.* In this event it becomes attenuated and in time the fibres break. *Nerve conduction then ceases.* This condition is known technically as *axonotmesis.*

If the damage severs the nerve the condition is known as *neuronotmesis.* For practical purposes these last two are the same.

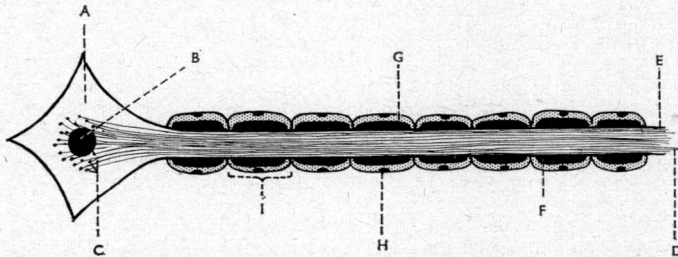

Fig. 97.—Structure of a nerve-fibre. A, Nerve-cell; B, Nucleus; C, Nissl bodies giving rise to D; D, Neurofibrils or axons; E, Axolemma containing axis-cylinder axoplasm and neurofibrils; F, Medullary or myelin sheath; G, Neurilemma; H, Nucleus of Schwann; I, Node of Ranvier.

PATHOLOGICAL CHANGES.—From the point of view of recovery the important factors are the integrity of the outer sheath of the nerve—the epineurium (*see Fig.* 118, p. 267)—and of the medullary or myelin sheath (*Fig.* 97), since it is by means of the myelin sheath that the nerve-impulses are conducted.

NEURAPRAXIA.—The nerve-cell and all the structures of the nerve-fibre are intact but the pressure has obstructed their function. As soon as this has been removed the nerve begins to recover.

AXONOTMESIS AND NEURONOTMESIS.—Whether the nerve itself has been severed or only the axons, the pathological changes are the same, and degeneration occurs (*Fig.* 98). The nucleus enlarges and the Nissl bodies disappear; the neurofibrils degenerate proximally as far as the nearest node of Ranvier. Distally, the axis-cylinder and neurofibrils completely disappear; the myelin sheath degenerates into fatty globules and finally disappears, until only the neurilemma and the nuclei of Schwann remain ('Wallerian degeneration').

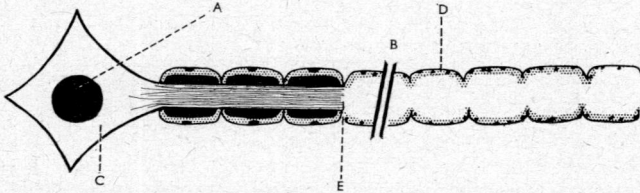

Fig. 98.—Wallerian degeneration following axonotmesis or neuronotmesis. A, Cell body empty of Nissl bodies; B, Level of lesion; C, Enlarged nucleus; D, Neurilemma and proliferating nucleus of Schwann; E, Degeneration of neurofibrils to nearest node of Ranvier.

Spontaneous regeneration occurs in axonotmesis and the prognosis is usually good. The nuclei of Schwann proliferate in the neurilemma distal to the lesion and, by the liberation of a chemical substance, attract the axons into the neurilemma sheaths. This rate of growth is 1 millimetre per day. In time, the myelin sheath and the axis-cylinder reappear and the nerve gradually returns to normal. In cases of severance no regeneration can occur until the epineurium has been sutured. Even so, the prognosis is often poor. Many peripheral nerves are mixed nerves, and the fibres may grow into the wrong neurilemma sheaths, e.g., a motor fibre may grow into a sensory neurilemma and vice versa, or there may be cross innervation. There is also considerable risk of scar tissue forming in the neurilemma which will impede the progress of the nerve; or the axons themselves may form a tangle of nervous tissue, i.e., a neuroma.

SIGNS AND SYMPTOMS.—

PARALYSIS.—This may be *partial* or *complete*, depending on the type and level of the lesion. The period of time for which the paralysis lasts will again depend on these factors. For example, a *neurapraxia* may give rise to complete paralysis, or to a variable degree of weakness. Since there is no actual structural damage, the time for which the disablement lasts will be relatively short. *Axonotmesis* or *neuronotmesis* involving the complex brachial plexus will, however, paralyse the entire arm and recovery will not be complete unless, and until, all the fibres have grown to their full length. On the other hand, either condition involving the ulnar nerve at the wrist will normally only cause paralysis of the interossei, the hypothenar eminence, the adductores pollicis, and the medial two lumbricals. The length of these nerves is relatively short and the paralysis will last for a comparatively short time.

SENSORY CHANGES.—Most peripheral nerves are of the mixed variety (i.e., they carry both motor and sensory fibres). In most cases of *axonotmesis* or *neuronotmesis* there is anæsthesia in the areas supplied by the nerves involved. *As the nerve regenerates* sensations of *pain*, *hyperæsthesia*, or '*pins* and *needles*' are usually experienced. The dividing line between such sensations and anæsthesia provides a useful aid in assessing prognosis. *Neurapraxia* may sometimes give rise to anæsthesia but more often the changes are those found in regenerating nerves.

TROPHIC CHANGES.—These are present in the affected areas, though they are more marked in some lesions than in others. They are present in muscles (which atrophy from disuse), the skin, and nails.

ELECTRICAL CHANGES.—In addition to the physical signs, changed responses to electrical stimulation will also be present. For details of these changes the student should consult one of the standard electrical text-books. Here it suffices to say that *so long as a conducting nerve is present all responses to stimuli are brought about by the nerve. Only in cases where the nerve has ceased to function will a contraction result from direct stimulation of muscle tissue*, and stimuli of a shorter duration than $\frac{1}{50}$ second will not stimulate muscle tissue (*Fig. 99A*). *The nerve* may be stimulated at the nerve-trunk or at the motor end-plates, *the muscle* can only be stimulated at the motor end-plate or by a longitudinal application of the

MULTI-TEST CHART for use with the

RITCHIE—SNEATH STIMULATOR AND MULTITONE TEN PULSE STIMULATOR.

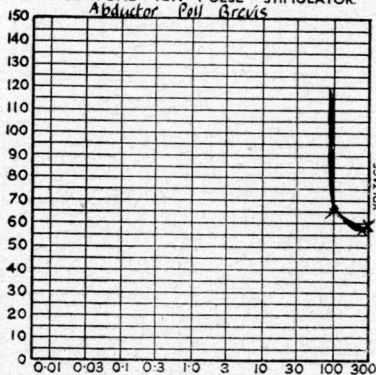

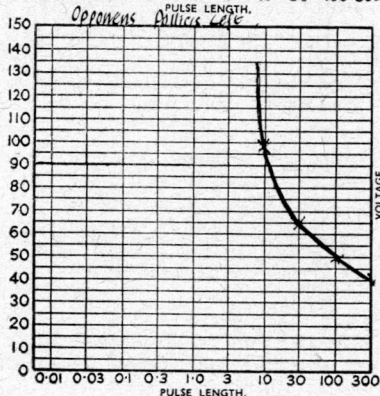

PATIENT Miss. H. aged 8.

DIAGNOSIS. Seq. Supracondylar fracture L. Elbow.

DATE.	REMARKS.
25/7/67	Shows CRD in Abductor pollicis brevis L. Opponens pollicis L. Normal curves for Flexor pollis Brevis.

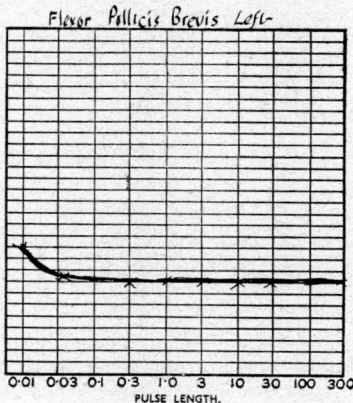

MULTITONE ELECTRIC CO. LTD. LONDON.

A

[See Legend overleaf

MULTI-TEST CHART for use with the

RITCHIE—SNEATH STIMULATOR AND
MULTITONE TEN PULSE STIMULATOR.

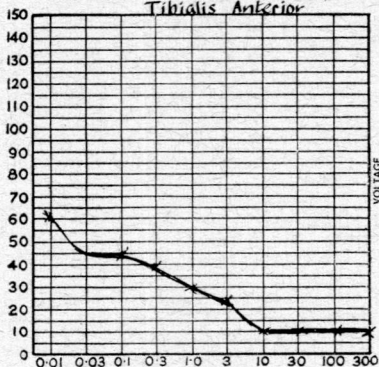

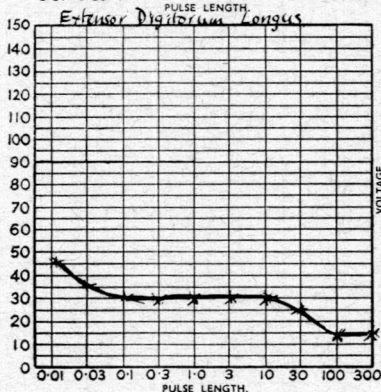

PATIENT Mr J.   aged 38.

DIAGNOSIS. Foot drop.

DATE.	REMARKS.
28. X. 66	Shows PRD in Tibialis Anterior. Ext. Digitorum longus. Ext. Hallucis longus.

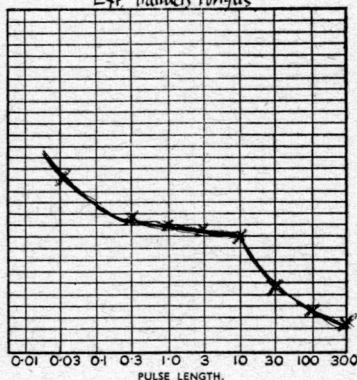

MULTITONE ELECTRIC CO. LTD. LONDON.

B

Fig. 99.—Showing normal conduction, complete and partial reaction of degeneration. A shows that the same voltage will stimulate the nerve up to $\frac{1}{10}$ sec., after which a slight increase is required in normal conduction. There is no response after 100 or 10 m. per sec. in denervated tissue. B shows the erratic nature of a partially conducting nerve, a much higher voltage being required to produce the same response than when all the fibrils are conducting.

current (from origin to insertion). The response to muscle stimulation is slower and more sluggish than the contraction resulting from stimulation through the nerve. From a diagnostic point of view the following points should be borne in mind.

1. *In neurapraxia* there will be electrical conduction *below* the level of the lesion, but not above it. The nerve-trunk, therefore, may or may not respond to stimuli but the motor end-plates will.

2. *In axonotmesis* there will be *no response to stimulation of the nerve-trunk*. For the first 14–21 days there will be *a response at the motor end-plate* to both a faradic and interrupted direct current, because the distal degeneration (Wallerian degeneration) is not established until then. After that there will be *no response through the nerve* but *the muscle will give its characteristic response to interrupted direct current*. The term *reaction of degeneration* is used to denote the response to electrical stimuli. It may be partial, complete, or absolute.

Partial Reaction of Degeneration.—There will be some response to both faradic and interrupted direct current, but the intensity required will be higher than that needed to stimulate normal nervous tissue (*Fig.* 99B). It indicates the presence of some conducting nerve-fibres, and is seen in the first 2–3 weeks following axonotmesis (for this reason a nerve-conduction test carried out before this time in such cases will not give an accurate picture); in cases of neurapraxia; and in cases of nerve regeneration.

Complete Reaction of Regeneration.—There is no response other than by the muscle tissue (*Fig.* 99 A). It indicates the absence of conducting nerve-fibres and is present at once in neuronotmesis and after 2–3 weeks in axonotmesis.

Absolute Reaction of Degeneration.—There is no response to any form of electrical stimuli, indicating complete fibrosis of muscle. It is to avoid this occurrence that treatment is given pending the regeneration of the nerve.

Principles of Treatment.—These are common to all forms of traumatic peripheral nerve lesions, and are as follows:—

1. PREVENTION OF CONTRACTURES.—This is essential, since denervated muscle will rapidly atrophy and contract. The application of *relaxed passive movements* in full range to all affected joints is usually sufficient to control this tendency, but care must be taken to avoid undue stretching of the nerve and the limb must be kept in a correct position during treatment. *Splints* may also have to be used, although many authorities feel that their use should be restricted as much as possible. When used they should be light and simple, and adequate padding is required to prevent pressure or friction on atrophic skin. 'Lively splints' are often helpful. These are hinged and elasticized to allow movement similar to that which occurs in normal muscle. They also prevent stretching of the denervated tissue following movement of the antagonists.

2. MAINTENANCE OF THE DENERVATED TISSUE.—The most important factor, common to all traumatic nerve lesions, is *maintenance of muscle bulk* pending regeneration of the nerve. Should this not be adequately maintained, *fibrosis* of the muscle will occur and any recovery of the nerve will be negated by the state of the muscle tissue. The application of interrupted direct current will effectively achieve this. Ideally, it should be given daily to all the affected muscles. It is not necessary to change to the faradic current as the nerve regenerates since, if a nerve-fibre is conducting, it will respond equally well to interrupted direct current. In the case of *complete paralysis of a limb* it is extremely important to control œdema. Because the supporting tone of the muscles is lost, the vessels dilate, and their permeability increases. Fluid therefore seeps out into the interstitial spaces. *Elevation, massage,* and *passive movements* can be used to combat œdema and in severe cases elastic or crêpe bandages should be worn. Adequate circulation must be maintained in order to keep up the nutrition of the tissues. *Massage and passive movements* will assist this to a certain extent and if anæsthesia is not too extensive to render such treatment dangerous, *heat* can also be applied. The most effective form is short-wave diathermy, applied by means of a coil and using a longitudinal field. *Contrast bathing* is also useful. If the tissues can be warmed before electrical and physical treatment is given, a greater response will be achieved in the way of contraction (Van't Hoff's Law).

3. RE-EDUCATION OF MUSCLE.—*As the nerve recovers and voluntary contraction again becomes possible this must be assiduously combined with electrical treatment.* It will follow the same lines as re-education in anterior poliomyelitis. The exercises will first be done with gravity eliminated and will gradually progress until resistance can be added (*see* p. 206). It should be noted that *a faradic response will be obtained some time before voluntary contraction is possible.* When considering *resisted movements* it should be remembered that the *strength of the contraction* depends not on the stimuli received at the anterior horn cell (as in anterior poliomyelitis) but *on the conducting power of the nerve-fibre itself.* For this reason Kabat techniques have little advantage over the other methods of applying resistance, but they may, of course, be used in re-education. An accurate knowledge of anatomy and a thorough understanding of the principles of treatment is essential to the physiotherapist in these cases. In examining these cases, it should be remembered that the muscular or cutaneous supply is not always that described in the text-books—for instance, sometimes the ulnar nerve supplies three or even four of the lumbricales, instead of only two; and the author has known one case of complete severance of the ulnar nerve just above the wrist, with no loss of sensation in the hand. Moreover, some nerves communicate so freely with others, that loss of sensation is often slight, or incomplete, if one of them is injured. Generally speaking, however, the nervous distribution is remarkably true to type.

Every nerve-lesion should be given an electrical-conduction test 2–3 weeks after the initial injury. The durations of the stimuli applied should range from 1 sec. through 1/10 sec., 1/50 sec., 1/100 sec., and 1/1000 sec. at least, and the results should be plotted on a graph. Only in this way can the nature and extent of the lesion be determined. Other similar tests should be given at regular intervals to assess progress.

METHODS OF TREATMENT applicable in these cases can be summarized as follows:—

1. A nerve-conduction test 2–3 weeks after injury followed by others at regular intervals.

2. Daily electrical stimulation with interrupted direct current over the motor end-plates of all affected muscles, and to the nerve-trunk if and when it can conduct impulses.

3. Full range passive movements to all affected joints to prevent contracture and possible œdema.

4. Active movements as soon as the muscles can be contracted voluntarily. These should form an integral part of all treatments of traumatic nerve-lesions. In addition the following methods can be used:—

a. Heat or contrast bathing to assist circulation and muscle activity. The possibility of burns arising because of anæsthesia must be carefully taken into account before this is given.

b. Splints to prevent contractures.

c. Massage to control œdema and assist circulation.

d. Bandages to control œdema.

Since treatment is common to all these cases it is not proposed to give further details of this. Only the main symptoms of each lesion and any special points will be discussed in the following pages.

We will consider first the lesions of the main nerves in the upper extremity—the ulnar, median, radial, and circumflex—then the two 'root-paralyses' of Erb (cervical 5 and 6) and Klumpke (cervical 8 and dorsal 1). In the lower extremity we shall describe the paralyses occasioned by lesions of the femora (anterior crural) and lateral popliteal nerves. Next we shall deal with the treatment of winged scapula and of facial paralysis. Finally, we shall discuss nerve sutures and the modifications of the treatment which are then required.

I. NERVE LESIONS OF THE UPPER EXTREMITY
ULNAR PARALYSIS

The ulnar nerve may be injured: (1) *In the axilla* (rarely), by a wound, by pressure (as of a crutch), or by the presence of a cervical rib (*see* p. 254). (2) *At the elbow*, where it may be torn or lacerated when a fracture or dislocation takes place, or later compressed by callus or scar tissue. (3) *At the wrist*, generally by direct injuries, such as cuts, wounds, etc. It may be injured in any part of its course by wounds or tumours.

SYMPTOMS.—

PARALYSIS IF THE INJURY IS AT OR ABOVE THE ELBOW.—

1. *In the forearm*, paralysis of the flexor carpi ulnaris and the inner half of the flexor profundus digitorum, resulting in weakening of adduction (ulnar deviation) of the wrist, and loss of flexion of the terminal phalanges of the fourth and fifth fingers.

2. *In the hand*, paralysis of the interossei, the two inner lumbricales, the adductores pollicis, and the adductor and flexor brevis minimi digiti, producing loss of abduction and adduction of the fingers, and inability to flex the metacarpophalangeal joints and at the same time extend the interphalangeal joints of the two inner fingers (sometimes of three or even four).

PARALYSIS IF THE INJURY IS AT THE WRIST.—The flexor carpi ulnaris and flexor profundus digitorum are uninjured. The changes mentioned above under (2) are the only ones present. This is a disabling form of paralysis, impairing the fine movements of hands and fingers.

ATROPHY OF ALL THE AFFECTED MUSCLES.—It is most evident on the inner side of the palm (hypothenar eminence), and in the hollows between the metacarpals on the dorsum of the hand.

POSITION OF THE HAND.—This is the well-known *main-en-griffe*, or claw-hand. It is due to paralysis of the interossei and two or more lumbricales which allows the unopposed action of the extensor digitorum and the long flexors to produce hyperextension of the metacarpophalangeal joints and flexion of the interphalangeal joints. As a rule, only the ring and little fingers are affected (*Fig.* 100).

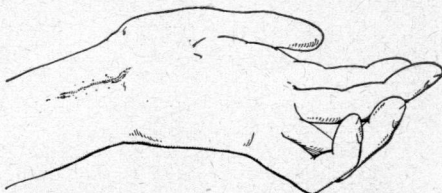

Fig. 100.—*Main-en-griffe* in ulnar nerve paralysis.

If the lesion is at or above the elbow, and the flexor profundus is paralysed, the last phalanges are flexed only slightly, if at all. The tendons of the flexores sublimis and profundus become visible, and stand out in the palm, owing to the wasting of the lumbricales and hypothenar muscles.

In *incomplete lesions*, fibrous changes often take place in the palmar fascia and the tendons become adherent to their sheaths. This produces an entirely fixed 'claw' position of at least the two inner fingers (Purves-Stewart*).

* *Peripheral Nerve Injuries.*

ANÆSTHESIA of the parts supplied by the nerve, i.e., the inner half of the palm, the dorsum of the hand, and one and a half inner fingers. If the lesion is at or only just above the wrist, the dorsal cutaneous branch escapes and sensation at the back of the hand and fingers is unaffected.

TROPHIC CHANGES, other than in muscles, are not marked.

Special Treatment Points.—The cause of the trouble, if still persisting, must first be removed by surgical means (e.g., callus, scar tissue, or cervical rib).

SUPPORT.—A special splint may be required. If so, one made of light metal and fitted with straps for each finger is preferable in these cases; if such is not available, an appropriately padded light plaster splint may be used.

POSITION OF THE HAND.—If the nerve is injured just above the wrist, the hand should be placed on the splint with the metacarpophalangeal joints flexed, the fingers straight, and the thumb in adduction close to the hand (*Fig.* 101). If it is

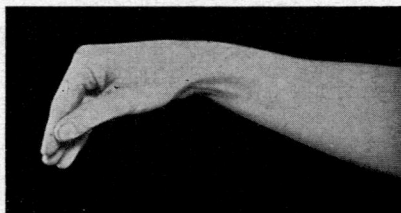

Fig. 101.—Position in which the hand should be splinted in ulnar paralysis. (Thumb should be more adducted than is shown in the figure.)

injured above the point where its branches to the two forearm muscles are given off, the wrist should also be slightly flexed and the hand adducted. *The corrected position must be maintained throughout treatment.*

PHYSICAL TREATMENT.—

MASSAGE.—*Hand massage* is specially important to prevent fibrous changes occurring in the palmar fascia in incomplete lesions. Effleurage should be given to the whole hand, and finger-kneading to all the muscles affected—that is, to the

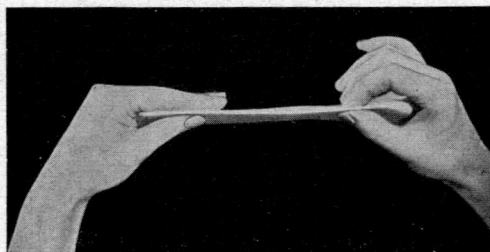

Fig. 102.—Grasping a sheet of paper with both hands. The left hand shows the position to be aimed at, the right hand that generally assumed by the patient in ulnar paralysis.

whole of the palm and hypothenar eminence, and the interosseous spaces at the back of the hand. Careful frictions should be given to all the fingers, especially the fourth and fifth.

ELECTRICAL STIMULATION.—*The indifferent pad* may be placed over the cervical or upper thoracic spine if the lesion is complete. If the lesion is at the elbow it is best applied to the nerve-trunk just above the elbow. The same position is often used for lesions at the wrist, but a better result may be obtained by placing the indifferent pad over the nerve-trunk at the wrist, or on the dorsum of the hand. Because the intrinsic muscles are so small the *active pad* should be correspondingly small.

ACTIVE MOVEMENTS.—The length of time elapsing before active movement is possible may be weeks, or months, depending on the injury. In some cases, of course, power may never have been completely lost.

'*Trick*' *Movements.*—It is necessary here to warn the physiotherapist against two 'trick' movements, which may lead her to suppose that power is returning before this is actually the case: (1) It is possible to produce a small amount of *abduction* of the fingers—plus hyperextension at the metacarpophalangeal joint— by using the extensor digitorum; and of *adduction*—plus flexion—by using the long flexors of the fingers. (2) She may find that there appears to be no loss of *adduction of the thumb*, because the flexor longus pollicis and opponens pollicis

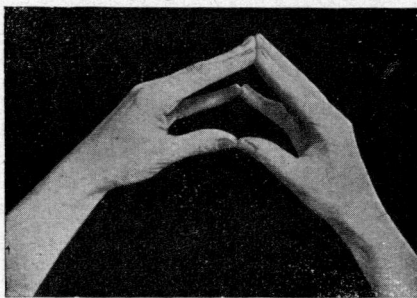

Fig. 103.

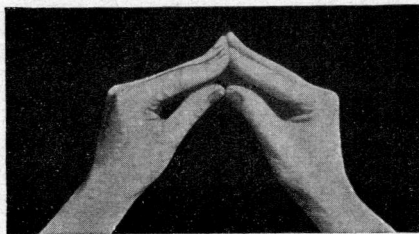

Fig. 104.

Figs. 103, 104.—'Old Gentleman'. In an early case the thumbs should not be so far abducted as in *Fig.* 103.

perform this action. But the flexor longus pollicis flexes the last phalanx at the same time and this flexion constitutes *Froment's sign*, which is typical of ulnar paralysis. To prevent the patient from abducting and adducting his fingers by means of the long flexors and extensor, the hand should be so placed that hyperextension is impossible during abduction, i.e., the metacarpophalangeal joints should be kept slightly flexed. During adduction, at least in the later stages, they should be kept in almost complete extension (though not, of course, in hyperextension), to avoid any possible flexion. *If there is no chance of the nerve recovering, trick movements may be encouraged, but if return of function is probable, they should not be allowed.*

As recovery progresses, the patient must be taught to use the hand normally; and he should practise the ordinary movements of everyday life—writing, sewing, tying knots, fastening buttons, etc. A few free and resisted exercises suitable for ulnar paralysis is given below.

EXERCISES.—

1. *Finger-parting and -closing* (hand in supination on table).—(*a*) Free, moving each finger separately. (*b*) Free, moving all fingers together. (*c*) Resisted, each finger separately; patient may push away weights with his fingers.

2. *Grasping a Sheet of Paper with Both Hands*.—Between thumb and first finger, keeping metacarpophalangeal joints flexed and interphalangeal joints extended (*Fig.* 102).

3. '*Old Gentleman*'.—Finger-tips and thumb of both hands placed together (hands in front of thorax), fingers slightly abducted, thumb between abduction and adduction (*Fig.* 103). Bring the four finger-tips close together, flexing the metacarpophalangeal joint, and bring thumb-tips into contact with index fingers (*Fig.* 104).

4. *Finger-stretching*.—Hands pronated on table, fingers flexed; stretch each finger forward in turn (*Fig.* 105). (Be careful not to hyperextend the metacarpophalangeal joints of the other fingers (*Fig.* 106).)

5. *Hands Side by Side on Table*, supinated. Approximate in succession, tips of two little fingers, two ring, two middle, and two index fingers.

6. *Place Index and Little Fingers* in front of middle and ring fingers (*Fig.* 107).

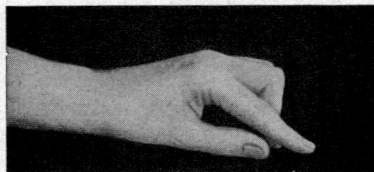

Fig. 105.

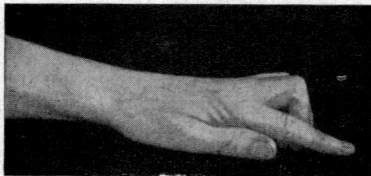

Fig. 106.

Figs. 105, 106.—Finger-stretching. Fig. 105, the exercise done correctly. Fig. 106, the exercise done incorrectly, with hyperextension of the metacarpophalangeal joints of the three inner fingers.

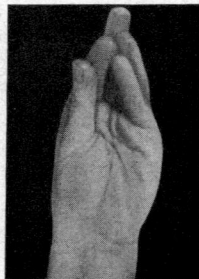

Fig. 107.—Exercise 6, ulnar paralysis. The index and little fingers placed in front of the middle and ring fingers.

MEDIAN PARALYSIS

The median nerve may be injured: (1) *In the axilla*, or *above the elbow*, although this is rare. (2) *At the elbow*, where it may be involved in a fracture, though far less frequently than is the ulnar nerve. (3) *Low in the forearm*, or *at the wrist*, the most common site of injury, since the nerve is in a superficial position.

SYMPTOMS.—

PARALYSIS IF INJURED AT OR ABOVE THE ELBOW.—

1. *In the Forearm*.—There is paralysis of the pronators and the wrist flexors, except flexor carpi ulnaris and one half of flexor digitorum profundus. The

forearm can only be pronated weakly to mid-position by the brachioradialis. The wrist can only be flexed very weakly, and is at the same time drawn to the ulnar side. The last phalanx of the thumb cannot be flexed. The index and middle fingers can only be flexed at the metacarpophalangeal joint (by the interossei), but not at either interphalangeal joint. The ring and little fingers can be flexed at all joints by the inner half of the flexor profundus, though less strongly because of the loss of the flexor sublimis. (Sometimes the ulnar nerve supplies rather more than half of the flexor profundus, and the middle finger can also be flexed.)

2. *In the Hand.*—There is paralysis of the thenar eminence (abductor pollicis, opponens pollicis, and outer half of flexor brevis pollicis) and the outer two lumbricales. The loss of the power of opposing the thumb to the fingers is the most serious feature of the injury, since the patient cannot use his hand for any fine movements unless he can do this. Abduction of the thumb, however, may be brought about by the abductor longus. The loss of the two outer lumbricales weakens flexion of the metacarpophalangeal joint of the index and middle fingers, and extension of their interphalangeal joints.

PARALYSIS IF INJURED AT THE WRIST, or below the point where the muscular branches are given off in the forearm.—The only loss is that of the intrinsic muscles of the hand—the thenar muscles and lumbricales.

ATROPHY of the front of the forearm and thenar eminence.

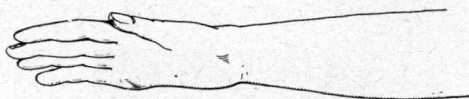

Fig. 108.—*Main-de-singe* in median nerve paralysis.

POSITION OF THE HAND.—The deformity is not obvious when the hand is at rest, except that the thumb lies back on the same plane as the fingers, producing the characteristic *main-de-singe* (monkey hand, *Fig.* 108), and that the atrophy of its muscles is marked. The hand is supinated, and the wrist in slight extension.

SENSORY CHANGES.—

Anæsthesia in the part supplied by the nerve—often incomplete.

Loss of Joint Sense in the affected fingers.

Hyperæsthesia to deep pressure in some cases.

Pain is specially common in lesions of this nerve. It may be spontaneous, or produced by pressure, and is known as *causalgia* or *thermalgia*. It is generally at the tips of the fingers, at the inner side of the thenar eminence, or at the junction of the palm with the index and middle fingers. It comes on suddenly and increases in intensity until it becomes almost unbearable. The patient may suffer from these pains for months, and so severe are they that he may become morbid and neurotic.

TROPHIC CHANGES are well marked, possibly because a large number of vasomotor fibres run in this nerve. The sweat-glands of the part may become more, or less active than normal, the skin may be reddened, and characteristic changes appear in the nails.

Special Treatment Points.—

SUPPORT: POSITION OF THE HAND.—A light plaster splint should be provided to hold the thumb abducted and opposed to the fingers, with the fingers semiflexed at all joints. The wrist should be flexed, and the hand supported in pronation in a sling. If the nerve is injured low down in the forearm, the wrist and radio-ulnar joints may be left free, unless a wound has to be considered.

PHYSICAL TREATMENT.—

ELECTRICAL STIMULATION.—Similar positions may be used for the indifferent pad as for the ulnar nerve, i.e., at neck, elbow, wrist, or hand.

MASSAGE may be required to prevent œdema which frequently occurs in this lesion. It should be given on the same principle as for the ulnar nerve, with special attention to the fingers and the dorsum of the hand. If there has been any sign of causalgia, the parts where it has been felt must be avoided. In some cases, it may contra-indicate massage of the hand altogether. Causalgia is sometimes treated by cold, wet, applications. In severe cases, injections into the nerve are sometimes tried.

ACTIVE MOVEMENTS.—

Trick Movements.—In order to bring about pronation of the hand, the patient slightly abducts the shoulder, so that the hand falls into pronation by gravity. This may be mistaken for a true active movement. He can also produce a similar movement by straightening the elbow and inwardly rotating the shoulder. Sometimes all the fingers may be flexed at all joints by the pull of that part of the flexor profundus which is supplied by the ulnar nerve, the contraction pulling the paralysed outer half with it. Flexion of each finger separately should, therefore, be practised.

The two inner fingers can be flexed at all joints by the deep flexor, which, having flexed the second interphalangeal joints, afterwards flexes the first. To work the flexor sublimis, the patient should practise flexing the first interphalangeal joints without having flexed the second (*Fig.* 109).

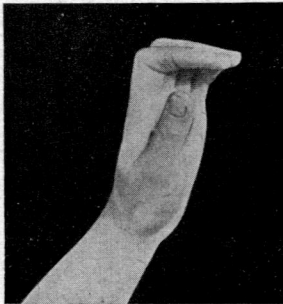

Fig. 109.—Flexion of first interphalangeal joints alone.

EXERCISES.—

1. *Grasping and squeezing a rubber ball*, not larger than a tennis ball. (*a*) Soft, (*b*) Hard. *Grasping and holding* objects of varying diameter. These exercises encourage gripping.

2. *Closing the hand*; *then opening gently*, not fully extending fingers or wrist when opening.

3. *Touching the tip of each finger in turn with tip of thumb*, making 'O's'.

4. *Touching the second phalanx of each finger with tip of thumb* (flexion of all joints of fingers).

5. *Piano-playing movements* of fingers with hand half-way between pronation and supination.

6. *Abduction of wrist.*—Hand on block or box, fingers flexed over edge; push away weight by abducting hand.

7. *Wrist-machine* for flexion and pronation when strong enough.

8. *Picking up and putting down* small objects—balls, dice, marbles, coins held by edges between fingers, etc.; also exercises with the sand-tray.

RADIAL (MUSCULOSPIRAL) PARALYSIS
(*Wrist-drop*)

The radial nerve, or its motor branch, the *posterior interosseous nerve* (deep branch of radial), may be injured: (1) *In the axilla*, generally by pressure, as of crutches; (2) *In the spiral groove (musculospiral groove)*, injury of elbow complicating fracture of the humerus (*see* p. 22); (3) *Near or below the elbow*, in injuries to that joint.

SYMPTOMS.—
PARALYSIS IF INJURED IN THE AXILLA.—

1. *In the arm and forearm.* There is paralysis of triceps and anconeus, brachioradialis and the supinator, and part of brachialis. Flexion of the elbow is weak and supination can only be performed in flexion by the biceps. There is complete loss of extension of the elbow.

2. *In the wrist and hand.* There is paralysis of all extensors of wrist, and long extensors of fingers and thumb with loss of extension of the wrist, metacarpophalangeal joints of the fingers, and all joints of the thumb.

PARALYSIS IF INJURED AT OR BELOW THE ELBOW (posterior interosseous nerve).—

All Extensors of Wrist, except Extensor Carpi Radialis Longus, which can only produce very weak extension of the wrist, if any.

Extensors of Fingers and Thumb.—As above.

Supinator.—Weakening of supination.

ATROPHY of these muscles; especially evident at the back of the arm and forearm. The wasting is, however, generally less marked than in median and ulnar lesions.

POSITION OF THE HAND.—*Dropped wrist*: the wrist hangs loosely in flexion and the metacarpophalangeal joints are also flexed, but contracture of the flexors is rare. The patient keeps the elbow semiflexed. The hand is pronated. When the patient attempts to extend the fingers, the wrist is flexed by the synergists.

ANÆSTHESIA is rare, because of the numerous communciations between the musculospiral and other nerves. If it is present, it is in the area supplied by the terminal cutaneous branch of the radial nerve.

TROPHIC CHANGES are not marked.

Special Treatment Points (of posterior interosseous paralysis—pure 'wrist-drop').—

SUPPORT.—The hand is flexed on a *short* cock-up splint, with the wrist in full, or almost full, extension. The metacarpophalangeal joints may also be supported in extension (not hyperextension) as well, but the other finger-joints should be left free; the thumb should be held in abduction and extension (*Fig.* 110). Various special splints have been devised, allowing the patient to move the thumb and fingers more than would be possible with a metal or plastic splint.

PHYSICAL TREATMENT.—

ELECTRICAL STIMULATION.—The *indifferent pad* is best placed over the musculospiral groove, or where the nerve emerges through the interosseous membrane.

PASSIVE MOVEMENTS.—Full extension of the wrist and fingers together should be given, to prevent any tendency to flexor contraction; extension of the thumb is also necessary.

EXERCISES for the later stages.—

1. For stretching movements, *see* free exercises for stiff wrist (pp. 123–5).

2. *Five-finger Exercises.*—Hand pronated on table, fingers flexed; raise each finger separately; later, all together (*Fig.* 111).

3. '*Piano-playing*'.—Position as No. 2. Same exercise, but done quickly, each finger in succession.

4. Hand pronated on table; raise fingers separately; later, all together.

5. *Finger parting.*—Starting position as in Exercise 3 for ULNAR PARALYSIS ('Old Gentleman'). Separate each pair of finger-tips in succession as far as possible from each other, keeping the others in contact (*Fig.* 112).

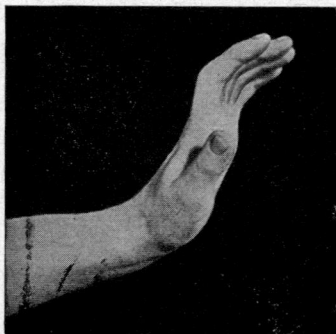

Fig. 110.—Position in which the hand should be splinted in radial paralysis.

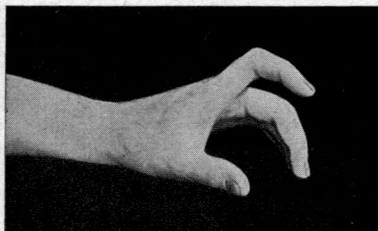

Fig. 111.—Five-finger exercise for radial paralysis.

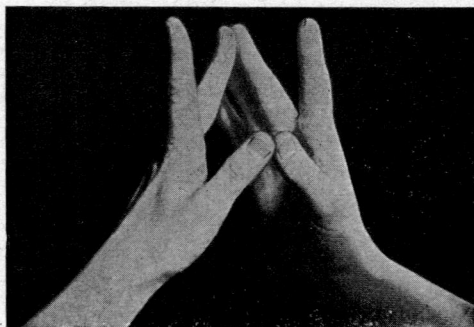

Fig. 112.—Finger-parting for radial paralysis.

6. Push away objects on the table by extending wrist and finger-joints.

7. Wrist machine, the bar being turned *towards* the patient's body.

The prognosis in radial injuries is much better than in those of the median and ulnar nerves, even after severance.

Detail of Re-education in the Use of the Wrist Extensors in a Case of Posterior Interosseous Paralysis

The following scheme shows the detail of the progressive re-education of a patient in the use of a single group of paralysed muscles. It is merely meant to illustrate the principles on which the re-education is carried out—especially as regards the use of gravity, the elimination of friction, and the type of muscle work to be required of the patient. The wrist extensors allow of fairly straight-forward treatment and have, therefore, been taken as an example. Other muscle groups present greater difficulties (*see* pp. 255–6). In most cases each muscle, or group of muscles must be studied for its own sake, and *in all cases due care must be taken to see that no paralysed group is brought into a harmful position or is unduly stretched,* while another is receiving attention.

Wrist Movements.—

I. GRAVITY ASSISTING.—
    POSITION.—Hand in supination over edge of table; wrist in full extension.
    EXERCISES.—1. Raise hand into a few degrees of flexion and drop (to relax antagonists).
        2. *Static holding*: Patient is told to try to hold wrist back in this position.

II. GRAVITY ELIMINATED.—
    FRICTION.—Eliminated by smooth surface, sling, or water.
    POSITION.—Between pronation and supination, i.e., hand in mid-position.
    EXERCISES.—1. *Static holding*: Wrist placed in full extension, patient told to hold it so.
        2. *Assisted movement*: Wrist flexed a few degrees, patient brings it to full extension with operator's assistance.
        3. *Free movement*: As (2), but unassisted.
    N.B.—The flexors may be used in the outer range.

III. GRAVITY RESISTING.—
    POSITION.—Hand in pronation.
    EXERCISES.—1. *Static holding*: Wrist held extended against gravity.
        2. *Eccentric movement*: Wrist lowered from full extension to mid-position.
        3. *Concentric movement*: Wrist raised from mid-position to full extension.
        4. *Concentric and eccentric movement*: (2) and (3) combined.

IV. RESISTANCE BY OPERATOR.—
    POSITION.—As convenient.
    EXERCISES.—*Concentric and eccentric movements,* in inner and full range to strengthen muscles.

V. GENERAL EXERCISES.—
    Whole range movements to both groups.
    Free exercises for mobility.
    Co-ordination exercises.

Extension of Thumb.—
The principles will be the same as those given above:—

I. GRAVITY ASSISTING.—
    POSITION.—Hand in pronation with arm abducted.

II. GRAVITY ELIMINATED.—
    POSITION.—Hand in pronation.

III. GRAVITY RESISTING.—
    POSITION.—Hand in mid-position.

PARALYSIS DUE TO INJURY OF CIRCUMFLEX NERVE

A lesion of the circumflex (axillary) nerve *alone* is rare, though it may occur as a complication of a dislocated shoulder, or of fractures in the region of that joint. Paralysis of the deltoid is more often due to a lesion of the *fifth cervical root,* when it is paralysed in conjunction with the other muscles having the same nerve-supply, the syndrome produced being then known as *Erb's paralysis* (*see below*).

SYMPTOMS.—Injury of the circumflex nerve alone results in:—

PARALYSIS AND ATROPHY of the deltoid and teres minor. The power of abducting the arm is almost lost, for the supraspinatus, though capable of lifting the arm, is unable to maintain it in the abducted position without the assistance of the powerful deltoid. External rotation of the shoulder is weakened.

ANÆSTHESIA over the deltoid area.

Special Treatment Points.—

SUPPORT.—An abduction splint of some kind may be used to prevent shortening of the adductors. If so, the shoulder may be put up in full abduction and external rotation, but nowadays it is more usual for the arm to be kept at the side and supported in a sling.

PHYSICAL TREATMENT.—

ELECTRICAL STIMULATION.—The arm should be supported in abduction by means of pillows, or can remain in the splint if one is worn. The *indifferent pad* may be placed on the cervical spine, or on the pectoral region. If the latter, *care must be taken to see that it does not impinge on the anterior fibres of the deltoid*. The *active pad* should be relatively large as the muscle is a coarse one.

ACTIVE MOVEMENTS.—The re-education of the abductors and external rotators is described under Erb's paralysis, and this is so similar to that of the deltoid and teres minor alone that it need not be described in detail here. *The only difference is that in circumflex paralysis the muscles performing elbow and radio-ulnar movements are unaffected.* These muscles do not need special treatment unless a splint is worn, in which case exercises should be given to maintain their strength.

ERB'S PARALYSIS

This is due to a lesion of the fifth cervical root, and sometimes of part of the sixth. It generally occurs as the result of an injury at birth through traction between the child's head and shoulder. The strain falls first on the upper roots of the brachial plexus, the fifth cervical root yielding first, and then the roots below it, in succession. It is rare for more than Cervical 5 and 6 to be injured.

A similar condition may be produced in later life by means of violence. The whole plexus may be torn or severed in these cases. A *cervical rib* (i.e., an extra rib attached to the last cervical vertebra, or an elongation of its transverse process) may cause much the same kind of trouble.

SYMPTOMS.—

PARALYSIS AND ATROPHY.—In the case of an injury to the *fifth cervical root alone*, there is paralysis and atrophy of the rhomboids, deltoid, supra- and infra-spinatus, teres minor, biceps, brachialis anticus, and the supinators. The result is loss of power to abduct or externally rotate the shoulder, flex the elbow, or supinate the forearm.

If the *sixth cervical root* is involved, some of the extensors of the wrist (those on the radial side) may also be affected.

POSITION OF THE ARM.—The arm hangs at the side with the forearm extended, while the palm of the hand faces outwards owing to the extreme pronation and inward rotation. Contractures are liable to occur in these cases if treatment is not given to prevent them, and the arm will then be fixed in this position by the subscapularis and the coraco-humeral ligament.

ANÆSTHESIA is rare. If present, it is found on the outer side of the arm and forearm, back and front, the area supplied by fibres from Cervical 5 (*see Fig.* 114).

TROPHIC CHANGES are absent or slight.

Special Treatment Points.—

SUPPORT.—In the case of a baby the arm is splinted in abduction to shoulder level, and external rotation, the elbow is semiflexed and the forearm supinated (*Fig.* 113). The wrist is usually extended as well, and if the wrist extensors are affected this *must* be done. In bandaging the arm of an infant to a splint of this kind, it is important to see that the hand is in a correct position, and not in a twisted or unnatural one. A plaster support may be used, but padded Kramer wire is preferable in these cases. The majority of cases treated in this way from birth recover in 3–6 months. Old congenital cases will require surgery.

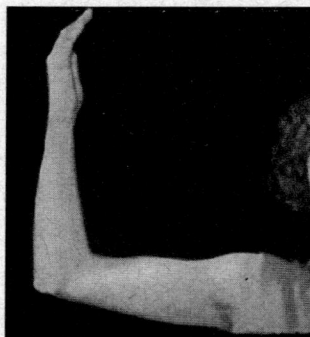

Fig. 113.—Position for splinting in Erb's paralysis.

Adult patients in whom the lesion is due to sudden violence may be treated by means of an abduction frame to hold the arm in the position described above, but it is usually held in a sling as for circumflex palsy.

PHYSICAL TRATMENT.—

TREATMENT OF INFANTS.—If treated from birth, there is usually little need for physical treatment other than to check the splint and alter it as the child grows. If physical treatment is required, gentle passive movements should be given to prevent contractures, and the baby must be encouraged to move the arm by reaching for objects which attract it. Older children who have not received early treatment will require operative treatment (*see below*).

TREATMENT OF ADULTS.—If the injury is due to sudden violence, physical treatment will be the same as for any other peripheral nerve-lesion, but it must be remembered that *a number of nerves are involved and each muscle group will require individual re-education.*

ELECTRICAL STIMULATION.—The patient should sit or lie with the arm in abduction as for circumflex palsy. The indifferent pad should be placed on the cervical spine.

PASSIVE MOVEMENTS.—Full movements are given to fingers, wrist, elbow and shoulder.

RE-EDUCATION EXERCISES.—

The Abductors.—In the early stages the patient is treated in the lying position on a plinth, which should be smooth and polished, or the arm is placed on a specially prepared polished board; alternatively, the arm can be supported in sling suspension, or in water. An adult should be required to perform successively static, assisted, free, and resisted abduction in the usual way. The arm should not be brought below shoulder level to begin with.

When a slight amount of power has returned to the muscles, the back of the plinth can be raised an inch or so. Static holdings are practised, and other active movements given in the same order as above. The back of the plinth is gradually raised more and more, so increasing the angle of the pull of gravity, until finally the patient can do his exercises sitting upright. In the later stages, the muscles are worked in their full range, the arm being brought down to the side.

The External Rotators.—The position of the patient is successively: (1) Lying (gravity assisting). (2) Side-lying on the sound side (gravity eliminated). (3) As (2) with resistance by the operator.*

The Supinators.—Positions: (1) Lying (gravity assisting). (2) Sitting, with the arm supported in abduction and the forearm semiflexed and held vertical (gravity eliminated). (3) As (2), resisted by the operator.

The Flexors of the Elbow.—Positions: (1) Sitting, the arm supported in abduction, the shoulder being outwardly rotated (gravity assisting). (2) Lying (gravity eliminated). (3) As (2) with slight resistance by operator.

At a Later Stage.—Pulley exercises to assist abduction may be added in older patients, the double pulley may be used so that the stronger arm assists the weaker (*see* Chapter XXIII). *Later still*, free and resisted shoulder and elbow exercises are added. Many of the exercises described in Chapter VI are suitable.

SURGICAL TREATMENT.—As has been said, treatment by physical means alone is rarely successful, except in the slighter cases among infants, or in adults where the severance of the nerve-root or -roots is not complete. In more serious cases, where the injury is extensive, or where the muscles and ligaments on the inner side of the joint have been allowed to shorten, treatment is by surgical means.

One of the following may be performed: (1) *Fairbank's operation*: division of the sub-scapularis and coraco-humeral ligament (the commonest operation). (2) Opening of the capsule, and correction of the position of the head of the humerus. (3) Suture of the divided nerves. The arm is afterwards immobilized in abduction and external rotation by means of a plaster spica for about 4 weeks.

Post-operative Treatment is on the same lines as that described above, but due attention must be paid to the scar. It should be remembered that young children will rarely tolerate electrical stimulation, and re-education in such cases is best achieved by purely physical means. Details of treatment after nerve suture are given on pp. 265–6.

KLUMPKE'S PARALYSIS

This type of paralysis is due to a lesion of the *eighth cervical* and *first thoracic roots*, produced by traction between the arm and the trunk. In adults it is due to violent injury, as when a man in falling from a scaffolding grasps at some support, such as a pole or beam, and the whole weight of his body falls suddenly on his arm; or as a complication of other shoulder injuries. It may also arise from a cervical rib or as the result of a birth injury, though less commonly than the Erb's type.

ANATOMY.—The *first thoracic root* supplies the intrinsic muscles of the hand, its fibres passing down in the median and ulnar nerves; the *eighth cervical root* supplies the long flexors of wrist and fingers.

The cutaneous supply of the first thoracic root consists of an area on the inner side of the forearm, back and front. This area is supplied through the medial

---

* Where a position in which gravity can be used as an assistance or resistance proves to be very awkward or inconvenient, it is better to regulate the amount of work done by means of assistance or resistance given by the operator, rather than by change of position.

antebrachial cutaneous (internal cutaneous) nerve. The supply of the eighth cervical root consists of two narrow strips down the middle of the upper extremity, one at the back and one at the front; the inner side of the hand; and one, or one and a half, inner fingers (*Fig.* 114).

SYMPTOMS.—

PARALYSIS.—If both these roots are injured there is complete paralysis and atrophy of *all the intrinsic muscles of the hand*, and of the *long flexors of the wrist and fingers*. This produces a condition similar to that caused by a lesion of both the median and ulnar nerves at the elbow, except that pronation is still possible. No movement at all is left in the hand, except extension of the metacarpophalangeal joints by the extensor digitorum and its accessory muscles, and extension of all joints of the thumb. Flexion of the wrists is also lost.

POSITION OF THE HAND.—This is a combination of *main-de-singe* and *main-engriffe* (*see Figs.* 100, 108, pp. 245, 249). The fingers are clawed—though the *flexion* of the last two phalanges is not so marked as in ulnar paralysis—and the thumb lies on the same plane as the fingers. The whole hand is flaccid and wasted.

ANÆSTHESIA is generally present in the area supplied by these roots, as shown in *Fig.* 114.

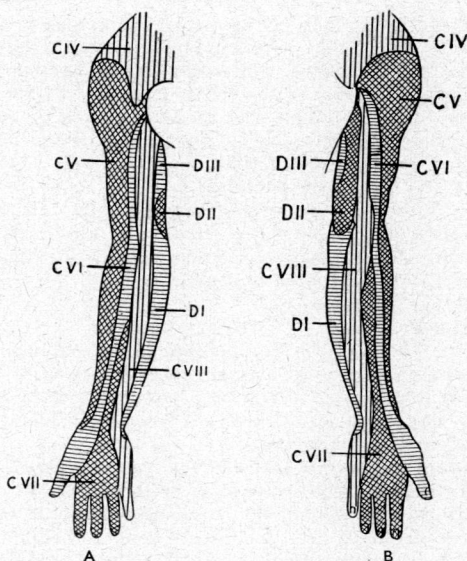

Fig. 114.—Cutaneous supply of nerve-roots in arm. A, Anterior; B, Posterior.

Special Treatment Points.—

SUPPORT.—A specially made splint is necessary to maintain the hand in the correct position. The metacarpophalangeal joints of the fingers must be flexed, the interphalangeal joints may be extended or slightly flexed, the thumb in flexion and opposition, half-way between abduction and adduction. The wrist should be partially flexed.

PHYSICAL TREATMENT.—

PASSIVE MOVEMENTS.—These are required for all joints of the hand: (1) All flexion movements of thumbs and fingers should be given to the limit, the wrist

9

being kept in the neutral position. (2) Opposition of the thumb is most important and abduction and adduction should both be given. (3) The fingers should be gently parted from each other, and each finger abducted and adducted. (4) The wrist should be fully flexed. (5) The interphalangeal joints should be extended, the metacarpophalangeal joints being flexed meanwhile.

ELECTRICAL STIMULATION AND MUSCLE RE-EDUCATION.—These will be as for median and ulnar nerve lesions. *When re-educating the hand the extreme importance of the opponens pollicis must never be forgotten.*

II. NERVE LESIONS OF THE LOWER EXTREMITY

Injuries to the nerves of the leg are usually the result of road accidents, or of some nervous disease such as poliomyelitis or multiple neuritis. We shall take as examples lesions of: (1) The femoral nerve, and (2) The lateral popliteal nerve.

FEMORAL (ANTERIOR CRURAL) PARALYSIS

This is rare as an isolated lesion, though the quadriceps often suffer in polio-myelitis or multiple neuritis.

SYMPTOMS.—

PARALYSIS.—There is paralysis of the quadriceps extensors and the sartorius. The loss of the latter muscle is not serious, but that of the quadriceps makes it quite impossible to extend the knee. Since these muscles are coarse fibred, atrophy is often extreme, especially that of the vastus medialis. Flexor contracture may develop at the knee. Only an injury near the beginning of the nerve in the pelvis would affect the branches to the iliacus, but in such a case, flexion of the hip would be weakened by paralysis of this muscle, as well as that of the rectus femoris, sartorius, and half of the pectineus.

ANÆSTHESIA is present in the area of distribution of the intermediate and medial cutaneous branches of the nerve—that is, on the inner side and front of the thigh, the inner side and front of the leg, inner ankle, and inner border of the foot; the region supplied by the saphenous nerve.

REFLEXES.—The knee-jerk is lost.

Special Treatment Points.—

SUPPORT.—The knee should be supported in full extension. A *back splint with a foot-piece* is generally worn at night and should be as light as possible. During the day, the patient may wear a *back splint* or a *walking caliper* (*see* p. 34). With the latter no weight is placed on the leg. Two points should receive attention when applying either splint or caliper:—

1. *The knee must be kept in full extension, but not in hyperextension.* If a hyper-extended position becomes established it is most difficult to correct later. To prevent this a *thin* pad of wool should be placed under the knee when on the splint. When a caliper is in use, the leather support behind the knee should be so arranged as to support both femur and tibia, but should not be so low down that it pushes the tibia too far forward.

2. Great care should be taken to *avoid pressure on the paralysed quadriceps* by bandaging or supports. When the leg is on a splint, the foot and lower leg can be bandaged to it, but the bandaging should stop immediately above the knee. A strap, or a few turns of bandage, should be applied over a layer of wool at the upper end of the splint.

PHYSICAL TREATMENT (for paralysed quadriceps only).—

ELECTRICAL STIMULATION.—A *large indifferent* pad should be placed under the thigh, *but should not impinge on the popliteal space.* A relatively large *active* pad should be used as the muscles are large. If there is a great deal of current leakage resulting in contraction of the flexors, a smaller pad can be placed on the nerve-trunk in the femoral triangle, but this is less practicable than the former position and is therefore best avoided if possible.

RE-EDUCATION EXERCISES.—Exercises are given successively in the following positions:—

Prone-lying on a Plinth (gravity assisting).—A thin, soft cushion should be placed on the plinth. The foot should hang over the end of the plinth. The physiotherapist should flex the knee about 10°, and let it drop on the cushion (to relax the antagonists). The patient should then try to hold the knee in this position.

Side-lying on the Sound Side.—A smooth, powdered board is placed between the legs, the knee is flexed to a right-angle, and the patient tries to extend it.★ The board may be so tilted that gravity is made to resist, or lightly assist, the movement. If held quite level, gravity is eliminated. The board is then removed and the patient asked to abduct the leg, keeping the knee stiff. This gives him the *sense* of holding his knee straight, although no actual muscle work is required in this position. As strength returns, he adopts an increasingly supine position, so that the pull of gravity on the knee is gradually increased. Finally, he should be able to raise his leg from the plinth with a straight knee from the *lying* or *half-lying position.*

Sitting Position.—In this position work can be done statically, eccentrically, and concentrically against gravity. The patient will then go on to resisted work.

Re-education in Walking.—When the muscles have sufficiently recovered, supporting apparatus will gradually be discarded. *Correct walking must be insisted upon, especially the bracing of the quadriceps when the weight is taken on the leg; neither must the leg be swung forward in an uncontrolled manner from the knee.* During the period of recovery, the other leg muscles should have been assiduously exercised and foot-drill practised, otherwise the patient may be in danger of flat-foot from inefficiency of the invertors. Weakness of the calf-muscles would also prove a serious handicap in walking.

LATERAL POPLITEAL PARALYSIS

This nerve, or its *anterior tibial* branch, may be injured in fractures of the upper extremity of the fibula. Occasionally, lesions occur before or during childbirth, from pressure in the pelvis on that part of the great sciatic nerve which contains the fibres destined for its lateral popliteal division (obstetrical paralysis).

SYMPTOMS.—

PARALYSIS AND ATROPHY OF THE INJURY OF THE LATERAL POPLITEAL NERVE.—There is paralysis and atrophy of the anterior tibial group, extensor brevis digitorum, and the peronei, with *loss* of dorsiflexion of the ankle, extension of the toes, and eversion of the foot, and *weakening* of inversion, which is possible only in plantar-flexion.

PARALYSIS IN INJURY OF THE ANTERIOR TIBIAL NERVE ONLY.—As above, except that the peronei are normal and eversion is possible.

ANÆSTHESIA is found on the lower two-thirds of the outer side of the leg, and on the dorsum of the foot and toes, except the last phalanges. If the anterior tibial nerve alone is injured, the only sensory loss is at the cleft between the first and second toes.

JOINT SENSE is lost in the joints of the foot and toes. If the whole nerve is injured it may affect the ankle as well.

TROPHIC CHANGES.—There are characteristic changes in skin and nails, and trophic ulcers are liable to occur.

★ Sling suspension apparatus or water may also be useful in these cases.

THE REFLEXES are unaffected, since the calf- and sole-muscles are sound.
Treatment.—
SUPPORT.—
FOR LATERAL POPLITEAL PARALYSIS.—A plaster splint or toe-spring will be used, with the foot in slight inversion, as well as in dorsiflexion.* A 'valgus wedge' is sometimes placed in the shoe to prevent the foot from being everted. It is raised about a quarter of an inch by means of a leather wedge inserted into the sole on the inner side.

PHYSICAL TREATMENT (e.g., of anterior tibial paralysis).—
ELECTRICAL STIMULATION.—A relatively small *indifferent pad* should be placed on the nerve-trunk as it winds round the head of the fibula. The *active pad* should also be fairly small.

PASSIVE MOVEMENTS.—Full movements should be given to the foot and ankle. Extension of the toes is important, but they should be flexed as well as extended. Care should be taken to see that mobility is maintained at the *metatarsophalangeal joint.*

RE-EDUCATION EXERCISES.—Unfortunately, we cannot invent such a variety of exercises for the foot as for the hand. *Extension of the toes and dorsiflexion of the ankle* should be given successively in:—

1. Forward-lying or kneeling, with the feet over the end of the plinth (gravity assisting); or side-lying with assistance from the physiotherapist.
2. Side-lying (gravity eliminated).
3. Half-lying (gravity opposing).

For *inversion,* the patient may be in half-lying throughout. Gravity is eliminated in this position, and assistance or resistance can be given.

Later, exercises should be given in *sitting* and *standing*, as for flat-foot.

Re-education in walking will be necessary.

III. WINGED SCAPULA

A deformity due to paralysis or weakness of the serratus anterior, often combined with similar weakness of the middle and lower trapezius, and of the rhomboids.

AETIOLOGY.—This type of deformity may be part of some general condition such as poliomyelitis, or the juvenile or infantile type of muscular dystrophy. More commonly, it is due to pressure on, or injury to, the nerve to serratus anterior (long or posterior thoracic nerve) resulting from shoulder or neck injuries. Some slight cases are merely due to poor muscular development and general weakness.

SYMPTOMS.—The patient is *unable to raise the arm above shoulder level,* having lost the power of outwardly rotating the inferior angle of the scapula; neither can he perform any forward pushing movements. On raising the arms forward to shoulder level, the *vertebral border of the scapula stands away from the ribs*, projecting backwards (*Fig.* 115).

Special Treatment Points.—
SUPPORT.—A most effective sling for these cases is in use in the Department of Physical Medicine at St. Thomas's Hospital. It consists of a length of 4-in.-wide flannel or webbing bandage, folded at one end to make a loop. The hand of the affected arm is placed in the loop so that the wrist is supported (*Fig.* 116). The remainder of the bandage is taken up over the *unaffected* shoulder and across the back, to pass through *in front of the forearm* close to the bend of the elbow (*Fig.* 116). The free end is then taken *behind the elbow,* so that *the full weight of the arm*

---

* Some authorities, however, prefer to keep the foot simply in dorsiflexion, without inversion or eversion.

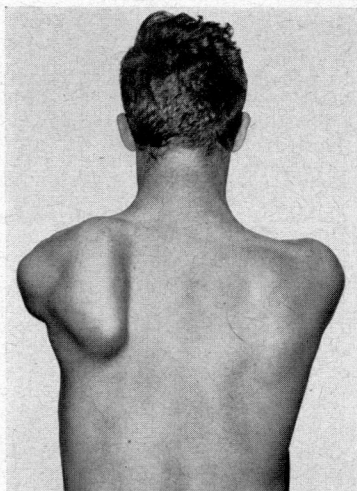

Fig. 115.—Winged scapula. The vertebral border stands away from the chest wall, during forward flexion of the shoulder while the inferior angle projects medially.

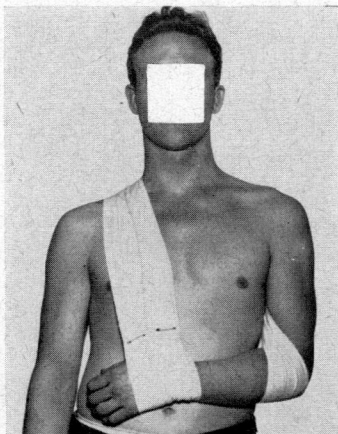

Fig. 116.—Anterior view of sling. Note that the weight of the arm is taken by the sling and that it holds the arm in elevation and external rotation.

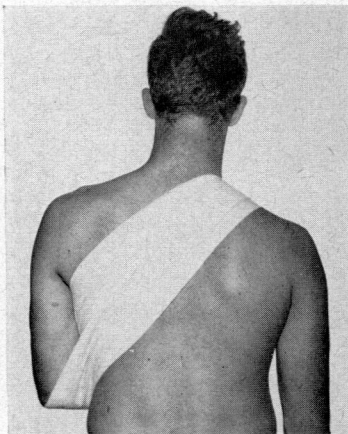

Fig. 117.—Posterior view of sling. Note direction of pull and double width of bandage holding the scapula in a correct position against the chest wall. *N.B.*—Any forward flexion movement whilst wearing the sling will enhance this effect.

is taken by the sling (*Fig.* 117). The sling is continued *across the back again, a strong upward pull being exerted the while* (*Fig.* 117). In this way the shoulder-girdle is pulled into *elevation* and *external rotation*, and *the scapula is thus held back against the chest wall. It is essential to see that the full weight of the arm is taken in the sling and that, once this is achieved, an upward pull is exerted until the sling is completed.* If this is not done the whole effect is lost.

The sling has the double advantage of leaving the fingers, hand and forearm relatively free, whilst not putting any weight on the affected shoulder, which might increase the tendency to depression and medial rotation caused by the serratus anterior lesion; nor is there pressure on the brachial plexus. In addition, *any movement towards forward flexion increases the effect of the sling.*

PHYSICAL TREATMENT.—

ELECTRICAL STIMULATION.—The patient should be treated in prone-lying with a *large indifferent pad* under the chest. The arm may either be completely abducted with the elbow flexed, or may remain loosely at the side.

PASSIVE MOVEMENTS.—Full elevation of the arm is most important.

RE-EDUCATION EXERCISES.—If the muscles are merely weak, it is not necessary to adhere quite so rigidly to the rules of re-education for paralysed muscles.

In the Early Stage: *Lying or Prone-lying Position.*—The foot of the plinth may be slightly raised, so that the patient's head is a little lower than his feet. A powdered board can be used if desired. The patient begins with his arms at shoulder level, or a little above, and practises raising them above his head (inner range). The elbow may at first be held in flexion, afterwards in extension. Later, the foot of the plinth is lowered, so that the patient is in a normal *lying* position. The head of the plinth is then raised till he is in the *half-lying*, and finally in the *sitting*, position. Movement may be successively static, assisted, free, and resisted. Suspension exercises and pool therapy can also be used.

Later Exercises.—

KABAT MOVEMENTS.—Repeated contractions may be used very effectively in cases of serratus anterior lesions. The shoulder patterns, known as 'flexion adduction' and 'flexion abduction', should be used. Free exercises should include:—

1. Reach-grasp-sitting or -standing; trying to keep scapula in position against chest wall.

2. Sitting 2-Arm-raising forward to shoulder level. This presents considerable difficulty. It may be tried first in lying or side-lying.

Many exercises in the list for stiff shoulders (*see* pp. 118–20) may be used in the later stages. Pulley exercises are also useful.

IV. FACIAL PARALYSIS

ANATOMY.—The seventh cranial, or facial, nerve supplies all the face muscles except the levator palpebræ superioris (supplied by the motor oculi) and the muscles of mastication (supplied by the trigeminal). It is therefore *the nerve of facial expression.* Its functions are not quite like those of other nerves, since the movements of the face muscles, although they may be voluntary, take place largely in response to *emotional stimuli*, and in such cases are purely reflex. The nerve has only one sensory branch, the chorda tympani, which supplies sensation to the anterior two-thirds of the tongue. Its nucleus—that is, the group of cells of origin of its lower motor neuron—is in the pons Varolii. It is connected with the cells of the cerebral cortex by fibres which form its upper motor neuron.

The facial nerve may be injured in various parts of its course:—

1. THE UPPER NEURON.—This may suffer in cases of hæmorrhage, thrombosis, tumour, etc. It then generally forms part of a hemiplegia (*see* pp. 182–3).

2. THE LOWER NEURON.—*The nucleus*—or its fibres within the pons—is occasionally attacked in acute anterior poliomyelitis, or injured by hæmorrhage, tumours, etc. There may or may not be injury to other nerves.

The peripheral fibres, after they have left the pons, may be injured or compressed either in their bony canal, or after they have emerged on the face. These are the cases with which we are most often concerned. They may be the result of otitis media (inflammation of the middle ear), accidental severance at operations on the ear, wounds, or fractures of the skull; or, most promising from our point of view, they may be due to inflammatory products which compress the nerve in the narrow stylomastoid foramen, causing a *neuritis*. Some cases may be due to a virus.

We shall here consider the symptoms and treatment of the *peripheral* form of facial paralysis only—the form commonly known as 'Bell's palsy'.

SYMPTOMS.—

IF THE NERVE IS INJURED AT THE STYLOMASTOID FORAMEN.—

Flaccid paralysis and atrophy of all the face muscles on one side, except the levator palpebræ superioris (which raises the upper eyelid) and the muscles of mastication. There is loss of *all* movement on that side, voluntary or emotional. Results:—

The eye can be opened, but not completely closed (paralysis of orbicularis oculi). Hence the blinking reflex is lost, the eye is not efficiently protected from dust or other injurious substances, and therefore tends to water. It may become inflamed (conjunctivitis).

The corner of the mouth drops, and the patient cannot raise it on the affected side in smiling.

Food collects between the teeth and the cheek when eating, because the tone of the latter cannot be maintained (paralysis of buccinator). Whistling becomes impossible.

Articulation is affected in the pronunciation of the labial consonants (*l*, *m*, *n*).

The power of wrinkling the forehead either vertically or horizontally is lost on the affected side. If the patient had wrinkles, they disappear.

The nasal fold is obliterated and the nostrils cannot be voluntarily dilated, though they move passively during breathing.

IF THE NERVE IS INJURED ABOVE THIS POINT.—In addition to the above symptoms there is loss of taste sensation in the anterior part of the tongue, or hypersensitiveness to certain sounds, according to the level of the injury. The auditory or other nerves may also be involved.

Treatment.—

MEDICAL AND SURGICAL TREATMENT.—Any treatment necessary for the actual cause of the palsy will be applied.

SUPPORT.—A hook attached to a piece of wire covered by narrow rubber tubing is sometimes used to support the corner of the mouth. Its other end is hooked round the ear.

PHYSICAL TREATMENT (of the inflammatory type).—The prognosis of this type is good, recovery generally taking place in 2–3 months, though in some cases it may be slow or incomplete.*

POSITION OF PATIENT.—The most comfortable arrangement is for the patient to lie down, the physiotherapist standing behind him. The patient's head should be supported on a small cushion.

ELECTRICAL TREATMENT.—In these cases *muscle stimulation should only be by interrupted galvanism*, whether or not there is reaction of degeneration. A *large indifferent pad* can be placed on the opposite arm and a *very small active pad* used. Faradism is inadvisable because it tends to produce *secondary contracture*; in

* In lesions af the nucleus or fibres within the pons, the prognosis is bad; and in the cases of severance during operation it is not very favourable. The treatment in these cases is similar to that given below.

addition most patients find it intolerable on the face. If secondary contracture should occur, all stimulation must be temporarily abandoned and the muscles very gently stretched. *Radiant heat* may be given during treatment, but the patient's eyes must be carefully protected. *Short-wave diathermy* or *erythemal ultraviolet radiation* at the point of emergence of the nerve on the face are sometimes recommended, the latter to act as a counter-irritant. *Potassium iodide or chlorine ionization* may also be given to the affected ear.

MASSAGE.—The patient often derives great comfort from massage, the face feeling less stiff afterwards. *Stroking* should be given from the chin upwards to the temple, and from the middle of the forehead downwards towards the ear. The technique should be gentle but at the same time firm and stimulating. Small, circular *finger kneadings* can be given all over the affected side of the face, care being taken not to stretch the muscles. *Tapotement* may be administered in the form of 'tapping' quickly and lightly with the finger-tips. It must be done very gently over the forehead and superciliary ridges, where only a thin layer of muscle covers the bone. *Frictions* are sometimes given at the point where the nerve enters the face, to soften any inflammatory deposits in this situation. This point may be found just below, and in front of, the lobule of the ear, over the neck of the condyle of the lower jaw. *Vibrations* performed with the tips of one or two fingers can also be used over the nerve-trunk at this point, or they may be administered by placing the whole hand flat on the affected side of the face.★

EXERCISES.—The patient should be in a room alone, or screened off from other patients, otherwise he will be self-conscious and unable to concentrate. A mirror is a useful adjunct. He should try to perform the following movements:

1. Closing the eyes.
2. Smiling.
3. Whistling, and blowing.
4. Closing the mouth tightly.
5. Smiling, showing the teeth, and raising the upper lip.
6. Wrinkling the forehead, vertically and horizontally.
7. Dilating the nostrils.,
8. Screwing up the whole face.
9. Pronunciation of words containing labials.

This part of the treatment can easily be made into a game when dealing with children. Later, it is possible to give gentle resistance to some of those movements.

SURGICAL TREATMENT.—In obstinate cases an operation is sometimes performed, consisting of *nerve anastomosis*, part of the spinal accessory, or hypoglossal nerve—generally the former—being joined to the distal end of the facial nerve. Sometimes the attachment of the temporal muscle may be so arranged as to move the facial muscles. Plastic operations may also be performed to improve the patient's appearance.†

POST-OPERATIVE TREATMENT is as described above.

V. OPERATIONS ON NERVES

Operations are performed on nerves for the following purposes:—

1. *To re-unite two ends of a severed nerve,* so that it may regenerate, the axons from the central end growing down into the sheath of the peripheral end (nerve suture).

★ This may be only *suggestion,* but it seems to be effective.
† Sir Harold Gillies, *Lancet,* Feb. 15, 1937.

2. *To free a nerve* that has been caught in forming callus, or is being compressed by displaced bone, scar tissue, or any other structure.

3. *To relieve pain in a nerve,* when this persists and cannot be lessened by other means. The operation consists of injections into the nerve, or even severance, or removal of some part of it.

4. *To join the central end of a healthy nerve to the peripheral end of a degenerate one.* This is known as 'nerve anastomosis'.

Nerve Suture

It often happens that we are asked to treat lesions of peripheral nerves after this operation. At the operation, the two ends of the nerve are located. There may be a considerable gap between them, or they may be deeply embedded in scar tissue, from which they have to be freed. The central end is cut back for a short distance in order to remove the degenerate part and the sheaths of the two ends are sewn up with small stitches. In some cases the nerve is wrapped in a piece of fascia to prevent adhesions from forming round it.

These operations are undertaken if the nerve is known to have been severed in an accident, paralysis having appeared immediately afterwards, or if a paralysis shows no sign of improvement about three months after its onset. If the operation is performed at once, it is known as *primary suture*; if after an interval, as *secondary suture*.

PROGNOSIS AND COURSE OF RECOVERY.—Some nerves regenerate more readily than others, e.g., the radial nerve recovers more satisfactorily than the median or the ulnar. Primary suture is more successful than secondary and the longer a nerve is left ununited, the worse are its chances of full recovery. The rate of recovery varies according to the site of the lesion; a nerve severed near its termination will recover much sooner than if it were severed high up. If sepsis is present, regeneration is delayed (Purves-Stewart).

As the nerve recovers, protopathic sensation returns first; then epicritic sensation and motor power almost simultaneously, but epicritic sensation is sometimes slightly in advance of motor power.

After a primary suture protopathic sensation may begin to return in about six weeks, epicritic sensation and motor power in about six months (Purves-Stewart).* If there is no return of power by the eighth month, there is not likely to be any later, and the nerve is sometimes re-sutured.

After secondary suture the prospects are not nearly so good. Epicritic sense and motor power do not return for nine months or a year, and their restoration is rarely perfect.

Treatment of a Case after Nerve Suture.—

SUPPORT.—The limb must be splinted in the correct position, with no drag on the nerve; for an ulnar nerve sutured at the wrist the metacarpophalangeal joint would be flexed, the interphalangeal joints extended, the thumb adducted, and the wrist slightly flexed. The surgeon will decide when physical treatment may begin.

MODIFICATIONS OF PHYSICAL TREATMENT.—

ELECTRICAL STIMULATION.—This will not be given until the surgeon permits it, and he usually waits until the wound has healed.

MASSAGE.—If this is requested, great care must be taken. *Any movements that could possibly drag on the nerve must be avoided.*

PASSIVE MOVEMENTS.—Any movements that do not stretch the nerve are permissible from the beginning, but *no strong movements are allowed for from*

---

* *Peripheral Nerve Injuries.*

6 weeks to 2 months. For example, in the case of suture of the ulnar nerve cited above, the fingers can be moved and the wrist may be further flexed, but *it should not be extended.* The elbow can be gently extended with the wrist in full flexion, but the movement must always be *relaxed,* and never *forced.* Gentle pronation and supination may be added once the wound is healed (10 to 12 days) and the shoulder-joint may be moved actively with the elbow flexed. Most of the above movements should be done actively rather than passively as soon as possible.

ACTIVE MOVEMENTS.—The physiotherapist must watch for the first signs of returning power, and as soon as these appear, re-education will begin. She will first look for the appearance of the protopathic sensation, and then the appearance and increase of epicritic sense. From that moment she can begin to expect the return of the power of movement. She must re-educate the patient in the use of *each* affected muscle, and finally restore the function of the limb by co-ordination exercises.

CHAPTER XIII

NEURITIS AND NEURALGIA: CRAMP: EPILEPSY

I. Neuritis and neuralgia: Brachial neuritis—Brachial neuralgia—Intercostal neuralgia or neuritis—Sciatica—Polyneuritis (multiple peripheral neuritis). II. Cramp. III. Epilepsy.

I. NEURITIS AND NEURALGIA

BEFORE considering neuritis and neuralgia we will briefly review the structure of a peripheral nerve.

STRUCTURE OF A PERIPHERAL NERVE.—A peripheral mixed nerve is composed of: (1) The axons of cells in the anterior horns of the spinal cord, i.e., *motor fibres*. (2) Fibres taking their origin in the ganglia on the posterior nerve-roots, i.e., *sensory fibres*.

Each of these fibres has its own medullary or myelin sheath and neurilemma. Between the fibres lies connective tissue called the *endoneurium* (Greek, *endon* = within); a delicate sheath binds the axons into bundles, and is known as the *perineurium* (Greek, *peri* = around); while another variety of connective tissue occupies the space between the bundles, and also forms the outer sheath of the whole nerve—this is the *epineurium* (Greek, *epi* = upon) (*Fig.* 118).

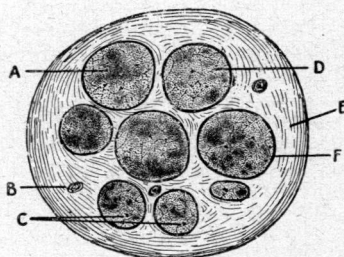

Fig. 118.—Diagram of a cross-section of a nerve, showing its sheaths. A, Axons; B, Artery; C, Arterioles; D, Endoneurium; E, Epineurium; F, Perineurium.

The two outer sheaths—perineurium and epineurium—are sometimes both included under the term 'perineurium'.

True *neuritis* (inflammation of a nerve) should be distinguished from *neuralgia* (pain, without pathological changes in the nerve), although their causes are similar. True neuritis, as distinct from neuralgia, is of two kinds: (1) *Interstitial neuritis*, that is, inflammation of the sheath and connective tissue of the nerve, the axis cylinders not being inflamed but only compressed; (2) *Parenchymatous neuritis*, that is, inflammation of the axis cylinders themselves.

Causes of Interstitial Neuritis and Neuralgia.—

1. PRESSURE.—This may be due to involvement of the nerve in callus following fracture; from a displaced bone or joint structure; from a cervical rib; from a tumour; or from an external agent such as axillary crutches or other aids or appliances. To cause neuritis or neuralgia the pressure must be prolonged.

Neuralgia may be a reflex manifestation, the pain being felt some distance from the actual cause.

2. TRAUMA.—Such injuries as fractures, dislocations, or sprains and strains may, at the time of the initial damage, cause bruising or laceration of a nerve.

Causes of Parenchymatous Neuritis.—

1. TOXINS AND POISONS.—These may be *intrinsic*, e.g., rheumatic or diphtheric products; or *extrinsic*, e.g., lead, alcohol, or arsenic.

2. METABOLIC DISTURBANCES AND VITAMIN DEFICIENCY.—Neuritis often complicates diabetes mellitus and is again due to toxic products, arising from the altered metabolism which accompanies the disease; vitamin deficiencies also give rise to altered metabolism, and to similar toxic products, the principal factor in neuritis being vitamin-B_1 deficiency (beri-beri).

NEURITIS.—

INTERSTITIAL NEURITIS.—The inflammation affects the epineurium, perineurium, and sometimes the endoneurium; only in very severe cases are the axons or their immediate sheaths involved. This form is therefore sometimes— more correctly—known as *perineuritis*. The commonest forms of interstitial neuritis are the *brachial, intercostal*, and *sciatic* varieties.

PARENCHYMATOUS NEURITIS.—The inflammation primarily affects the axons, though the interstitial tissue generally shares in the inflammatory reaction. Neuritis of a purely motor nerve is generally of the parenchymatous type (*see* FACIAL PARALYSIS, p. 262). Polyneuritis or multiple neuritis (affecting all or most of the peripheral nerves) is also of the parenchymatous type. It is described on p. 278.

GENERAL SYMPTOMS.—

Interstitial Neuritis.—The predominant feature of interstitial neuritis is *pain*, more or less intense according to the severity of the inflammation. It is due to pressure exerted on the sensory fibres by the congested tissues of the sheath. It may be acute, or dull and aching in character. There are usually tender points on the trunk of the affected nerve, and swelling of the nerve itself, if superficial, can sometimes be felt. The pain may be worse in the final distribution of the nerve, or it may be of equal intensity all along its course. *Other disturbances of sensation*, such as paræsthesiæ, arise in serious cases. If motor fibres are irritated, there may be *twitchings* of muscles. *Reflexes* are normal in a simple interstitial neuritis. *Trophic changes* may occur in skin and nails.

Parenchymatous Neuritis.—In addition to the above symptoms *atrophy* and *paralysis* will occur in parenchymatous neuritis.

NEURALGIA.—Neuralgia ('pain in a nerve'—Greek, *neuron* = nerve, *algos* = pain) is not due to inflammation of the nerve itself, but either to pressure upon it, or to unhealthy conditions of the blood on which it depends for its nourishment. Thus we see how the same causes can give rise to either condition; it is important to remember that *what begins as neuralgia may end as neuritis*, particularly if the cause is chronic in nature.

GENERAL SYMPTOMS.—The *pain* is of a shooting, throbbing variety, more intermittent than that of neuritis. There is *tenderness* in the affected part, but the nerves are not thickened or swollen. There may be *muscular twitching or tremor*, due to irritation of motor fibres, *but never paralysis*. *Trophic changes* are sometimes seen if the vasomotor nerves are involved. These consist of excessive perspiration in the affected part and redness, or pallor of the skin.

GENERAL PRINCIPLES OF TREATMENT.—In the case of *interstitial neuritis* and *neuralgia*, treatment is chiefly directed towards the cause and the relief of pain. *Parenchymatous lesions* fall into the category of paralytic conditions and will be treated accordingly.

MEDICAL AND SURGICAL TREATMENT.—The causative agent will be treated by appropriate medical or surgical measures.

PHYSICAL TREATMENT.—*Heat, massage*, and certain forms of *electrotherapy* may be employed for the relief of pain in cases of interstitial neuritis and neuralgia.

In parenchymatous lesions the prevention of contractures and atrophic sores, and the re-education of paralysed muscles are the principal aims of treatment. The methods used, and the principles which apply, have already been discussed in earlier chapters dealing with paralysis due to peripheral nerve, or lower motor neuron lesions. In this chapter it is proposed to deal first with interstitial neuritis and neuralgia, and then with the parenchymatous form.

BRACHIAL NEURITIS

This is an intensely painful form of neuritis which needs great care in treatment. One or more nerves in the arm may be affected, and tender spots are found at various points on their course: over the brachial plexus in the posterior neck triangle; in the ulnar nerve as it passes between the internal condyle and the olecranon process; in the median nerve in the cubital fossa; or in the radial nerve as it leaves the musculospiral groove. The patient is not infrequently neurotic, but it is often difficult to say whether the neurosis is partly the cause, or wholly the result, of the neuritis. There are many causes, but it is frequently due to some form of compression.

CAUSES.—

1. Osteo-arthritis and/or spondylosis of the cervical spine.

2. Herniation of a cervical disk or disks.

3. Presence of a cervical rib, causing pressure on the brachial plexus in the thoracic outlet (*thoracic outlet compression syndrome*).

4. Faulty posture leading to sagging of the shoulder-girdle, with resultant thoracic outlet syndrome. The cause of this faulty posture may be habit, general debility and poor musculature, chronic muscle strain, 'fibrositis', or muscular rheumatism.

5. Some form of toxic product.

The onset may be *acute* or *subacute*, the pain first appearing in the neck and thence spreading to the arm.

Treatment.—

MEDICAL OR SURGICAL TREATMENT.—This consists of a search for, and treatment of, the cause. It may be necessary to remove a cervical rib, or to perform a laminectomy for a prolonged intervertebral disk (*see* p. 71). Alternatively, traction may be applied in cases of disk lesions. Sometimes specific septic foci (e.g., teeth or tonsils) are removed.

PHYSICAL TREATMENT.—

THE ACUTE STAGE

REST AND SUPPORT.—The arm will be rested by supporting it in a large sling. The patient may be in bed for a time, in which case the arm may be supported in a sling or merely rested on pillows.

WARMTH.—All sufferers from neuritis are intensely sensitive to cold, and the arm and shoulder must be kept warm.

ELECTRICAL TREATMENT.—*Heat* may be applied in the form of *radiant heat* or *short-wave diathermy*. If the latter is used it is best administered by means of a coil wound round the arm from shoulder to wrist, if it can be tolerated. When giving heat treatment it should be remembered that, *although the initial response is one of relief, a later effect may be exacerbation of pain.* For this reason the dose should be kept to a minimum in the early days, and a careful note made of the patient's reaction to a gradual progression in dosage. *If there is any tendency to an increase in pain the dose should be reduced immediately.* Some patients gain considerable relief from anodal galvanism. The forearm is placed in a bath, and a large pad applied over the brachial plexus, the *anode* being connected with this pad, and the *cathode* placed in the bath. *Ionization* may be given for the relief of pain, the drug used being a form of analgesic such as calcium or novocain.

The Subacute Stage

This may be the onset of the condition, or a progression from the acute stage. In either event, when the inflammation has subsided sufficiently for the patient to be able to bear it, massage should be tried in addition to the treatment outlined above.

POSITION OF PATIENT.—The arm should be supported by pillows, the patient sitting or lying down. Warmth during treatment is essential and no part of the limb should be unnecessarily exposed. Except for the performance of effleurage or stroking, the massage can well be carried out under a light shawl, so that the arm is kept covered during almost the whole of the treatment. The room should be warm and without draughts.

MASSAGE.—At first, vibrations may afford most relief.* They should be given with the flat hand, and should cover the whole arm, beginning in the neck over the brachial plexus. Reflex stroking, from shoulder to hand, may next be added if the patient finds it soothing, but many patients are unable to tolerate any form of stroking at this stage. If this is the case it should be omitted, and careful kneading tried instead. The latter must be a very gentle movement, light and slow, but not of a stretching type. It cannot be too strongly emphasized that, *if pain increases instead of diminishing, treatment should cease immediately.*

The Chronic or Convalescent Stage

ELECTROTHERAPY AND MASSAGE.—This should be continued as long as it is of benefit to the patient. At this stage frictions can be given to the shoulder and neck muscles if required.

PASSIVE MOVEMENTS.—As a case of neuritis improves, passive movements should be added to prevent stiffness in the joints. At first these should be given very gently and by the *relaxed* method. '*Stretching* movements', if necessary, are only given in the final stages, and with the greatest care.

ACTIVE MOVEMENTS.—Light active movements should begin as soon as possible, though no exact time can be given for their commencement. The physiotherapist must use her own judgement, and consult the doctor. Assisted movements, within the limit of pain and in small range, will be given first. They should be very gradually increased in range, and others added in due course. Later the movements will be free, and exercises of the 'pendulum' type can be added. Finally, if all goes well, the patient should proceed to general arm exercises, both free and resisted, to strengthen the muscles and reduce any stiffness due to immobilization of the limb. *It is particularly important to exercise the shoulder-girdle muscles, especially those which raise the shoulders.*

Treatment of brachial neuritis is, unfortunately, not always successful. If the pain increases instead of diminishing, treatment should cease, possibly to be resumed at a later stage. Careful inquiries should be made as to the patient's sensations, say half an hour after the end of the treatment. In the later stages, some pain on active movement may be inevitable, though even then nothing should be done which could cause the inflammation to flare up again; but during

---

* Possibly mainly a form of suggestion, but often effective. However, only a physiotherapist who can perform these movements finely and in perfect rhythm should attempt to see them for this type of patient.

the early stages treatment is meant to soothe, *and anything which causes pain must be avoided.* To take any risks with an inflamed nerve is to court disaster.

BRACHIAL NEURALGIA

Many cases of pain in the arm are forms of *neuralgia* rather than of neuritis. Such cases are often due to thoracic outlet syndrome, osteo-arthritis of the cervical spine, a displaced intervertebral disk in this region, long-standing 'fibrositis', or muscular rheumatism of the shoulder or neck muscles.*

Brachial Neuralgia due to Compression in the Thoracic Outlet
(*Thoracic Outlet Compression Syndrome*)

AETIOLOGY AND ANATOMICAL ABNORMALITIES.—The lower cord of the brachial plexus may be compressed between the first rib and the clavicle; stretched over the first rib—or a cervical rib if present—behind the insertion of scalenus anterior; compressed between the scalene muscles; or compressed by membranous bands, etc. The subclavian vessels may also be compressed. Whatever *actually* produces the pressure, the *exciting cause* of the symptoms is a *lowering of the shoulder-girdle.* This is undoubtedly the result of weakness and loss of tone in the elevator muscles, which is caused by general fatigue, the carrying of heavy weights, and too strenuous use of the arms. It is especially common in middle-aged housewives who stand in queues, carry heavy shopping baskets, or who do much washing of clothes, etc., entailing considerable strain on the arms.

SYMPTOMS.—These may be primarily those of neuritis, with pain as the predominant symptom. There may be wasting in the intrinsic muscles of the hand, and paræsthesia of the fingers; but if the subclavian vessels are involved, there will also be circulatory symptoms not unlike those of Raynaud's disease—cold, dusky, or pallid hands, with some swelling (*see* p. 431).

Treatment.—

GENERAL TREATMENT.—The primary aim in this type of case is to strengthen and improve the tone of the shoulder muscles, especially the elevators (upper trapezius and levator scapulæ), and to correct the posture of the shoulders, raising the level at which they are habitually carried. (This must not be exaggerated, of course, otherwise we merely substitute one bad posture for another.) Dr. Cyriax emphasizes the fact that it is useless to give exercises to the trapezius muscles unless the patient is taught to keep the shoulders very slightly shrugged all the time. "Strengthening a muscle in no way hinders it from relaxing when not in use. . . . Before lifting anything heavy she must shrug her shoulder right up and maintain this position of her scapula all the time she is carrying the weight. So far as possible she must avoid wearing an overcoat."† It should not be forgotten, however, that if pain is a serious factor, it must be relieved before attempting to re-educate the muscles.

PHYSICAL TREATMENT.—

MASSAGE.—If required, effleurage and kneading may be given to the muscles of the shoulder and neck regions, to relieve pain and induce relaxation. To massage the arm is valueless since the origin of the pain is not there.

PASSIVE MOVEMENTS.—*Relaxed* passive movements may be required for the shoulder if there is any tendency to stiffness. They may also be used as an introduction to active movement.

ELECTRICAL TREATMENT.—Radiant heat, infra-red radiation, short-wave diathermy, anodal galvanism, or ionization may be given to reduce pain.

---

* It must be remembered, however, that *continued* pressure or irritation may transform a neuralgia into a neuritis.

† James Cyriax, *Text-book of Orthopædic Medicine*, Vol. I, Chapter VIII, p. 187. Students are recommended to study this section.

EXERCISES.—Relaxation exercises for arm and shoulder are helpful, *but no downward drag should be allowed* and for this reason suspension apparatus is frequently used. Exercises which raise the shoulder-girdle should be practised, especially such as are done with the arm above shoulder level. Shoulder shrugging movements are particularly useful. The exercises should be graduated. Movements are generally free at first, and later resisted—either by the physiotherapist or by springs, weights, medicine balls, etc. Movements of head and neck (flexion and extension, lateral flexion, and rotation) should be included.

Brachial Neuralgia due to Osteo-arthritis of the Cervical Spine with or without Displaced Intervertebral Disk

Treatment.—

GENERAL AND PHYSICAL TREATMENT.—The treatment in the case of *osteo-arthritis* alone is similar to the above. Exercises to strengthen the neck muscle should be included in the treatment.

In cases of *disk herniation* the patient may be treated by head traction, either manual or by means of head suspension apparatus; by manipulation; or, in some intractable cases, by operation. Exercises similar to those given for a thoracic outlet syndrome may be included in the treatment.*

CASES DUE TO FIBROSITIS† OR MUSCULAR RHEUMATISM

There may be palpable 'nodules' in the muscles of the shoulder-girdle, especially the upper trapezius. Whatever these 'nodules' are the patient will probably benefit from heat, massage, and deep transverse friction, but it is inadvisable to begin treatment with very deep massage, especially on the sensitive trapezius. The area at fault should be identified before treatment is begun and the patient placed in an appropriate position for massage (Cyriax)—prone-lying for the trapezius and splenius. The painful areas in the arm need not be touched. It is important that the patient should learn to relax, and treatment should include exercises of the shoulder-raising type, and neck movements as described above.

INTERCOSTAL NEURALGIA OR NEURITIS

This is generally encountered in the form of *neuralgia*, and may be due to muscular rheumatism, fibrositis, or trauma of the deeper layers of the back or intercostal muscles, though such conditions may, of course, exist in either of these muscle groups without producing a neuritis or neuralgia. In some cases the pain is caused by a prolapsed thoracic disk.

SYMPTOMS.—The principal symptom is a *sharp neuralgic pain*, especially noticeable when the patient takes a deep breath, since the act of inspiration stretches the intercostal nerves. The pain is generally unilateral, or worse on one side of the body than on the other. In severe cases, backache may be troublesome. In 'fibrositic' cases there are *tender nodules in the muscles*. In the traumatic variety there is a definite area of tenderness. *Tender points are also to be found on the nerves*, especially at the places where their cutaneous branches emerge: (1) Near the spinous process (posterior primary divisions). (2) In the mid-axillary line (lateral cutaneous branches of intercostal nerves). (3) Near the sternum (anterior cutaneous branches of intercostal nerves).

Treatment.—

PHYSICAL TREATMENT.—This is similar to that described for brachial neuralgia of 'fibrositic' origin.

---

* K. N. Lloyd (1948), "Shoulder-raising and Neck Exercises in the Treatment of Brachial Neuralgia", *Brit. J. phys. Med.*, 11, 85.

† It is not proposed to discuss the nature of fibrositis here. This is considered in Chapter IV.

POSITION OF PATIENT.—The patient should lie on the sound side, in a comfortable position, supported by pillows. If both sides are affected, he may lie first on one side and then on the other. Warmth is important.

MASSAGE.—This should begin with *soothing strokings* over the painful area. It is most convenient to begin the strokings from the region of the sternum, carrying them as far as the mid-axillary line—the mammary gland in women being, of course, avoided—after which the back of the thorax is similarly treated, the stroking being carried from the vertebral column to the mid-axillary line. This should be followed by careful *kneadings* over the whole region. Since the condition is generally due to an inflammatory condition in the muscles, these should be as deep as the patient can bear them, though their strength may have to be modified in some cases. As soon as they can be tolerated, *frictions* should be given from end to end of each intercostal space. The movement should be a transverse one across the intercostal muscles, except, of course, where this is impossible because of the overlying scapula. The deep muscles on either side of the thoracic spine should also be treated, as well as any others in the neighbourhood in which 'fibrositic' nodules can be detected. Special attention should be given to the points of exit of the nerve branches. After the frictions *kneading* or *effleurage* may be given. Effleurage should be towards the axillary glands and may be followed by stroking, or fine *vibrations*.

EXERCISES.—Free side-bendings (to both sides), trunk rotations, and back-raisings should be employed. *Deep breathing* will be added as the pain decreases, but should not be required of the patient in the early stages. Later, *stretching exercises*, such as 2-arms-stretching-upward, and half-stretch (or half-neck-rest) stride-standing or -sitting, side-bending, with the other hand on the ribs, are of benefit. When the pain has gone, *mobility* exercises for the thorax, and breathing exercises of all kinds should be given before the patient ceases treatment.

ELECTRICAL TREATMENT.—*Radiant heat, infra-red radiation*, or *short-wave diathermy* are often of great benefit.

In the case of thoracic disk lesions manipulative treatment may be tried.

SCIATICA

The name sciatica is commonly given to any painful condition along the course of the great sciatic nerve. It may, in fact, be a *neuralgia* or a *neuritis*. The former is due to some form of pressure on the nerve; the latter consists of an inflammation of the sheaths or connective tissue surrounding the axons themselves. It is most commonly an interstitial neuritis, but in some very severe cases the inflammation may spread to the axons, and set up a parenchymatous neuritis. Either form of neuritis constitutes a *true clinical sciatica*, distinguished by definite neurological signs. Like brachial neuritis it may be acute or subacute in onset.

CAUSES.—The causes of *neuralgic pain* may be any of the following: (1) *Osteo-arthritis* of the lumbar spine; (2) *Muscular rheumatism* or *fibrositis* in the lumbar muscles or those in the gluteal region and the thigh; (3) *Sacro-iliac strain*; (4) *Osteo-arthritis* or other *bone diseases* of the hip-joint; (5) *Chronic deformity of the lumbar spine* (lordosis or scoliosis); (6) A *gravid uterus* or *pelvic tumours*; (7) *Rectal tumour* or *chronic constipation*.

There is much controversy as to the actual cause of *true sciatica*. During the past few years *prolapse of lumbar or sacral intervertebral disks** has been widely accepted as an important factor, and today many authorities regard this as the chief cause of true sciatica. Others believe that *lumbar spondylitis* or *sacro-iliac lesions* are essential factors.

---

* See p. 70.

Parenchymatous lesions may result from any of the above causes and are also seen as the result of bacterial, chemical, or metabolic toxins. They are often present in such diseases as gout and diabetes.

SYMPTOMS OF SCIATIC NEURITIS (true sciatica).—The condition may develop suddenly with an acute attack of 'lumbago' (pain in the lower back), followed within a few days by pain radiating along the course of the sciatic nerve; or it may develop more insidiously, periods of pain being experienced when the nerve is stretched in walking, etc. This gradually increases in frequency and intensity until it reaches a climax.

CLINICAL SIGNS.—

PAIN.—The patient complains of pain, coming on suddenly or gradually. He may describe it as 'gnawing', 'tingling', or 'burning' pain, which may be continually present, or may occur in paroxysms. It is often extremely severe, especially at night. It is worse in any position that causes *pressure* on the nerve (e.g., in sitting), or which *stretches* it (e.g., standing erect with the heel on the ground). When in bed, the patient lies on his side, with hip and knee flexed and ankle plantar-flexed.

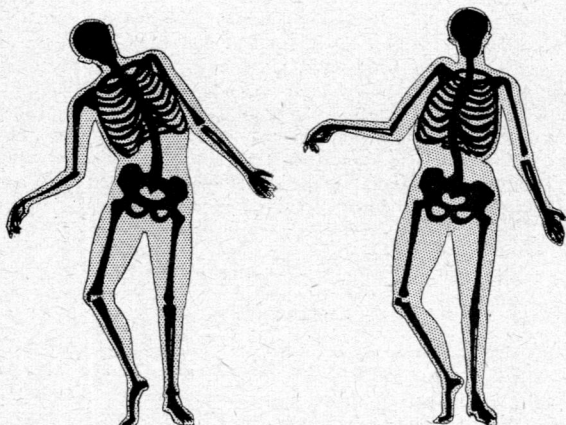

Fig. 119.—To avoid stretching the nerve the patient flexes hip and knee and stands on the toes. The pelvis tilts up, producing a lumbar curve convex to the unaffected side.

Distribution of Pain.—The pain often begins in the lumbar region or in the hip-joint, and tends to spread downwards. It may never reach below the knee, and is generally worse at the back of the hip and thigh, but it may involve any, or all branches of the nerve in its whole course.

GAIT.—To avoid stretching the nerve in a severe case, the patient walks on the toes of the foot of the affected side, with plantar-flexed ankle, the hip and knee being kept bent. This produces a limp and he may suffer great pain while walking. Often the only positions in which the patient is at all comfortable are kneeling, and lying on his side with hip and knee bent, and foot plantar-flexed. Because of his altered stance, the pelvis is tilted up on the affected side and a compensatory scoliosis may develop (*Fig.* 119).

NEUROLOGICAL SIGNS.—

TENDERNESS.—Specially tender points may be found as follows: (1) The point where the nerve emerges through the greater sciatic foramen (great sacro-sciatic notch) at the junction of the lower and middle thirds of a line from the posterior superior iliac spine to the outer part of the tuberosity of the ischium. This point can generally be found by looking for the highest point of the gluteal mass as the patient lies prone. (2) Half-way between the ischial tuberosity and the great trochanter, where the nerve emerges from beneath the gluteus maximus, lying over the neck of the femur. (3) Sometimes all along the back of the thigh, as far as the popliteal fossa (popliteal space). (4) There may, in cases of very extensive inflammation, be tender points on the lateral popliteal nerve (at the head of the fibula), the medial popliteal nerve (in the popliteal fossa), the posterior tibial nerve (below the medial malleolus), the sural or external saphenous nerve (alongside the tendo Achillis), or the plantar nerves (in the sole of the foot). The muscles supplied by these nerves may also be tender to pressure and stretching, as well as to voluntary contraction.

LASÈGUE'S SIGN.—If the knee is kept in full extension and the foot dorsiflexed, the hip cannot be flexed to any extent without causing great pain, this being brought about by the direct stretching of the nerve. It is the same if the trunk is the part moved—the patient cannot bend forward from the hips when standing, or assume the long-sitting position.

In *parenchymatous lesions*, be they acute or chronic, there may be considerable *wasting of muscles*, and *weakness* of the leg. Occasionally there may be *cramp* and *fibrillary tremors*. *The ankle-jerk may be lost*. The knee-jerk may be increased or normal, but is rarely lost. In very rare cases there is *reaction of degeneration*. All these symptoms denote an extension of the trouble in the axons. There may be numbness and impaired objective sensation along the outer side of the foot and leg, but a definite paralysis or anæsthesia is very unusual.

COURSE OF THE DISEASE.—This varies according to the cause. A mild attack may clear up completely in a few weeks. The majority of cases are far more troublesome, however, and the trouble may persist for months or years. Some cases become chronic and are punctuated with occasional acute attacks.

Treatment.—

GENERAL AND MEDICAL TREATMENT.—In severe cases, the patient may be ordered bed-rest for a time in the most comfortable position possible but nowadays it is more usual to immobilize the back in plaster and to let the patient remain up and about. *Sedatives* will be administered as required, and *injections* into the nerve of various substances (mainly analgesic) are often given. *Counter-irritation* (blistering over the nerve) is sometimes tried.

PHYSICAL TREATMENT.—From the point of view of physical treatment the most important principle is the strengthening of the muscles in the lumbar region, and the correction of posture. Since there is so much difference of opinion regarding these cases the physiotherapist must scrupulously obey the wishes of the physician or surgeon in charge of each patient with whom she deals. Neuritis caused by prolapsed disks has been dealt with on pp. 70–72. Here we will deal briefly with neuralgia or neuritis in which there are no marked signs of a parenchymatous lesion, but which is not, apparently, caused by a disk lesion.

Sciatica due to Neuralgia, or Neuritis not caused by a Disk Lesion (in which there are no Marked Signs of a Parenchymatous Lesion)

Both these conditions may be treated in much the same way as already described for brachial neuritis, but cases of brachial neuralgia can be treated earlier and more vigorously than those of sciatic neuritis. Whilst pain is still present, these cases should not be treated by massage or exercises at all. In the *acute stage* radiant heat, galvanism, short-wave diathermy, or other forms of electrical treatment may be possible, but the nerve itself should be given complete rest. Massage may be possible in the sub-acute stage, but it must be very gentle and light, and *must not cause pain.* A medical man, in a lecture to the Chartered Society of Physiotherapy, once suggested that any physiotherapist, asked to treat a case of true perineuritis, should immediately take influenza, and hand the case over to her dearest enemy! There is still much wisdom in this advice, and these cases should be treated with the greatest caution.

When all inflammation has gone from the tissues and the pain has ceased, i.e., in the *late* stages of an acute case, or in a *chronic* condition, deep massage and exercises can be given.

MASSAGE.—This should include the *lumbar* and *gluteal* regions, and the *back of the thigh.* Both sides of the back should be treated, since some degree of inflammation may be present in the muscles on both sides. Any tender thickenings in the muscles should now be sought. They are often found round the iliac crest, near the spines of the ilium where so many muscles have their origin, or near and over the sacrum, but they may also be scattered throughout the fleshy parts of the muscle. Deep transverse frictions should be given to these thickenings and to any nodules in the muscle over the nerve as it leaves the notch, or as it emerges from under the gluteal fold. (Students should make sure of the position and surface marking of the nerve.) Finally, kneading and effleurage should be given to accelerate blood- and lymph-flow.

ACTIVE MOVEMENTS.—These should include exercises for the glutei and quadriceps, as well as free and resisted exercises to mobilize and strengthen the lumbar region. *Relaxation exercises* should not be forgotten, because anyone who has had neuritis or neuralgia, or indeed muscle inflammation of any kind, tends instinctively to hold his or her muscles in contraction. In the first place this is a protective reflex, designed to immobilize the part and thus minimize the pain, but it very easily becomes a habit and may then give rise to persistent low backache.

EXERCISES.*—

A suitable early scheme would be as follows:—
1. Gentle breathing exercise.
2. Quadriceps contractions, ankle and foot exercises.
3. Prone-lying Head-raising and Head-rotation.
4. Prone-lying Gluteal contractions.
5. Neck-rest-prone-lying Bracing shoulders back.
6. Breathing exercise.

Later.—The following may gradually be added to the above scheme.
1. Prone-lying Alternate Leg backward-raising.
2. Prone-lying Alternate Knee-bending and stretching, at first free, then with resistance (progressing to 2-Knee-bending and stretching, free and resisted).
3. Foot-support-prone-lying, hands clasped behind back Head- and Shoulder-raising (assisted).
4. Lying Back-arching. The shoulders are raised from the couch, the spine hollowed from head to buttocks.
5. Prone-kneeling Alternate Leg-raising backwards and lowering.
6. Prone-lying Trunk-rotation in small range.
7. Prone-kneeling lumbar contractions (hollowing spine).
8. Prone-kneeling Trunk-rotation with Arm-stretching. The patient turns to right or left, raising the corresponding arm sideways and upwards.
9. Crook-lying Abdominal contractions (later + Gluteal and Adductor contractions). Static work only should be done at first and the patient should neither raise

---

* These exercises are intended only as a guide and the numbering does not imply that they are necessarily to be added in this exact order. The physiotherapist must study the individual patient when choosing exercises. They are also suitable for disk lesions and other back injuries.

the buttocks from the bed, nor tip the pelvis backward. A small hard cushion may be put beneath the lumbar spine, or the patient may place his hands there and be told to press the back into them. Later, the exercise may be done in the usual way.

10. Prone-kneeling Alternate Leg- and Arm-backward, raising (i.e., left arm and right leg together).

11. Prone-lying 2-leg-raising (with assistance if necessary).

12. Foot-support-prone-lying Head- and Shoulder-raising (free).

Strong Exercises.—

1. Kneeling Trunk-backward-falling (hollowing lumbar spine). This is abdominal work, but only in the outer range.

2. Forward-bend sitting Trunk-rotation with Alternate Arm flinging.

3. Prone-kneeling Abdominal and Lumbar contractions ('donkey'), performed quietly and without jerk.

4. Prone-lying Head- and Shoulder-lifting+2-Leg-lifting.

5. Prone-lying Raising to Prone-falling position.

6. Stride-standing Trunk-falling-forward and -raising (with straight back). This is an exercise to stretch the hamstrings, which are often short. The spine should not be flexed and no overpressure is to be given.

7. Games, especially such as entail spinal extension. Medicine-ball exercises, etc. (*See* Chapter XXIII.)

8. If these are allowed spinal flexion exercises can now be carefully introduced beginning with Back-raisings vertebra by vertebra.

ELECTRICAL TREATMENT.—Faradism may be ordered in the later stages; to strengthen the quadriceps.

Other Varieties of Sciatica

Forms of sciatica caused by pregnancy, tumours, or constipation, tend to disappear as soon as the cause is removed by natural, medical, or surgical means. In such cases the patients, if sent for placebo treatment, will require massage and active exercises to strengthen the muscles. Relaxation exercises should also be included in the treatment.

If the cause is osteo-arthritis of the hip or spine, the affected joint may be manipulated, or an open operation performed on it. The physiotherapist who undertakes the post-operative treatment should ascertain the exact intentions of the surgeon with regard to the joint, e.g., whether it is to be fixed or mobile, and, if the latter, to what extent. She should then scrupulously carry out any instruction he may give as to the nature and range of the movement permitted. Apart from any modifications thus required, the treatment will be on much the same lines as that described above (*see also* OSTEO-ARTHRITIS, pp. 148–51).

POLYNEURITIS
(*Multiple Peripheral Neuritis*)

This consists of an inflammation of the peripheral nerves due to some form of poisoning. Both motor and sensory fibres are involved.

AETIOLOGY.—Neuritis of this type is always due to some kind of poison in the blood. These poisons may be: (1) *Bacterial, or infective,* of which the commonest form is *acute infective polyneuritis,* probably due to a virus. (2) *Extrinsic,* consisting of poisonous chemical substances which enter the body in various ways, as by ingestion or inhalation, such as alcohol, arsenic, lead, etc. (3) *Such as are formed in the body as the result of disordered metabolism,* in such diseases as gout, vitamin-B_1 deficiency, or diabetes. Neuritis of this kind may also occur after long periods of over-exertion, or in connexion with anæmia or debility.

PATHOLOGICAL CHANGES.—This form of neuritis is both *interstitial* and *parenchymatous,* that is, it attacks not only the sheaths but the axons as well.

The sheaths are acutely inflamed and press on the sensory fibres, causing intense pain. The axons undergo degenerative changes, resulting in paralysis of the muscles, and anæsthesia.

VARIETIES.—The type most commonly encountered in hospital work is the acute infective type, and even so it is comparatively rare. We may also meet with alcoholic and lead-poisoning cases, those due to diabetes, etc., and still more rarely with those due to arsenic. Cases of neuritis due to overwork and debility may appear occasionally.

Prognosis is good in all these forms, complete recovery being the rule, though occasionally one or more muscles remain weak or powerless. The recovery is often very slow, however, and a year or more may elapse before it is complete. Vagus involvement is the chief danger. Death sometimes occurs from respiratory or bulbar paralysis, especially in the acute infective form, but, except for such cases as these, the outlook is good.

It is proposed to describe the clinical features and treatment of the acute infective type, and then to deal briefly with the salient features of other forms.

Acute Infective Polyneuritis

This type begins abruptly with *vomiting, headache, fever,* and *pain in the back and limbs. Paralysis* follows in a few hours or a few days, generally in all four limbs, though the legs may be affected first. The cranial nerves and those supplying the trunk muscles may be involved, as well as the respiratory muscles. *Anæsthesia* may spread from the limbs to the trunk. *Reflexes are lost,* and there may be *sphincter trouble.* A tracheotomy, or treatment in an artificial respirator, will be required in the early stages if the respiratory muscles are involved, but, as has been said, prognosis is good, complete recovery being the rule.

Order of Recovery of the Muscles.—Of the extensors in the forearm, those of the wrist generally recover first, then the extensor digitorum, and, finally, the extensors of the thumb. In the legs, either the extensor longis hallucis or the tibialis anterior may be the last to regain power.

Principles of Treatment.—The principles are the same for all cases of polyneuritis.

GENERAL TREATMENT.—The patient is kept in bed during the early period and is given appropriate medical treatment. (In alcoholic neuritis and some other forms, the administration of vitamin B has a favourable result.)

PHYSICAL TREATMENT.—The principles of physical treatment resemble those which apply in anterior poliomyelitis, transverse myelitis, or any other lower motor neuron disease. In the early stage the aims are: (1) *To prevent contractures and deformity* by affording proper support to the limbs, and maintaining mobility in the joints. (2) *To relieve pain.* (3) *To assist respiration,* if this has been affected, and to maintain the patient's general health at the highest possible level pending recovery. The methods used will be similar to those already described for lower motor neuron or peripheral nerve lesions and for interstitial neuritis.

SUPPORT.—Appropriate splints should be provided, *cock-up splints* being used for the hands, and suitably padded, light, plaster splints for the feet. As a rule, these need not come above the knee. The splints will be retained for as long as necessary and the feet should be splinted *at night* until the muscles are quite strong, although the hand splints may be removed much sooner. *Sand-bags* are often used to support the feet, but these are unsatisfactory for, if the patient turns on to his side or pulls himself up in the bed, the feet may be left unsupported. If they have to be used temporarily, a cradle should be provided. Great care should be taken to see that the toes are not pressed down, as this could result in a rigid hallux flexus, as well as trouble with the other toes. A small pillow or roll should be placed under the knees to prevent hyperextension.

ELECTRICAL TREATMENT.—Heat in any of its forms, anodal galvanism, or ionization may be used to relieve pain. In some cases interrupted direct current may be required to maintain muscle bulk pending recovery of the nerves.

MASSAGE AND RELAXED PASSIVE MOVEMENTS.—As soon as the patient can bear it, very gentle massage, similar to that given in brachial neuritis or sciatica, can be given. The depth will be increased as the patient improves, and a wider selection of manipulations may be used. This progression must not, however, be hurried, and *the massage must never cause pain*. Full range passive movements should be given as soon as possible, especially to the lower extremity. Contractures are rare in the arms, but can be very troublesome in the legs, feet, and toes. All the joints of the toes should be moved and the ankle brought into full dorsiflexion (the calf muscles are rarely paralysed). Inversion and eversion should also be given, but the foot must be kept in the mid-position between treatments. When the muscles are sufficiently recovered to protect the joints against over-stretching, forced movements can be used to regain the last degree of mobility.

RE-EDUCATION EXERCISES.—These must begin as soon as possible in order to treat the patient successfully, and the physiotherapist must know exactly how things stand. An accurate knowledge of anatomy is essential, for she has to determine which muscles are paralysed, and which nerves, or nerve branches, are out of action. No two cases are alike, nor are the two arms, or legs, of the same patient always similarly affected. For instance, though the extensors of the wrist and fingers are nearly always involved, the muscles supplied by the median nerve may be affected in one hand, and those supplied by the ulnar nerve in the other. Another vagary is for both these nerves to suffer on one side, and one on the other. Having ascertained precisely what is wrong, decided on the grade of contraction present in each muscle, and, ideally, performed an electrical test, the physiotherapist will proceed with her re-education programme as described for peripheral nerve lesions, anterior poliomyelitis, etc. It is advisable to make out a muscle chart, not only for her own benefit and the better to assess progress, but also to encourage the patient who may well be depressed and discouraged by the length of the illness.

Exercises suggested for individual nerve lesions (Chapter XII) will be suitable in the later stages.

CO-ORDINATION EXERCISES.—When the recovery of individual muscles is well advanced, the patient must be taught to co-ordinate his movements, and use the limbs normally.

The Hands.—The fine movements of the hands are the most difficult to regain. In addition to specific exercises, the patient should practise the following actions: Writing; handling of small objects; tying shoe-laces; doing up buttons; threading beads; tying knots; knitting and crocheting; threading beads with needle and cotton; using a knife and fork. In the case of a woman, sewing should be practised, at first with wool on coarse canvas, using cross stitch and a blunt wool needle; then with a large darning needle on soft material. Progress should be made to finer sewing; using scissors; making button-holes; threading needles; cutting out pictures, etc.

Re-education in Walking.—It is important to wait until the inverters have regained sufficient strength to prevent an incorrect standing position before beginning re-education in walking. Thereafter it follows the usual lines. A 'valgus wedge' may be needed in the shoes, and the patient should be carefully watched for signs of flat-foot.

A course of general exercises should conclude the patient's treatment.

Other Forms of Peripheral Neuritis

ALCOHOLIC NEURITIS

This form of neuritis is connected with vitamin-B deficiency, because vitamin B is readily destroyed in the abnormal conditions prevailing in the upper part of the alimentary canal.

SYMPTOMS.—The onset is generally *gradual*, though there is an acute form which is far less common, and is often fatal, the patient dying of respiratory or cardiac failure.

The terminal branches of the nerves are first affected, so that the hand and forearm muscles, and those of the foot and lower leg, are the first to be paralysed. The *extensor* muscles are more seriously affected than the *flexors*, producing wrist-drop and foot-drop. The feet are involved before the hands, and recover much more slowly. *Reaction of degeneration* is present and may be complete or partial; the *reflexes are lost in the affected areas*; *and trophic changes* occur in the skin and nails.

LEAD NEURITIS*

This occurs in those occupied in trades where lead is much used, e.g., painters, plumbers, etc.

SYMPTOMS.—*The extensors of the wrist are principally affected*, producing wrist-drop. This may be because in many of these workers there is constant strain on these muscles entailed by the use of brushes and hammers (Purves-Stewart). The brachioradialis and abductor longus pollicis, for some unknown reason, are rarely affected, though supplied by the same nerve as the others. The feet generally escape. There is hardly ever any *pain* in this form.

ARSENIC NEURITIS*

This occurs in workers in trades in which arsenic is used, or occasionally, when too much of the drug has been taken in medicine. It may also be ingested through adulterated beer or sweets.

SYMPTOMS.—Arsenical paralysis resembles the alcoholic type in many ways. *Marked sensory symptoms* (paræsthesia, anæsthesia, and pain) are a feature of this form. The feet are more affected than the hands, though both may suffer, and *skin eruptions* are a prominent feature.

NEURITIS DUE TO DEBILITY, ANÆMIA, ETC.

This closely resembles alcoholic neuritis.

II. CRAMP

A spastic condition, due to over-contraction of the muscles without relaxation—in other words, a *tetanus*. The name 'cramp' is generally given to the *tonic* variety of spasm—that is, to a condition of fixed spasm—rather than to a series of spasmodic jerks (*clonic* spasm).

AETIOLOGY.—Cramp is a symptom, not a disease in itself (*see also* Chapter XIX). It is due to irritation of a nerve by pressure, or to increased excitability in a motor nerve.

Cramp very frequently occurs in the calf-muscles, or in the sole of the foot (interossei). It may occasionally occur in the quadriceps, or the abdominal muscles. Other muscle-groups are sometimes attacked, but far less commonly.

---

* Both lead and arsenic poisoning have many symptoms other than those of neuritis; but with these we are not concerned.

Patients suffering from nervous diseases, or recovering from peripheral nerve lesions or neuritis, may suffer acute attacks of cramp. For this reason, it will be briefly considered here.

GASTROCNEMIUS CRAMP

Gastrocnemius cramp, or cramp in the calf-muscles, is the commonest form and one which has been experienced by most people at some time or another, generally while in bed at night. It is brought about by *an over-strong plantar-flexion of the foot*, either passive—produced by the pressure of heavy bedclothes—or active. (A similar condition is the very dangerous cramp which is sometimes the cause of a bathing fatality. Strong work of the leg muscles and the coldness of the water produce cramp of some muscle-group in the leg, and disable the swimmer.)

SYMPTOMS.—There is *intense tonic spasm of the gastrocnemius*, which feels as hard as iron. *The pain is very severe* during the attack. The muscles are sometimes tender in the intervals between the attacks.

Treatment during the Attack.—When an attack of cramp occurs, anyone present should try to stretch the affected muscle-group. In gastrocnemius cramp *the knee should be straightened and the ankle dorsiflexed*. The patient is generally unable to reach his foot to do this for himself, and it is impossible for him to dorsiflex it actively against the spasm of the powerful calf-muscles. (Anyone subject to this form of cramp at night generally rises and tries to walk, since, when he is putting his foot to the ground the ankle is dorsiflexed by the weight of his body.) Soothing strokings and rhythmic kneading may also help to relax the muscles and relieve the pain. In cases of persistent cramp calcium ionization may be tried in an attempt to raise the threshold of irritability of the nerve.

III. EPILEPSY

We are not called upon to treat epileptics as such and the causes and changes do not concern us as physiotherapists. The occurrence of a 'fit' in the physiotherapy department is, however, not impossible, since epileptics often come to be treated for other ailments. A note should always be made on the letter or card of such a patient, and the physiotherapist in charge of the treatment should be informed of the disability, and, if necessary, told what to do should an attack take place.

THE EPILEPTIC FIT.—There may, or may not, be an *aura*—that is, a peculiar sensation preceding the attack and acting as a warning. The aura may be a sensory perception of sound, light, or smell. There may be twitchings of the limbs, numbness, a feeling of intense fear, nausea, palpitation, or giddiness. It only lasts a few moments and the actual 'fit' follows immediately. It has two phases: (*a*) the tonic and (*b*) the clonic stage.

THE TONIC STAGE.—The patient falls to the ground with a characteristic cry, and becomes unconscious, passing at once into a condition of rigidity. The legs and arms are completely rigid, the former in extension, the latter with bent elbows and clenched hands, the thumb generally flexed across the palm. The face is first pale and then livid. The breathing is almost arrested by the contraction of the thoracic muscles. This stage lasts about half a minute, and is followed at once by the clonic stage.

THE CLONIC STAGE.—This consists of violent convulsions, which begin in the muscles of the face and spread to those of the limbs and trunk. It is at this stage that the tongue is often bitten. The patient foams at the mouth, and the face becomes cyanosed. This phase lasts about three minutes. Then the muscles relax, the cyanosis disappears, the respiration improves, and the patient may recover consciousness, or fall into a deep natural sleep. When he wakes he feels exhausted and irritable.

Treatment.—The only part of the treatment which concerns us is that which is required during an attack. There is little we can do, but that little is important. If the patient has an aura, and we thus get a warning of the approach of an attack, he should be placed flat on a couch or on the floor with a low cushion under his head, well away from furniture or anything with which he might come into contact during the convulsive stage. If the fit comes on without warning, he must be left where he fell. As soon as possible, something should be put between the teeth to prevent the tongue from being bitten in the clonic stage—a spoon, or a pencil or piece of wood wrapped in linen or a bandage will serve the purpose. If there is time, any tight clothing should be loosened. During the clonic stage, the patient must be prevented from injuring himself—any objects round him, such as chairs and tables, should be moved out of the way. The convulsive movements should be restrained, but not forcibly prevented. In a hospital department, screens should be put round the patient, especially if children are present, but no attempt should be made to move him until the convulsions have ceased. When they are over, he should be put to bed or covered up warmly and allowed to sleep. If a patient *must* go home after a fit, he should be sent in a car, or at least accompanied by some responsible person in case a second attack should occur.

It is obviously not advisable that patients subject to fits should be given electrical treatment, be placed in the head suspension apparatus (e.g., for scoliosis), allowed to climb high on ladders, walk on a boom high above the floor, or take up any position which might be dangerous or fatal should a fit occur at that time.

CHAPTER XIV

DISEASES OF MUSCLE

The dystrophies (Pseudo-hypertrophic muscular dystrophy; Erb's juvenile type; Infantile type)—
Amyotonia congenita—Thomsen's disease—Myasthenia gravis.

ALL these conditions have certain features in common. There is gross and progressive *muscular weakness.* *Contractures* and *deformities* are very liable to occur, and all are *incurable.* Death usually follows some pulmonary complication (e.g., pneumonia). The expectation of life varies with the different forms of disease. Some are rapidly progressive and death intervenes early; others are more insidious and the victims reach adult and even middle life. The same principles of treatment apply to all.

Principles of Treatment.—

GENERAL.—Every effort should be made to enable the patient to lead as active and happy a life as possible. Where benefit can be expected from them, suitable drugs will be administered. Warmth, nourishing food, and hygiene are important.

PHYSICAL.—This is probably the most valuable form of treatment, though it can only be palliative. The aims are *to prevent contracture and deformity; to maintain as much muscle power as possible*; and *to help the patient to lead as active, happy, and healthy a life as possible, for the maximum period of time.*

THE DYSTROPHIES

Muscular dystrophy, or myopathy, is a disease of the muscles themselves, and not of the nervous system, although the symptoms in some ways resemble those of paralysis. The word 'dystrophy' means a condition of impaired or faulty nutrition (Greek, *dys* = hard, difficult, bad, and *trophe* = nourishment) and the disease is, in fact, a degeneration of muscle. It produces atrophy of some muscles, and enlargement—but not true hypertrophy—of others. There are three principal varieties: (1) The pseudo-hypertrophic type; (2) Erb's juvenile type; (3) The infantile or facio-humeroscapular type.

1. PSEUDO-HYPERTROPHIC MUSCULAR DYSTROPHY

AETIOLOGY.—This is an *hereditary* and *familial* disease. Like hæmophilia, it descends in the female line through the mother to the sons, appearing as a rule in two or more boys in a family. Girls are only rarely affected. The age of onset is childhood (5–8 years).

PATHOLOGICAL CHANGES.—Some muscles atrophy, and others increase in size but this *pseudo-hypertrophy* does not make the muscles stronger, for their enlargement is due to increase of interstitial substance. The fibres degenerate, the degeneration being partly fatty and partly fibrous. Hence the muscles, though large, are weak. *There are no neurological changes.*

SYMPTOMS.—There is *atrophy* of the latissimus dorsi, the lower part of trapezius and pectoralis major; the biceps, triceps, serratus anterior, and the flexors of the hip. The hamstrings and adductors are also affected.

There is *pseudo-hypertrophy* of the glutei, the calf muscles, deltoid, and infra-spinatus. The large calf muscles often attract attention first, being sometimes very noticeable. In fact, the mother is often proud of the boy's well-developed legs (*Fig.* 120).

The child's *powers of walking* suffer, he stumbles and is easily tired. The *gait* is waddling and awkward, and the feet are placed wide apart in order to broaden his base. Owing to the weakness of the gluteus maximus he throws his body backwards from the hips, the abdomen protruding. This produces a marked

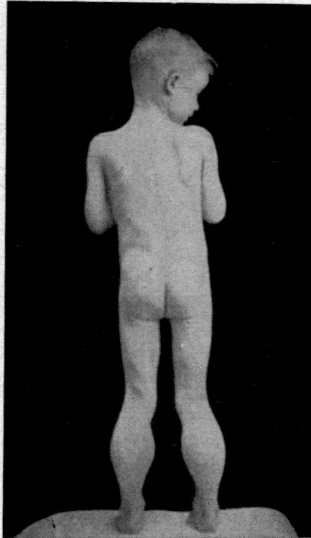

Fig. 120.—Pseudo-hypertrophic muscular dystrophy, showing pseudo-hypertrophy of the calves. (*Case of Dr. Patterson's from French's 'Index of Differential Diagnosis'*.)

lordosis which is one of the characteristics of this condition. His *manner of rising from the supine position is diagnostic.* If he is lying on his back on the floor, he first turns over and gets on to his hands and knees. He then extends his knees, working his hands gradually closer and closer to his feet. Then, placing his hands alternately one above the other on his thighs, he raises his trunk to an upright position. As the disease progresses he is unable to rise without pulling himself up by catching hold of surrounding objects, and he is finally prevented, either by weakness or by deformities, from rising at all. Some patients adopt a frog-like mode of progression, with hips and knees flexed.

Contractures.—These develop late in the course of the disease, the calf muscles being particularly prone to this. The hips and knees become flexed, and the foot strongly plantar-flexed (talipes equinus or equino-varus). The lordosis produced by weakness of the gluteus maximus has been referred to above. In the later stages of the disease, when the spinal muscles become involved, kyphosis takes the place of lordosis, and scoliosis may follow.

Reflexes.—The tendon-jerks decrease gradually as the muscles degenerate.

Electrical Changes.—There is no R.D., but the response to electrical stimuli gradually diminishes and finally disappears.

DISEASES OF MUSCLE

DISEASES OF MUSCLE 285

PROGNOSIS.—The patient rarely survives the age of 20. The power of standing is generally lost between the ages of 10 and 14 years, and the disease progresses more rapidly after this period.

2. ERB'S JUVENILE TYPE

AETIOLOGY.—This form appears later than the pseudo-hypertrophic type, usually between the ages of 12 and 16, but sometimes even later. It is more slowly progressive than the pseudo-hypertrophic type, and affects both sexes.

SYMPTOMS.—*The muscles of the shoulder-girdle and upper arm* are affected first, those of the *pelvic girdle and spine* later. In this type all the muscles atrophy. Those chiefly affected are the latissimus dorsi, serratus anterior, pectoralis major, trapezius, the rhomboids, biceps, triceps, and brachio-radialis. The deltoid and the muscles of the hand escape. The shoulders fall forward, and the scapulæ are winged. Later, deformities develop, similar to those of the pseudo-hypertrophic type.

PROGNOSIS.—The patient may live for many years, the general heath being good as a rule. The power of walking is retained much longer than in the preceding form, and the patient can often follow some light occupation well into adult life.

3. INFANTILE TYPE (FACIO-HUMEROSCAPULAR)

AETIOLOGY.—This form generally attacks infants, but is occasionally delayed until adolescence.

CHANGES.—Atrophy and pseudo-hypertrophy may both be present.

SYMPTOMS.—The *facial muscles* are affected first. The eyelids cannot be closed; the lips become thickened, weak, and flaccid; and the mouth hangs open, which interferes with distinct speech. The intrinsic muscles of the eyes and tongue escape. Later, the disease spreads to the muscles of the *shoulders and arms*.

PROGNOSIS.—As in the pseudo-hypertrophic type, this is bad, but the progress of the disease is slower, and the patient may live for some time.

Treatment.—The specific aims of treatment are: (1) *To maintain the strength of the muscles* and *to improve their blood-supply* in an attempt to delay degeneration as long as possible. This applies to all the muscles, *particularly the respiratory muscles*. (2) *To improve the patient's general health* in order to increase his resistance to infections, especially such as attack the lungs.

GENERAL TREATMENT.—Medical treatment will consist of tonics, cod-liver oil, etc. As yet, no effective drugs have been found.

PHYSICAL TREATMENT.—It should be stressed that these diseases cannot be cured, but their progress may be delayed by treatment. Erb's juvenile type is the most hopeful from a therapeutic point of view, but it is rarely encountered.

MASSAGE.—This should be stimulating in order to assist circulation. Effleurage, kneading, and picking up can all be given, but the treatment should not be a long one. *General massage* may prove helpful.

PASSIVE MOVEMENTS.—Attention must be paid to the condition of the joints, passive movement should be given to prevent contractures. Dorsiflexion of the foot, extension of the hip and knee, and extension of the elbow are especially important. The condition of the joints of the shoulder should be carefully watched, since it must not be allowed to stiffen.

EXERCISES.—A short table of exercises should be given, the patient being made to use all the affected muscles. Resistance should be given where practicable, and to this end the Kabat method of re-education may be tried in the early stages. At first, however, it may be better to teach the patient to perform simple movements in lying or side-lying, for example:—

1. Side-lying Hip-flexion and -extension (for gluteus maximus, and the flexors of the hip).

2. Side-lying 2-Foot-bending and -stretching (calf muscles and anterior tibial group).

3. Lying 2-Arm-raising sideways and upwards and -lowering (serratus anterior and deltoid; latissimus dorsi).

4. Lying Alternate arm-flexion across chest (pectoralis major).

5. Sitting (or half-lying) 2-Arm-rotation-out with breathing (infraspinatus and teres minor).

6. Half-lying (or side-lying) 2-Forearm-bending and -stretching (biceps).

7. Lying (or crook-lying) 2-Arm-bending and -stretching. Assistance may be required at first, either manually, in water, or using suspension apparatus, but resistance should be added later.

If any muscles are very weak, the patient should be taught to contract these muscles individually, without producing any movements of the joints. Static contractions of the glutei, quadriceps, biceps, and deltoid, for instance, are not difficult to obtain.

Later, it may be possible to attempt the exercises in standing, and efforts should be made to improve posture and gait, although improvement is not likely to be more than temporary.

Abdominal contractions and trunk flexion movements may be given to strengthen the abdominal muscles, and to prevent the lordosis from becoming fixed. Other easy trunk exercises can also be attempted.

Breathing exercises are most important and should never be omitted.

ELECTRICAL TREATMENT.—General ultra-violet irradiation may be ordered for its tonic effect.

Precaution.—The patient should be warmly covered during massage and should be adequately clothed while doing exercises. If he becomes hot, great care must be taken to prevent his catching cold afterwards. A chill might well be the cause of a tragedy. It is also important not to tire the child.

AMYOTONIA CONGENITA

A congenital disease affecting the muscles and resembling a flaccid paralysis. It is *familial* and often *hereditary*.

SYMPTOMS.—The *muscles are flaccid*, soft, and toneless; they do not harden in contraction like ordinary muscles, although there is no actual paralysis (the nervous system not being involved) and there is no wasting. The *legs* are generally most affected, but the *back muscles* are weak and the child cannot sit up or hold its head erect, until well beyond the usual age (second year or later). The patient is often unable to stand or walk, though the ability to do so sometimes develops later. The joints are flail, owing to the hypotonia of the muscles and consequent relaxation of the ligaments; the limbs can therefore be placed in all sorts of abnormal postures (*Fig.* 121). The sphincters are normal.

Electrical Changes.—The response to electrical stimulation is diminished and children, and even infants, can bear strong faradic currents.

The *deep reflexes* are lost owing to lack of muscle tone, but the *superficial reflexes* are normal (Purves-Stewart).

PROGNOSIS.—Improvement often takes place, but there is no cure.

Treatment.—The specific aims of treatment are: (1) *To improve the tone and nutrition of the muscles*; (2) *To teach the child to use his limbs*, sit up, and walk.

Treatment should be carried out on much the same lines as for a flaccid paralysis. A long course of treatment will be necessary, and the child should be under supervision as growth continues. Splints are not required as a rule.

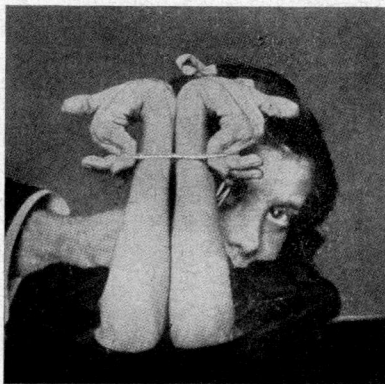

Fig. 121.—Amyotonia congenita.

THOMSEN'S DISEASE
(*Myotonia Congenita*)

A rare condition in which the voluntary muscles go into spasm when movement is attempted, and in which relaxation is delayed.

AETIOLOGY.—It is an *hereditary* disease which is also *familial*. It generally affects more than one of a family and appears in early childhood.

PATHOLOGY.—It is caused by some congenital defect in the muscles, which have too great a proportion of sarcoplasm to fibrils. The muscular fibres are greatly enlarged and hypertrophied.

SYMPTOMS.—The *muscles go into tonic spasm* when the patient attempts to perform voluntary movements. This condition is most marked in the *leg muscles*. For instance, the spasm comes on when he begins to walk, but decreases if he continues to do so. If he stops, it returns when he starts again. If he rests, the stiffness makes it very difficult for him to rise. He cannot voluntarily relax his muscles. The *muscles of face, eye,* and *tongue* may be similarly affected, and spasm of the latter may make speech difficult. The *sphincters are normal. Respiration and other vital functions* are not disturbed, nor is there much actual weakness.

Electrical Changes.—The reaction to electrical stimulation is peculiar. The contraction induced by the interrupted direct current does not consist of a single quick twitch but is unduly prolonged, the muscle only relaxing gradually. The same is the case with faradism. The constant current produces a series of rhythmic contractions. This peculiar response is known as the *myotonic reaction*.

PROGNOSIS.—The disease is incurable, but is neither progressive nor fatal.

Treatment.—The specific aims of treatment are *to reduce the spasm and to assist more normal use of the muscles.*

GENERAL TREATMENT.—Like most victims of muscular disease the patients are very sensitive to cold, which, in this case, increases the spasm. They should wear warm clothes and have nourishing food. Warm baths, or whirlpool baths if they can be obtained, help to reduce the spasm.

PHYSICAL TREATMENT.—

MASSAGE AND EXERCISES.—The patient may be treated in much the same way as a case of hemiplegia (*see* pp. 85–8).

MYASTHENIA GRAVIS

This is a rare condition in which the voluntary muscles are weak and easily exhausted. Even slight exertion produces such fatigue that the muscles cannot work at all unless rested. There is rarely any muscular wasting.

AETIOLOGY.—Both men and women are affected, though women are slightly more susceptible. The disease comes on in youth or early middle age. The cause is unknown, but the thymus gland seems to be involved in some way, a persistent thymus often being found. In some cases an exophthalmic goitre also exists.

PATHOLOGY.—There are no constant changes in the nervous system, nor are there marked degenerative changes in the muscles themselves. *Apparently the main defect is in the neuromuscular junction, nerve impulses failing to pass to the muscle-fibres.* This is thought to be due to some failure in the liberation of acetylcholine, or to its premature distribution.

SYMPTOMS.—The *facial muscles* are most affected, especially those of the eyes, lips, and tongue, the latter interfering with eating and speaking. The patient cannot keep the eyes open, or hold the head erect, for long at a time. All the affected muscles are temporarily improved by rest, but grow worse and worse during repeated movements, so that they are always at their best in the morning and at their weakest in the evening. Gradually, the *muscles of the arms and legs* and the *respiratory muscles* become involved, and a tracheotomy or some form of respirator may be required in the later stages.

Reflexes.—The tendon-jerks are present and may be slightly increased.

Electrical Changes.—The reaction to stimuli is normal at first, but this gradually decreases and finally ceases. This is known as a *myasthenic reaction.*

PROGNOSIS.—The disease is incurable and in many cases is slowly progressive, though there may sometimes be fairly long periods of remission. In other cases the disease proves rapidly fatal, death usually resulting from cardiac or respiratory failure.

Treatment.—As yet no completely satisfactory treatment has been found. Rest is indicated, and the patient should not exert herself to the point of fatigue. Prostigmin, given by mouth or by injection, has been found to have good results. This may be combined with atropine. The thymus gland is sometimes removed in patients who do not respond to the treatment by drugs.

From the point of view of physical treatment little can be done. Massage, passive movements, and gentle exercises may improve the patient's comfort, but great care must be taken not to tire her. In the later stages treatment similar to that given in cases of cardiac failure (*see* Chapter XX) may be required. It may also be necessary to assist respiration and clear the lungs and respiratory tract.

CHAPTER XV

DEFORMITIES OF THE UPPER AND LOWER EXTREMITIES

Types and causes of deformity; General principles of treatment. I. Deformities of the upper extremity: Sprengel's shoulder—Club-hand and congenital absence of radius, ulna, or other bones—Dupuytren's contracture—Contracted fingers. II. Deformities of the lower extremity: Congenital dislocation of the hip—Coxa vara—Genu valgum—Genu varum (bandy-legs) and bow-legs—Flat-foot and weak foot—Pes plano-valgus—Metatarsalgia—Talipes—Pes cavus—Hallux valgus—Hallux rigidus and hallux flexus—Hammer-toe.

A DEFORMITY is a malformation of any part of the body, due to a distortion of the bony skeleton, or to an alteration in length of some of the soft tissues. Deformities may be divided into two classes: (1) *Congenital* and (2) *Acquired.*

1. The Congenital Deformities are caused by the retention of the fœtus in some incorrect position before birth, or by some failure, or abnormality, of development. They may, or may not, be hereditary.

A congenital deformity is one actually present *before* birth. A deformity caused by an injury *during* birth is not a congenital one.

2. The Acquired Deformities may be due to one of many causes, the most common of which are: (1) *Bone disease,* e.g., tubercle infection, carcinoma, rickets, etc. (2) *Joint disease,* e.g., various kinds of arthritis, gout. (3) *Paralysis,* from whatever cause, leading to muscle imbalance and alteration in joint structures. (4) *Muscle disease,* e.g., muscular dystrophy. (5) *Trauma,* e.g., injuries at birth or in later life, fractures, separated epiphyses, burns, scars, etc. (6) *Mechanical strain,* such as is imposed by certain occupations which put undue strain or pressure on some parts of the body, e.g., on the spine, in those whose trade necessitates the carrying of heavy weights; by habitual poor posture; or by incorrect distribution of body-weight due either to loss of correct postural sense resulting from some defect of the postural reflex (*see* p. 341), or to altered joint mechanics following fractures, etc., involving joint surfaces (e.g., fracture-dislocation of ankle leading to flat foot).

Degrees of Development of Deformities.—In most acquired deformities, three degrees or stages are recognized. The characteristics of these are as follows:—

1. FIRST DEGREE.—

CHANGES IN MUSCLE TONE AND HABITUAL POSTURE: NO BONY CHANGE.—The patient can himself correct the position of the affected part.

2. SECOND DEGREE.—

DEFINITE CONTRACTURE OF SOFT TISSUES, i.e., muscles and ligaments, with a *Slight Degree of Bony Change.* The patient cannot himself correct the deformity, but it can be corrected to some extent by the physiotherapist.

Intermediate between these two degrees comes a stage in which there is definite spasm or even shortening of the muscles, etc., without any appreciable alteration in the bone.

3. THIRD DEGREE.—

SERIOUS BONY CHANGES.—Very little correction, if any, can be obtained by the physiotherapist.

10

The first-degree deformities are *curable*; those of the second degree may be *improved* by treatment. For those of the third degree little can be done, unless they exist in some part where surgical interference is possible.

GENERAL PRINCIPLES OF TREATMENT

Whatever the degree of acquired deformity, the broad principles of treatment remain the same, namely (1) *to direct appropriate medical or surgical treatment to the cause where this can be beneficial;* (2) *to prevent the formation of a possible secondary deformity;* (3) *to restore the balance between stretched and contracted structures as far as possible;* (4) *to strengthen weakened muscles so that they can maintain the correct position;* (5) *to re-educate postural sense;* (6) *to attend to the general health and nutrition of the patient where this is unsatisfactory.* In the case of congenital deformities much depends on whether or not the skeleton or musculature is deficient. In cases in which the bones are present, though malformed, the principles of treatment are similar to those outlined above. In cases where the bones are mal-developed or absent every effort must be made to reduce the inevitable deformity to a minimum by any appropriate operative treatment, by stretching tightened structures, and by increasing muscle power. Having done this, the child must be taught to compensate for the loss of bone or muscle as fully as possible by re-education of movement and, if necessary, by artificial aids.

I. DEFORMITIES OF THE UPPER EXTREMITY

Acquired deformities of the upper extremity, other than those of paralytic origin, are rare, and few call for treatment by physical means. Improper distribution of body-weight is the determining factor in most acquired deformities, and since this factor is not operative in the case of the upper extremity, except in children at the crawling stage, such deformities are less common than in the lower extremity. *Congenital* malformations, also, are found far less frequently in the arms than in the legs. The acquired deformities which do occur are mostly the result of paralysis, bone diseases, or injuries.

SPRENGEL'S SHOULDER

A rare congenital condition in which one scapula (or occasionally both) is in an abnormally high position on the thoracic wall.

AETIOLOGY.—

CAUSE.—The deformity may be caused by a constrained position of the fœtus in utero, thus preventing the descent of one or both scapulæ, which are much higher in the early stages of fœtal development than at birth.

HEREDITY is often a factor, and other deformities are often present in the same patient.

UNILATERAL cases are much more common than bilateral.

SEX.—The sexes are affected about equally.

DEFORMITY (*Fig.* 122).—

1. In unilateral cases *the position of one scapula is abnormally high.* The condition is generally accompanied by scoliosis in the thoracic region, the convexity being *towards* the side of the raised shoulder. In bilateral cases, both shoulders are raised, and the thoracic and lower cervical vertebræ stand out prominently.

2. The scapula is not only *raised* but *rotated*, generally in such a way that the upper angle is nearer the spine than the lower. Sometimes the rotation is in the opposite direction, when the inferior angle may even overlap the vertebral column.

3. The *superior angle* shows prominently in the neck.

4. The *clavicle* may be shortened to the extent of one inch, so that the scapula is nearer to the spine on the affected side.

5. The *mobility* of the shoulder is much reduced because of the fixation of the scapula, abduction and elevation being limited.

6. The *upper part of the chest* may be poorly developed.

COURSE.—The deformity generally gets worse as the patient grows older.

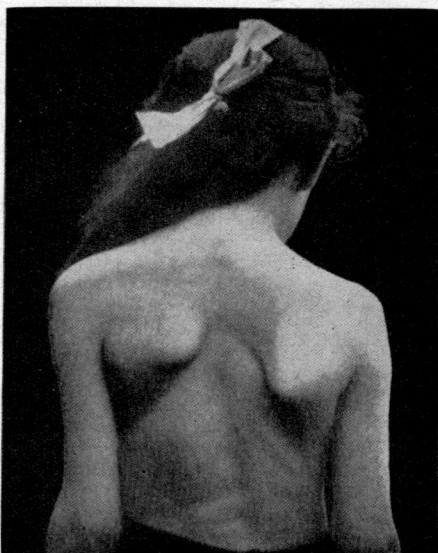

Fig. 122.—Congenital elevation of the left scapula (Sprengel's shoulder

PATHOLOGICAL CHANGES.—
BONES.—

1. *The scapula is malformed*, being broader and more curved than normal and the long axis of the bone is horizontal instead of vertical.

2. *A bar of bone*, or *fibrous bands*, often connect it to the vertebral column, generally to one of the cervical vertebræ.

3. *One or more of the vertebræ may be absent* or *a cervical rib may be present*.

MUSCLES.—The trapezius is always weak and defective. Various other muscles attached to the scapula may be abnormal or absent—the levator anguli scapulæ, serratus magnus, infraspinatus, latissimus dorsi, teres major, pectoralis minor, rhomboids, etc. The sternomastoid and pectoralis major have also been found to be defective or absent in some cases.

Treatment.—Little can be done in the way of correction, and most attempts to replace the scapula are unsuccessful. There is also grave danger of *stretching the brachial plexus by altering the position of the scapula*. Shoulder range can, however, be improved following surgical intervention.

SURGICAL TREATMENT.—The incision is made along the vertebral border of the scapula (sometimes also along part of the superior border). Any fibrous bands holding the scapula to the vertebræ are divided and a bony bar, if present, removed. Some surgeons divide any muscles which hold the scapula in an abnormal position, others concentrate only on fibrous or bony bands for reasons given above.

PHYSICAL TREATMENT.—When the wound is healed treatment designed to regain mobility is begun. *Massage* may be given to improve the circulation and so assist in preventing the formation of adhesions which would counteract the effect of the operation, but *movement* is the most important factor. *Passive* and *active movements* should be given to all the joints of the shoulder-girdle, special attention being paid to *abduction* and *elevation* of the arm, and to *rotation of the scapula*. It is important to learn from the surgeon which muscles are defective or absent, and if any were divided at the operation. Complications such as torticollis or scoliosis must also be treated. The shoulder-girdle muscles should be treated in the same way as muscles recovering from paralysis (*see* pp. 206, 253). In the early stages the use of a pool or suspension apparatus is helpful. In many cases, however, the result is disappointing.

CLUB-HAND AND CONGENITAL ABSENCE OF RADIUS, ULNA, OR OTHER BONES

The long axes of forearm and hand should be in a line with one another—any deviation from this line constitutes 'club-hand'. The condition may be congenital or acquired. (1) *Congenital* cases are far less common than similar deformities in the foot. They are most often associated with congenital absence of radius or ulna, the former being the commoner. Cases in which the bones are normal are very rare. The condition is often *bilateral* and other deformities may be present elsewhere in the body. (2) *Acquired* cases are due to paralysis, arthritis, bone disease, or trauma.

CHANGES AND SYMPTOMS (congenital form).—

1. As in club-foot, the hand is in a *position of exaggeration of one or more of its normal movements*—flexion, extension, adduction, or abduction. Two of these are often combined. The position of flexion is much commoner than that of extension, and the commonest of all is that in which the hand is *flexed* and *adducted*.

2. *If the radius is absent* the hand deviates to the radial side, and the ulna is excessively bowed. The thumb may also be absent, or its metacarpal bone wanting, the phalanges being attached to the carpus only by soft tissues.

3. *If the ulna is absent* there is ulnar deviation, and one or more fingers on the inner side of the hand may be missing.

Treatment.—

CASES WITHOUT BONY DEFECT.—These are treated by wrenching, and are put up in plaster or specially made splints which keep the hand in an over-corrected position.

PHYSICAL TREATMENT is similar to that for club-foot (*see* p. 320), i.e., passive stretchings in conjunction with active exercises as soon as the child is old enough to perform them.

CASES WITH BONY DEFECT (e.g., absent radius).—

SURGICAL TREATMENT.—This is designed to correct the bowing of the ulna and to attach it to the carpus, in order to prevent radial deviation. The ulna may be split to make two bones and articulated at the wrist with the carpus, or a wedge osteotomy may be performed. The bone may either be inserted into the carpus, or fixed to the carpus by means of a bone-graft. Another form of operation includes a bone-graft from the tibia which is mortised above into the ulna about its middle, and inserted below into the radial side of the dorsum of the carpus (*Albee's Operation*). If the first metacarpal bone is missing, the thumb may be amputated, being quite useless, or an attempt may be made to articulate the first phalanx to a carpal or metacarpal bone (Tubby).

PHYSICAL TREATMENT.—

Pre-operative.—Little can be done until operative measures have been carried out, but it may be possible to begin muscle re-education and so prepare the patient for post-operative treatment.

Post-operative.—During immobilization, treatment should be given along the usual lines and following the usual rules. *Passive* and *active movements* for the wrist and hand will begin as soon as the surgeon allows. It is important to understand exactly what was done at the operation in order to make an accurate assessment of the possible range of movement.

For acquired forms of hand deformity, *see* description of ARTHRITIS, PARALYSIS OF NERVES OF ARM (Chapters VII, XII).

DUPUYTREN'S CONTRACTURE

A flexion deformity of the fingers due to contraction of the palmar fascia. It most commonly affects the ring and little fingers, and is usually bilateral.

AETIOLOGY.—The deformity occurs much more frequently in men than in women, and appears in middle life or old age.

CAUSE.—There is some uncertainty about what actually causes the contracture but heredity appears to be a factor, the condition often being familial. Gout, rheumatism, and metabolic diseases have also been blamed for its appearance.

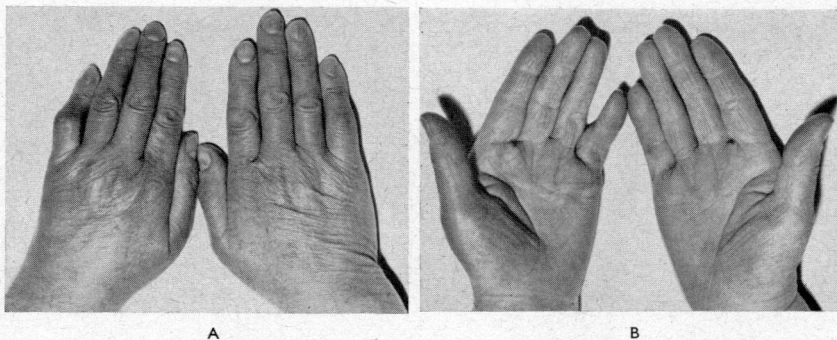

Fig. 123.—A, Dorsal and, B, Palmar aspects of early Dupuytren's contracture. The little fingers are primarily affected. Note ridging of skin on the palmar aspect, particularly the left, which is the more seriously affected.

In many cases, injury to the tissues of the palm seems to be an *exciting* cause, since the contracture is often found in people whose occupations entail constant over-use or pressure on this part of the hand.

PATHOLOGY.—

1. The seat of the trouble is the *palmar fascia*, which becomes thickened and nodular, in accordance with a chronic inflammatory reaction. Later, it contracts, and bands of fascia draw the fingers down into the palm of the hand. The *skin* also becomes contracted. The ring finger is most frequently affected and later the little finger, but sometimes the latter is the first to suffer (*Fig.* 123). The other fingers are far less commonly involved, and the thumb very rarely.

2. The finger is first drawn down at the metacarpophalangeal joint, then at the first and second interphalangeal joints (*Fig.* 123), so that finally the fingers are flexed into the palm (*Fig.* 124).

3. The joint structures become contracted and arthritic changes occur in the joints (*Fig.* 125). Finally, the tendons become shortened as well.

SYMPTOMS.—

1. The *position* of the fingers is as described above. As they are drawn down, the shortened bands of fascia stand out like cords in the palm. They also radiate up to the second phalanges. The skin, which adheres to them, is thrown into wrinkles (*Fig.* 123).

2. The patient may complain of *neuralgic pain* in the hand. Equally there may be no pain unless the fingers are forcibly extended, or the fascia subjected to pressure.

Treatment.—In the early stages or in very slight cases, it may be possible to improve the condition by giving frictions and deep massage to the palm of the hand, by stretching the shortened structures, and by active exercises for the extensors.

ELECTRICAL TREATMENT is sometimes effective and is designed to soften the fibrous tissues. To this end ultrasonics or iodine, chlorine, and sometimes histamine ionization may be given to the palmar aspect of the hand, to produce a fibrolytic effect.

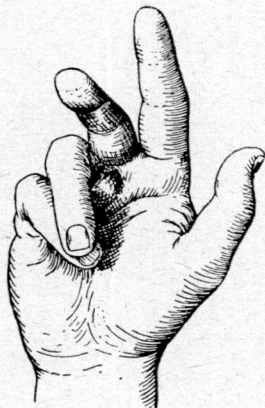

Fig. 124.—Dupuytren's contracture in later stages.

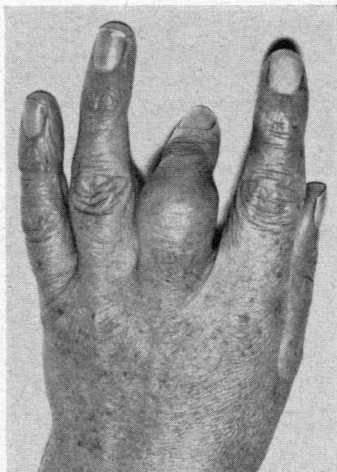

Fig. 125.—Dupuytren's contracture affecting middle finger showing marked arthritic changes in the joint.

An operation is generally necessary to effect a cure.

SURGICAL TREATMENT.—The operation consists of severance of the contracted bands of fascia by various methods, or removal of the fascia itself.

POST-OPERATIVE TREATMENT.—Support: The finger, or fingers, are put up in extension by means of a splint applied to the palm of the hand, including the affected fingers. The length of time for which it is worn continuously depends on the views of the surgeon. It is usual nowadays to discontinue day-time splintage as soon as possible (1–2 weeks) in order to avoid stiffening of the hand, and to rely on passive and active movements to maintain the correction; or to substitute rigid splinting with 'lively' splints. A night splint is generally required for some months after the operation.

PHYSICAL TREATMENT.—

MASSAGE.—Again, whether or not this is allowed depends on the views of the surgeon. Some allow the palm to be massaged, as well as the rest of the hand and forearm, as soon as the wound is quite securely healed. Others will not allow massage under any circumstances. Certainly movements constitute the most important form of treatment.

MOVEMENTS.—Stretching movements must be given to the fingers, and active movements practised by the patient, particularly extension. The patient should also be taught to do the passive stretching himself, after soaking the hand in hot water. Wax baths and hot soakings form a useful preliminary treatment.

General hand, finger, and arm exercises should also be given.

In some cases, the correction obtained at the operation is not quite complete, and is continued afterwards by serial splintage.

CONTRACTED FINGERS

This deformity is congenital and hereditary.

DEFORMITY.—The fifth finger is most often affected, or sometimes the fourth and fifth fingers together. The condition gets progressively worse after birth. It is due to contraction of fascia and skin, and exists only in the fingers, not in the palm of the hand as in Dupuytren's contracture. As a rule, the *first phalanx is extended*, the *second flexed*, and the *third extended*. There is no muscular wasting.

Treatment.—

PHYSICAL TREATMENT.—A special splint is used to keep the fingers straight, and they should be manipulated daily, if possible several times a day (*see* notes on manipulation of stiff fingers, p. 123).

SURGICAL TREATMENT.—In more severe or neglected cases, the contracted bands of fascia are divided, the fingers being put up in extension on a small splint.

POST-OPERATIVE TREATMENT.—This consists of *passive* and *active movement*, and *massage* may also be given if the surgeon agrees. The patient should be under supervision for some time, as recurrence of the deformity is common.

For VOLKMANN'S ISCHÆMIC CONTRACTURE, *see* p. 25; for the results of sepsis in the upper extremity, *see* pp. 157, 158; and for deformities due to paralysis of peripheral nerves, *see* Chapter XII.

II. DEFORMITIES OF THE LOWER EXTREMITY

CONGENITAL DISLOCATION OF THE HIP

In this condition one or both of the femoral heads are found to be partially or wholly displaced from the acetabulum at birth.

AETIOLOGY.—

SEX INCIDENCE.—The condition is much commoner in girls than in boys (80 per cent). The reason for this is unknown.

SIDE AFFECTED.—The dislocation may be *unilateral* (generally of the left hip) or *bilateral*; the former being much more common.

HEREDITY appears to be a factor in some cases.

CAUSE.—Congenital dislocation is due to defective pre-natal development of the acetabulum.

PATHOLOGICAL CHANGES.—

BONES.—

1. The *acetabulum is more shallow than normal* and often takes the form of a small triangular depression, the posterior and upper lip being deficient. Even if almost perfect at birth, it fails to develop further, and fills up with fibrous tissue and fat. The head of the femur, by exerting pressure on the ilium, makes

a new acetabulum, though this is rarely deep enough to form a safe socket for the head. Sometimes more than one of these depressions may be seen if the head has moved from one part of the bone to another.

2. The *head of the femur* is generally displaced *backwards* and *upwards* on to the posterior (external) surface of the ilium. Less commonly it is displaced anteriorly, and lies below the anterior superior spine. It becomes more or less deformed, either flattened at the points where it lies against the ilium, or ultimately destroyed by the friction against that bone. The angle of the neck may be decreased (coxa vara) or the neck itself may be twisted. Sometimes the deformity is so serious as to render the replacement of the head in the acetabulum very difficult.

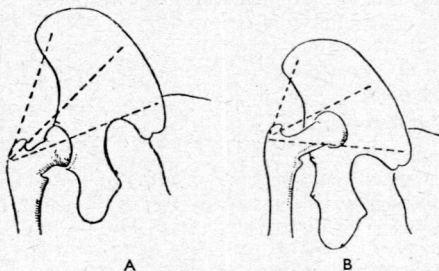

Fig. 126.—Direction of fibres of gluteus medius and minimus. A, Normal; B, In congenital disloca- tion of the hip. The broken lines indicate the direction of the muscle-fibres.

LIGAMENTS.—

1. The *ligamentum teres* is gener- ally rudimentary or missing.

2. The *capsule* is *stretched* by the displacement of the femoral head. The weight of the body falls not, as normally, on the head of the femur, but on the capsule, which becomes hypertrophied, especially antero-inferiorly. This anterior portion is stretched across the acetabulum, finally becoming ad- herent to its rim, leaving only a small opening, which makes reduction difficult. This difficulty may be increased by the position of the psoas tendon (*see below*).

3. The *glenoid labrum* is *partially absent* and the *joint cartilage may also be defective.*

MUSCLES.—These changes are most important. For the purposes of description we may divide them into two groups. (1) *The long muscles, passing from the pelvis to the shaft of the femur, or to the tibia or fibula,* viz., the hamstrings, sartorius, rectus femoris, the adductors, gracilis, and tensor fasciæ femoris. These muscles all become more or less shortened, and offer a good deal of resistance to reduction. (2) *The short muscles, passing from the pelvis to the upper extremity of the femur;* the glutei, obturators, quadratus femoris, and psoas. These muscles are not shortened, but owing to the changed position of the upper part of the femur in relation to the pelvis, they are altered in direction, and therefore, also as regards their function.

The Glutei.—Owing to the higher position of the great trochanter, gluteus medius and minimus, instead of passing *obliquely* downwards and outwards to their insertion, become much more *horizontal* in direction (*Fig.* 126). This puts them at a mechanical disadvantage and makes their pull ineffective, not only as abductors of the hip but also in their most important function of keeping the pelvis level during weight-transference, when one leg is off the ground. It will be remembered that in this position the abductors on the side of the supporting leg act from their insertion on the femur to their origin on the ilium, thus counter- acting the tendency for the pelvis to drop towards the non-weight-bearing leg, Because of the mechanical disadvantage *the patient cannot keep the pelvis straight when standing on the affected side* and it *drops towards the sound side* (*see below*). Gluteus maximus is also displaced and no longer covers the ischial tuberosity, which lies beneath the gluteus medius and minimus only.

The Psoas.—In posterior dislocations the tendon of this muscle is displaced as it crosses the brim of the pelvis, so that it compresses the capsule of the hip-joint, producing an 'hour-glass' shape. It thus stretches from its origin to its insertion like a sling, and the pelvis is supported on it, and on the capsule. This weight drags the muscle downward, away from its origin, so that the lumbar spine is pulled forward and a lordosis is formed. The position of the tendon may also make reduction difficult.

SIGNS AND SYMPTOMS.—These are not usually noticed until the child begins to walk, although its presence can sometimes be detected in infants by a difference in level of the gluteal folds and the creases on the medial aspect of the thigh.

1. *Trendelenburg's Sign.*—As described above, the patient cannot hold the pelvis level when standing on the affected side, because the abductors are at such a disadvantage that they cannot function effectually. This dropping of the pelvis towards the sound side when the patient stands on the affected side constitutes Trendelenburg's sign, and accounts for the peculiar gait.

2. *Gait.*—In unilateral cases there is a very marked *limp*, the patient dropping the pelvis towards the sound side every time the weight is placed on the affected limb. In order to counteract this the trunk is jerked in the opposite direction (i.e., towards the affected side). In bilateral cases the gait is an exaggerated *waddle*, the pelvis being dropped alternately on either side, and the trunk jerked correspondingly from side to side.

3. *Lordosis* occurs in *posterior dislocations*, partly for the reason given above, and partly because the pelvis is tilted forward and the back hollowed to compensate for this. It disappears when the hip is flexed. It is much less marked in the unilateral cases than in the bilateral.

4. *Scoliosis develops in unilateral cases*, the *convexity* of the curve being *towards the sound limb*, because the pelvis is dropped on this side (*see* p. 343).

5. There is *apparent shortening* of the leg (1–1½ in.) because the head of the femur is too high on the hip-bone. This can be demonstrated by placing the child in crook-lying with the feet on the plinth, when the affected knee will be found to be lower than its partner. In small children there is increased mobility of the limb, and the head of the femur can be drawn downwards by traction on the leg.

6. The *great trochanter is above Nélaton's line* (i.e., a line drawn from the anterior superior spine to the tuberosity of the ischium), instead of on the line. Since it protrudes above the upper border of the gluteus maximus it is prominent, though this is more noticeable in adults than in children.

7. In bilateral cases the buttocks are *broad, flat, and somewhat triangular in shape*, owing to the altered position of the gluteus maximus and, as already mentioned, the tuber ischii is no longer covered by this muscle. Also, in bilateral cases, the perineum is wider than normal.

8. Children suffer *no pain* as a rule, but as they grow older there is *fatigue on exertion*, especially in bilateral cases. Spasm of muscles may also cause considerable pain. The symptoms tend to become worse as the patient advances in age.

Treatment.—This is directed towards replacing the femoral head in the acetabulum and maintaining it in position until normal development of the latter occurs. The earlier it is begun the better. Results are not good after six years of age.

SURGICAL TREATMENT.—Reduction may be closed or open: the former is only possible up to the age of six years in unilateral cases (four years in bilateral cases); the latter being used for children over six-years, and on those in whom closed reduction has failed.

CLOSED REDUCTION

1. DIVARICATION.—This is suitable for cases under eighteen months old in which the head is not too high up on the ilium. It consists of gradual abduction of the legs over a period of two or three weeks until they are almost in a straight line. This position is maintained by means of a plaster cast for about nine months,

after which the angle is decreased and the limb fixed in a plaster spica until X-rays reveal development of the acetabulum (9–18 months).

2. THE MANIPULATIVE METHOD: THE LORENZ OPERATION.—This, or some similar manipulation, is suitable for children under 6 years of age in unilateral cases, or under 4 years in bilateral cases. Generally speaking, the younger the child, the better is the chance of a successful result. After the age of 4 years, it is much more difficult to reduce the dislocation. The child is anæsthetized, and the shortened muscles are stretched. The adductors sometimes require a tenotomy. The surgeon then flexes the hip, thus bringing the head of the femur down behind the acetabulum; he then carries the leg backwards into a position of abduction to a right angle, sometimes even carrying it behind the plane of the body, and thus forcing the head over the back part of the rim of the acetabulum.

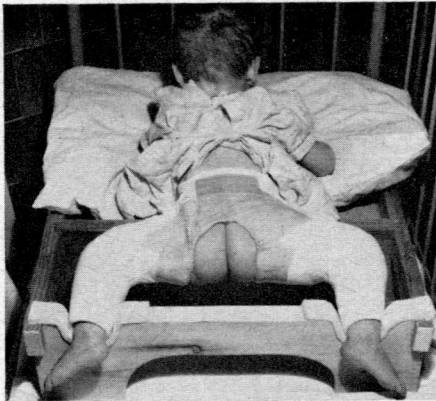

Fig. 127.—Child with congenital dislocation of right hip, in plaster fixation in 'frog position', being nursed on a frame. Note the increased angle of right leg compared with left.

Fixation.—Reduction is maintained by means of a plaster spica or cast as above, the leg being held in abduction to 90°, outward rotation, and sometimes slight hyperextension (*Fig.* 127). In bilateral cases both hips are reduced at the same time. The 'frog' position is most usually adopted nowadays, the child lying in a frame to facilitate nursing. The knee may or may not be included in the bandage. The period of fixation lasts until X-rays reveal definite signs of acetabular development. Broadly speaking, it lasts from six to eighteen months. It is usual to change the plaster every three months. Some surgeons bring the limb down a little more from the abducted position each time a new bandage is applied. Others keep it in the fully abducted position during the whole period of fixation. Sometimes a plaster is applied which allows of limited movement in the hip while preventing any possibility of adduction. In unilateral cases, the child is generally encouraged to try to walk with the plaster still on, as the pressure and friction thus caused are thought to help deepen the acetabulum. The heel has to be raised on the affected side. Even in bilateral cases the child can sometimes get about with the help of sticks.

3. THE OPEN OPERATION.—This is carried out in the case of patients too old for manipulative reduction, or in cases where the latter has been tried and has failed. The acetabulum is deepened, and the head of the femur replaced; or other operations designed to stabilize the head are performed. (For Gill's 'shelf operation', *see* Walter Mercer, *Orthopædic Surgery*, p. 36. A flap of the outer layer of the ilium above the acetabulum is turned down to make a better upper rim for the latter. Weight-bearing is generally allowed after 3 months.)

PHYSICAL TREATMENT.—

AFTER THE MANIPULATIVE OPERATION

1. DURING THE PERIOD OF FIXATION.—The lower leg may be massaged

and movements should be given to the foot and ankle, and to the knee if it has been left free.

2. AFTER FIXATION.—As has been said, some surgeons bring the limb down gradually from the abducted position by a series of plaster bandages, while others maintain full abduction throughout the fixation period. In the case of full abduction being maintained throughout the fixation period, the child's limb will be more or less fixed in this position.

Massage.—This is advisable in the early stage to improve circulation and to ease tension. Gentle *heat* may also be given before, or during, massage. The child may be placed in the lying position and the lower limbs vigorously massaged. She should then be turned over into the prone position and the posterior muscles treated, special attention being paid to the glutei. The back may also receive a dose of effleurage and kneading.

Exercises.—If the limbs are able to be brought side by side, or almost so, *active* exercises will be needed for strengthening purposes, and correct walking must be taught.

Even if the limb, or limbs, are more or less fixed in the abducted position, it is, as a rule, better to avoid *forced* movement, and trust to *free* active movements to bring the leg gradually to the normal position. Passive stretching of the hamstrings may be carefully given if the knee cannot be fully extended. If an attempt *is* made to mobilize the hip passively, great care is necessary, since too forcible adduction might redislocate the joint, even after months of fixation. Gentle hip-rolling is the best movement to give, the pelvis being fixed so that the movement takes place in the hip-joint, not in the joints of the spine.

In older children, the contracted tissues may have to be stretched under an anæsthetic, after which passive, as well as active movements must be given to preserve the mobility obtained.

Active Movements.—*Abduction* is, of course, the principal movement to be practised. For some time after the end of the fixation period the patient should be able to reproduce the position in which the limbs were put up, and should rest and sleep in this position. Abduction should at first be done in the lying position; afterwards—in unilateral cases—it may be tried in side-lying; later still, in standing, the patient abducting the affected hip. Resisted movements and free exercises should both be given. Later, as a preparation for walking, the patient should stand on the affected hip and first flex, and later abduct, the sound leg slightly, keeping the pelvis level in the meantime.

Extension of the hips should also be practised in the forward-lying position, and should again be resisted and free.

Adduction, and with it *internal rotation*, should be given very carefully, and are best confined to free movements.

Exercises for the abdominal and back muscles are also necessary, since lordosis is a feature of all cases, especially the bilateral type, and scoliosis is a complication of the unilateral.

Re-education in Walking.—This is undertaken as soon as permitted by the surgeon. The patient will have to be taught not to drop the pelvis on the sound side in unilateral cases, or on each side in the bilateral; that is, the limp or the waddle has to be eliminated. This is often no easy task. The patient walks at first with the feet wide apart, and this must be gradually corrected. The spine must be carefully watched for signs of scoliosis.

AFTER THE OPEN OPERATION

Treatment is on similar lines but the surgeon will decide when it is to begin. The plaster is generally retained for 6–9 months.

COXA VARA

This is a deformity consisting of a decrease of the normal angle between the neck and shaft of the femur.

AETIOLOGY.—

SEX INCIDENCE.—Males are more often affected than females.

AGE INCIDENCE.—Coxa vara appears most commonly in early adolescence, because at this time of life the still growing bone is subjected to increased strain, the patient leaving school and going to work. It may, however, be congenital, or occur in infants or in adults.

SIDE AFFECTED.—It is more often unilateral than bilateral.

CAUSES.—

Congenital Form.—The cause of this deformity is unknown. It is sometimes associated with congenital dislocation of the hip.

Acquired Form.—

1. *The adolescent* (*static*) *form* is due to the weight of the body—increased by the carrying of heavy objects—falling on bone that is not sufficiently hardened to bear it.

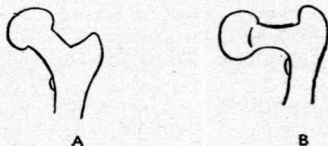

Fig. 128.—Showing deformity of neck in coxa vara. A, Normal angle of head with shaft—about 130°; B, Angle in coxa vara—about 90°.

This leads to sudden, or more often gradual, slipping of the upper femoral epiphysis. If no treatment is given the epiphysis reunites in an abnormal position.

2. *Other causes are:* (*a*) *Injury*; fractures of the femoral neck. (*b*) *Bone disease*, e.g., osteomyelitis; osteochondritis; rickets. (*c*) *Joint disease*; e.g., arthritis; tuberculosis of the hip.

PATHOLOGICAL CHANGES.—

BONES.—

1. *The neck of the femur*, which normally forms an angle of about 130° with the shaft, is *depressed* so as to form a much smaller angle, e.g., 90° (right angle) or less (*Fig. 128*).

2. The neck, besides being depressed, may also be *distorted*; it is most commonly bent backwards, that is, it forms a curve with the convexity forward.

3. *The head is often deformed*, and its lower part is subluxated—no longer contacting the acetabulum.

MUSCLES.—Because of the downward bending of the neck, the great trochanter is correspondingly raised. The same kind of changes are found in the position of the glutei as in congenital dislocation (*see above*), but not as a rule to such a great extent. The *abductors*, however, are always weak and tend to atrophy, while the *adductors* become shortened.

SYMPTOMS.—Many symptoms are similar to those found in congenital dislocation.

1. *Limitation of Movement, and Position of Leg.*—

a. In the commoner form, where the neck is depressed and has a forward convexity.

i. *Abduction* is extremely limited. Not only do the muscles and ligaments limit movement through adaptive shortening, but owing to the lowering of the head of the femur and the depression of the neck, the latter comes into contact with the upper part of the acetabular rim as soon as abduction begins. *Adduction* is increased, and the leg is held in an adducted position.

ii. *Flexion* is limited, and *extension* slightly increased because of the forward convexity of the neck.

iii. *Internal rotation* is increased and *external rotation* limited, for the same reason.

iv. The patient stands with the leg *adducted*, the hip *externally rotated*, and the foot *everted*; the pelvis is tilted *down* on the affected side.

b. In the less common form where the neck is simply depressed, but not otherwise bent, abduction is even more limited than in the case where there is a forward convexity, but there is little loss of flexion, and the rotary movements are normal.

2. *Gait.*—In *unilateral cases* there is a pronounced limp, since the abductors work at a disadvantage, as in congenital dislocation (*see above*). In *bilateral cases* there is a waddling gait, very clumsy and ungraceful, the patient sometimes even crossing his knees as he walks, owing to the exaggerated adduction in the hip-joint.

3. As in congenital dislocation *the great trochanter is above Nélaton's line*, and is prominent. This is due partly to its elevated position, and partly to the atrophy of the muscles covering it.

4. The leg is *shortened*, because of the decrease of the angle of neck and shaft. This is *true shortening*.

5. *Trendelenburg's sign* is occasionally present.

6. *Pain, weakness*, and *stiffness* are felt in the affected hip in the early stages. In some cases the patient may complain of pain in the knee. The pain may become very severe later.

7. *Complications.*—Lordosis is present in some, but not all, of the bilateral cases, and scoliosis in the unilateral, the lumbar curve being *towards the affected side*. Compensatory knock-knee and flat-foot may also be present.

Treatment.—This is directed towards relieving the strain on the epiphysis in slight cases, or towards gaining reduction in more severe cases.

SURGICAL TREATMENT.—If the onset of the disease is detected at an early stage the patient will be ordered to rest in bed for a time, in order to relieve the strain on the epiphysis. If there is definite slipping of the epiphysis traction is applied in abduction, in order to obtain reduction. It is maintained for about four to six weeks. Following bed-rest or traction, the patient is fitted with a weight-relieving caliper or plaster, which may be retained from twelve to eighteen months. Some surgeons pin the epiphysis following reduction, but this is not always successful, since it is difficult to maintain. In some cases no external fixation is required and movements can begin at once. Later, it may be advisable for the patient to change his occupation, at least temporarily, *if* it is a laborious one.

PHYSICAL TREATMENT.—

1. EARLY ADOLESCENT CASES (EPIPHYSEAL COXA VARA, i.e., cases due to slipped epiphysis).—Physical treatment will be similar to any case involving prolonged bed-rest, or traction for the lower extremity. *Heat* and *massage* may be given, particularly if there is much pain or spasm, but the most important form of treatment consists of movement.

Passive and active movements can begin as soon as the surgeon allows. Suspension apparatus is often very helpful.

Abduction must be practised, but *no active adduction should be allowed*. Abduction may be given both as a resisted and a free movement, but the physiotherapist should passively carry the limb back to the midline of the body. *Internal rotation* and *flexion* must be practised in the same way, if they are limited. Foot and knee exercises should also be included in the treatment.

The exercises are best performed in *lying or half-lying*. If the side-lying position is assumed for hip flexion, care must be taken to prevent the hip falling into adduction. Even in half-lying the patient is liable to adduct the thigh during flexion of the hip, and this must be prevented. Side-lying must not be used for cases with bilateral deformity. All these difficulties can, however, be obviated by the use of suspension apparatus.

2. Cases where there is Definite Softening or Yielding of Bone, as in Bone Diseases such as Rickets.—

Support.—The leg is put up in plaster in *full normal abduction*. This corrects the deformity, because, while the head of the femur is held in position by the lower part of the capsule, the upper border of the acetabulum presses on the neck, straightening it out and increasing the angle between neck and shaft.

3. Cases where the Bone has Hardened in the Deformed Position, e.g., cases due to old injury, etc.—

Surgical Treatment.—These cases are generally treated by *osteotomy*, a wedge being cut from the outer side of the upper extremity of the femur, opposite the lesser trochanter, and the opening closed. After this, or any similar operation, the limb is fixed in an *abduction plaster* or in some special splint for about 8 weeks. The limb is then brought down parallel to the other, and following another period of from 4 to 8 weeks, during which a short plaster spica or caliper is worn, the patient is allowed to walk without support.

Post-operative Physical Treatment.—This is on the same lines as that for any patient immobilized in plaster. More active treatment, on the same lines as that described for congenital dislocation of the hip, can commence as soon as the plaster is removed.

Later Treatment of All Cases.—

Re-education in walking.—As in congenital dislocation of the hip, the patient must be taught how to keep the pelvis level, so as to eliminate the limp or waddle. The physiotherapist must pay careful attention to the position of the feet, an everted position being common, and leading ultimately to 'weak' or 'flat' foot. Foot-drill (*see* pp. 313–16) should therefore be given.

General Leg Exercises should also be practised, but the patient should not do many exercises in standing at first.

Balance Exercises and Free Exercises of all kinds should finally be given to improve posture.

COMPLICATIONS such as knock-knee, flat-foot, scoliosis, or lordosis must, of course, be treated.

GENU VALGUM

(*Knock-knee*)

This is not a congenital deformity, but one which usually develops a few months after the child begins to walk.

AETIOLOGY.—The principal causes of knock-knee are: (1) *Rickets* in infancy; thus it is much less common in these days than formerly, rickets itself being less prevalent; (2) *More rapid growth of the internal than the external femoral condyles.* This occurs in some children, causing the line of the knee-joint to slope slightly outwards, instead of being horizontal;* this form of knock-knee is very common in children, but tends to right itself spontaneously, as the growth of the external condyles catches up with that of the internal. (3) *Muscular and ligamentous weakness* in adolescents (static form), at a time of life when increased work is required of them.

Other causes are fractures or injuries in the region of the joint, or operations for genu varum; paralysis (generally infantile paralysis) of the semimembranosus and semitendinosus, or of the quadriceps; or disease of the joint itself. Genu valgum may be secondary to coxa vara, flat-foot, or spinal curvatures.

PATHOLOGICAL CHANGES.—There are two degrees of this deformity: (1) Those in which there are *muscular and ligamentous changes only*; e.g., adolescent

---

* Philip Wiles, *Essentials of Orthopædics*, p. 27.

(static) cases in their early stages; (2) Those in which there are *bony changes* also, e.g., in old rachitic, or neglected static cases.

The bony changes are most marked in the rickety form of knock-knee, and are therefore most noticeable at the epiphyses, which are enlarged.

BONY CHANGES.—

1. *The medial condyle of the femur is hypertrophied and lengthened.* Even in a normal knee, the greater weight falls through the lateral condyle. In a patient with genu valgum, the pressure on the outer side is intensified, while hardly any falls on the inner side.

2. The shafts of the femur or tibia may be curved, particularly in cases of rachitic origin. The lower third of the femur may be convex inwards; the tibia may be curved with the convexity inwards, outwards (bow-legs), or forwards; or there may even be a double curve in this bone.

LIGAMENTOUS and MUSCULAR CHANGES.—

1. There is *shortening* of the *lateral ligament* and *stretching* of the *medial ligament*.

2. The semimembranosus, semitendinosus, sartorius, and vastus medialis become elongated.

3. The tendon of biceps femoris and the iliotibial band of fascia become contracted.

As a result of this relaxation of important ligaments and muscles, the stability of the joint is affected and the following changes also occur:—

1. There is *increased mobility* at the knee-joint. Rotation of the knee, normally possible only in semiflexion, can now take place to some extent when the knee is extended. Sometimes the knee is hyperextended.

2. The *patella* may be displaced outwards, or even dislocated.

3. The *tibia is rotated outwards* on the femur by the contracted biceps tendon. The femur may be rotated inwards.

If the condition is complicated by flat-foot, the latter is often peculiar in that the front part of the foot is twisted inward.

SIGNS AND SYMPTOMS.—

1. If the patient's knees are placed together, there is a space between the feet, varying from two to twenty inches. If the feet are placed together, the knees become crossed.

2. The angle between the thigh and ankle is decreased.

3. The deformity is more marked when the patient stands, because the body-weight, falling on the weak muscles and ligaments, leads to further yielding. It disappears when the knee is flexed, although it is not very clear how this happens.*

4. The *gait* is clumsy and uncertain because of the weakness of the ligaments and instability of the joints, also because the knees tend to cross. A small child generally turns the toes in, and later a peculiar form of flat-foot supervenes.

Complication.—Besides flat-foot, the patient may develop scoliosis if the deformity is unilateral, or worse on one side than on the other.

Treatment.—The patients may be divided into two classes: (1) The first class comprises all children under four years of age, the adolescent cases, and any others in whom bony change is absent or negligible. (2) The second contains *old* rickety cases, in which the bones have hardened and in which bony deformity is considerable; also *neglected* 'static' cases in which bony change has ultimately developed.

---

* Sir Robert Jones points out that in knock-knee due to rickets, the deformity disappears in flexion because only the lower ends of the femoral condyles are distorted, and not their posterior surfaces (*Orthopædic Surgery*, Chapter XV).

GENERAL TREATMENT.—

CLASS 1

Adolescents, and children who are weak but not rachitic, require rest, and appropriate medical treatment will be administered.

If the cause is *rickets,* and the bones are still soft, the condition itself must be treated (*see* p. 445). From the point of view of the specific deformity, rest is essential. The child must be kept off his feet and prevented from walking.

SUPPORTS.—These are required in all but very slight cases.* They usually take the form of calipers applied to the *outer* side of the leg so that the convexity of the curve, which is maximal at the knee-joint, is gradually drawn towards the support.

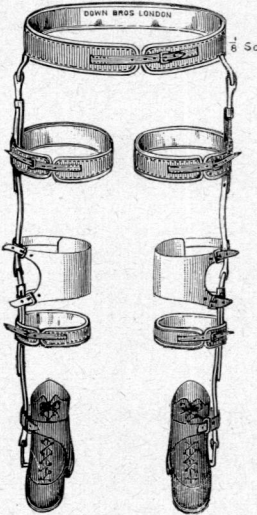

Fig. 129.—Support for genu valgum.

The caliper consists of a band round the pelvis, from which a metal rod passes down the outer side of the leg to the foot, where it is secured to the sole of the boot.

The support is fastened to the leg by straps or metal bands (*Fig.* 129). The knee is kept in extension, but the ankle is free to move. The supports prescribed by different surgeons vary in their details, but they are all on the same principle. Sometimes a long lateral splint is worn at night, the knee being drawn towards it by a bandage. The splints may have to be worn for about 2 years.

CLASS 2

Operative treatment is required for these cases, the structural changes being too far advanced to benefit from any other form of treatment.

PHYSICAL TREATMENT.—

CLASS 1

Cases in Class 1, corresponding to *first degree* deformities, are treated on the same lines as other similar conditions, but physiotherapy alone is not very effective.

Position of Patient.—The most suitable position is half-lying, with the knees in extension.

MASSAGE.—*The whole limb* may be treated with stimulating massage in order to improve the circulation and soften the structures on the outer side of the thigh. *Stretching techniques* should be given to the iliotibial band, to the biceps and its tendon, and to the lateral ligament of the knee-joint, *but care must be taken not to stretch structures on the medial aspect.*

PASSIVE MOVEMENTS.—These take the form of *passive pressure* which is given with one hand on the inner side of the knee and one on the outer side of the leg just below the knee, or, alternatively, on the outer side of the ankle. The latter grasp gives the better leverage, but must not be used if the knock-knee is complicated by bow-leg, or if the bones are soft.

---

* Philip Wiles considers that treatment by splints or operation is desirable when the deformity has produced a distance of 3 inches between the malleoli by the age of 3 years, and continues to progress during the next year. He thinks operation preferable to prolonged splinting in most cases, because the latter interferes gravely with the child's activity, and may cause him to acquire the cripple's mentality (*Essentials o f Orthopædics,* p. 29).

In *bilateral cases,* with the same exceptions, the ankles may be tied or strapped together, a firm pad or sand-bag being placed between the knees. The patient may then be left in that position for ten minutes or so. The physiotherapist must be careful to see that the straps are comfortable and not over-tight. This form of stretching is not suitable for little children, unless someone can remain to amuse them.

ACTIVE MOVEMENTS.—Knock-knee is a difficult problem to tackle, differing from most deformities in that the position of the knee is not that of an exaggeration of one of its normal movements. It cannot, therefore, be corrected by use of the muscles which perform the opposite action. Outward movement (*abduction*) does not exist in the normal knee, and there are, therefore, no muscles which directly produce inward movement (*adduction*). However, *the stability of the knee,* and therefore the maintenance of its correct position, *depends on the surrounding muscles,* and we must do all we can to strengthen these muscles, particularly those which are stretched—the vastus medialis, gracilis, sartorius, and semitendinosus.

Since the trouble arises from laxity of ligaments, and since flexion further relaxes them, it is obvious that the proper position in which to give exercises is one of *full extension.*

This, of course, limits the choice of exercises to a great extent. We want to strengthen all the muscles of the thigh, but *we must be careful not to produce greater contracture of biceps and the iliotibial band.*

The following are suitable:—

1. *Half-lying, Leg-adduction and -outdrawing.*—This should shorten the gracilis, and relax the tensor fascia femoris. *Leg-abduction and in-pressing, with outward pressure on the knee and inward pressure on ankle* is a much-used exercise. It simply works the abductors of the hip, the knee being held meanwhile in the corrected position. An objection to it is that the use of the tensor fascia femoris must surely lead to further shortening of the iliotibial band, and, provided the physiotherapist presses firmly inward on the ankle (or higher on the tibia) all the time, and resists the movement with the hand on the inner side of the knee, the former seems a better exercise.

2. *Quadriceps contractions.* These are easily taught, even to small children. It is important to get inner range contraction in vastus medialis.

3. *Half-lying external rotation of the hip, with the knee firmly supported.* It should be done concentrically and eccentrically. This counteracts the medial rotation of the femur and uses the sartorius, but *external rotation must not be allowed to take place in the knee.*

When the patient is allowed to walk without support, general leg exercises should be employed. *Treatment for flat-foot* must be given if necessary. To begin with, a knock-kneed child must be allowed to walk with his feet apart, and should not be required to stand or walk with the feet together. If and when the deformity is cured, re-education in correct walking will be necessary.

CLASS 2

As has been said, these cases cannot be cured by support and manipulations alone. They represent second- and third-degree cases and surgical treatment is necessary.

OPERATIONS.—The operation performed is either (1) osteotomy or (2) osteoclasis.

OSTEOTOMY.—This is the more usual operation. It generally consists of cutting a wedge from the inner side of the femur above the knee-joint, and bringing the cut surfaces together, although some surgeons prefer to take the wedge from the inner side of the upper end of the tibia (*Fig.* 130).

OSTEOCLASIS.—This consists of fracture of the lower end of the femur, or slight displacement of its lower epiphysis. It is rarely performed now.

FIXATION.—The leg is either splinted, or put in plaster for 6 to 8 weeks, after which the patient is allowed to get about on crutches.

POST-OPERATIVE TREATMENT.—During immobilization, treatment will be similar to that given for fractures immobilized in plaster.

When the leg is out of plaster the knee can be gently mobilized. Active flexion and extension of the knee should be given, together with exercises for the hip and foot. Strong passive (lateral) pressures are no longer necessary. They would, in fact, be dangerous, since they might produce the opposite deformity (genu varum) by over-correction.

When the patient is allowed to walk, he must be taught to do so correctly.

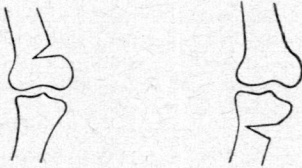

Fig. 130.—Showing two forms of osteotomy for genu valgum.

GENU VARUM (BANDY-LEGS) AND BOW-LEGS

These are conditions in which a line drawn from the head of the femur to the middle of the ankle-joint falls inside the centre of the knee-joint (MacEwen). Genu varum, or 'bandy-legs', is a deformity of the whole limb, 'bow-legs' of the lower leg only, although the term *genu varum* is often applied indiscriminately to either.

AETIOLOGY.—Genu varum is a more common deformity than knock-knee; it starts in childhood and is generally bilateral. Formerly the chief cause was rickets, but the deformities are still found in small children who are not rickety, but who have been allowed to walk too soon, the body-weight being too much for the bones which are still soft. This is specially the case in fat, heavy children. Sitting cross-legged on the floor may also be a factor.

PATHOLOGICAL CHANGES AND PHYSICAL SIGNS.—In both these deformities there is always some measure of bony change.

GENU VARUM.—

Bones.—The shafts of the *femur*, *tibia*, and *fibula* are all *curved outward*, the maximum convexity of the curve being at the knee. When the patient stands with his feet together the knees are widely separated.

Muscles and Ligaments.—The ligaments on the *outer side of the knee are lengthened*, and those on the *inner side shortened*. The muscles on the *outer side of the thigh* and leg—biceps femoris and the peronei— *are stretched; the adductors are shortened*.

Postural Defect.—There is internal rotation at the hip-joint, and hyperextension at the knee.

BOW-LEGS.—Only the shafts of the tibia and fibula are bent, with the convexity outwards, the peronei alone being stretched. The lower end of the tibia is usually rotated inwards on the long axis of the femur, since the tibia "is a flexible three-cornered rod, and cannot on that account be bent laterally without rotating" (Mercer). The patient, therefore, turns his toes in. Forward bending of the tibia is also found, with shortening of the tendo Achillis.

GAIT.—This consists of a waddle, not unlike that of bilateral congenital dislocation of the hip.

PROGNOSIS.—The condition tends to spontaneous improvement, the growing bone filling up the concavities, but complete cure does not always take place and the patient loses in height.

Treatment.—It is unusual in these days to treat these conditions unless the deformity is obviously increasing. Treatment of the postural defect in mild cases can considerably lessen the appearance of deformity, and to this end a course of exercises may be prescribed. *Physical treatment* will follow the same lines as that for *genu valgum*, but the treatment will be in reverse. The most important exercises are gluteal contractions and external rotation of the hip, to counteract the internal rotation of the femur which tends to enhance the deformity. These exercises also reduce hyperextension at the knee to a certain extent. The table should include general leg exercises and re-education in walking, particularly if the patient turns his toes in.

Should a case be due to rickets the patient will require general treatment (*see* Chapter XX) and may in addition be treated by supports, massage and exercises. The support for *genu varum* is the reverse of that used for knock-knee—the steel rod being on the *inner* side of the leg, and the convexity of the curve being drawn inwards towards the support. (For *bow-legs*, the support extends only from the internal condyle of the femur to the internal malleolus.) The supports may well have to be worn for 6 or 8 months in young children. Unless the rickets is still active the child is usually allowed to remain active.

SEVERE CASES

These include cases in which the deformity is increasing and those of rickets. They are treated by operation.

SURGICAL TREATMENT.—This again consists of osteotomy or osteoclasis.

OSTEOTOMY.—A wide wedge is cut from the outer side of the femur above the exterior condyle, or from the maximum convexity of the curve of the tibia. Sometimes both bones are so treated.

OSTEOCLASIS.—The bone is broken at the point of greatest curvature, and set in an over-corrected position.

For an *anterior* curve of the tibia, the tendo Achillis is divided in addition to osteotomy or osteoclasis.

POST-OPERATIVE TREATMENT.—This follows the same principles as that of genu valgum. Re-education in walking is very important in the later stages. The patient needs careful watching for some time. A relapse is possible, and occasionally the opposite deformity (genu valgum) may result from over-correction, insufficient support, or inadequate after-treatment.

FLAT-FOOT AND WEAK FOOT

Under this heading may be grouped many different varieties of foot troubles. 'Flat-foot' is generally defined as a *collapse of the internal longitudinal* and *transverse arches of the foot*, combined with *eversion*. There are, however, many kinds of 'weak foot' (a better name for the condition) of which the following are the most common: (1) *Pes planus*, or flat-foot pure and simple, consisting of dropping of the arch without eversion of the foot. (2) *Pes valgus*, the everted foot, without dropping of the arch. (3) *Pes plano-valgus*, the everted foot, with collapsed arches.

A *flat* foot may cause little or no inconvenience, provided that it is mobile; an everted foot is always productive of trouble.

Anatomy and Functions of Foot

THE ARCHES OF THE FOOT

These may be classified as follows: (1) *The longitudinal arch*—(*a*) Internal; (*b*) External. (2) *The transverse arch*—(*a*) Posterior; (*b*) Anterior.

1. THE LONGITUDINAL ARCHES.—

The Internal Longitudinal Arch is composed of the os calcis, talus, and navicular, the three cuneiforms, and the three inner metatarsal bones. It is supported by muscles and ligaments, the most important of which are the inferior calcaneonavicular (or 'spring') ligament, which passes like a sling below the talus; the plantar fascia, the interossei, and intrinsic muscles of the foot; the tendon of tibialis anticus, inserted beneath the inner border of the foot; that of tibialis posticus, which keeps the navicular in close contact with the head of the talus; and that of flexor digitorum longus. The latter, passing along almost the whole length of the sole and pulling on the toes (provided that they are not 'clawed' but held firmly in extension by the intrinsics when weight is taken on the foot), supports the whole of the longitudinal arch, especially at its two weakest points, viz., behind and in front of the cuneiform bones.

The inner arch is much higher than the outer, and on its maintenance depends the existence of the 'spring' in walking. It will be noticed that the posterior pillar of the arch, the os calcis, being fitted for weight-bearing passes straight down to its point of contact with the ground, i.e., the centre of the heel. The anterior pillar, however, slopes gradually, and being formed of several separate bones connected by ligaments, provides the elasticity which breaks the jar when the foot comes in contact with the ground, and gives the spring to the gait.

The External Longitudinal Arch is made up of the os calcis, the cuboid, and the two outer metatarsals. It rests on the ground, and is much stronger and less mobile than the inner arch. It has, moreover, strong ligamentous and muscular supports—the long and short plantar ligaments, the tendon of the peroneus longus, the plantar fascia, and the small muscles of the foot.

2. THE TRANSVERSE ARCHES.—

The Posterior Arch consists of the talus, cuboid, navicular, and the cuneiform bones, its summit being the second cuneiform. It is supported by the tendons of peroneus longus and tibialis posticus, the plantar fascia, and the intrinsic muscles of the foot.

The Anterior Arch consists of the five metatarsal bones, the third and fourth forming its highest part. This is the most mobile part of the transverse arch. It is flattened out when weight is taken on the front of the foot, and is very liable to collapse permanently, causing the front of the foot to spread. Many people, whose longitudinal arches are quite good, have collapsed anterior arches. This arch is normally maintained by the small muscles of the sole, especially the interossei and the transverse fibres of adductor hallucis.

MAINTENANCE OF THE ARCHES

The real supports of the arches are the *muscles*. The ligaments alone would soon give way under the strain imposed by the weight of the body—as indeed they do, if the muscles, from weakness or disease, fail in their work. "It is not the function of ligaments to withstand continuous strain; this is a function of muscles" (Bankart).

The weight of the body tends to produce *abduction and eversion of the foot*. It is the function of the muscles to counteract this tendency, since *eversion is the position of weakness*, the whole weight of the body being thrown on to the internal longitudinal arch, which is not fitted to sustain it. *The position of strength* for the foot is that of *adduction and inversion*, the weight falling on the outer arch, so that it is distributed to those parts of the foot which are meant to bear it, that is, to the os calcis, the outer border, and the heads of the five metatarsal bones.

It will be remembered, of course, that the movements of abduction and adduction, together with those of inversion and eversion, take place at the sub-taloid and mid-tarsal joints. The only movements in the ankle-joint are plantar- and dorsiflexion, though occasionally a very small amount of lateral movement occurs when the foot is in full plantar-flexion. A certain degree of plantar- and dorsiflexion also takes place in the mid-tarsal joint, at the end of the corresponding movements in the ankle.

FUNCTIONS OF THE FOOT

The foot is used in two ways: (1) As a *support* in standing; (2) As a *lever* in walking.

1. AS A SUPPORT.—Many people feel that the '*position of rest*' of the foot—that is, the position maintained while standing, as distinguished from that assumed when walking—should be one of slight abduction and eversion. We do undoubtedly tend to keep our feet slightly abducted and everted when 'standing at ease'. If, however, this position is allowed to persist, not only when at rest, but during activity, the result will be a *permanently* everted foot, with limitation of the power of inversion. Equally, if this position is habitually *exaggerated* while standing, whether from fatigue, weakness of muscles, excessive body-weight, or a defective postural reflex, the same unfortunate results follow. The danger in this 'position of rest' is that, while *normal muscle tone* would prevent overmuch eversion of the foot, the ligaments would be put on the stretch if the muscles fail to perform this function efficiently. The foot would then fall into a position of *extreme* eversion and abduction. For this reason many authorities now say that, in all cases, the 'resting position' should be one of *slight adduction and inversion*.

2. AS A LEVER IN WALKING.—In walking, the foot is used as a second-order lever to raise and propel the body forward. When taking a step, the heel of the back foot is raised from the ground, and the weight of the body transferred to the front leg. The final 'push off' is given by all the toes, but especially by the big toe. The *fulcrum* of the lever is considered to be at the heads of the metatarsal bones, the *power* (the calf muscles) being applied at the point of attachment of the tendo Achillis to the os calcis. The *weight of the body* falls in front of the ankle-joint, between the fulcrum and power, so that the lever is one of the second order. This is the one sometimes known as the 'power lever', because of the great mechanical advantage it gives to the working force, since the power arm must always be longer than the weight arm.

Since the inner side of the lever (i.e., the first metatarsal) is longer than the outer when walking correctly, the strain is thrown outward on to the stronger side of the foot, relieving the weak inner border (*Fig.* 131).

CORRECT WALKING

When the foot is put down on the ground after the leg has been swung forward, it first rests on the heel, then the front part of the foot is put down firmly. As the weight falls on the foot, the arches, especially the internal longitudinal and anterior transverse arches, are flattened to some extent, and there is a tendency to eversion. Normally the arch is re-formed and the everted position corrected by the muscles and by the elasticity of the ligaments, as soon as the weight of the body is removed. If people habitually walk with their feet everted, restoration of the arches and the inverted position eventually becomes impossible, because, in time, the muscles weaken and the ligaments stretch. *Such people must be taught to walk with the feet pointing straight forward, and the toes pressed firmly on the ground* as described above, to prevent undue spreading of the anterior arch. (*See also* RE-EDUCATION IN WALKING, p. 49). The tendency to eversion of the foot, when the weight falls, may be counteracted by a slight movement of inversion, which transfers the strain to the outer border.

ERRORS IN WALKING

1. If the feet are *everted* while walking, the strain is thrown onto the weaker, inner side of the foot, and the arch is thus depressed. The big toe is also forced

into abduction, since the patient 'pushes off' with the inner side of the under-surface of this toe instead of with the under-surfaces of all five toes. The advantages of the leverage are, thus, lost. In such cases hallux valgus may complicate flat-foot, the two conditions forming a 'vicious circle', each making the other worse.

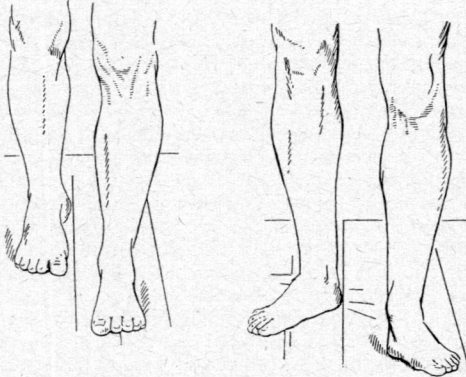

Fig. 131.—Proper (left) and improper (right) attitudes in walking. (*After Whitman.*)

2. Another error is that in which the ankle is either not extended at all, or only very slightly, and the foot is not used as a lever at all. The person walks in a stiff and ungraceful manner, coming down heavily on his heels—as if, in fact, his feet were in splints. Patients with weak or flat feet often combine these two incorrect methods of walking.

3. The toes may be held flexed, i.e., 'clawed', when extending the ankle (*see below*).

FUNCTIONS OF THE TOES IN WALKING

ACTION OF THE FLEXOR LONGUS DIGITORUM.—The late Mr. Lambrinudi,* of Guy's Hospital, pointed out that the function of this muscle had not been fully understood. It had been regarded purely as a flexor of the toes; but at no time during the act of walking—at least on smooth ground—are the toes *flexed*. He showed how the muscle, when it contracts, acts as a support for the metatarsal heads. Passing beneath them like a sling, it distributes the weight of the body, which would otherwise fall on these alone, to the whole of the toes as well. By so doing it also enlarges the area of the fulcrum of the lever which has been described above. This can only take place, however, if the interphalangeal joints are held in extension by the lumbricales and interossei; hence the necessity for healthy intrinsic muscles, and correct co-ordination among them. If through some failure of this mechanism the toes do not remain flat on the ground but are 'clawed', the metatarsal heads alone take the weight. This explains the connexion between 'claw-toes' and metatarsalgia. For this reason, exercises for the intrinsic muscles are essential in all cases of weak foot or lowered arches.

PES PLANO-VALGUS
(*The Flat and Everted Foot*)

Such a case may be regarded as a typical case of flat-foot. The condition is usually bilateral.

* *Guy's Hospital Gazette.*

AETIOLOGY.—

AGE.—A form of flat-foot, with very low or dropped arches, but no eversion, is common, and may be seen in both children and adults. It is generally painless, and causes little or no trouble. The *painful* everted foot is commonest (1) during adolescence, when increased strain is put on the feet, and (2) after the age of 30 or 35, when the muscles grow weaker.

SEX.—Flat-foot is commoner in women than in men.

CAUSES.—The causes of this very common type of deformity are many and varied. It may be due to *special causes*, such as: (1) *Paralysis* or *paresis* of any of the muscles which invert the foot or support the arches. In this connexion it should be mentioned that a very common cause is slight spasm, or shortening, of the tendon of tibialis anticus. This holds the inner border of the foot in slight dorsiflexion and inversion, so that the big toe does not rest on the ground unless the foot is slightly everted. (2) *Traumas*, including any injury to the lower extremity, but especially Pott's fracture. (3) *Other deformities*; it may be compensatory to genu valgum or varum, or hallux valgus. (4) *Arthritis*. (5) *Œdema*. (6) *Rickets*.

General ill health, anæmia, debility, etc., may predispose to the *static* type but the actual causes are:—

a. *Unsuitable foot-wear.*

b. *Habitual bad posture*, either in walking, or, worse still, in standing, the foot being allowed to remain for long periods in extreme eversion. This is due to a defect of the postural reflex (*see* p. 341), unless there is definite muscle-weakness, which constitutes a special cause.

In some cases there may be a definite *exciting cause*—an increase of the body-weight, due to obesity or pregnancy, overstrain, the habitual carrying of heavy weights, or much standing. The last-mentioned accounts for its prevalence in nurses, policemen, waitresses, and shop assistants.

PATHOLOGICAL CHANGES.—Muscular changes occur first, as stated above; next come ligamentous changes, leading to displacement of bones, and lastly actual bony changes. The latter are not marked in the average case, however.

MUSCULAR AND LIGAMENTOUS CHANGES.—Besides weakness of the interossei and intrinsic muscles of the foot these consist of:—

1. *Stretching of ligaments* on the inner side of the foot; the inferior calcaneonavicular ('spring') ligament; the internal lateral (deltoid) ligament of the ankle, the small ligaments and plantar fascia on the medial side of the sole.

2. *Shortening* of those on the outer side; external lateral ligament of the ankle, etc.

3. *Stretching*—and later, in severe cases, *atrophy*—of the tibialis anticus and posticus, and the intrinsic muscles of the foot, especially of the interossei.

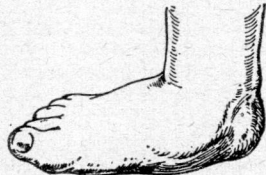
Fig. 132.—Talipes valgus with flat-foot.

4. *Spasm* and, later, *structural shortening* of the peronei, from overaction of these muscles.

5. *Shortening* of the Achilles tendon, with contraction of the calf muscles, sometimes occurs. Some surgeons say that this is *always* the case, and is indeed the original factor in the condition, the patient trying to compensate for her inability to obtain complete dorsiflexion at the ankle by extension and abduction at the midtarsal joint and eversion at the subtaloid.

DISPLACEMENT OF BONES: DEFORMITY.—

1. The *talus* rotates downwards and inwards in normal eversion, but if the foot is weak this position is exaggerated, and in time becomes an actual deformity,

the bone remaining permanently out of place. It can be seen as a prominence on the inner side of the foot (*Fig.* 132).

2. The *navicular* is carried down with it, and the tuberosity can be felt under the foot.

3. The *longitudinal arch* is thus lowered, and, in severe cases, rests entirely on the ground. The inner side of the foot loses its concave appearance, and becomes convex inwards (i.e., towards the middle line of the body).

4. The *os calcis* is also rotated downward and inward, the patient walking on the internal tuberosity.

5. The *posterior part of the foot* is therefore turned *downward* and *inward*, whilst the *front of the foot* is turned *downward* and *outward* in an everted position.

6. At the same time, the foot is *spread out*, appearing much wider at the part where the arch should be (*Fig.* 132). The front of the foot also spreads from collapse of the *anterior arch* (*see also* p. 368).

7. The *heel* projects, the *external malleolus* being less prominent than usual, whilst the *internal malleolus* is lowered and becomes much more prominent than in the normal foot. If looked at from behind, the tendo Achillis may be seen to describe a curve with the convexity inwards.

BONY CHANGES.—

1. The bones are subjected to pressure on the outer side of the foot, and hence become *wedge-shaped*, this being especially the case with the cuboid. On the inner side they become wider.

2. *The neck of the talus* is lengthened.

3. A small facet may form on the outer side of the os calcis, for articulation with the external malleolus.

SIGNS AND SYMPTOMS.—

1. There is a sensation of *weakness and strain* on the inner side of the foot.

2. *Pain* is a prominent symptom in severe cases. It consists of fatigue and aching while the foot is at rest, which increases when the patient stands or walks. It is most commonly found under the inner border of the foot, where the ligaments are stretched, or at the heads of the metatarsal bones (METATARSALGIA, *see* p. 318). In some cases it is felt round either malleolus, over the dorsum of the foot, up the calf or the front of the leg. In a few cases it may occur in the knee, hip, or even the lumbar region.

3. *Mobility: Inversion* is limited because of the displacement of the talus; *extension and flexion* may also be incomplete. *The movements of the toes* are often limited also, because the whole foot is held stiffly in walking, with little movement of the toe-joints. In the later stages all the joints of the foot become stiff.

4. *Loss of spring in walking*: the gait is awkward and ungraceful, the patient bringing the heels down heavily and walking with the feet turned out.

5. The *position and appearance* of the foot are as described above.

6. *Circulatory symptoms* may also be present—coldness, numbness, or increased perspiration, of the feet.

> In examining such a case, the patient's shoes should be inspected, to see in what places they are worn down. Not only the state of the heel, but also that of the sole, should be observed.

DEGREES.—

This deformity, like others, may be divided, roughly, into three degrees, for purposes of description.

FIRST DEGREE.—(*a*) Mere postural deformity; the patient can correct the position. (*b*) Transition stage. Alteration in muscular and ligamentous structures, with displacement of bone, and probably pain; the position of the foot cannot be self-corrected.

SECOND DEGREE.—Stage of slight bony change, marked spasm and contracture of muscles; complete correction not possible.

THIRD DEGREE.—The arthritic foot; changes in bones; marked changes in joints; almost complete rigidity.

Principles of Treatment.—The aims of treatment, as in all deformities, will be to mobilize the joints of the foot if necessary; to restore the arches as far as possible; to strengthen the muscles, and to re-educate the patient in their correct use. It will also be necessary to re-educate postural sense in some cases, and all cases require re-education in walking. Methods of treatment will therefore be somewhat as follows:—

FIRST DEGREE.—In cases of *postural deformity* attention must be paid to the prevention of too much standing and to the wearing of correct footwear. General exercises and re-education in correct posture may be required, as well as foot-drill and walking exercises. In the *transition stage* passive movements may be required in addition to the treatment outlined above, to restore mobility.

SECOND DEGREE (Rigid Flat-foot).—Wrenching will be necessary to achieve mobility. Following this, proper supports should be worn for varying periods. The patient will require intensive foot-drill. If in an occupation entailing much standing, a change may be advisable.

THIRD DEGREE (The Arthritic Foot).—A complete cure cannot be expected, though an open operation may afford relief. Permanent supports will be necessary, and post-operative foot-drill and re-education in walking are essential. In some cases wrenching may be tried before operative measures are decided on.

FIRST DEGREE (POSTURAL DEFORMITY)

FOOTWEAR.—Special footwear is not necessary at this stage, provided the patient wears comfortable, well-fitting shoes. Many women, particularly young women and adolescents, are horrified at the thought of 'sensible' shoes, but attractive footwear can still measure up to the following requirements. The front of the shoe should not compress the toes; that is, the sole should be wide enough for the whole of the foot and toes to rest on it, and the upper should in no way press upon them. The inner side of the shoe should be straight from the waist to the tip, and the waist should fit closely to the foot. The sole should be flat, not convex, in order to avoid crowding the toes into the central hollow. A heel should be worn, but it should not be so high that the foot slides forwards in the shoe, thus pressing the toes against the end of it (1–2 in. is reasonable). Moreover, it should form a support for the heel of the foot; a high and narrow heel is unsuitable for much standing or walking. The shoes should be sufficiently large to accommodate the foot comfortably (if the toes are pointed, a larger size should be worn). (For other defects in shoes, *see* p. 318.)

PHYSICAL TREATMENT.—In treating this type of patient the following points should be taken into consideration:—

1. Postural sense is very often defective. If this is so it will affect the whole body, not only the feet. The posture of the head, shoulders, trunk, pelvis, and knees should all be examined and receive attention if necessary. Any special cause must, of course, receive treatment as well.

2. It is highly probable that muscles other than those of the lower legs and feet will be weakened through disuse, or incorrect use. This is especially true of the glutei and the quadriceps, and may also apply to the spinal and abdominal muscles. These groups may therefore require exercises.

3. From the point of view of the feet, the lumbricales and the intrinsic muscles are the most important, and require intensive physiotherapy. Flexor digitorum longus, tibialis posticus, and tibialis anticus should not, however, be neglected,

but if tightness of the latter is a primary cause of the condition it should not be specifically strengthened. A simple test for a tight tibialis anterior is as follows:—

The patient should sit or lie with the leg supported and the foot completely relaxed. The physiotherapist then grasps the heel and places it in line with the tibia. She then notes the position of the fore-foot. If it is *adducted* (i.e., rotated in) the tibialis anterior is tight.

If the tendo Achillis is tight, similar care must be exercised with regard to tibialis posticus, to avoid increasing the flexion at the ankle.

ELECTROTHERAPY.—Faradic foot-baths are invaluable in the treatment of flat-foot or weak foot. Not only do they strengthen the muscles, but they help the patient to regain the feeling of movement and to understand what movements are possible. The foot should be stimulated longitudinally and transversely and specific stimulation should be given to the lumbricales and interossei. The posterior tibial muscles and tibialis anterior may also be stimulated during the treatment. *Faradic treatment should always be used in conjunction with exercises and must not be used as a substitute for active exercises.*

EXERCISES.—These may be given in sitting and standing.

In Sitting.—It is often better to begin the exercises in this position, since it enables the patient to concentrate on the foot movements, particularly when attempting lumbrical action.

1. Heel-raising and -lowering, either with both feet together or alternately.
2. Sitting with feet crossed, resting on outer borders.
*3. Sitting with heels resting on ground, flex toes and adduct fore-foot.
4. Heel-raising, first onto ball of foot, then onto toes, and lowering. The movement should be done in stages to begin with, then in one smooth movement.
5. Tailor-sitting, or sitting with leg crossed over knee, foot-circling. This may require modification if tibialis anterior is at fault.
*6. Drawing the sole of one foot up the shin of the opposite leg. The foot must be kept dorsiflexed, and the hip must not be abducted.
7. Leg crossed over knee, Toe-flexion and -extension. The physiotherapist may give support behind the metatarsal heads as the patient flexes his toes. This may also be done with the feet in dorsiflexion, the heels resting on the ground.*
8. Picking up objects with the toes—pencil, marble, towel, etc.
9. Sitting Toe-separating.
10. Abduction of the big toes, if possible.
11. Pressing the toes on the ground, the metatarsal head not being raised. This is a useful prelude to lumbricales exercise.
12. Lumbricales exercise. *This is the most important exercise*, and also the most difficult. It requires careful teaching and much practice. The toes must be *flexed at the metatarsophalangeal joints* and *extended at the interphalangeal joints*. The following methods may be helpful in teaching the exercise.

a. The patient tries to do the movement with the help of electrical stimulation in the faradic foot-bath.

b. The physiotherapist does the movement herself and the patient tries to copy it.

c. A thin book or platform is placed under the toes. The patient presses down onto this and lifts the metatarsal heads off the ground.

d. The physiotherapist holds the toes down while the patient tries to lift the metatarsal heads up.

e. The patient presses his toes down as in Exercise 11, then shortens the foot, keeping the toes pressed down throughout the movement. This may also be done as a separate exercise, when lumbrical action has been mastered (*see below*).

---

* These exercises are not suitable if tibialis anticus is tight.

When unilateral exercises are being performed the resting foot must be held in a corrected position, or resting on the outer border, as in Exercise 2.

In Standing.—Many of the above exercises can be done in standing.

1. Correct standing. The patient should stand with the feet parallel, and about 3 in. apart at the heels. She must then be taught the correct weight-bearing areas of the foot. She must learn to throw the weight onto the outer border of the foot by a slight movement of inversion, but, at the same time, *the whole length of the toes must be kept pressed firmly against the ground.* As has been mentioned on p. 308, this is a strong position of the foot, which counteracts the natural tendency to eversion and flattening of the arches when weight bearing. In this position tibialis anticus not only acts as an invertor to throw the weight outwards, but also as a synergist to the long flexors of the toes. It fixes the ankle, enabling the long flexors to expend all their power on the toes, and in so doing it raises the medial longitudinal arch. This gives the interossei and small muscles of the sole a mechanical advantage, so that they can prevent flattening of the transverse arches.

2. Standing Foot-shortening, re-forming the arch (*Figs.* 133 A, B). This is really only a stronger form of the above, the inversion being carried slightly beyond what is required for correct weight bearing, and the toes being pressed

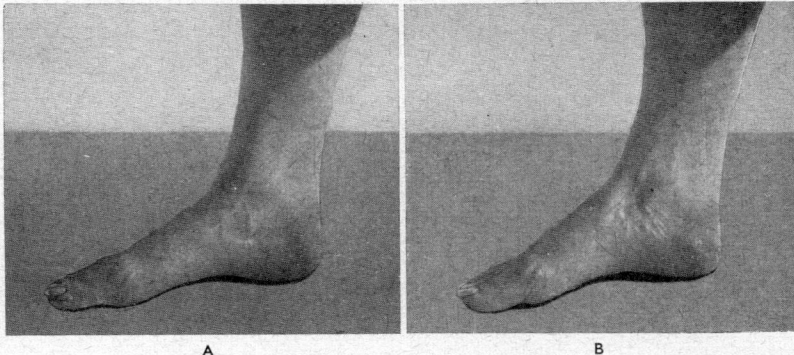

Fig. 133.—A, Standing Foot-shortening, re-forming the arch. B, Shows the increase in height of the arch.

very hard on the ground. If the foot is mobile the tibialis anterior draws the arch up very strongly, and the whole foot may be shortened about half an inch. After the position has been held for a few seconds the muscles should be relaxed, *but the foot must not be allowed to fall back into the everted position.* The exercise should be frequently repeated, but the position should not be held for more than a few seconds at a time. Both in this and the previous exercise, the knees should be firmly braced.

3. Close-standing, or standing with the feet 2 or 3 in. apart, gluteal contraction with external rotation of the hips, as for genu varum (p. 307). This also re-forms the arch, provided that the toes are firmly pressed on the ground as in the two previous exercises.

4. Walking on the inclined board (*see* p. 129).

5. Standing at edge of plinth, toes over the edge. Flexion and extension of the toes of both feet.

6. Correct walking (*see* 'RE-EDUCATION IN WALKING', pp. 49–50).

The exercises outlined above are intended as a basis from which the student may compile schemes of her own, making any necessary modifications or progressions. Patients with first degree flat-foot or weak foot may be treated in classes, but individual treatment should always be given at first. It should continue until the patient has really learnt to do the exercises correctly.

Unnatural Forms of Walking.—Since the main object of the treatment of this type of patient is to re-educate postural sense, the author does not personally consider it a good plan to teach any form of walking which is *unnatural*, e.g., walking on the outer borders of the feet, tip-toe walking, pointing the toes and putting them down before the heels, or rising on the toes between steps. Such activities may be employed as variations in class-work, but in individual work the aim is to restore the correct manner of walking by impressing it upon the patient's mind, not to replace one incorrect form by another equally incorrect. (In walking on the outer borders, for instance, the patient fails to extend the ankle, never flexes the knees, and holds the spine rigid.)

Tip-toe Exercises.—These are obviously as inadvisable in cases where the Achilles tendon is shortened, as are strong inversion exercises in cases where tibialis anterior is tight. If the tendo Achillis is shortened, it must, of course, be stretched. This, however, is best done manually rather than by active exercise, to ensure that the stretching really takes place in the *ankle*, and does not merely farther extend the *mid-tarsal* joint (*see* p. 328 and *Fig.* 136, p. 322). Even in straightforward cases, tip-toe exercises are probably best left until the later stages of treatment, and *care must be taken to see that tibialis anterior is not unduly stretched*. Running and dancing exercises mobilize and strengthen the foot and may be used when the patient has regained the correct sense of posture. Neither should be indulged in to excess, however.

Home Exercises.—Most of the above are suitable for home exercises, *provided the patient thoroughly understands how they should be done*. She should be told to sit either with crossed feet resting on their outer borders, or with the feet in the correct position for weight bearing. This position must always be adopted when standing, and when walking the feet must be kept straight, not turned out.

First Degree (Transition Stage)

The patient should rest the feet as much as possible. The housewife should sit to do as many chores as possible, and those whose occupations entail standing should rest with the feet up as often as possible when off duty.

FOOTWEAR.—This should be as described above, but it may be advisable to raise the heel and sole of the shoe about a quarter of an inch* on the inner side by inserting a leather wedge. This is known as a 'valgus wedge', and has the effect of tipping the foot over towards the outer border, thus preventing eversion during standing and walking.

Other forms of support may be used to hold up depressed arches, but they should always be prescribed by the doctor. Many patients attempt to treat themselves by buying ready-made supports. They should always be discouraged from doing this, as many of these supports are quite unsuitable, or at all events inappropriate, for their particular trouble.

PHYSICAL TREATMENT.—

MASSAGE.—If the foot is painful, massage may afford relief by improving the circulation and removing the products of fatigue or inflammation from the muscles. Effleurage should be given to the whole leg to promote drainage, though concentrated treatment should be reserved for the foot. *The dorsum of the foot and*

---

* Or three-sixteenths of an inch. Some authorities state that, in practice, they have found it better to raise the sole only for women, and both sole and heel for men.

malleolar region should receive finger-kneadings and effleurage and *the sole* should be given effleurage, stroking, kneading, and frictions provided the patient can tolerate the treatment. It is sometimes possible to replace a slightly displaced talus by means of pressure during massage. It will not, of course, remain corrected, but it can thus be mobilized and prevented from becoming fixed in a position of deformity. Wax baths, hot soaking, and contrast bathing can be used as a preliminary to massage, and help to relieve pain. The two latter can be self-administered at home.

PASSIVE MOVEMENTS.—These will be required to increase the mobility of the foot, attention being paid to the following:—

1. Inversion.
2. Dorsiflexion and plantar flexion of the ankle. *Care must be taken to see that no eversion occurs during dorsiflexion.*
3. Foot-rolling. This must be given in an inward direction, and the foot should not be carried outward beyond midline.
4. Mobilization of the joints between the metatarsal bones. It is important that each metatarsal bone should in turn be grasped and steadied by the fingers and thumb of one hand, while the adjacent bone, similarly grasped, is moved backwards and forwards upon it.
5. Flexion and extension of the toes. During this movement the metatarsus should be firmly supported with one hand, and traction applied to the toes with the other.

In addition to general toe movements, toe-rolling and abduction should be given to the big-toe.

ACTIVE MOVEMENTS.—The following should be practised, after mobilization, both as free and resisted movements:—

1. Inversion of the foot.
2. Flexion and extension of the ankle.
3. Flexion and extension of the toes, free.

Electrotherapy and exercises should be given as for the less severe cases, the exercises being performed first in sitting, then in standing.

SECOND DEGREE (RIGID FLAT-FOOT)

Mobility must be restored before any re-education is possible, and this can only be achieved by surgical means.

SURGICAL TREATMENT.—

WRENCHING.—This is performed under an anæsthetic, the foot being mobilized in every direction. All adhesions are broken down, and the Achilles tendon divided if shortened. Foot supports are usually worn for varying periods after the operation.

PHYSICAL TREATMENT.—This is begun immediately after the operation.

PASSIVE MOVEMENTS.—These are most important, since the correction obtained by the surgeon's manipulation must be maintained. The movements are given on the same lines as those described above.

RE-EDUCATION follows on the usual lines, but the exercises must be off-weight to begin with.

THIRD DEGREE (THE ARTHRITIC FOOT)

This is an unsatisfactory condition to treat. If the surgeon decides to operate, the treatment to follow depends entirely on the nature and purpose of the operation chosen. In cases in which no operation takes place, the patient will probably be given permanent supports. *Active exercises* and *re-education in walking* may be attempted though in many cases it will be unwise to allow the patient to walk without the supports. *Passive (forced) movements* will be inadvisable.

METATARSALGIA

(*Morton's Disease*)

A condition in which, as the name implies, there is pain in the metatarsal region. It is usually felt beneath the metatarsal heads, or in the region of the fourth toe. The latter is sometimes known as 'Morton's disease'. It is due either to collapse of the whole of the anterior arch of the foot, or to displacement of the head of one of the metatarsal bones which compose it. The former leads to splaying out of the metatarsal heads, which in turn stretches the transverse ligaments and causes the pain. The latter causes direct pressure on nerves.

AETIOLOGY.—

AGE.—Metatarsalgia generally occurs in middle-aged people.

SEX.—It is more common in women than in men, probably because the former often wear harmful shoes.

CAUSES.—These are very similar to the causes of flat-foot, namely:—

1. *Weakness of the intrinsic muscles*, which causes the metatarsal heads to drop.

2. *Foot deformities*, particularly talipes equinus, or pes cavus.

3. *Unsuitable footwear*, e.g., too high a heel which causes the foot to slide forward, and the weight to be taken on the metatarsal heads; the toes are often compressed in a narrow space, which further depresses the metatarsal heads, and the ligaments are stretched. Shoes which have a convex sole also force the metatarsal heads downwards; those which are too narrow as well, exert pressure on the displaced bones and cause pain. Whitman* lays great stress on the danger of the 'rocker sole', by which he means one which is convex anteroposteriorly, and which therefore keeps the toes in extension, pushing down the metatarsal heads and preventing the interossei (the chief supports of the anterior arch) from being used (Whitman; Tubby).

4. *Traumatic or inflammatory conditions*, e.g., fracture of metatarsal bone, arthritis.

PATHOLOGICAL CHANGES.—The heads of all the metatarsals, or of one alone, become depressed. The ligaments stretch and the muscles become weakened. There is pressure on nerve-endings which gives rise to pain. If there is a specific cause there will also be pathological changes consistent with that condition.

SIGNS AND SYMPTOMS.—

1. Pain. If the whole arch is deformed it may be dull and aching in character, or take the form of intermittent periods of excruciating pain. If one joint only is affected the pain is usually severe in the region of the joint. It is relieved when footwear is removed. In both cases the pain radiates through the foot and may even extend to the calf.

2. The affected area is acutely tender to pressure.

3. Passive plantar-flexion of the metatarsophalangeal joints often leads to acute pain.

4. The metatarsal heads are prominent in the sole of the foot.

5. Callosities form over the metatarsal heads, and may later become inflamed.

Principles of Treatment.—It is necessary to rest the foot, to relieve the strain on the metatarsal heads, to relieve pain, to strengthen the intrinsic muscles, the interossei, and lumbricales, and to re-educate walking.

SUPPORTS AND FOOTWEAR.—

1. *Suitable shoes must be worn*. They must be of sufficient width and length, with flat soles and not excessively high heels. Unless the patient is prepared to be sensible in this matter, treatment will be of little use.

---

* *Journal of Orthopædic Surgery.*

2. In order to take pressure off the metatarsal heads a pad or bar is placed across the sole of the foot *behind* the metatarsal heads, following their shape exactly. It may be made of felt, but cork or a firm material is preferable. The support should be about a quarter of an inch thick and have bevelled edges, so that it fits comfortably to the foot. It may be fixed to the foot by adhesive strapping, or a band of wide elastic.

In slight cases, adhesive plaster strapping applied round the fore-foot separates the heads of these bones and so relieves pressure and friction.

In addition a leather bar may be fixed across the sole of the shoe (the 'metatarsal bar'), or the sole thickened behind the metatarsal heads. More elaborate arch supports are sometimes prescribed for use within the shoe.

PHYSICAL TREATMENT.—

HEAT.—This is given for the relief of pain. It may be given in the form of *short-wave diathermy, wax baths,* or *infra-red* or *luminous radiation* applied to the sole of the foot, though this is a less practicable form of treatment than the preceding forms. Relief can be afforded at home by the use of hot soaking or contrast bathing.

In other respects treatment is the same as for flat-foot, faradic foot-baths, active exercises, and re-education in walking being given. *Flexion of the toes* is the chief movement for the collapsed anterior arch, or a displaced bone in that arch, since it brings into action the interossei, lumbricales, and other small muscles of the sole which are its principal supports.

Tip-toe exercises are not advisable, since they produce hyperextension of the toes, depress the metatarsal heads, and put further strain on the anterior arch.

SURGICAL TREATMENT.—Very severe cases of Morton's disease are sometimes treated by operation, the head of the fourth metatarsal being removed. The foot is put up in plaster, and walking—with an appropriate support (*see above*) —is allowed in about 2–3 weeks. Sometimes, instead of this operation which weakens the foot, relief is obtained by dividing the affected digital nerve or nerves. Foot exercises and re-education in walking are indicated.

TALIPES

(*Club-foot*)

The foot has, as we know, four principal movements: flexion and extension at the *ankle*; inward movement, including inversion and adduction; and outward movement, consisting of eversion and abduction. The side-to-side movements take place at the *sub-taloid* and *mid-tarsal joints.* A fixation of the foot in any of these positions, or in an exaggerated form of one of them, constitutes the deformity of *talipes.* It is usually combined with inability to carry out the opposite movement, or at least with great limitation of that movement. The name of 'club-foot' is applied either to the whole group of these deformities, or, more especially, to talipes equinovarus, the commonest type.

VARIETIES.—As might be expected there are four principal varieties: (1) *Talipes equinus,* in which the foot and ankle are in extension (plantar-flexion); (2) *Talipes calcaneus,* in which they are in dorsiflexion; (3) *Talipes varus,* in which it is adducted and inverted; (4) *Talipes valgus,* in which it is abducted and everted. In addition to these there are cases in which the arches are depressed or obliterated (PES PLANUS OR PES PLANO-VALGUS, *see* pp. 307, 310) or abnormally high (PES CAVUS, *see* p. 332).

These malformations exist in varying degrees of severity, from slight limitations of movement to obvious, and fixed, deformities. In neglected cases the foot may become twisted and distorted in an extreme degree, and callosities form at points where undue pressure is exerted. Frequently, two of the above-mentioned varieties are combined. Thus we may have *talipes equinovarus*, the commonest type of all, in which extension is combined with inversion; *talipes calcaneovalgus* and *calcaneovarus*. Each may, of course, exist alone, although this is far less common, particularly in the *equinus* or *calcaneus* form. In about 50 per cent of cases the deformity is bilateral. In unilateral cases the right foot is more commonly affected.

CAUSES.—These deformities may be: (1) Congenital; or (2) Acquired.

1. The *congenital form* is due to an abnormal intra-uterine position. It may possibly be due to increased mechanical or hydraulic pressure in utero, and in some cases heredity appears to be a factor.

2. The *acquired forms* are due to flaccid paralysis (especially acute anterior poliomyelitis), spastic paralysis, injuries or diseases of bones, joints, or soft tissues, or the formation and contraction of scar tissue. Hysterical forms of the contracture are also seen. The commonest cause of acquired forms is flaccid paralysis. In such cases trophic changes, attendant on this form of paralysis, are present to a varying degree.

In describing the various kinds of talipes we shall give most attention to the congenital variety. The treatment of the congenital and of the paralytic forms is similar, but in the latter the rules for treating paralysed muscles must be observed (*see* p. 205). The pathological changes occurring in all these varieties will not be described in detail—they must be studied in the orthopædic text-books dealing with the subject.

General Principles of Treatment.—These are the same for all types of deformity, namely:—

1. *To reduce the deformity.*
2. *To maintain the reduction.*

Reduction.—This can be achieved either by manipulation, or by operative measures. From birth until the age of about 3 months, reduction can usually be obtained by daily manipulative stretching. In infants from 3 months to 2 years old, forcible manipulation under anæsthetic is required. Over the age of 2 years operative treatment is necessary.

Maintenance of Reduction.—In very young babies strapping, to hold the foot in an over-corrected position, is often all that is required. If, however, the deformity is not corrected within eight weeks, some more definite form of support is necessary.

The most usual form is a Denis Browne splint, or a modification of it. Plaster splints may sometimes be used.

Denis Browne Splint (Figs. 144, 145).—This consists of an L-shaped piece of aluminium. It should be suitably padded and one limb bent up and applied to the outer side of the leg, the other limb to the sole of the foot. It is kept in place by adhesive plaster. The splints are applied to *both* feet, and the foot-pieces are connected by a cross-bar. If the club-foot is unilateral, the normal foot is fixed to the cross-bar in such a way as to be turned outward at an angle of 20° (that is, in normal eversion), and the club-foot to an angle of 90° from the sagittal plane. This fixation should be maintained for about 9 months (Denis Browne). The child should be encouraged to kick, and may stand up in it when possible. When the foot is fully mobile, and can be held in the corrected position, the splint may be discarded. Its place is taken by special boots riveted to the cross-piece, which hold the feet in the same position as they were in on the splint. These 'boots' have open toes, and unlace completely from one end to the other, so that they allow for the growth of the child's feet and need not be constantly changed as he grows.

PHYSICAL TREATMENT.—In infants, from birth until the age of 3 months, the physiotherapist may be responsible for the reduction of the deformity. In children over the age of 3 months the responsibility for reduction does not rest on her. In all cases, however, physical treatment plays a very large part in the maintenance of the reduction. It will consist mainly of stretching manipulations to the affected structures, where these are appropriate.

Pre-operative treatment may be requested in more severe cases, to ensure that the muscles are in as good a condition as possible to withstand the period of immobilization.

Talipes Equinus

The congenital form is rare, the paralytic form more common. It is frequently seen in cases of cerebral palsy.

DEFORMITY.—The heel is raised from the ground, and the patient walks on his toes, the weight falling on the heads of the metatarsal bones. *The deformity involves the ankle-joint only*, the foot being in full extension; the position of *the mid-tarsal joint is quite normal.* The longitudinal arch

Fig. 134.—Talipes equinus.

is increased, but the forefoot is broadened, because the heads of the metatarsal bones are spread out in consequence of the weight which falls on them. Both feet may be affected. In congenital cases the deformity is often slight. It is more marked in paralytic cases because the foot is dropped, not only at the ankle but at the mid-tarsal joint as well, the arch being very much increased in height (*Fig.* 134). The toes later become clawed.

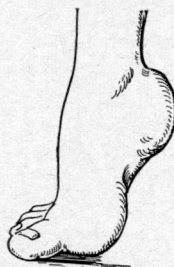

PATHOLOGICAL CHANGES.—

BONES.—The changes are not marked.

LIGAMENTS.—There is *stretching* of the anterior ligament of the ankle, the anterior parts of the lateral ligaments, and all the ligaments on the dorsum of the foot, with *shortening* of the 'spring' ligament, the long and short plantar ligaments, the small ligaments of the sole, and the plantar fascia.

MUSCLES.—There is *lengthening* of the anterior *tibial group*, and *contraction* of the calf muscles and tendo Achillis, long flexors of toes, and peroneus longus.

Treatment.—

EARLY CASES IN INFANTS.—These are treated by manipulation and fixation.

FIXATION.—The following methods may be adopted:—

1. An aluminium or light metal splint is often applied, and kept in position by straps, bandages, or adhesive plaster. It should be padded in the usual way, and covered with waterproof material in the case of very young infants. The foot is dorsiflexed to a right angle, or as near this as possible. The splint is bent to the same angle, and applied to the back of the leg and the sole of the foot.

2. The Denis Browne splint may be applied, but the foot will not be placed in eversion.

3. The foot is sometimes put in a plaster splint, but this is inadvisable in the case of young babies because of the danger of it becoming softened through soiling.

4. In slight paralytic cases, where the child is old enough to walk, some form of apparatus which prevents plantar-flexion beyond a right angle is sometimes used.

PHYSICAL TREATMENT.—The splint is removed for treatment, but the foot should be kept in as correct a position as possible until it is replaced. In paralytic cases, this is, of course, absolutely essential.

Passive (Forced) Movements.—The foot must be pressed up into dorsiflexion. This should be done several times a day, if possible, and the mother should be taught how to do it, so that she can give home treatment. If the ankle-joint

11

alone is affected, the physiotherapist should grasp the heel with one hand, pulling it downwards, while with the other she takes hold of the instep and forces it upwards (*Fig.* 135). If, as in the acquired form, the foot is also dropped at the mid-tarsal joint, the heel grasp remains similar, but the other hand should be placed along the length of the sole, so that the upward pressure produces movement in both the ankle and mid-tarsal joints (*Fig.* 136).

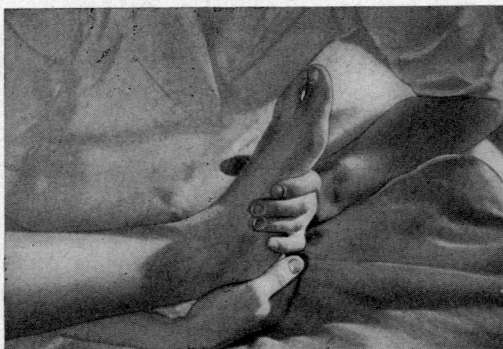

Fig. 135.—Manipulation of the foot in talipes equinus (congenital form).

Active Movements.—Dorsiflexion of the ankle must be practised as soon as the child is capable. Foot exercises must also be given. The child will require careful watching when beginning to walk.

SEVERE CASES (e.g., neglected cases in older patients).—These have to be rectified by operation.

SURGICAL TREATMENT.—The Achilles tendon and the plantar fascia are divided. If the toes are clawed the tendons of both the flexors and extensors of the toes are also divided. The foot is put up on a splint, or in plaster. The former has the advantage of allowing movements to be continued at an earlier period. The latter is more likely to be used in paralytic cases, and may then have to be worn for several months because of the spastic element.

PHYSICAL TREATMENT (POST-OPERATIVE).—This will begin as soon as the surgeon allows. If the position of the foot is maintained by a splint, treatment can begin when the tendon can stand strain, usually in 2–3 weeks. If a plaster is worn treatment may be given as for any limb immobilized in plaster, but more specific treatment will have to be delayed until the plaster is removed.

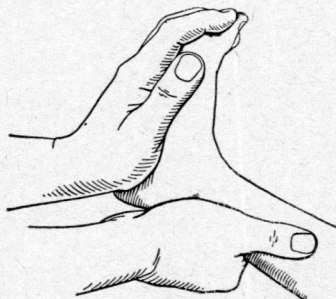

Fig. 136.—Manipulation of talipes equinus (acquired).

Massage may be required after removal of the plaster, in order to improve the condition of the skin. Otherwise it is not usually necessary.

Passive movements are most important, for the tendon must not be allowed to re-unite in a shortened position. At the same time care must be taken not to overstretch the tissues (producing talipes calcaneus), and *the movement of dorsiflexion must not be carried beyond the normal limits.*

Active movements must also be given. As soon as the patient is allowed to walk, he must be taught to do so correctly. Exercises for dorsiflexion of the foot are continued, and the patient should be given movements to stretch the calf muscles such as curtsey-standing, lunge position, etc. These are, of course, added gradually.

PARALYTIC FORM.—The type of paralysis must, of course, be taken into consideration when dealing with these cases, and treatment given accordingly.

Talipes Calcaneus

This is not such a common deformity in either the congenital or acquired form as talipes equinus or equinovarus. The acquired form is generally the result of anterior poliomyelitis, but it may sometimes occur after an operation on the tendo Achillis, in which there has been too much stretching or lengthening.

Congenital Form

POSITION OF THE FOOT.—The foot is not affected, but the *ankle-joint is dorsiflexed*. The cases vary in severity. Some hardly amount to more than a slight limitation of plantar-flexion, while in others the foot forms an acute angle with the leg (*Fig.* 137).

PATHOLOGICAL CHANGES.—

Bones.—The deformity only affects the ankle-joint, and there is very little displacement or deformity but occasionally, the tibia, fibula, or certain bones of the foot may be defective or absent.

Ligaments.—The *anterior ligament*, and the *anterior portions of the internal and external lateral ligaments* of the ankle are *contracted*; the *posterior portions* of the *lateral ligaments*, and the *posterior ligaments*, are *stretched*.

Muscles.—The *anterior tibial muscles* are *contracted* and the *calf muscles* are *stretched*.

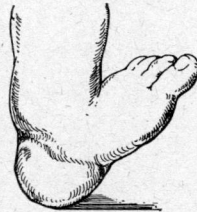

Fig. 137.—Talipes caclaneus.

Treatment.—

SLIGHT CASES.—In many cases in infants, the deformity corrects itself when the baby begins to walk and the calf muscles gain strength. Slight deformity in older children can usually be corrected by the application of a light aluminium splint which holds the foot in plantar-flexion, and by the use of passive stretching for the contracted structures, together with active movements and exercises to regain plantar-flexion. Similar splintage and stretching is sometimes given to infants before they begin to walk.

SEVERE CASES AND THOSE IN OLDER CHILDREN.—If the deformity persists in infants, or in neglected cases in older children, surgical treatment is required. This consists of *tenotomy of all anterior tibial muscles*.

Fixation and Post-operative Treatment.—The principles are exactly the same as for talipes equinus, but the foot is put up in *plantar-flexion* and physical treatment is devoted to re-educating this movement. For the grip and method used for passive stretching of the anterior tibial muscles, *see* p. 324 and *Fig.* 138.

Paralytic Form

POSITION OF THE FOOT.—This differs from the congenital form in that *the arch is also exaggerated*, sometimes to an extreme degree. The heel is lengthened, for reasons given below, and its tuberosities stand out prominently. The patient walks on the back of the heel, which becomes callous because of the undue weight placed on it. With improved methods of treatment for paralysis such severe deformities are rarely seen nowadays but it is very important to guard against this possibility when treating patients with paralysed posterior tibial and calf muscles.

PATHOLOGICAL CHANGES.—There is far more displacement in this type, since the deformity affects *both the ankle and the mid-tarsal joints.*

BONES.—

1. The *calcaneum* drops, since both the calf muscles and deep posterior tibial group are out of action. It becomes oblique, or even vertical, in direction.

2. *The longitudinal arch of the foot is much increased in height,* because, although the ankle-joint is dorsiflexed, it drops at the mid-tarsal joint, the navicular and cuboid bones having slipped downwards and forwards. This happens partly because the force of gravity draws the forefoot down, and partly because the patient, in walking, tries to get his toes to the ground. Finally, the muscles and fascia of the sole contract, and the mid-tarsal joint, abnormally mobile at the beginning of the trouble, is held down by these structures. Since the heel is completely dropped, even the pull of the extensors of the toes only serves to draw the forefoot and heel closer together, thus enhancing the deformity.

3. The *talus* is displaced backwards.

LIGAMENTS.—The anterior ligaments of the ankle, and the small ligaments on the plantar aspect of the foot, become *contracted,* and the posterior ligaments of the ankle-joint are *stretched.*

MUSCLES AND FASCIA.—Because of the paralysis and atrophy of the calf muscles and posterior tibial group, there is *contraction* of the anterior tibial group, the muscles of the sole and the plantar fascia.

SKIN.—The trophic changes typical of paralysis are present. Callosities form under the heel, and the skin is often abnormally thin under the forefoot.

SYMPTOMS.—

1. *Position of the foot;* as described above.

2. *Gait.*—The patient may be quite lame. He brings the heel down first, and the front part of the foot drops down afterwards.

Treatment.—Some cases, in which the deformity is not too severe, respond quite well to physical treatment.

PHYSICAL TREATMENT.—

FORCED PASSIVE MOVEMENTS.—

1. *To stretch the contracted structures in the sole.* The hind-foot should be held firmly in one hand, in such a way that the ankle-joint remains steady during the movement. The front part of the foot is forced upwards with the other hand (*see Fig.* 136). Movement should take place only in the mid-tarsal articulation.

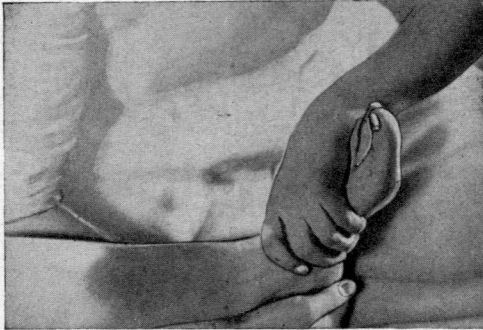

Fig. 138.—Manipulation of talipes calcaneus.

2. *To stretch the contracted structures on the front of the leg and foot.* The foot should be grasped as near the ankle as possible, and an endeavour made to plantar-flex it; the other hand should grasp the os calcis and draw it upwards (*Fig.* 138). Care must be taken *not to increase the plantar-flexion at the mid-tarsal joint* during this movement.

Active Movements will be given as in any lower motor neuron lesion, the same rules being applicable.

SEVERE CASES: SURGICAL TREATMENT.—These cases require surgical intervention, and are treated by one of the following operations:—

1. FASCIOTOMY AND WRENCHING.—Division of the plantar fascia, and manipulation of the foot into shape, followed by fixation in plaster until the tissues are sufficiently healed to withstand strain.

2. SHORTENING OF THE ACHILLES TENDON.—

3. WHITMAN'S OPERATION.*—This operation is used in cases of talipes calcaneovalgus, and in severe cases of talipes calcaneus. It consists of removal of the talus, and backward displacement of the foot. Sometimes tendon transference is also required. The talus is entirely removed, together with the sustentaculum tali. The whole foot is then moved backwards, until the internal surface of the external malleolus lies against the calcaneo-cuboid joint, and the outer surface of the internal malleolus against the inner surface of the calcaneum, behind the navicular. The cartilage is stripped off these surfaces of the malleoli, and a thin layer of bone cut from the parts of the os calcis and cuboid beneath them, so that they grow together. The tendons of the peronei are sometimes used to supplement the Achilles tendon.

The patient remains in bed for three weeks, with the foot in plaster, in a slightly equinus position. A new plaster is then applied and walking is allowed. In two to four months the new joint will have become stable and the plaster is discarded, but some form of walking apparatus will be necessary for a year or more.

POST-OPERATIVE PHYSICAL TREATMENT.—The result of this operation is to do away with *lateral* movement of the foot, while preserving flexion and extension at the ankle. Dorsiflexion, however, is now limited by contact of the navicular with the tibia, so that the deformed position cannot be reproduced. Moreover, the weight of the body falls nearer the middle of the foot, and the heel is not pressed downward. The shortening of the leg, occasioned by removal of the talus, is compensated by the slightly equinus position of the foot. *It is most important to remember these points when giving movements.*

Massage may be required for the skin once the plaster is removed. If so, it is given in the usual way.

Passive Movements.—Plantar- and dorsiflexion of the ankle must be given, but *no lateral movement should be attempted.* The toes must be kept mobile.

Active Movements.—Ankle and toe movements will be required, particular attention being paid to plantar-flexion.

Re-education in Walking.—When the patient begins to walk, he must be taught to do so as correctly as possible, taking equal steps, and bearing weight on the front of his foot. When the retentive apparatus is removed he will be provided with a shoe which keeps the foot in a slightly equinus position. It is then necessary to teach him to walk *without undue tipping of the pelvis, and without a limp.* In cases of extensive paralysis, in which supports will have to be worn permanently, the foot is kept at a right angle to the leg.

The possibility of a scoliosis developing should not be overlooked.

ROBERT JONES'S OPERATION.—This produces *arthrodesis* (fixation) of both the ankle and mid-tarsal joint. It is used in very severe cases of talipes calcaneus or calcaneovalgus. A wedge of bone is cut from the tarsal bones on the dorsum of the foot, to get rid of the cavus deformity, and at a subsequent operation part of the upper surface of the talus is removed, together with the articular cartilage from the tibia and fibula. The ankle-joint is then fixed with the foot at a right angle. This operation is performed if there is complete loss of power in the calf muscles. If any remains, the second operation (arthrodesis of the ankle) does

---

* These operations on bone are not carried out before the age of 9 years, preferably later.

not take place, but, instead, the tendo Achillis and posterior ligament of the ankle are shortened.*

Post-operative Treatment.—

Passive Movements may be given to the toes, but not, of course, to the ankle or mid-tarsal joints.

Active Movements.—To begin with, the patient, if old enough, should sit on a chair or stool, with his feet resting on the ground. The calf muscles and posterior tibial group are probably both useless, but the long extensors of the toes and the interossei and short muscles of the foot should be exercised, if they are still in action. If the toes can be pressed down hard on the ground, the tibialis anticus will contract, acting as a synergist to them. The peroneus longus and brevis will similarly come into action if the toes are strongly extended.

The patient will not be allowed to walk until the union of the bones is quite secure. If the leg is shortened, a raised sole will be necessary, since the shortening cannot be compensated by plantar-flexion of the foot. As the ankle is stiff, walking can never be normal, but with re-education much can be done to overcome this disability.

If the ankle-joint has *not* been fixed, movements are given as soon as the foot is out of plaster.

Talipes Varus

This is slightly more common than are either talipes calcaneus, or equinus alone. Details of its symptoms, treatment, etc., can, however, easily be worked out from the account of talipes equinovarus which follows.

DEFORMITY.—The foot is in a position of exaggerated *inversion* and *adduction*, so that the patient walks on its outer border. The skin therefore becomes thickened, and callosities develop.

PATHOLOGICAL CHANGES (*see also* TALIPES EQUINOVARUS).—In pure varus there is no change in the ankle-joint, *the deformity occurring only in the subtaloid and mid-tarsal joints*.

The *contracted* muscles are the tibiales anticus and posticus. The peronei become *stretched*. Similarly, the ligaments on the outer side of the foot and ankle are lengthened, and those on the inner side shortened.

Treatment.—This follows the same lines as that for talipes equinovarus, except that no stretching of the tendo Achillis is required. A small aluminium splint may be applied to the outer side of the foot and leg to reduce the deformity, or, alternatively, the foot is fixed by plaster or adhesive strapping.

SEVERER CASES.—

SURGICAL TREATMENT.—The following operations may be performed:—

1. *Wrenching of the foot*, under an anæsthetic.

2. *Tenotomy* of the tibiales anticus and posticus, with division of the internal lateral ligament.

3. *Osteotomy.*—In very severe cases, a wedge of bone is cut from the outer side of the tarsus, so that the foot can be straightened.

Post-operative Treatment.—See TALIPES EQUINOVARUS.

N.B.—Hysterical contracture may simulate this form of talipes.

Talipes Equinovarus

This is by far the most common type of talipes, affecting the *ankle, subtaloid*, and *mid-tarsal joints*.

---

* Dunn's operation has a similar result—arthrodesis of the mid-tarsal and subastragaloid articulations, and sometimes of the ankle also. Fixation in plaster is maintained for 4 months, and the patient walks in the plaster after 4 weeks. Other arthrodesing operations of the ankle and foot are *Lambrinudi's* and *Hoke's*. These and others are described in *Orthopædic Surgery* by Walter Mercer (4th edition, 1950).

DEFORMITY.—

CONGENITAL FORM.—The foot is *plantar-flexed* at the *ankle-joint*, and the heel is raised. It is also *adducted* and *inverted* at the *subtaloid and mid-tarsal joints* (*Fig.* 139). In very severe cases the intertarsal, talo-metatarsal, and metatarsophalangeal joints may also be affected.

Signs and Symptoms.—

1. *The inner border of the foot is raised and shortened*, and its natural concavity greatly increased.

2. *The longitudinal arch* is generally *exaggerated*.

3. *The outer border of the foot is convex*, and weight is taken on it if the patient is of an age to walk. In very severe cases weight may even be taken on the dorsum of the foot.

4. *The skin in these regions is thickened*, and callosities and false bursæ develop. These may become inflamed, or even suppurate (Tubby).

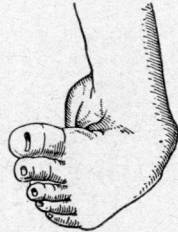

Fig. 139.—Congenital talipes equinovarus.

5. *The heel remains small*, not developing as the patient grows. The skin under it remains thin, never having been subjected to pressure.

6. *In untreated cases* the whole foot fails to attain its proper size, although the forefoot appears broad.

7. *In unilateral cases* the affected foot is smaller than its fellow, and in some cases the leg on the affected side may be shorter than the other.

8. The *gait* is awkward and waddling if the deformity is bilateral. The patient walks on the outer borders of the feet and, in severe cases, has to lift one foot over the other in walking.

9. *There is gross limitation of movement.* Even in a newborn infant, force is required to dorsiflex the foot. *This limitation of movement is an important diagnostic point*, as many infants hold their feet in an equinus position. Only if movement is limited is treatment required.

PARALYTIC FORM.—This is rarely seen nowadays, but the appearance of the foot is similar to that of the congenital type. In addition there are characteristic changes in muscles, skin, nails, etc.

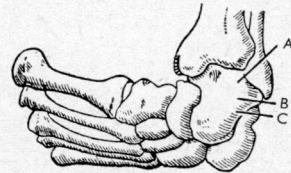

Fig. 140.—Bony changes in severe congenital talipes equinovarus. A, Bony ridge on talus which locks against tibia and prevents reduction; B, Abnormal quadrilateral surface on outer aspect of talus; C, Prefibular tubercle.

PATHOLOGICAL CHANGES.—

BONES.—The most important are as follows:—

The *talus is displaced forwards* to such an extent as to be almost out of its socket. The head and neck are directed downwards, and forwards, and the neck becomes elongated. The front of the bone enlarges owing to a lack of pressure from the malleoli. This fact renders subsequent reduction very difficult, the bone being too large to be easily fitted into the mortice of the ankle-joint.

The *calcaneum is raised* because of the extended position of the ankle. It is also *tilted inwards* and *rotated medially around its vertical axis*.

The *navicular, cuboid, and the other tarsal bones are drawn upwards and inwards*, the navicular lying on the medial side of the head of the talus. In some cases the navicular is absent. Sometimes the tibia is rotated medially around its own axis, so that the lateral malleolus is advanced. It may even lie anterior to the medial malleolus. The bones on the inner side of the foot are unduly compressed, while those on the outer side are released from the normal pressure. Hence overgrowth takes place. For further details of bony changes the reader is referred to Mercer's *Orthopædic Surgery*, McMurray's *A Practice of Orthopædic Surgery*, or Whitman's *Orthopedic Surgery*.

LIGAMENTS.—Those on the dorsum and lateral side of the foot are *stretched*; those on the medial side are *contracted*, especially the 'spring' ligament, and the posterior and internal lateral ligaments of the ankle. The plantar fascia and ligaments are also contracted.

MUSCLES.—

The *calf muscles* atrophy, and the tendo Achillis contracts. The *muscles of the anterior tibial group* and, in addition, the *tibialis posticus* are all *shortened*. The *peronei* are *stretched*.

Treatment.—

INFANTS FROM BIRTH TO 2–3 MONTHS.—These are treated by manual manipulation and fixation or support. Treatment should begin as soon as the condition is diagnosed, preferably

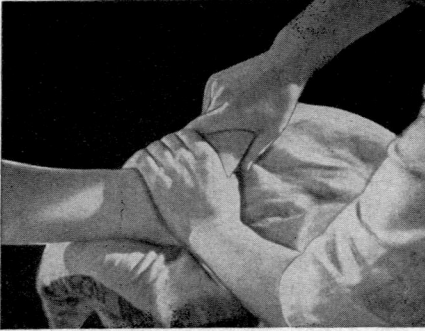

Fig. 141.—Manipulation of pes cavus.

within a week or ten days of birth. The foot is maintained in the correct position, or in as correct a position as is obtainable for the time being. In the latter case, the fixation is altered as the correction progresses.

MANIPULATION: (PASSIVE MOVEMENTS).—This must really be seen to be properly understood. *Each component of the deformity must be treated*, i.e.: (1) Pes cavus, the exaggeration of the arch; (2) Adduction and inversion; (3) Plantar-flexion of the ankle. The physiotherapist stands on the outer side of the deformed foot, or sits with it on her knee.

1. *Pes Cavus.*—The foot should be grasped at the back and front, and the contracted structures of the sole stretched (*Fig.* 141) (*see also* p. 324).

2. *Adduction and Inversion.*—The thumbs of both hands are placed over the talus and the fingers encircle the leg and foot. The talus thus becomes the fixed point, or fulcrum, round which the stretching movement takes place. The *forefoot* is then *everted*, the *sole* being *turned downwards* and *outwards*, its external border being raised. Steady pressure must be exerted on the talus throughout (*Fig.* 142).

3. *Plantar-flexion of the Ankle.*—The procedure is as described on p. 322 (*Fig.* 135). Each component has been described separately for ease of under-

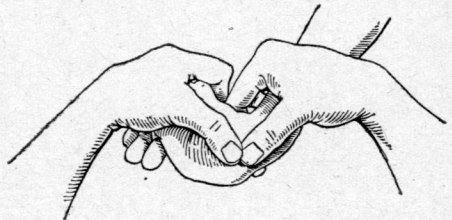

Fig. 142.—Manipulation of congenital talipes equinovarus to overcome the inversion.

standing. Many people, in fact, prefer to give each manipulation separately, some leaving the plantar-flexion deformity until the varus deformity has been rectified, but in infants all these movements can be combined in one operation, as the foot is so small. The heel can be pulled down, and pressure given to the head of the talus with one hand, while, with the other, the foot is everted and the ankle dorsiflexed. When manipulating a baby's foot it is very important to see that *the length of the sole is well supported* in order to avoid the possibility of producing a 'boat-shaped' foot, by over-stretching the mid-tarsal joint.

In slight cases the manipulation is easily done. In more resistant ones it will cause some pain, but this ceases as soon as the stretching is over. In either case the baby will scream so that it is best done quickly.

FIXATION (*Fig.* 143).—Following manipulation the foot can be fixed in the corrected position by means of adhesive strapping applied in the following way:—

1. A strip of adhesive plaster is taken from the medial condyle of the tibia, and passed under the heel, to pull it into a valgus position. It is continued up the outer side of the leg, as far as, and over, the knee.

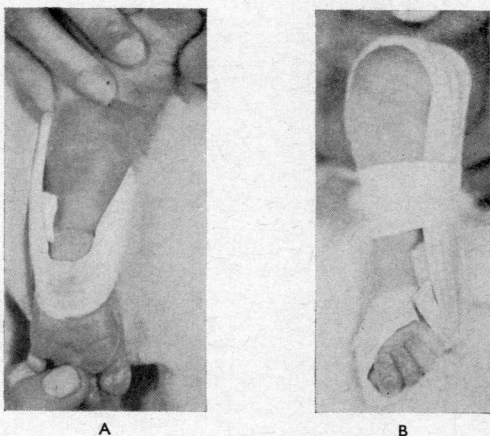

A   B

Fig. 143. Fixation of talipes equinovarus. A, The first length of adhesive plaster is applied to the heel, and B, the second to the forefoot ; both are carried around the knee. (*Reproduced by kind permission from 'Essentials of Orthopaedics' by P. Wiles.*)

2. Another strip is taken from below the lateral malleolus, across the dorsum of the foot and under the big toe, to pull the foot into a valgus position. It, too, is taken up the outer side of the leg to finish over the knee. A pad may be placed over the talus before this strapping is begun. It is usual to apply this method of fixation for very young infants, but if the deformity is not corrected within 2 months some definite form of support is required.

SUPPORT.—The following are most commonly used.

A simple aluminium splint, suitably bent and padded (*Fig.* 144). This is applied to the *outer* side of the leg and foot, and is gradually bent more and more until the over-corrected (valgus) position is attained. The splints are not very easy to apply, and are liable to become displaced unless firmly bandaged. The physiotherapist must, therefore, make quite sure that there is no interference with the circulation before letting the child go. When the varus deformity has been completely corrected, the splint is applied as for talipes equinus.

Denis Browne splint, see p. 320 and *Fig.* 145.

A succession of plaster bandages is sometimes applied. These are not suitable for very young babies because of their liability to become soiled, and because their weight tends to immobilize the whole leg.

Various other kinds of supports may be used, ranging from simple 'tin shoes' to specially made metal splints, furnished with pads and straps. Many are hinged on the principle of the Denis Browne splint, so that the position of the foot can be altered as required. If the Denis Browne splint, or similar apparatus, is used, strapping may be dispensed with. The mother should be taught to apply the strapping or splint, so that she can do this at home.

INFANTS FROM 2 MONTHS TO 2 YEARS.—After the age of 2 months, forcible manipulation (wrenching) under anæsthetic is required to effect a reduction. The foot is then maintained in the corrected position by plaster fixation or some form of splint. If plaster is used, it is usually changed every 2 or 3 weeks* and if necessary a better correction obtained. If a splint is worn, passive movements are continued. As soon as the child is old enough, active movements in the desired directions must be encouraged. Later, correct walking is taught.

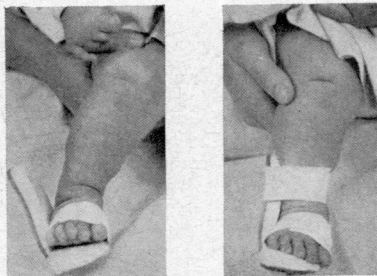

Fig. 144.

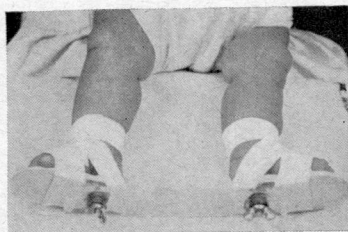

Fig. 145.

Figs. 144–5.—Applying Denis Browne splint to an infant with bilateral talipes equinovarus. First the foot is strapped to the sole-plate, then the leg to the side-plate, and finally the cross-bar is fixed in position. Sometimes a splint similar to that shown in Fig. 145 is used alone. (Reproduced by kind permission from 'Essentials of Orthopaedics' by P. Wiles.)

CHILDREN OVER 2 YEARS OLD.—

SURGICAL TREATMENT.—This is now the only means of obtaining reduction. The operations performed may be: (1) Brockman's operation for division of the contracted structures; (2) Osteotomy for the tarsal bones. This cannot, however, be performed until the child is over 8 years old, as ossification is not sufficiently advanced until then.

Brockman's Operation.—This consists of: (1) Division of the contracted ligaments on the medial side of the sole and foot, and freeing of all structures from the inferior and medial surfaces of the calcaneum: from the head of the talus, and from the navicular and cuneiform bones. The talonavicular joint is opened and the foot fixed in as much correction as is safe. After 2 weeks it is fixed in full eversion. The foot is put in plaster for about 10 to 12 weeks, or supported on an appropriate splint. It may subsequently be necessary to divide the Achilles tendon, and the posterior ligament of the ankle-joint, by means of a tenotomy.

Post-operative treatment: If the child has walked, he is usually allowed to continue walking in plaster, and supervision is required to see that this is as correct as possible. Otherwise little can be done in the way of physical treatment until the plaster is removed. Then massage and passive movements may be given, if required. Active exercises and re-education in walking must, of course, be given. The child

* Different surgeons have different ideas as to the length of time of fixation necessary, and as to replacement of plasters, etc. Physiotherapists must adapt themselves to the methods of the surgeon under whom they are working.

DEFORMITIES OF THE LOWER EXTREMITY 331

will probably require a T-strap and medial iron, with the shoe raised on the outer side, for some time after the removal of the plaster and should wear a splint at night.

Osteotomy.—A wedge of bone may be cut from the tarsal bones on the outer side of the foot (calcaneum, cuboid, and talus) and the talo-navicular and deltoid ligaments divided. The foot is then manipulated into the correct position and kept in plaster for about 6 weeks. This is known as *cuneiform tarsectomy. Dunn's operation* (*see* p. 326) is also used for this condition. *Pending osteotomy it is essential to maintain any correction that has been achieved, and to keep the foot as supple as possible.* During this period the child usually wears an iron and shoe similar to that used after Brockman's operation.

Post-operative treatment will be required as described above. The exact nature of the treatment depends on the operation performed and the physiotherapist should make sure that she knows what was done at the operation, so that she can carry out the surgeon's instructions intelligently.

AFTER-CARE: IMPORTANCE OF SUPERVISION.—Although correction may be obtained in a few months, the patient will need supervision for years, as relapse is not uncommon. He should continue to receive treatment once a week for some months after he appears to be completely cured, and should periodically attend for examination by the surgeon for some years after the operation. The importance of this should be most strongly impressed on the parents, and they should be told to report *at once* if there is the slightest sign of anything wrong with the child's foot or manner of walking. If seen immediately, the relapse can be prevented; if it is neglected, the damage may be irreparable.

In paralytic cases, when all, or nearly all, the muscles acting on the foot and ankle-joints are useless, the surgeon sometimes *arthrodeses* the foot. In such cases re-education in walking will be required post-operatively. The toes should be moved passively, and, possibly, actively, if the intrinsic muscles of the foot are in action, or if any long flexor or extensor has escaped.

Talipes Valgus

The congenital form of this deformity is fairly common; the acquired forms, apart from pes plano-valgus, are rare.

DEFORMITY.—The position of the foot is similar to that seen in ordinary flat-foot (*see Fig.* 132, p. 311). The deformity varies greatly in severity, from a slight limitation of inversion with an abnormal amount of eversion, to a fixed and rigid position of the foot. There is pain under the inner border when the child walks.

PATHOLOGICAL CHANGES.—

CONGENITAL FORM.—The changes are similar to those present in flat-foot (*see* pp. 310–12). Talipes valgus is sometimes complicated by partial or complete absence of the fibula, or some other abnormality of the leg bones.

ACQUIRED FORM.—This is usually caused by paralysis, or bone injuries. Insufficient re-education in walking following a Pott's fracture may sometimes account for it. The changes are as described on pp. 311–12. In the *paralytic form* the tibialis anticus will be paralysed, and other muscles may be involved as well.

Treatment.—

SLIGHT CASES.—The treatment is the same as that for flat-foot or 'weak foot', together with appropriate fixation. A small padded aluminium splint may be applied to the *inner* side of the leg and foot in the case of an infant. *Plaster bandages,* or *adhesive strapping* may also be used.

For treatment of paralytic cases, see ANTERIOR TIBIAL PARALYSIS, p. 259.

SEVERE CASES.—These are treated operatively.

For Congenital Cases.—

a. Without Absence or Defect of Bone.—Tenotomy of the peronei.

b. Very Severe Cases with Absence of Fibula.—(i) Arthrodesis of foot and ankle. (ii) Amputation of the foot (since pain and discomfort are always present).

For Paralytic Cases.—

a. Tendon transference, e.g., of the peroneus brevis to the inner side of the foot.

b. Arthrodesis of the ankle and foot.

c. Dunn's operation (*see* p. 326, footnote).

d. Whitman's operation (*see* p. 325).

Post-operative Treatment.—

1. *After tenotomy* treatment is carried out on the lines described for talipes equinus.

2. *After arthrodesis*: Re-education in walking, no attempt at mobilization being permitted.

3. *After tendon transference*: Passive movement, faradism, and re-education of the peroneus brevis in its new function. Later, re-education in walking will be required.

4. *After Dunn's and Whitman's operations*: See pp. 325, 326.

Talipes calcaneovalgus is uncommon and *talipes calcaneovarus* still more so. *Talipes equinovalgus* is also rare. The changes, symptoms, and treatment may be worked out from those present in the simple varieties. Whitman's operation, or that of Robert Jones, is used for talipes calcaneovalgus.

PES CAVUS

(Hollow or Contracted Foot)

In this condition the *longitudinal arch of the foot is exaggerated*, so that it is abnormally high. This exaggeration of the arch is due to *dropping of the tarsus*, rather than to actual raising of the arch. The condition is usually accompanied by clawed toes. It is generally an acquired deformity, but is sometimes, though rarely, congenital. It may itself be the only deformity, or may accompany talipes, especially in the equinovarus or calcaneal forms.

CAUSES.—The chief causes of the *acquired* form are: (1) *Paralysis or weakness of the lumbricales and interossei muscles* (idiopathic claw-foot, the most common type, which develops during childhood). (2) *Paralysis of the long flexors of the toes*, enabling the foot to be drawn into strong dorsiflexion by the unopposed anterior tibial muscles. The *calcaneum* is directed *upwards* and the *tarsus* is *angulated*. (3) *Boots, shoes, or socks which are too short* and therefore cramp the foot. (4) As already mentioned it may accompany *talipes*.

DEFORMITY AND CHANGES.—In paralytic cases the foot drops slightly at the mid-tarsal joint, as the result of an alteration in the position of the calcaneum or in that of the metatarsal heads. In time the plantar structures become so contracted that the deformity becomes fixed.

Paralysis of the Long Flexors.—The changes are similar to those described for acquired talipes calcaneus (p. 323). The unopposed pull of the anterior tibial muscles raises the anterior part of the calcaneum, and the forefoot drops at the mid-tarsal joint. The *anterior transverse arch* is depressed by the strain put on it, and in time becomes convex. The toes are hyperextended at the metatarsophalangeal joints (claw-foot), partly because of the pull of the long extensors, and partly because of the lowering of the metatarsal heads. The first phalanx points upwards and the distal phalanges become flexed (*Figs.* 146–149).

Paralysis of the Lumbricales and Interossei.—Here the changes occur in reverse order. Normally the lumbricales and interossei act synergically during action of the long flexors, to prevent flexion of the interphalangeal joint during contraction of the long flexors in walking. If this synergic action is lost, the long flexors are unopposed and the toes become clawed. The proximal phalanx exerts pressure on the metatarsal heads, forcing them down. In this way the *transverse arch drops* and the angle of the forefoot is altered, it being, in effect, dropped.

SYMPTOMS.—*Pain* develops in the sole of the foot because of pressure on the metatarsal heads, and may radiate into the dorsum of the foot and up the front of the leg, but this rarely occurs until the age of adolescence. *Corns* may form beneath the metatarsal heads, or over the first phalanx of the toes, and may also become very painful.

Treatment.—Since the pain develops so late, these patients rarely seek treatment during the early stages, so that it is almost always too late for physical treatment, alone, to be of any use.

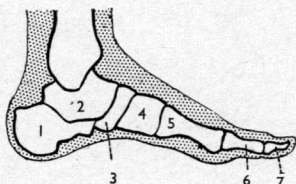

Fig. 146.—Normal foot. 1, Calcaneum; 2, Head of talus; 3, Navicular; 4, 1st cuneiform bone; 5, 1st metatarsal; 6, Proximal phalanx; 7, Distal phalanx.

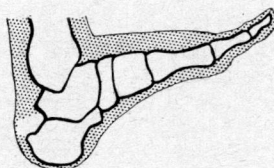

Fig. 147.—Calcaneum raised owing to pull of anterior tibial group. Forefoot unable to reach ground.

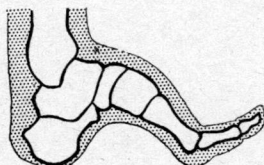

Fig. 148.—Forefoot drops, transverse arch drops with hyperextension of metatarsophalangeal joint. Pes cavus.

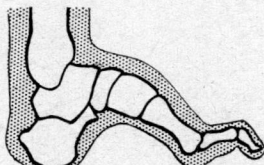

Fig. 149.—Toes become flexed. Pes cavus and claw-foot.

If treated in the early stages, stimulation with the faradic current, and re-education of the intrinsic muscles, may arrest the deformity. Special shoes with sloping soles may also help to correct the deformity.

SURGICAL TREATMENT.—Operative measures are required in severe cases. Among the operations performed are:—

1. FASCIOTOMY.—This consists of division of the plantar fascia and stretching of the foot, with severance of the extensor tendons of the toes if these are contracted. This is followed by fixation for about 3 to 4 weeks, though some surgeons keep the foot immobilized for a longer period. The patient is allowed to weight-bear in the plaster, as this helps to flatten the longitudinal arch.

Post-operative Treatment is carried out on the usual lines. If the scar becomes painful, gentle frictions may be given to the area.

2. STEINDLER'S OPERATION.—This is sometimes used in the more severe cases. It consists of 'stripping' of the whole of the under-surface of the calcaneum, the plantar fascia, the abductores hallucis and minimi digiti, and the flexor brevis

digitorum all being divided.* The foot can then be stretched and the cavus position corrected to the desired extent. Although the immediate results are good there is a tendency for the deformity to recur.

Post-operative Treatment is on the usual lines, consisting of stretching, active exercises, and re-education in walking.

3. LAMBRINUDI'S OPERATION.—This effects a redistribution of muscle power, and consists of arthrodesis of the interphalangeal joints of the toes. This corrects the 'clawing' of the toes, since the long flexors now flex the toes at the metacarpophalangeal joints, and therefore support the metatarsal heads. The functions of the whole foot are improved, and the painful corns and callosities disappear. This operation is contra-indicated if there is dislocation of the metatarsophalangeal joints, or if the long flexors are paralysed.

Post-operative Treatment is as described above, special attention being paid to movements of the metatarsophalangeal joints.

HALLUX VALGUS

A deformity of the great toe, in which the *first metatarsal* is in a position of *abnormal abduction, the phalanges being adducted*. The condition is very often familial, and is usually bilateral.

AETIOLOGY.—

AGE.—Although the defect is present in early life it may not give rise to trouble until middle age or later.

CAUSES.—The primary cause is the varus deformity of the first metatarsal bone but the following may aggravate the conditions: (1) *Badly shaped shoes*. They may be too pointed, too tight, or too short, so that the toe itself may be forced into a valgus position; or the heel may be too high, so that strain is thrown on the first metatarsophalangeal joint, thus enhancing the varus deformity of the first metatarsal, and the valgus position of the toe itself. Often all four faults are combined in one shoe. (2) *Injury or disease*, such as gout or arthritis.

DEFORMITY.†—The toe is in a valgus position, the space between the first and second metatarsal heads being wider than in a normal foot. In some cases the toe lies under or over the second toe. The first metatarsal head becomes prominent forming the well-known 'enlarged joint'. A 'false bursa' forms over it and a painful corn develops on the skin. The whole area is thickened and inflamed and may even suppurate. This enlargement constitutes the condition known as a 'bunion' (*Fig.* 150).

PATHOLOGICAL CHANGES.—Besides the alteration in the position of the bones, arthritic changes occur in the metatarsophalangeal joint. The joint space is increased medially, and decreased laterally, the medial structures becoming *stretched* in consequence, while those on the lateral side are *contracted*. The first phalanx is subluxated, and may even dislocate. The articular cartilage atrophies, and becomes eroded where it no longer contacts bone. New bone is laid down on the inner side of the metatarsal head, leading to the formation of bony 'spurs' (exostoses). The tendon of the extensor longus hallucis is displaced laterally and becomes shortened. Thus it increases the deformity when it pulls on the already displaced second phalanx. The adductor hallucis is also shortened, and there is interference with the intrinsic muscle action because of these changes.

---

* The muscles are divided near their origin on the calcaneum. They slide forward, and become re-attached to the bone in their new position.

† The student should make sure she understands the terminology involved. The first metatarsal is *abducted*, i.e., directed away from the midline of the foot. It is in a *varus position*, i.e., directed towards the midline of the body. The great toe (the phalanges) is *adducted*, i.e., directed towards the midline of the foot and is in a *valgus position*, i.e., directed away from the midline of the body.

The foot becomes everted, and the arch may drop, owing to inadequate support of its anterior pillar.

COMPLICATIONS.—

1. *If pain is present*, a varus position may result, the patient tending to throw his weight onto the outer side of the foot in order to avoid weight on the painful joint.

2. Metatarsalgia may develop as a result of interference with the function of the intrinsic muscles of the foot.

3. The 'bunion' may suppurate.

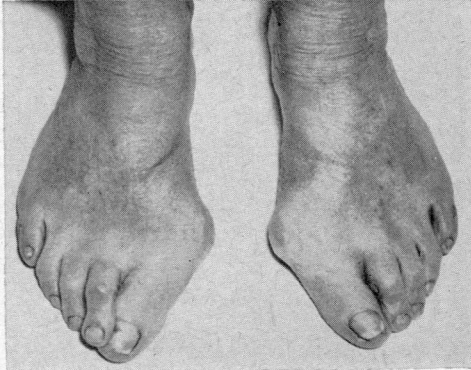

Fig. 150.—Bilateral hallux valgus showing bunion formation. Note enlarged space between 1st and 2nd metatarsal heads. The great toe lies under the second toe on the right foot and a corn has developed on the 1st interphalangeal joint.

Treatment.—

FOOTWEAR AND SUPPORT.—Correct shoes of sufficient size *must* be worn. The inner border should be *straight*, not curved, and the heels must not be too high. Sometimes a valgus wedge (*see* p. 316) is advisable. Various contrivances are advocated to relieve pressure on the bunion, such as a bunion ring or pad. A splint along the inner side of the foot and toe may be worn at night, but it must be so shaped as to avoid pressure on the painful joint. It is, however, doubtful whether this has much effect.

SLIGHT CASES.—These may respond to physical treatment.

Passive movements should be given at least twice a day, and the patient should be taught to do this himself. Particular attention must be paid to abduction of the toe.

Faradic foot-baths may be given, and *active movements*, consisting of flexion, and, if possible, voluntary abduction of the toe, should also be taught. If the foot is weak or flat, appropriate treatment and support must be provided for the arches.

SEVERE CASES.—Most cases are too advanced to be greatly benefited by the above treatment. In these cases operative measures are required.

SURGICAL TREATMENT.—The following operations are most commonly performed: (1) *Arthroplasty*. This consists of removal of the bunion and exostoses, with division of shortened structures, so that the joint can be replaced in the correct position. This operation is only suitable if the function of the foot is good, and very often there is a recurrence. (2) *Keller's operation*. This consists of removal of the proximal two-thirds of the proximal phalanx, together with the bunion and the medial portion of the metatarsal head. (3) *Mayo's operation.* Here the proximal phalanx is untouched, but the metatarsal head is removed together with about five-sixths of the bone. Following these operations the position is usually maintained by means of firm dressings and bandages, but some surgeons apply plaster fixation for 2–3 weeks. In some cases traction is applied by means of a wire through the pulp of the toe.

A palliative measure consists of removal of the 5th metatarsal (Perkins). This in no way affects the joint but by narrowing the foot enables a shoe to be worn in comfort, thus relieving pressure on the bunion.

Post-operative Treatment.—This is usually allowed from about the third day onwards. To begin with it consists of gentle passive movements only, which continue until the stitches are removed (10th–14th day). *Gentle active movements* begin as soon as the stitches are removed, and are progressed to active foot and toe exercises, in sitting, and later in standing, together with re-education in walking. *Faradic foot-baths* may also be given. The patient is usually allowed to take weight on the foot in 2–3 weeks. If the joint becomes hot and swollen the foot must be rested until the inflammation subsides but gentle active movements can usually be continued. If plaster fixation is used, treatment is given within the limits of the plaster until it is removed.

The following operation is sometimes performed if the condition is diagnosed in children. A wedge of bone is dissected from the lateral side of the base of the first metatarsal. It is then re-inserted on the medial side and the toe straightened. Plaster fixation is applied for eight weeks until union occurs. Thereafter, post-operative treatment is given as described above.

HALLUX RIGIDUS AND HALLUX FLEXUS

Hallux rigidus is a condition in which there is partial or complete *limitation of movements of the great toe at the metatarsophalangeal joint.*

CAUSES.—These are not fully understood. It may be due to: (1) *Injury,* e.g., kicking the toe against a stone. (2) *Tight shoes.* (3) *Focal sepsis.*

PATHOLOGICAL CHANGES.—These are very variable. The head of the metatarsal bone may be enlarged, though not to a great extent, and the cartilage bruised or even eroded. The synovial membrane and peri-articular structures may be acutely inflamed, and the cause of much pain, especially in hallux flexus. There may be tenosynovitis of the extensor longus hallucis. In its early stages the muscles are in protective spasm. Later, permanent shortening of soft structures may occur and, finally, osteo-arthritic changes may take place.

DEFORMITY.—The toe may become partially or completely rigid, all extension beyond a straight line being lost. In the latter case the power of flexion is also lost. Sometimes the first phalanx is fixed in a position of *flexion* on the metacarpal bone (hence the name 'hallux *flexus*'), but more often it is in a line with the metacarpal bone. Movement at the interphalangeal joint is usually unimpaired.

SIGNS AND SYMPTOMS.—(1) There is *severe pain* on using the foot and walking is difficult. (2) *The metatarsophalangeal joint is tender,* pressure increasing the pain. (3) There is *spasm and rigidity of the toe.*

Treatment.—This must be commenced at an early stage, before the cartilage erodes and the joint becomes ankylosed. It is designed to rest the foot and relieve pressure and, therefore, spasm.

REST AND RELIEF OF PRESSURE.—Special shoes may be prescribed, designed to relieve the joint of all pressure by the insertion of a 'valgus wedge', together with a 'metatarsal bar'. Sometimes a below-knee plaster is applied.

PHYSICAL TREATMENT.—This consists of re-education of the intrinsic muscles of the foot, and of walking.

SEVERE CASES.—These require operative treatment. This consists of arthroplasty, with removal of the proximal half of the first phalanx. The tendon of the extensor longus hallucis is not divided, since the phalanges are not abducted and there is no displacement.

Post-operative Treatment.—This is the same as for hallux valgus, but the most important movement is *extension*. Re-education in walking is most important, and the patient must be taught to 'push off' with his toes, which entails *extension* of the metacarpophalangeal joint.

HAMMER-TOE

A *contraction of the second toe*, consisting of *extension* of the *first phalanx* and *flexion of the second.*

AETIOLOGY.—(1) This deformity may be *congenital*, and heredity is a marked factor. (2) In the *acquired form*, tight or short shoes are to blame. The second toe, which is most often affected, is often the longest. It is pressed backward and kept in a position of flexion, by too short a shoe. Lateral pressure from one that is too narrow forces the big toe over the others, compressing the last two phalanges of the second toe in particular.

DEFORMITY: CHANGES.—The first phalanx of the toe, as mentioned above, is in extension, the second is flexed; the third may be flexed, extended, or in a straight line with the second.

A *corn* forms over the prominent first interphalangeal joint, and this corn, which may become inflamed, is the most troublesome symptom of the deformity.

The *lateral ligaments* of the joint are *shortened*, holding it in the deformed position. Both the long flexor and extensor tendons are *contracted*, as is the skin underneath the toe.

Treatment.—Correct shoes must be worn, and care must be taken, in the case of growing children, to see that neither shoes nor stockings are too short. The toe requires frequent manipulation, and a small splint may be worn within the shoe, or the toe may be kept flat by strips of adhesive plaster. These are placed *over* the affected toe, and *under* those on either side. The toe should always be splinted at night.

SEVERE CASES.—These require surgery.

SURGICAL TREATMENT.—(1) The toe may be forcibly straightened by manipulation under an anæsthetic. (2) Contracted ligaments and tendons may be divided, with removal of the corn. (3) The first interphalangeal joint may be excised, in order to produce ankylosis. This is usually the method of choice.

Post-operative Treatment.—

If the joint is mobilized passive movements may be given. After simple manipulation they begin at once, active exercises and re-education in walking following in 10–14 days.

If the joint is to be ankylosed no movements must be given until union is firm. Exercises for the other joints of the toe are then begun. The patient is generally allowed to walk soon after the operation, but wears a small toe-splint inside the shoes until the ankylosis is quite firm.

CHAPTER XVI

DEFORMITIES OF THE SPINE

Posture—Postural Deformities—Deformities. I. Anteroposterior curves; II. Lateral curves; III. Principles of Treatment; Kyphosis; Lordosis; Kypholordosis; Sway-back; Flat-back. Scoliosis; Torticollis.

POSTURE

By posture we mean the alinement of the head, neck, shoulders, trunk, pelvis, and limbs. If this is correct an imaginary plumb-line dropped from the side of the head should pass through the middle of the ear, shoulder, hip, knee, and lateral malleolus (*Fig.* 151).

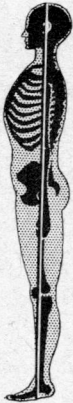

Fig. 151.—Correct posture showing line passing through ear, shoulder, hip, knee, and lateral malleolus.

The Importance of Posture.—Of late years much attention has been given to this very important matter. It has been increasingly realized that bad posture, so common in these days, is responsible not only for actual deformities, with their attendant psychological disabilities, but for many other troubles, particularly those attributable to inadequate abdominal support. Dr. J. Goldthwait* pointed out in this connexion that, although in many adults various adaptations of muscles, ligaments, and bones have taken place as the result of faulty body mechanics, so that complete correction is impossible, yet in almost every case of chronic muscular, neurological, or visceral trouble (other than those definitely due to disease) re-education in correct body mechanics may be expected to effect an improvement, if not a cure, while even in many cases of visceral damage or disease, a certain measure of relief can be obtained by this means.

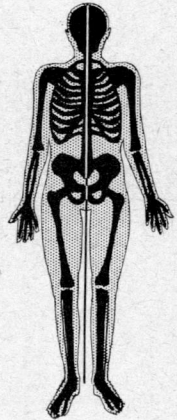

Fig. 152.— Line of gravity.

MECHANICS OF POSTURE.—The line of gravity of the human body is an imaginary line drawn vertically through the centre of the body from the crown of the head to a point between the two feet, on either side of which line the weight is equal (*Fig.* 152). The weight is also equal in front of and behind it (*Fig.* 151). The line represents the direction of the pull of gravity.

If the body is to balance properly and without effort, the line of gravity must fall well within the base, or supporting area—that is, the space occupied by the two feet upon the floor. For perfect balance in the erect position, the line should fall right through the centre of the base.

* *Body Mechanics in the Study and Treatment of Disease.*

If, in inclining the body to the right or to the left, it were simply bent to the side by movement at the intervertebral joints only, the line of gravity would no longer fall within the area covered by the feet, but outside this area on one side or the other. Similarly, if the body were bent forward or backward, either at the hip-joints or at the intervertebral joints, the line of gravity would then fall in front of or behind the base. In none of these positions could the balance of the body be maintained without support. In order to maintain our balance in stoop-standing, arch-standing, or side-arch-standing we have to counteract the effect of moving one part of our body, by moving another part as well. To maintain stoop-standing we fall backward at the ankle-joint, thus the hip and gluteal regions are also carried backwards, the body-weight is redistributed, and balance maintained. In arch-standing the opposite movement takes place at the ankle, and the abdomen and pelvis are carried forwards. In bending to the side we carry the opposite hip outward, e.g., when bending to the right, the left hip moves outwards, producing *abduction* in the right hip, *adduction* in the left (*Fig.* 153).

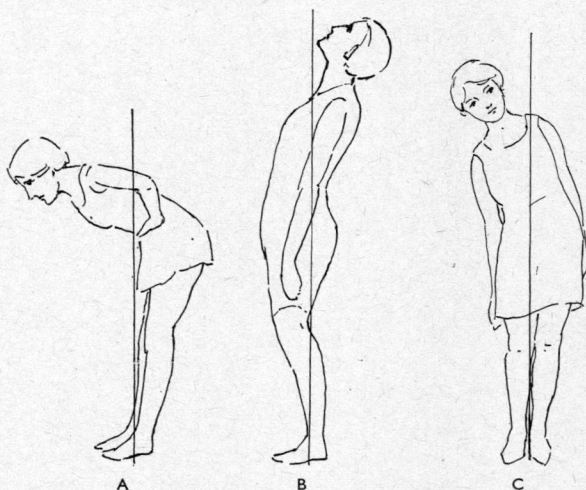

Fig. 153.—Position of line of gravity in bending: A, Forward;
B, Backward; C, Sideways.

MAINTENANCE OF POSTURE.—Normally the body is kept in the correct posture by the beautifully balanced action of opposing muscle groups, and by the efficient working of the nerves which control this type of muscular activity. Such activity is, in effect, an anti-gravity reaction. It is known as *postural tone*, and exists throughout the body. This form of work does not, however, produce fatigue in the same way as do voluntary contractions of the same muscles. If a man be asked to extend his spine, or even his knee, repeatedly, the muscles will soon tire; yet he can remain in a sitting or standing position for a very long time. Although the muscles are in a state of contraction, and although the impulses producing this condition are carried by the same nerves which initiate voluntary movement, the contraction is a *static* (isometric) one, and the stimuli reach the muscle-fibres at a much slower rate—only about 8 or 9 per second, instead of the 50 or so per second required to bring about a *tetanic* (isotonic) contraction. Moreover, each stimulus reaches only a small number of muscle-fibres, one set contracting, and then relaxing as another set contracts, so that no single fibre is in action for long at a time.

Before studying the exact mechanism by which postural tone is maintained it is important that the student should understand the principles governing general muscle tone.

Muscle tone may be described as *a state of awareness of skeletal muscle*, which enables it to respond to motor unit activation. Provided the muscles are in normal connexion with the central nervous system all have tone, and this is brought about by their special sense organs, the *muscle spindles*.

The muscle spindle appears to be suspended longitudinally in the muscle between the normal muscle-fibres (*Fig.* 154 A). The spindle contains special muscle-fibres (*intrafusal fibres*), around each of which are wound special *sensory* nerve-endings (*Fig.* 154 B). Each of these nerve-endings connects to form one

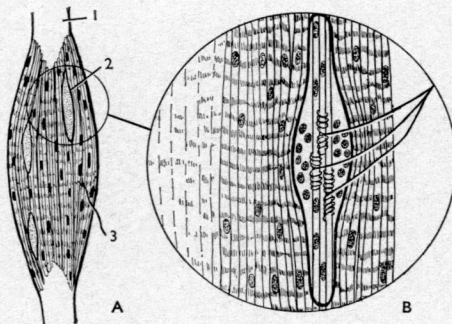

Fig. 154.—A, Position of muscle spindle. 1, Tendon; 2, Spindle; 3, Motor-unit fibre. B, Specialized intrafusal cells and nerve-endings.

afferent nerve-fibre which passes to a posterior root ganglion, whence the afferent impulses may either travel to higher centres, or direct to the anterior horn, thus forming part of the *reflex arc* concerned with muscle tone.

This reflex arc is known as the *servo loop* or *spindle circuit*. From the posterior root ganglion *afferent sensory* fibres connect with the anterior horn. It is now known that two kinds of cell exist in the anterior horn; large anterior horn cells which activate the motor unit, and small *spindle-circuit cells* which activate the intrafusal cells (*Fig.* 155). All influences playing on the large anterior horn cells also play on these small cells.

FUNCTION OF SERVO LOOP.—Because of its position in the muscle, the spindle is acutely sensitive to any alteration in its tension. Just as postural tone represents balance between opposing muscle groups, so *muscle tone represents balance between the motor unit fibres and the intrafusal fibres*, the tension between the two being equalized.

Suppose the muscle is stretched for some reason. This immediately increases the tension in the spindle, and to restore the balance the motor-unit fibres must be brought into contraction. To this end *afferent* impulses ('distress signals') leave the spindle and travel by way of the posterior root ganglion to the *large* (motor-unit) *anterior-horn cells*. *Efferent* stimuli travel thence to the *motor end-plate*, and a contraction ensues. As the muscle-fibres contract the tension on the spindle relaxes, so that a point can soon be reached at which the muscle-fibres have contracted to such a degree that the spindle, instead of regaining its equilibrium, hangs slackly between the contracted fibres. *Afferent* stimuli again leave the intrafusal fibres, but this time they pass from the posterior root ganglion to the *small cells in the anterior horn* (spindle-circuit), and a contraction of the *intrafusal fibres* ensues. In this way muscle tone is maintained, any alteration in tension being instantly recorded and adjusted.

The muscle spindle's sensitivity to stretching is known as the *stretch reflex* and it is of paramount importance in the maintenance of posture. It is also one of the prime factors in proprioceptive neuromuscular facilitation. It should now be possible to see that if the trunk falls slightly forward, the muscle spindles in the glutei and hip extensors will be stretched and their tone will be increased. At the same time, any tendency to overtone will be counteracted by similar activity in the hip flexors.

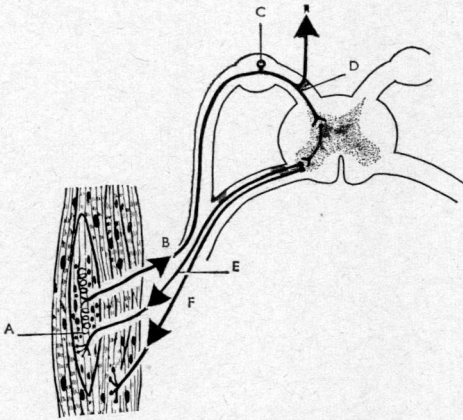

Fig. 155.—A, Spindle with intrafusal cells and fibres; B, Afferent fibre from spindle; C, Posterior root ganglion; D, Nerve loop to large motor-unit cells and spindle-circuit cell; E, Efferent to intrafusal cells; F, Efferent to motor-unit cells.

THE POSTURAL REFLEX.—The mechanism whereby the correct position of the body is maintained, at rest or during activity, is known as the *postural reflex*. It also has a *sensory* (afferent) and a *motor* (efferent) component, like all reflexes. The afferent stimuli reach the brain from the eyes, the labyrinth of the ear (semi-circular canals) the skin, tendons and joints, as well as from the muscles. The position of the head has particular significance in relation to the postural reflex. Afferent stimuli are also received from the cerebellum, particularly with regard to the position of the head in space, and to group action of muscles. Stimuli from muscles and joints and from the skin of the soles of the feet, pass up the fasciculi gracilis and cuneatus to the nuclei of the same name in the medulla. From there most of the conducting fibres cross and go up via the optic thalamus to the cerebral cortex, enabling us to *know* in what position our limbs are. Others, on which the maintenance of postural control really depends, do not reach conscious level, travelling only to the pons or midbrain. Perhaps the most important centre is *Deiters's nucleus* in the pons, which receives labyrinthine stimuli in addition to many others, and which gives rise to the *vestibulospinal tract*. Visual stimuli reach the midbrain, whence *efferent* stimuli travel via the spinotectal tract to the anterior-horn cells. The fascinating subject of the linkage between the various tracts and centres involved in postural control cannot be discussed in detail here, but it is important to remember that the postural reflex is also influenced by the cerebral cortex and corpus striatum (lentiform nucleus), the red nucleus in the midbrain, and the cerebellum. The *afferent* fibres to the latter pass from skin and muscles up the spinocerebellar tracts, being joined by some from the nuclei gracilis and cuneatus; the *efferent* fibres go via the red nucleus and rubrospinal tract to the anterior-horn cells.

POSTURAL DEFORMITIES

Even though we have the means of maintaining balance in any position, to stand with the body bent, even slightly, in any direction, imposes a strain on the muscles on the side from which the bending takes place. This is because the force of gravity, instead of falling through the centre of the body, pulls at an angle on the flexed upper part. The more the body is bent, the greater is the angle of its pull, and the greater the strain on the muscles (*Fig.* 156). If this bend is *fixed* for any reason, the patient will tend to relieve the strain by bending the spine in the opposite direction at a higher or a lower level. In other words, she *compensates*.

These facts have to be borne in mind when considering the causation and development of all postural deformities.

TYPES OF DEFORMITY.—Alteration in posture may occur in an anteroposterior or lateral direction, but it is important to realize that *the reason for either is an alteration in the angle of pelvic tilt away from the normal*; also that *the fault does not necessarily lie in the spine.*

ANTEROPOSTERIOR CURVES.—If, for some reason, a person holds the pelvis tilted forwards, e.g., by keeping both hips fixed in a slightly flexed position, the body assumes a curve with its convexity backward. In order to keep his body upright he compensates by bending his spine backward, thus

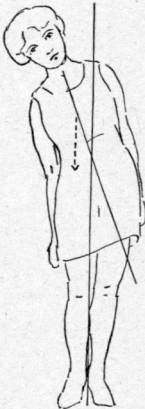

Fig. 156.—Angle of pull of gravity on the flexed spine.

producing a curve with an exaggerated *forward convexity* in the lumbar region (lordosis). This, in its turn, is compensated by a curve with an exaggerated *curve backward* in the thoracic region (kyphosis). Sometimes there may even be a final, exaggerated *forward convexity* in the cervical region (*Fig.* 157). Alternatively, anteroposterior curvatures may begin in the upper part of the spine, producing compensatory curves below them. In all cases of spinal deformity the principal condition is known as the *primary curve*, and subsequent compensatory curves as *secondary curves*.

LATERAL CURVES.—These are known as 'scoliosis' and, again, the trouble need not begin in the vertebral column itself. It may well have its origin in the feet, knees, hips, or even in the arms. If a person has one leg shorter than the other, or if he habitually puts weight on one foot, bending the knee of the leg so that it is relatively *shortened* so long as this position is maintained, the pelvis will be lower on one side. Let us assume that the right leg is shortened in some way. If the spine were kept in its normal relationship to the pelvis, i.e., at right angles, the whole body would be carried over to the right. This constitutes a curve with *the convexity to the left*. To obviate this, and to keep the head in a line with the sacrum and bring the line of gravity back to its median position, the patient compensates by flexing the lumbar spine to the *left*, thus forming a second curve with *its convexity to the right*. This lumbar curve in turn may produce a third (thoracic) curve above it with *its convexity to the right* (*Fig.* 158). As in anterolateral curves the process may take place from above downwards, beginning with the cervical spine or shoulder-girdle.

BODILY TYPES AND POSTURES.—

There is really no 'normal' type of posture, since no two human beings are alike in skeletal, muscular, or neurological make-up; nor do any two people use their bodies in the same way. Generally speaking, individuals may be divided into three main types—the slender, the heavy, and the so-called 'normal' or intermediate—each having its own characteristic make-up.

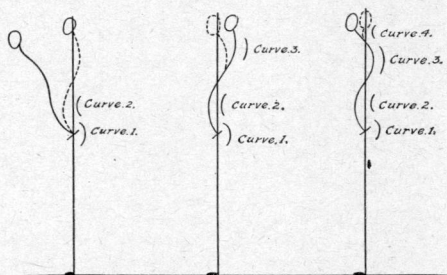

Fig. 157.—Diagram to illustrate development of compensatory curves in kypholordosis. A, Shows flexed hip, with pelvis tilted forward. This constitutes *Curve 1*, with convexity backward. This is compensated by *Curve 2*, hyperextension of lumbar spine (lordosis). B, The lordosis compensated by *Curve 3*, flexion of thoracic spine (kyphosis). C, The kyphosis compensated by *Curve 4*, a curve with convexity forward in cervical region.

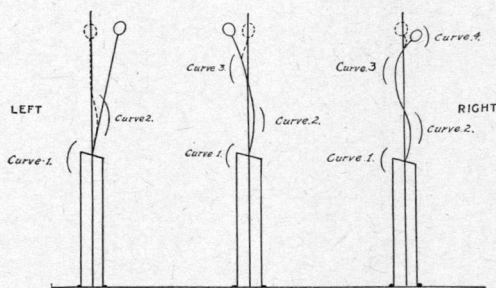

Fig. 158.—Diagram to illustrate development of compensatory curves in scoliosis. A, Shows shortened leg on the *right* side; pelvis tilted downwards on this side. Pelvis and spine at right angles to it constitute *Curve 1*, convex to *left*. This is compensated by *Curve 2*, a lumbar curve convex to *right*. B, The right lumbar curve compensated by *Curve 3*, *left* thoracic. C, The left thoracic curve compensated by *Curve 4*, *right* cervical.

The slender type is most inclined to faulty posture, especially to *lordosis*. The spine of such a patient has a tendency to bend back from its lowest part, the pelvis being tilted forward at the same time, thus forming a forward curve with the maximum convexity in the mid-lumbar region. Following this the compensatory kyphosis develops, the chest droops, the ribs become more vertical, the costal angle is increased, the head is carried forward, and the cervical fascia loses its tension. This may ultimately lead to cramping, and possibly even to displacement of organs, producing visceral disturbances, or aggravating any such troubles if they already exist.

The heavy type also tends to bend backwards, but at the *lumbodorsal junction*, the pelvis thus being tilted backwards. People of this kind tend to develop kyphosis and rigidity of the thorax. Lordosis is uncommon in this type.

The intermediate type varies according to which of the others it most nearly approaches. The spine may bend back at a point between those characteristic of the other two types.★

Because of these varieties in postural types, the characteristic physical make-up of each patient should be taken into consideration when assessing his or her special disability.

DEGREES OF DEFORMITY.—These may be *postural* (Arvedson's 'first degree curves') or *structural* (Arvedson's 'third degree curves'). In the *postural* curves, occurring in children and young people, there is no bony change: there may not even be muscular weakness. There *is* a defective postural reflex, and in many cases there is also a psychological or nervous factor. Any form of nervous disturbance or imbalance, in greater or less degree, may cause faulty posture in children, adolescents, and adults, and in such cases, unless the psychological condition is set right, it is unlikely that we shall fully correct the postural defect. This only applies, however, to defects complicated by psychological factors.

The structural curves.—It used at one time to be assumed that all, or almost all, postural defects would, if neglected, develop into structural ones. It is, however, probably only very rarely that this occurs, but this is no reason for neglecting such postural cases, or failing to keep them under supervision. In such postural curves as do become structural there would appear to be a *transition stage* between the two, when some degree of alteration has only taken place in the length of soft structures (muscles and ligaments), the bones not yet being affected. At this stage treatment can be of great value.

Serious structural curves have other causes than mere faulty posture or nervous upset. They may be due to unilateral lung disease, tuberculosis, paralysis, etc., or the cause may be unknown, as in idiopathic scoliosis. In structural cases, the bony changes may be slight (Arvedson's 'second degree') or serious (Arvedson's 'third degree').

I. ANTEROPOSTERIOR CURVES

The Pelvic Tilt.—As already mentioned, these deformities usually depend on the increase, or decrease, of the pelvic tilt beyond the normal, which, in its turn, depends on a general laxity of the muscles controlling the pelvis, namely, the *glutei* and the *abdominals*. The normal inclination of the pelvis is about 30°, and at such an angle the anterior superior iliac spines are on the same vertical plane as the symphysis pubis. In conditions in which the pelvis is tilted *forward*, the inclination is *increased* to about 40°, while in those in which the pelvis is tilted *backward* the inclination is *decreased* to about 20°. This can be measured by an instrument called an inclinometer.† The deformities are produced by the patient's attempt to keep the centre of gravity above the feet, and there are four varieties of anteposterior deformity.

VARIETIES.—(1) *Kyphosis*; (2) *Lordosis*; (3) *Sway-back*; (4) *Flat-back*.

1. In *kyphosis*, or 'round-back', the vertebral column is bent forward in the lower lumbar region to compensate for the *backward pelvic tilt*. This eliminates the normal lumbar concavity, and leads to the formation of a *long curve with its convexity backwards*. This may also include the cervical region although the

---

★ Besides Dr. Goldthwait's book, the student is advised to read two pamphlets by Dr. Armin Klein: *Posture Clinics* and *Posture Exercises*, published by the U.S. Department of Labor; also Philip Wiles, *Essentials of Orthopædics*, Chapter I, and John Colson, *Postural and Relaxation Training*.

† For a description of this instrument and explanation of its use, *see* Philip Wiles, *Essentials of Orthopædics*, Chapter I.

maximum convexity is in the thoracic region. The legs are inclined slightly backwards at the ankles, and the *line of gravity falls in front of the hip-joints.* A second type is also described, in which the legs are inclined forwards and the trunk is bent backwards, causing a sharp angle in the lower lumbar region, the line of gravity falling behind the hip-joints. The student should not confuse this type of curve with sway-back, which it resembles in appearance (*see below*). Kyphosis is invariably accompanied by '*round shoulders*', while other signs of defective postural reflex are often present—for example, inwardly rotated hips and flat-foot.

2. In *lordosis,* or 'hollow-back', the *pelvis is tilted forward.* The patient compensates by bending backwards in the lumbar region, thus *increasing the normal lumbar curve.* A compensatory kyphosis may develop above this level though it is often not very marked. Such a deformity constitutes *kypholordosis.*

3. In *sway-back,* the *pelvis* is again *tilted forward,* but the patient, instead of compensating by means of a lordosis, *bends the spine sharply backward at the lumbosacral angle.* There is often an existing thoracolumbar kyphosis which, however slight, precludes compensation by lordosis. The legs are inclined slightly forward at the ankle-joints, so that the pelvis projects forward, and *the line of gravity falls behind the hip-joints.*

4. In *flat-back,* the *pelvis is tilted backward* to 20°, and the normal lumbar lordosis is flattened out. Both *lumbar* and *thoracic curves* are, in fact, *diminished,* and the spine is often nearly straight.

II. LATERAL CURVES

These consist of: (1) *Scoliosis*; and (2) *Torticollis.* The latter, though not strictly a spinal deformity, may end by producing one.

SCOLIOSIS

By the term *scoliosis* is meant a bending of the vertebral column to one side combined with *rotation of the bodies of the vertebræ towards the convexity* of the curve, the *spinous processing being directed towards the concavity.* Apart from the infantile idiopathic form (*see below*), it is more common in girls than in boys.

Children of school age are most liable to develop scoliosis and the school medical services now provide regular inspections of children's backs. In many cases a cure can be obtained by detecting the curvature at its very beginning, and severe structural curves, once common, are now rare. A slight curve developed in childhood or adolescence may remain stationary or right itself and cause no further trouble, and many adults have slight curves without being aware of the fact but this should not provide an excuse for the neglect of scoliosis in children or young people. Idiopathic scoliosis does not clear up of itself, and will certainly get worse unless adequately treated.

Any pathological condition which is at the root of the trouble must be dealt with, medically, surgically, or by physical measures. Most forms can be dealt with by exercises, but in certain cases supports for the back may be necessary. All cases of scoliosis should be thoroughly examined before treatment is begun.

VARIETIES.—The varieties of scoliosis may be classified as follows:—

1. SIMPLE CURVES, consisting of a single curve in one direction only; (*a*) *Cervical*: (*b*) *Thoracic*: (*c*) *Thoracolumbar,* a single curve including the lower thoracic and upper lumbar regions, with its maximum convexity at the eleventh or twelfth thoracic vertebra: (*d*) *Lumbar*: (*e*) *Long* C curve, involving the whole, or a large part, of the spine (*Fig.* 159 A). The simple curves are generally—though not always—postural, since as soon as a simple curve becomes fixed, it usually compensates above or below.

2. COMPOUND CURVES, consisting of two or more curves in different directions. Thus we may have: (*a*) *Double curves* (S curves), e.g., left cervical and right thoracic; or right thoracic and left lumbar (*Fig.* 159 B); (*b*) *Triple curves*, e.g., left lumbar; (*c*) *Quadruple curves* (rare), which consist of four curves distributed over the three regions of the spine.

CLASSIFICATION AND CAUSES.—As regards their cause, cases of scoliosis may be divided into two classes—*primary* and *secondary*.

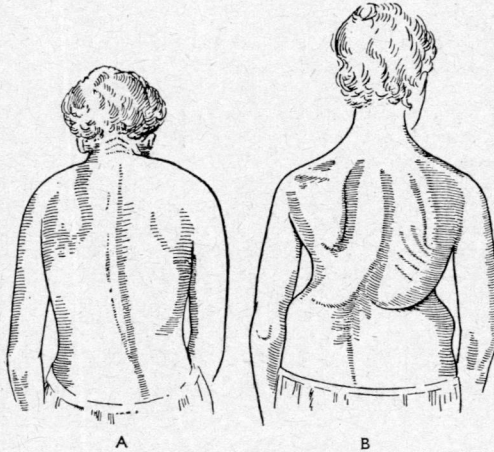

Fig. 159.—A, Scoliosis. Long C curve; B, Scoliosis. S curve.

1. PRIMARY SCOLIOSIS arises spontaneously, not as the result of any previous known disability. It may be due: (1) To some deficiency of the postural mechanism, or to general muscular weakness. This is the *postural*, or 'first degree' type (which may—but usually does not—develop into a structural scoliosis); or (2) It may be due to a quite unknown cause. This is known as *Idiopathic Scoliosis*, which accounts for most of the structural curves other than those caused by other diseases or injuries.

Idiopathic Scoliosis.—There are two groups, *infantile* and *adolescent*.

Infantile idiopathic scoliosis (*Figs.* 153 and 160) is generally noticed during the baby's first year, especially if the curve is thoracic. It is commoner in boys than in girls. The curve is usually convex to the left. It is slowly, but inexorably, progressive, and may be very severe by the time the patient is adolescent. Even so, *pain* rarely occurs until the patient is middle-aged, when *backache* may be severe. There may be surprisingly little interference with *function*, even when the deformity is marked.

Adolescent idiopathic scoliosis: This is the commoner form, occurring between the ages of ten and fifteen years. Girls are affected much more frequently than boys. The curve is generally convex to the right.

Thoracic curves have the worst prognosis. They develop more quickly, especially if they first appear before the age of twelve, and the final deformity is more severe than in any other region. *Lumbar* and *thoracolumbar* curves compensate well, are far less noticeable, and do not interfere with function. *Compound* (S) curves may be fairly severe, especially if the thoracic is the primary curve, but, since the curves compensate each other, the deformity may not be very obvious when the patient is dressed. She will, of course, lose height.

2. SECONDARY SCOLIOSIS is the result of some previously existing deformity or disease. Some of the commonest causes are as follows:—

i. *Deformities in other Parts of the Body (Compensatory Scoliosis).*—The curve may be compensatory to other deformities of neck, arm, leg, or trunk—especially to any which cause the lower extremities to be of unequal length. These deformities may be congenital, paralytic, rachitic, or static.

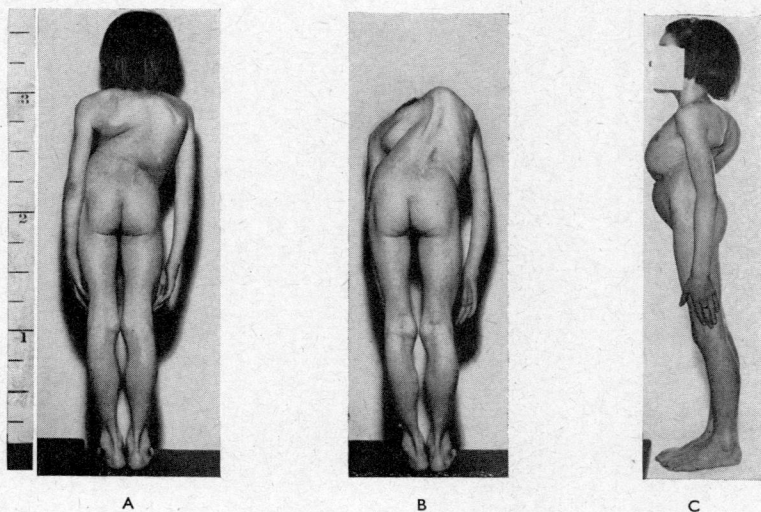

Fig. 160.—Gross idiopathic scoliosis: A, Right dorsal, left lumbar curves. Note exaggeration of deformity, particularly rotation and lateral deviation of vertebræ and bulging of thorax. Trunk displaced to right, but there is no inclination of the pelvis. The buttocks are level and the weight is taken equally on both legs. B, Same patient in flexion. Deformity markedly increased. Note dorsal kyphos and pull of subcutaneous tissues. C, Same patient, lateral view. Note gross deformity of thorax in anteroposterior plane. Sharply defined vertebral border of left scapula and flattening of ribs on left. Dorsal kyphos formed by posterior angles of right ribs. Increased lumbar lordosis and 'pot-belly'.

ii. *Tuberculous Disease of the Hip.*—If the hip is shortened by being fixed in *flexion* only, the convexity of the curve is to the side of the *shortened* leg, the pelvis being lower on this side. If, however, the hip is also *adducted*, the convexity is towards the *sound* side because the patient, in trying to get the affected leg to the vertical position, raises the pelvis on this side (since no movement can take place in the hip-joint), walking on the toes of this foot (*Fig.* 161).

iii. *Unilateral Paralysis of Abdominals, Back Muscles, or Ilio-psoas*, the concavity of the curve being toward the healthy side, owing to the unopposed pull of the normal muscles.

iv. *Injuries to the Spine.*

v. *Unilateral Lung Disease* (pleurisy, empyema, etc.) in which either one side of the thorax is bound down by adhesions, or else one lung has collapsed altogether. This may produce a curve *convex* either to the sound or to the affected side (*see* p. 395). The same thing may occur following thoracic surgery.

iv. *Congenital Causes.*—There is a form of congenital scoliosis due to malformation of some of the vertebræ.

vii. *Hysteria.*—Hysterical scoliosis is occasionally seen.

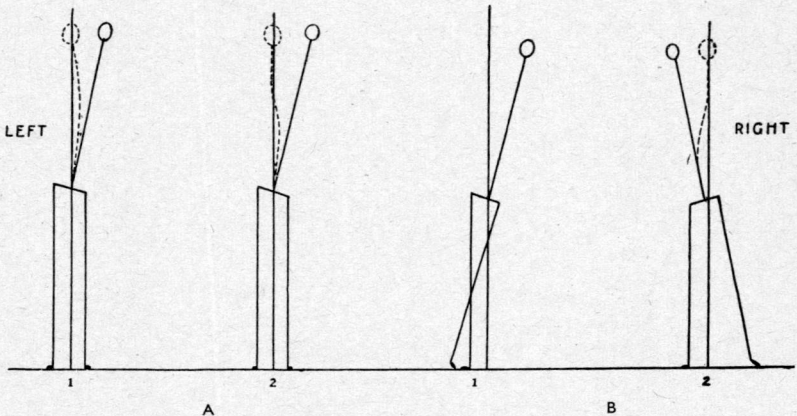

Fig. 161.—Diagram to illustrate scoliosis resulting from tuberculous disease of the hip.
A, Right hip fixed in flexion only. The result is a long C curve convex to the *right* (1) or a
simple lumbar curve in the same direction (2). B, Right hip fixed in flexion and adduction
(1). The result is a lumbar (or long C) curve convex to the *left* (2).

EXAMINATION OF A CASE OF SCOLIOSIS.—The patient, suitably undressed,* should be placed in a good light with her back to a window. The
whole of the back should be visible to the examiner. She should stand with the
feet a little apart and the feet and legs should be bare.

The physiotherapist should wait a few minutes before beginning her examination, to give the patient time to assume her natural posture. The patient should
not be told to 'stand straight'.

The following points should be carefully noted:—

1. THE FEET.—Look for signs of *flat-foot, or any other deformity* of foot or toes.
Note if unilateral or bilateral.

2. THE LEGS AND KNEES.—Look for signs of *bow legs, genu valgum,* or *varum,*
etc.

3. THE HIPS.—Look for *coxa vara,* or signs of *fixed flexion* or *adduction* of either
hip. Notice if there is any *wasting of muscles* in leg, thigh, or buttock. This may
point to a slight attack of paralysis in the past. Notice also if the hips are internally
rotated and whether or not the patellæ look straight forward.

4. THE PELVIS.—

a. See if the pelvis is *tilted laterally.* This suggests a difference in the length of
the legs. Note this, and measure later.

b. Look for *rotation* of the pelvis, often present in a lumbar curve. The hip
may be rotated forward, either on the side of the convexity or on that of the

---

* Little girls, especially those of a shy and nervous temperament, often become acutely
uncomfortable and upset if required to stand up before others in a minimum of clothing. This
makes it impossible for the physiotherapist to discover what her ordinary posture is, as she will
stand stiffly with her muscles in contraction. Shorts or knickers, and a special garment covering
the chest but leaving the back exposed, are suitable for purposes of examination.

concavity. This depends on the position of the last lumbar vertebra and of the sacrum. If they form part of *the existing lumbar curve, the pelvis will be rotated forward on the side of the concavity*; if they form the beginning *of a compensatory curve, the hip will be forward on the side of the convexity*. If the curve ends with the fourth vertebra and there is no compensatory curve below, the pelvis will be normal in position.

5. THE LUMBAR REGION.—Notice:—

a. Any obvious signs of *lateral deviation*.

b. The comparative prominence of the iliac crests. That on the concave side will *appear* the higher, because the soft structures are drawn away from that side.

c. The width of the back on the two sides of the spine. It will sometimes appear wider on the concave side.

d. The contour of the body at the waist-line; the angle is accentuated on the concave side, decreased or obliterated on the convex.

6. THE THORACIC REGION (*Figs.* 162–3). Notice:—

a. Any obvious signs of *lateral deviation*.

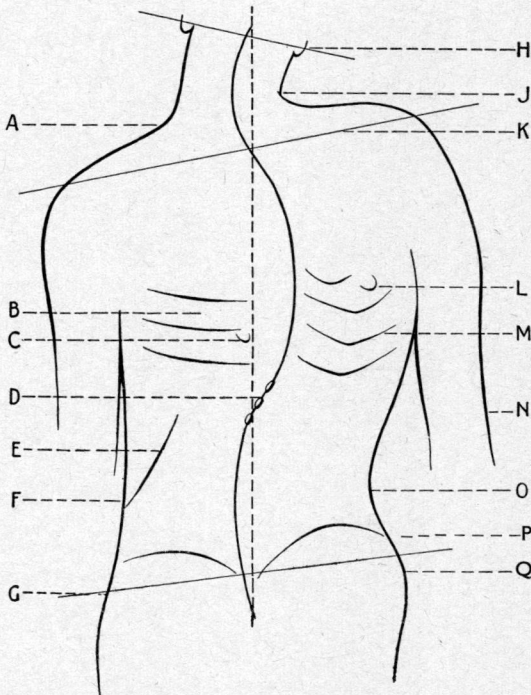

Fig. 162.—Examination for scoliosis.—A, Angle of neck and shoulder increased; B, Flattened ribs on thoracic concavity; C, Position of inferior angle of scapula; D, Prominent vertebra at the junction of the two curves; E, Fold of flesh following line of thoracic concavity; F, Angle at waist obliterated; G, Inclination of pelvis; H, Level of ears; J, Angle of neck and shoulder decreased; K, Level of shoulders; L, Position of inferior angle of scapula; M, Bulging ribs on thoracic convexity; N, Position of arm, denoting displacement of trunk to side of thoracic convexity; O, Angle at waist accentuated; P, Iliac crest raised on side of concavity; Q, Prominent hip on side of concavity.

b. The *relative level* of the shoulders; that on the *convex* side is *higher,* unless there is a marked cervical curve in the opposite direction.

c. The *contour of the ribs,* which bulge *backward* on the *convexity* of the curve, and are *flattened* on its *concavity.*

d. The relative position of the scapulæ, as regards their height, rotation, and distance from the vertebral column. On the side of the *convexity of a thoracic curve,* the *scapula is raised* and its *inferior angle rotated out.* It lies farther from the vertical column than it would if the spine were normal, since it slips

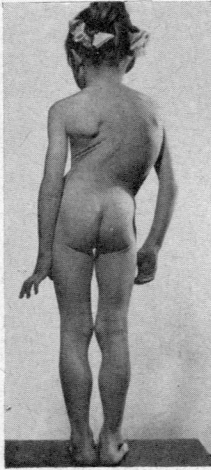 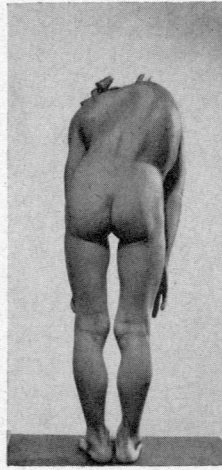

Fig. 163 A   Fig. 163 B

Fig. 163 A.—Right dorsal, left lumbar scoliosis. This demonstrates points in *Fig.* 162. As yet cervical curve not marked. In addition note difference in level of buttocks (pelvic tilt); rotation of pelvis (left hip forward, denoting compensatory nature of lumbar curve); tendency to bow legs (more pronounced on left); medial displacement of tendo Achillis (more marked on left); weight taken on right leg; varus position of forefoot (big toe does not contact ground).

Fig. 163 B.—Same patient in flexion. Note that lateral deviation and rotation of vertebræ more pronounced, also bulging of ribs on side of convexity. Pelvic tilt has corrected to a certain degree but rotation more pronounced. Space increased between thighs and knees. Weight has shifted to left leg and varus position of forefoot now seen on right foot.

outwards over the sharply bent angles of the ribs. The scapula on the concave side is lower, lying vertically, and closer than normal to the vertebral column, having been carried inwards over the flattened ribs.

e. The width of the back. The back appears wider on the convex side owing to the bulging ribs.

f. Folds in the flesh of the back. In an S curve a fold is seen passing upwards from the region of the waist, and following the line of the thoracic concavity.

7. CERVICAL REGION.—The following points should be noted:—

a. *The position of the head,* and the *contours* of the two sides *of the neck.* In a cervical curve, the angle between neck and shoulder is *increased* on the *convex* side, *decreased* on the *concave* side.

b. The relative level of the ears.

8. ANY PROMINENCE OF THE VERTEBRÆ in any region should be noted. They often appear prominent at the junction of two curves.

9. DISPLACEMENT OF THE TRUNK.—Notice whether one arm hangs farther away from the body than the other, and whether the whole body is carried over to one side. This is most markedly so in fixed thoracic curves, when the whole trunk is displaced towards the side of the convexity.

10. ACCOMPANYING KYPHOSIS OR LORDOSIS should be noted.

11. EXAMINATION OF THE WHOLE SPINE IN FLEXION.—For this the patient is asked to bend forward with the back rounded, the arms hanging loosely, and the head down. The physiotherapist stands in front of her, and looks along the spine. The *lateral deviation* and the *rotation of the vertebræ* are much more obvious in this position. (This may form the first part of the examination in order to get a general idea of the nature of the curve or curves.)

12. THE FRONT OF THE THORAX.—

a. Notice if the bulging of the ribs on one side, and the flattening on the other, correspond to the deformity observed when examining the back.

b. Watch the patient's breathing, and note any peculiarity.

PALPATION AND MEASUREMENTS.—First place the patient on a plinth in the prone position and feel for any tender spots in the muscles, especially on the side of the convexity. Press each vertebra and see if any pain is caused anywhere by the pressure. If so, mark the vertebra and report it to the doctor.

Now place the patient in the supine position.

1. VERIFY THE ROTATION OF THE PELVIS by measuring the distance between the umbilicus and the anterior superior spine on either side. (This is not an *entirely* reliable test, as the umbilicus is not always exactly in the midline.)

2. MEASURE THE LENGTH OF THE LEGS.—The measurement may be taken from the anterior superior spine to the medial malleolus, or from the great trochanter to the external malleolus. The latter gives the actual length of the leg from the great trochanter downwards, but would not show such differences in length as would be occasioned by abnormalities of the neck of the femur, such as coxa vara; or of the hip-joint, such as tuberculosis or congenital dislocation. The former measurement is therefore the more reliable.

TESTS FOR MOBILITY.*—

1. Let the patient bend forward in the flexed position, and then to both sides, noting any limitation of movement.

2. Place her in the head-suspension apparatus, if one is available, and see if the curve is partially or completely obliterated.

3. If the curve proves mobile, test the patient's ability to correct her own position.

I. Postural Curves (First Degree)

These cases are treated on the same principle as any other postural deformities, the *aims* being *to re-educate the patient's postural sense, to restore muscle tone* on both sides of the back, and *to obtain relaxation* in tense patients (*see below*).

Relaxation will follow the same lines as that described for kyphosis.

Postural Correction.—As in any postural deformity the patient must first be taught to correct her posture in simple lying, sitting, and standing positions, and she must practise this until she regains the *feeling* of correct posture. Thus she learns to assume, and deliberately keep, a good posture until its maintenance becomes automatic. It is better to begin with passive correction, the physiotherapist putting the patient into the correct attitude—straightening the pelvis (this *must* be the first step), pressing down the high shoulder, correcting the spine on one side or the other—and then asking the patient to hold it for

* For further details, *see* E. M. Prosser, *Manual of Massage and Movements.*

a few seconds. Later the patient must learn to correct her posture by means of *verbal instructions*.

Exercises.—Most of the exercises should be double-sided. They should be free and resisted. The former, being more natural and spontaneous, will assist mobility, but resistance is needed to strengthen the muscles. It is sometimes forgotten that the muscles on the posterior aspect of the body are not the only ones acting on the spine. The abdominal muscles are equally important, both as flexors and side-flexors. Abdominal contractions should be practised, and, indeed, most 'straight' abdominal exercises are useful, provided that they are not too strong. *Alternate* side-bendings should also be included as should arm and leg exercises and, of course, breathing exercises. In fact, *the body as a whole should be treated* and all its muscles exercised. *Mobility exercises*, as such, are rarely necessary, but it is as well to include a few, in order to prevent the development of any stiffness.

II. Structural Curves (Second Degree)

(i.e., *Moderately Severe Curves*)

PATHOLOGICAL CHANGES.—

MUSCULAR AND LIGAMENTOUS CHANGES.—There is *stretching* of all structures *on the convex side* and *shortening* of all those *on the concave side* of the curve.

BONY CHANGES.—These are present in varying degrees in all structural curves. It must be remembered that the *bending of the spine in scoliosis is always accompanied by rotation of the bodies of the vertebræ towards the convexity of the curve*; the more marked the curve, the greater the rotation (*Fig.* 164).

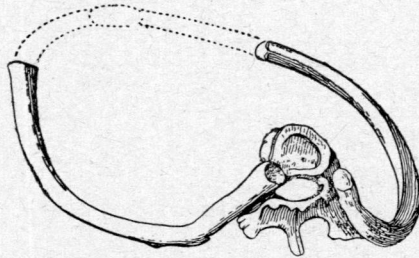

Fig. 164.—Horizontal scheme of vertebræ and ribs in scoliosis.

Changes in the Vertebræ.—

The vertebral bodies become wedge-shaped owing to constant pressure on them on the side of the concavity.

The pedicles on the *convex* side become more *anteroposterior* in direction than is normal; those on the *concave* side are more *transverse* in direction and, being compressed, become smaller than is normal.

The laminæ on the *convexity* of the curve lie more *transversely* than is normal and those on the side of the *concavity* in a more *anteroposterior* direction but they are not much altered in shape.

The transverse processes are also altered in direction, those on the *convex* side being more *anteroposterior*, those on the *concave* side more *transverse* in direction. Those on the convexity of the curve are carried farther backward than their fellows and therefore lie closer to the spinous processes.

The spinous processes are less altered in position than the bodies, or any other part of the vertebræ. These processes may be almost, or entirely, in the midline, so that the severity of the curve may not be apparent from their position. They are, however, generally curved in such a way that the tip points to the convex side.

The articular processes may become ankylosed with those above and below.

Changes in the Ribs and Thorax.—The ribs on the side of the convexity of a thoracic curve become more sharply bent at their angles, and *bulge backwards*, owing to the rotation of the vertebral bodies to that side; also, they slope downward more vertically. There is a flattening of the angles on the concave side, and the ribs are more horizontal in direction. At the foot of the thorax, there is a compensatory flattening of the ribs on the side of the convexity, and a bulging on the side of the concavity. This produces what is known as the 'diagonal thorax' (*Fig. 164*).

Changes in the Pelvis.—In lumbar curves, rotation of the pelvis may similarly cause a 'diagonal pelvis'.

THE VISCERA.—In severe cases there may be pressure on, or displacement of, thoracic, abdominal, or pelvic organs.

EXERCISES FOR MOBILITY.*—When a patient with scoliosis of this degree first comes for treatment it must be directed towards mobilizing the spine as much as possible within the limits of the structural change. For the first month or more, therefore, many of the exercises will be directed to the attainment of this result. Hanging in head-suspension apparatus is sometimes used, head or trunk rolling being used according to whether it is designed to mobilize a cervical, thoracic, or lumbar curve. Treatment continues as described above for first degree curves.

III. Structural Curves (Third Degree)

(i.e., *Very Severe Curves*)

Treatment is much the same as for the 'second degree' types, but far less improvement can be expected.

SUPPORT.—At this stage, the patient may possibly be provided with some kind of plaster jacket, which may be succeeded by some form of removable support strengthened by steel bands, but surgical treatment is more usual nowadays.

SURGICAL TREATMENT; OPERATIVE FUSION OF VERTEBRÆ.—This is performed in order to prevent the deformity from increasing, and to relieve the patient from having to wear supports for the rest of her life. The curve is corrected as much as possible by manipulation or plaster jackets, and the necessary number of vertebræ are fused by arthrodeses of their posterior articulations, and by bone-grafts from the tibia applied along the sides of the spinous process. Thus no further bending or rotation can take place in this area. A plaster support is worn for 6 to 18 months. The operation is not as a rule performed on children. Careful postural training should follow the removal of the support.

PRINCIPLES OF TREATMENT

I. POSTURAL OR FIRST DEGREE CASES

General Principles.—

1. The general health must receive attention, since poor health is often either the cause or the effect of the deformity. Any predisposing causes will be treated by the physician or surgeon, and any psychological factors must receive attention.

---

* *General strengthening of muscles and postural re-education* should accompany, or even precede, any definite attempts to restore mobility. In certain cases, "to mobilize a rigid curve before building up the muscles is to court disaster" (Forrester-Brown), since, if the muscles cannot support the spine, and the patient has no idea of the correct position, the greater the mobility the greater the danger.

12

Rest is also an important factor since fatigue is at the root of many cases of postural deformity in all age-groups.

2. The patient's *habitual posture* must be corrected, and those in charge of a child should be made to understand the importance of this.

Physical Treatment.—The aims of physical treatment in any postural deformity are as follows: (1) *To correct the deformity* and habitual posture, and *to re-educate postural sense*; (2) *To stretch any tightened structures*; (3) *To strengthen the muscles concerned in postural control* so that they can maintain the corrected position; (4) *To improve ventilation*—this is particularly important in kyphosis and scoliosis. With regard to the deformity it will be appreciated that the amount of correction possible will depend on the degree of deformity and its cause.

Heat and massage are not usually given unless there is pain, in which case effleurage, kneading, and frictions may be given as for any case of backache. Unaccustomed exercise may lead to an accumulation of fatigue products which give rise to backache, particularly if the muscles are weak, and this may enhance the postural defect.

RELAXATION.—In many children and adolescents, the muscles are in a state of tension, and no permanent postural correction can be hoped for, unless relaxation is first obtained. 'Shortened' muscles are often merely muscles in a state of tension. If they are 'passively stretched', they may respond by increased contraction, the stretch reflex having been evoked. There are various methods of reducing this state of overtone, whether by attempting to relax the whole body, or by relaxation of some specially tense group of muscles.

1. *Total relaxation* may be achieved by laying the patient in a comfortable position, e.g., lying (or crook-lying), half-lying, prone-lying, or side-lying, with the body supported, where necessary, by pillows. Relaxation is then taught in the usual way. Another way of achieving total relaxation is by use of the Guthrie-Smith suspension apparatus.

2. *Local relaxation* need not necessarily be taught in lying, though it is generally best for the patient to practise first in this position. The patient is required to contract the affected muscles fully, and then 'let go'.

POSTURAL CORRECTION.—*This is the most important part of the whole treatment*—more important even than teaching exercises designed to strengthen the back muscles, *since a defective postural sense, rather than muscular deficiency, is at the root of the trouble.* It should begin as soon as relaxation is achieved. The first step in postural correction is to make the patient *appreciate postural sense*, so that she can feel the difference between right and wrong. This is often best achieved by starting with passive correction, the physiotherapist putting the patient into the correct position. This must begin from the pelvis, since the position of the pelvis governs posture. Any deviation from normal, however slight, must be corrected and care must be taken to see that the knees and feet are kept in the mid-position throughout. Next, the shoulder-girdle must be brought into alinement with the pelvis, and finally the head is brought into line with the rest of the body. This corrected position will feel strange to the patient who will be convinced that the new position is wrong, and in this way an awareness of postural sense is created. To emphasize this awareness, the patient should be allowed to adopt her former posture, and then be corrected passively again, or asked to attempt active correction for herself, any deficiencies being made good by passive correction. When the feeling of correct posture has been absorbed the patient must begin to learn *postural control*. At this stage mirrors are invaluable aids. At first verbal instructions are helpful, e.g., 'Tuck your tail in', 'Lower your shoulder', 'Draw in here' (indicating the muscle group), but in time the patient must be able to correct herself without directions, and this self-correction must be constantly practised. Having achieved simple postural control, movements must be performed in the correct posture until its maintenance becomes habitual and automatic, that is, until the postural reflex is fully re-established.

EXERCISES.—Here a difference of opinion exists. Some believe that treatment should be based on Dr. Arvedson's methods of treatment of deformities, i.e., the strengthening of particular weak and stretched muscle groups by means of resisted exercises, as well as the stretching of their shortened antagonists by so-called 'passive movement' (the latter really being a form of *forced* movement), and that besides special exercises for specific muscle groups, mobility exercises, balance, and breathing exercises should be included. Others feel that all the exercises should be free.

Mobility Exercises.—If there is any real stiffness of spine or shoulders, these should be added. They should consist of rhythmic swinging movements, head and trunk rollings, active side-bendings, and rotations. Even if there is no actual shortening, these movements promote relaxation of the tense muscles by reciprocal innervation. Whether or not passive (forced) stretchings should be given is a matter of opinion, but it is perhaps better to rely on mobilizing exercises rather than to risk the possibility of increasing the tendency to contracture by initiating a stretch reflex through passive movement.

Balance Exercises.—These may include such exercises as:—
1. Marching with a book on the head.
2. Marching with a stick held behind the head (arms in heave-grasp position).
3. Balance walking on the balancing form or boom.

Breathing Exercises are needed to stretch the pectorals, expand the chest, and increase the range of respiration. The emphasis should therefore be on inspiratory movements.

POSTURAL TREATMENT BY FREE EXERCISES ONLY.—Many people now believe that it is more satisfactory, on the whole, to treat these cases by free rather than by resisted exercises. It is felt that the posture of the body *as a whole* needs attention, rather than any single muscle group, since, as has been emphasized above, the trouble is caused as a rule not so much by definite muscle weakness as by some defect in the postural reflex. If the exercises are to be free, class-work can be employed, but it is advisable, if possible, to treat children in *small classes*, so that they may have the stimulus of each other's presence, and of movements carried out in harmony with others, but can receive at the same time a due share of the physiotherapist's attention. Class-work has the advantage that rhythm, activity, and marching and running exercises will stimulate children, and music may well be used as an auxiliary. Time can also be saved in a busy department, *but it should be emphasized that bad posture must be carefully corrected throughout the treatment.*

Exercises designed to increase, or to preserve, mobility of the spine and thorax, and to correct the posture of the head, back, and shoulders will, of course, be a special feature of the table. (*See* Chapter XXIII for Children's Classes.) Ideally, this form of treatment should be followed by relaxation and individual postural training. If this is not possible, relaxation should be practised in class and some time given to individual correction. The tables should have plenty of variety, movement and activity, and, in the case of children, should appeal to their imagination and play instinct, as well as to their love of movement (*see* Chapter XXIII). Games and dancing can also be made use of (*see below*).

THE IMPORTANCE OF RHYTHM is increasingly realized in these days. All the processes of the body are normally rhythmic—the heart's beat, the respiratory movements, the peristaltic action of the unstriated muscle tissue. Failure of the postural reflex brings about a loss of rhythm in the body—a loss of harmonious co-operation between the different parts of the nervous system, and between groups of muscles. This sense of rhythm has to be won back as well as postural sense, though its gradual restoration may be a long process. There are many different systems in use today designed for the perfecting of bodily movement in men, women, and children, and many of them are adaptable to the needs of scoliotic or kyphotic patients, or those suffering from various other deformities of limbs or trunk. Folk-dancing (English or foreign), dances modelled on those of Greece, ballet movements, rhythmic exercises like those based on the teachings of Madame Agnete Bertram or Margaret Morris* offer a wide field of choice to the worker. Space forbids any description of these systems here. Moreover, they should be studied at first hand. The experienced physiotherapist may perhaps take something from each, or even work out a system of her own, but she must bear in mind the limitations of her patients, and not ask more of them than they are able to perform.

II. Second and Third Degree Curves (Structural Deformities)

Aims of Treatment.—These vary from postural cases in that when a patient with a second degree structural deformity comes for treatment, the first requirement is to *mobilize the spine* as far as possible in an attempt to lengthen the contracted soft parts. Only when this is achieved can we begin to *correct the deformity* as far as possible, *strengthen weak muscles*, and *improve the posture generally*.

Obviously, we cannot correct a *bony* deformity. In third degree cases, therefore, little improvement can be expected. What mobility is left in the spine and thorax must be maintained and, if possible, increased. *Breathing exercises* are most important. The patient must be taught to establish new postural reflexes, maintaining as erect an attitude as possible, and holding the shoulders and pelvis as level as she can. Exercises to strengthen the muscles should be given, but special exercises for correction of curvature are probably of little use.

KYPHOSIS

(Kyphosis Arcuata; Round Back)

This deformity may make its appearance at any period of life, but is most common in childhood, adolescence, or old age. The back is rounded, the head carried forward, and the chest flattened. The shoulders, also, are round, the scapulæ being too far forward on the chest wall. Kyphosis is commoner in girls than in boys, and a *primary* kyphosis is commoner in the heavier type of individual.

CAUSES.—

In Infancy and Childhood.—Probably the commonest cause is habitual bad posture, often acquired at school. The child may be suffering from undetected defects of sight or hearing, or nasal obstructions which, by causing a flat or pigeon chest, produce a correspondingly round back and shoulders.

There may be an emotional factor. Mental or physical fatigue may be at the root of the trouble.

Naturally, such children must be predisposed to the deformity by muscular weakness or reflex deficiency, since many children and adults constantly assume extremely bad postures without ever acquiring an actual deformity. Weakness or paralysis of longitudinal back muscles may be the cause, as may failure of development of the normal curves of the spine. It will be remembered that at birth the spine has one long backward curve; the other curves develop later. Rickets was at one time responsible for many deformities, but with the higher

---

* Readers are advised to study the methods of Dr. Goldthwait, *see Body Mechanics in the Study and Treatment of Disease*; also John H. Colson, *Postural and Relaxation Training in Physiotherapy and Physical Education*.

standard of living and improved dietary knowledge in Britain today this condition is now rare.

IN ADOLESCENCE AND ADULT LIFE.—Besides habitual bad posture, the condition may be brought about by certain occupations; by arthritis or rheumatism; by lung affections in which both lungs are involved (e.g., emphysema); and by various paralytic conditions. A brief description of a specific form of adolescent kyphosis is given on p. 360.

IN OLD AGE.—This may be the result of causes operative at an earlier time of life, or may, in some cases, be due simply to muscular weakness. More often, however, it is due to degeneration of the intervertebral disks or bodies of the vertebræ.

PATHOLOGICAL CHANGES.—This deformity, like any other, may be divided into three degrees. In the early stages, no change is present except laxity and poor tone in the muscles. *In time, the pectoral muscles become shortened.* This interferes with the mobility of the thorax, and hence with respiration, especially with full inspiration. *The longitudinal back muscles are stretched and weakened in their upper parts* and the *transverse back muscles,* especially the rhomboids and the middle part of the trapezius, also suffer in this way. *The posterior ligaments* of the vertebral column are lengthened, and those on the *anterior aspect* are correspondingly shortened. In the late stages, the *vertebræ* may become wedge-shaped, being much narrower in front than behind, owing to the pressure on the anterior margins. This is uncommon, except in adolescent kyphosis.

To begin with, then, we must concentrate on relaxation, mobilization, and breathing. Correct diaphragmatic and costal breathing must be taught, special prominence being given to inspiratory exercises, and general relaxation may help. In kyphosis, the tense muscles are the pectorals. To relax these the patient may be asked to round the shoulders as much as possible, crossing the arms over the chest, and then to drop the arms to the side; to press the upper arms against the sides of the chest, and then relax; or to circle the shoulders (with arms by the side), first carrying them forwards and upwards, and then allowing them to drop downwards and backwards. For this exercise, a small, hard cushion should be placed between the patient's spine and the back of the plinth or chair, so that the shoulders are free to drop backwards. The most suitable starting positions are half-lying or sitting with the back well supported. At a later date local relaxation may be given in standing. If there is tension in the neck muscles, head-rolling should also be performed.

The patient should lie down for a short time before and after treatment. She may lie prone or supine, or each in turn. Since few children will lie still for long, their rest includes a certain amount of exercise: in the prone position, the back muscles are used in raising the head; in the supine position, the abdominal muscles (Forrest-Brown). Crook-lying is a better position than lying.

The precise treatment necessary to gain mobility will depend on the state of the tissues. Transitional and mild cases may respond to mobility exercises alone, e.g., such movements as active Trunk-rolling, or 'Sawing', quick Trunk-rotation, Alternate side-bending, Back-raising, and 2-Elbow-backward-carrying or -circling, and more serious changes will require some definite form of stretching. In some cases hanging in head-suspension apparatus may prove effective, because the whole spine is stretched in this position. Most cases, however, require more stringent measures.

When a *decided improvement in mobility has taken place,* definite corrective exercises may be given, mobility and relaxation exercises being followed by active contractions of the weak muscles.

Abdominal and gluteal contractions must be taught, and the movements combined to produce pelvic rocking. In this way the patient learns control of the pelvic tilt so that she can assume the correct position at will, and maintain it for increasing periods of time. The patient's own weight will tend to correct the thoracic kyphosis during pelvic rocking, but extremes of movement should not be allowed, since this may produce a tendency to lordosis. Breathing exercises should be given in the corrected position, the patient pushing out the ribs in the lower costal region as far as possible to encourage active chest expansion. She may also perform simple movements of arms and legs. Later, double-sided exercises may be added, *but they must not be so hard as to make her abandon the corrected position, or only be able to maintain it with a good deal of strain.* Having mastered postural correction in crook-lying, the patient may proceed to correction in sitting or knee-sitting (first with and then without back support), the position of the pelvis being corrected as before. As she now has to maintain the correct posture from the hips upward she must be shown how to flatten her back and 'draw herself up'.* The position of head and neck needs attention, and the patient must learn to move in all the joints of the cervical spine, and not merely the occipito-atlantal joint. When this position has been mastered, simple exercises are performed in it, as above.

Exercises for the feet should not be neglected, and these should be given in sitting at first, later in standing, and finally walking, until the patient is able to maintain the correct position during activity.

SPECIAL EXERCISES FOR THE BACK MUSCLES.—

1. *For the longitudinal back muscles* exercises should include (*a*) *Head-extensions* and (*b*) *Back-raisings.*

2. *For the transverse back muscles* movements should include (*a*) 2-*Arm-parting,* (*b*) *Forward-bend* 2-*Elbow-backward-carrying,* and (*c*) 2-*Arm-bending* and -*stretching outward and backward.*

3. The above groups may be arranged to provide *combined exercises for both longitudinal and transverse back muscles.*

Some specific *mobility exercises* should always be retained in the scheme, and breathing exercises in lying, sitting, and standing must be practised.

HOME EXERCISES.—A short scheme of home exercises should be taught, but they will only be of value if they are carried out conscientiously and intelligently. This fact must be impressed on the patient, or the parents in the case of children.

PRECAUTIONS AGAINST OVERCORRECTION.—When correcting the pelvic tilt, care must be taken not to over-correct the deformity, producing a *lordosis,* or, in the case of a *high* kyphosis, a *kypholordosis.* In a kyphosis with some stiffness, over-correction might even result in a *sway-back.* One must not allow the patient to replace one fault of posture by another equally bad, but must teach her to take, and hold, the *right* posture. To avoid over-correction of the pelvic tilt in performing special exercises for kyphosis, starting positions should be carefully considered. *Crook-sitting* and *tailor-sitting* are suitable, and also *long-sitting,* provided that the hamstrings, which in the kyphotic patient are often short, do not prevent the patient from sitting upright. This would be disastrous for the kyphosis. Crook-lying should always be preferred to lying (*see above*). The abdominal muscles need to be strengthened and trained, but should not be worked in the outer range without counteracting movements. In any case, such movement as strong backward bendings to arch position which involve outer-range abdominal work should not be given to a kyphotic patient, unless the pelvis is fixed, as in prone-lying.

---

* Miss M. Gardiner, in *The Principles of Exercise Therapy,* says, as regards the position of the head, "An upward thrust of the vertex in the erect positions may be sufficient to achieve satisfactory alinement of the whole body, provided no unnecessary tension is allowed to develop elsewhere." I am sure this is true, and that such an "upward thrust" often brings about a correction of the pelvic tilt automatically. The patient should also be taught to take her weight correctly on her feet—heels, toes, and outer borders.

Strong static abdominal exercises, e.g., Foot-support-long-sitting Trunk-falling-backward-and-raising, should also be avoided. Hollowing of the lumbar spine must be corrected if it occurs during the performance of any exercise. *It is particularly liable to occur during any movement which entails raising the arms above shoulder-level.*

Second and Third Degree Cases

Even in a structural case, some slight improvement can be expected, though such cases are difficult to treat, and often prove disappointing in their results.

STRETCHING AND CORRECTION BY SUSPENSION EXERCISES.—In the so-called 'passive' stretchings—really forced movements—it is not possible to get the patient to relax. The pectorals are very sensitive muscles, and the discomfort, or even pain, caused by the stretching, makes the patient contract them strongly, however much she might wish to relax. This type of movement is certainly not

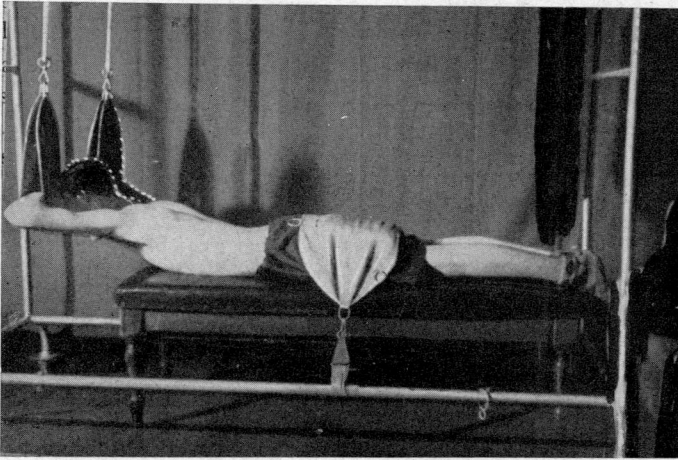

Fig. 165.—Correction by suspension exercises. (Note, additional slings should support the upper arms or the chest; they were removed for purposes of photography.) (*From 'Rehabilitation, Re-education and Remedial Exercises'. Baillière, Tindall, & Cox, by permission of O. F. Guthrie-Smith.*)

'passive', therefore, and becomes an active movement for the very muscles it is designed to lengthen. In certain cases relaxation of the pectorals can be achieved far more satisfactorily by means of *active movements* for the back muscles, because as these come into action the anterior muscles relax by reciprocal innervation, but in more severe cases it may not be possible for the patient, with her weak back muscles, to stretch them sufficiently by her own unaided efforts. It is here that *suspension apparatus* can be of great value. To use this the patient lies prone on a plinth, a wide band being carried over the buttocks and thighs to fix them to the couch. The arms are supported by slings placed under the upper arms and forearms (*see Fig. 165*). The ropes to which the slings are attached are then adjusted in such a way as to bring the thoracic spine into a slight arch position, the weight of the patient's trunk between the two fixed points tending to reverse the curve. This position is maintained for several minutes (the time being gradually lengthened as the course of treatment proceeds), and the patient is taught to adapt herself to the stretching, and relax. Both the pectorals and the anterior ligaments of the spine are thus lengthened. In this position the patient must learn to contract and strengthen both the longitudinal and transverse back muscles by localized contractions and movements. *Mobility exercises, e.g.*, Trunk side-swingings, passive or active, may also be given in suspension apparatus.

OTHER STRETCHING AND MOBILITY EXERCISES.—

1. *Stretch-grasp-knee-sitting Chest-down-pressing.*—This is a well-known exercise. The patient sits on her heels, grasps a wall-bar, or some other fixed object about eighteen inches from the ground, and tries to force the chest downward to the floor. She should, at the same time, attempt to flatten her back by contracting the extensor muscles. The exercise is corrective as well as productive of mobility. Moreover, the danger of lordosis when rising to the erect position is eliminated. It must not be *assisted* by the physiotherapist, but she should indicate *where* the contraction of the muscles is to take place. It should not cause pain.

2. *Klapp's Stretching Exercise.**

3. *Mr. Bellis Clayton's Crawling Exercises.*—These are designed both to obtain mobility and also to exercise the weak muscles. An account of them will be found in the final chapters of his *Physiotherapy in General Practice.*

4. *Strap Exercises.*—These are rarely used now, being only really suitable for small, light patients, with a minimal degree of structural change. The patient lies on her back on a low narrow plinth, and, with arms raised above her head, grasps a wall-bar or some other form of support. One strap is placed across the abdomen, and the physiotherapist, standing astride the patient, places one foot on either end of it. This holds the abdomen down, and prevents lordosis. Another strap is passed under the maximum convexity of the kyphosis, and is pulled upwards, thus correcting the curve by pressure.

POSTURAL CORRECTION.—This should be carried out on the same lines as for the postural cases; but, naturally, a full correction cannot be obtained. The aim is to help the patient to acquire as good a posture as is possible in the circumstances. *Precautions against Lordosis* are even more necessary than in postural cases because, the thoracic spine being rigid, the patient often confuses extension of the lumbar spine with contraction of the transverse back muscles. Abdominal exercises must be assiduously practised.

Adolescent Kyphosis

(Scheuermann's Disease. Vertebral Epiphysitis or Osteochondritis)

This disease usually occurs in boys between the ages of 12 and 16 years. The middle and lower parts of the thoracic spine are implicated. The cause is uncertain but for some reason the spine appears to be unable to support the load it has to bear. There is inflammation of the upper and lower epiphyses of the body of the vertebra; the latter become fragmented at the epiphysial line and the surfaces of the body become uneven. The body becomes wedge shaped, being narrower at the front. Later, spontaneous recovery takes place, but the wedging remains. There may also be prolapse of the nuclei of several intervertebral disks. Backache is common but there is rarely any actual pain. Three to five vertebræ are usually affected, and there is rigidity and increase in the normal anteroposterior curve in the area of the lesion. The condition is slowly progressive up to the age of about 21 years when ossification of the bones is complete. The deformity then becomes permanent. It is therefore only amenable to treatment in its earliest stages, and this should begin as soon as the condition is diagnosed.

The aims of treatment, as in all cases of epiphysitis, are to relieve the strain on the epiphyses, and to prevent or correct the deformity, pending spontaneous

---

* For a short account of Klapp's Crawling Exercises, *see* Miss M. Gardiner, *The Principles of Exercise Therapy*, 2nd edition, p. 100.

recovery. *Recumbency*, on similar lines to that of early Pott's disease, is essential (*see* p. 165). At the end of the period of recumbency, the patient begins exercises. These consist of *hyperextension* exercises, and careful movements for the posterior shoulder muscles and the head and neck muscles. They should be given at first in prone-lying. If desired the suspension apparatus may be used. Correct posture should be taught in lying, sitting, and standing. General spinal exercises, similar to those for a fractured vertebral body, are added gradually. *Flexion* of the spine must never be forced, and the movements should be smooth and rhythmical. The patient must be watched for any sign of fatigue or backache; the latter, if it occurs, must be reported to the doctor immediately, as it may mean that the deformity is again increasing.

LORDOSIS

The causes are similar to those leading to kyphosis, namely: habitually incorrect posture, or defective postural sense (the pelvis is tilted forwards, and the patient compensates for this by hollowing the lumbar spine, *see Fig.* 157, p. 343); it may be a compensatory mechanism, the lordosis being a compensatory deformity to a high kyphosis, or to conditions involving the hip-joint,* e.g., bilateral congenital dislocation of the hip, or tuberculosis of the hip involving the fixation of the joint in flexion, etc. (*see* p. 343 and *Fig.* 157); weakness or paralysis of the abdominal muscles, the flexors of the lumbar spine; or even careless treatment of kyphosis.

PATHOLOGICAL CHANGES.—

The *abdominal muscles* are stretched, the *lumbar muscles* contracted, and the *ligaments* on the front of the spine are lengthened, those on the back shortened. The *glutei* are weakened and the *hamstrings* may be lengthened. Bony change is uncommon in lordosis.

It rarely falls to our lot to deal with lordosis alone. In most cases it is seen in connexion with kyphosis or some other deformity, or as the result of weak abdominal muscles after pregnancy, long illness, etc. If it is present alone, we must, of course, guard against the development of a compensatory kyphosis.

The aims of treatment are similar to those which apply in kyphosis, but in lordosis it will be necessary to mobilize and stretch the *lumbar* spine if its range of movement is diminished, and to strengthen the *abdominal muscles*, and hamstrings if required.

Massage is not usually needed unless backache is a symptom but *relaxation* should be taught, as in other spinal conditions.

The patient should first be taught to correct the position of the pelvis, and shown how to tilt it backward by contracting the lower part of the abdominal muscles and the glutei. This should be done successively in lying, sitting, and standing. The position of the thorax is then corrected. The chest is raised, and the shoulders pressed back, the head held well up, and the chin in (but not drawn back into an unnatural position). The correct position of the pelvis must be carefully maintained. When standing, the patient is told to 'make herself as tall as possible'. Exercises should then be performed, after which posture should be checked, and corrected if necessary. Long-sitting is the position *par excellence* for lordosis, since it is impossible to hollow the lumbar spine in this attitude. Crook- or tailor-sitting may take its place if the hamstrings are long. Crook-lying and stoop-sitting are also good starting positions, though it is possible for the

---

* The *original* trouble may even be lower down the limb, e.g., in some deformity of knee, ankle, or foot. In cases where the forefoot is, or has been, painful, the patient may throw the weight back to the heels in standing, and incline the legs backwards, tipping the pelvis forward in order to compensate. This may happen in cases of metatarsalgia, or hallux rigidus, or even of weak foot or flat-foot.

patient to hollow the back in either. *All the inner range 'straight' abdominal exercises* are excellent for lordosis—that is, those in which these muscles act as flexors of the spine, but *strong* static abdominal exercises should not be used. It must not be forgotten that there may be marked weakness or diminished tone of the hip extensors as well as of the abdominals, and special exercises for these muscles should be included in the scheme. They are, after all, the muscles that control the pelvic tilt, and since our principal aim in lordosis is to *decrease* the tilt, i.e., tilt the pelvis further backwards, their importance is obvious. All quick, strong trunk movements round the transverse (frontal) axis mobilize the lumbar spine, but the physiotherapist must see that the lumbar spine is not *hyperextended* at the end of any of these movements. This is particularly liable to happen as the patient raises herself after the downward movement of 'Hewing' or Forward- and downward-bending, because of the raised position of the arms.

PRECAUTIONS AGAINST KYPHOSIS consist in giving exercises in positions corrective of that deformity, e.g., heave-grasp, neck-rest, or yard-sitting or -standing; in careful supervision of the posture of the patient's head and shoulders during exercise; and in special movements for the back and shoulder muscles.

KYPHOLORDOSIS

This being merely a combination of the two preceding conditions, it does not need further description. The lordosis is generally the primary curve.

Since, in many cases, a treatment for kyphosis or lordosis is practically a treatment for kypholordosis, little more need be said on the subject except that exercises for the back muscles should be given with the lumbar spine held corrected; those for the abdominals, with the thoracic spine extended and the shoulders held well back. Stretch-grasp-stoop-stride-standing Shoulder-pressing plus Holding is one of the best exercises for this deformity. It is useful both in postural and structural cases. Crook-sitting with back support is a good early exercise.

SWAY-BACK

This deformity is treated on the same lines as the others, in fact much as kypholordosis. The patient must be taught to tilt the pelvis *backward*, and to hold it in the right position, to eliminate the backward bend at the lumbosacral angle, and to correct, as far as possible, the kyphosis. This is of the thoraco- lumbar type and is probably the result of a localized form of adolescent kyphosis (Wiles). The patient should practise 'drawing herself up' and special exercises for the longitudinal and transverse back muscles, hip extensors, and abdominals are necessary.

FLAT-BACK

This condition, the reverse deformity to lordosis, is too uncommon to appear often in our departments. The pelvis is tilted backwards and the hamstrings are shortened. The normal lumbar curve is flattened, and if the thoracic spine is mobile and there is no kyphosis, this curve also is diminished. Stiffness and back- ache may appear in later life.

In these cases the *aim* is to try to *increase*, instead of *diminish*, the normal curves. The patient must be taught to tilt the pelvis forward, and hollow the lumbar spine. It may be a good plan to start postural training in *lying* rather than in *crook-lying*, in order to obtain a lordosis, and early exercises may include 2-leg-lifting in outer range. In sitting and standing the patient should bend forward slightly at the hips, and then backward in the lumbar region, contracting the extensors strongly. If the position of the pelvis and lumbar spine can be rectified, the thoracic region may right itself, or will at least be easier to correct. The position of the head may need attention. *Mobility exercises* are important because stiffness in the spine may develop later, and an attempt should be made to stretch the hamstrings. *Corrective exercises* should consist of lumbar contraction performed slowly, arch positions and backward-bending, also exercises for the hip flexors, to correct the pelvis and relax the hamstrings.

SCOLIOSIS

CORRECTION OF CURVE.—Nowadays, stretching, when necessary, is usually produced by means of the suspension apparatus. *Passive (forced) stretchings* of the soft structures on the concavity of the curve (without relaxation) are not likely to be of much use, and manual pressures are rarely, if ever, used. In the first place, no physiotherapist can give them forcibly enough, nor maintain them long enough to rectify the deformity to any appreciable extent. Secondly, they tend to induce forcible contraction of the very muscles which we wish to lengthen. In addition, many of these pressures require special apparatus or the co-operation of one or more skilled assistants, and, for this reason, prove impracticable.

The Guthrie-Smith apparatus is now in common use in hospitals, and the objections to manual pressure, as stated above, do not apply to this form of correction. It can be maintained for as long as is suitable for the patient at the stage she has reached, and it imposes no strain on the physiotherapist. The discomfort is not great, and the patient can gradually be taught to relax while in suspension. This type of exercise is not purely passive, and the patient can be taught to build up the strength of her muscles by repeated small contractions. A broad sling is placed under the maximum convexity of the curve, e.g., in the thoracic region, and is attached by ropes to the upper bars of the apparatus. This provides *the fixed point from which the stretching is to take place, and the ropes must be so adjusted that the rotation as well as the lateral flexion will be corrected, forward, upward, and inward pressure being exerted on the rib angles.* The head, pelvis, and lower limbs are also supported in slings suspended from above, but springs are included in the attaching cords. The upper and lower parts of the body on either side of the fixed point are then lowered, so that the curve is reversed, or at least decreased. The patient must first be taught to relax in this position, and later to contract her muscles over the fixed point, and to make small downward movements of the head and legs. In this way the treatment constitutes a combined passive stretching with active contraction.

Strap Exercises (see p. 360, KYPHOSIS) can be adapted for use in scoliosis, with the strap under the maximum convexity, and the patient suitably rotated.

RELAXATION EXERCISES.—If suspension apparatus is not available, the patient can be taught to relax in prone-lying. She should be put into as correct a position as can be assumed without discomfort, and should be taught relaxation in this position. A small pillow should be placed under her forehead if the head is kept in the central position, or under the temple if it is turned to one side.

ACTIVE CONTRACTIONS OF MUSCLES should follow immediately on the passive stretchings, because the shortened structures on the concave side, having been stretched to their utmost, will offer least resistance to movement, and the weak muscles of the convex side will therefore be working under the best possible conditions. To begin with, the muscles should only be worked in their *inner range of contraction,* or the movement performed concentrically and eccentrically. The exercises consist of active side-bendings, trunk-rotations, etc., the patient bending towards the convex side, and then relaxing. *It is necessary that the origin of the working muscles should be firmly fixed. Static holdings,* in which the patient takes, or is placed in, a corrected (or over-corrected) position, and is required to maintain that position for a certain time, may also be performed.

PRECAUTIONS.—

1. The 'holdings' must not be continued beyond the point of fatigue. (The appearance of tremor indicates the necessity of rest.)

2. Throughout the performance of exercises the patient's position must be watched and carefully corrected. Self-correction before a mirror should be taught to older children and adults.

3. Patients with deformities involving differences in the length of the legs which necessitates the wearing of apparatus should keep it on during treatment. If this is not possible a book or some object of suitable height should be placed under the foot of the short leg when exercises are given in standing. Most exercises should be given in sitting, lying, or hanging, or in one of their derived positions and the all-fours position is sometimes useful, since in it the spine is supported at both ends.

Supervision and treatment are specially necessary during the period of growth, but even after this is over the patient should continue periodic check-ups. The general health of these cases needs care, and their occupation should be in accordance with their strength.

The question of how best to deal with structural deformities is a difficult and controversial one, to which at present no entirely satisfactory answer has been found. The tendency today is to treat the body as a whole, but a physiotherapist who wishes to specialize in orthopædics will do well to acquaint herself with the best features of all systems, and adapt them to the needs of the individual cases with whose treatment she is concerned.

TORTICOLLIS

(*Wry-neck*)

A malposition of the head and neck due to a unilateral shortening of the sternomastoid and sometimes of other muscles as well. Torticollis may be *congenital* or *acquired*.

The Congenital Form.—The deformity is slightly more common in girls than in boys, and is more often found on the left side than on the right. Occasionally, *both* sternomastoids are contracted. The cause may be malposition in the uterus, or some developmental defect in the affected muscle.

PATHOLOGICAL CHANGES.—

1. The sternomastoid on one side is *shortened*, and there is a sclerosis or hardening of the muscle tissue (i.e., a degenerative change), especially in the sternal portion. Occasionally other muscles are affected (the scalenes, platysma, splenius, or trapezius).

3. If the case is untreated, bony changes arise, as in a cervical scoliosis.

DEFORMITY.—

POSITION OF THE HEAD.—In accordance with the function of the sternomastoid, the head is fixed in *side flexion to the same side as the affected muscle and rotated to the opposite side*, e.g., in a *left* torticollis, the head is bent to the left, and the face rotated towards the right. The left shoulder is raised, and the whole head is displaced towards the sound side. The contracted muscle feels hard, and may have a localized swelling near its centre, but there is no pain. The deformity increases as the patient grows, and it is therefore important that it should be corrected as early as possible. Scoliosis, of course, is present in the cervical region, the convexity being towards the sound side. In neglected cases, this may produce a compensatory curve or curves lower down. This generally, though not always, rights itself after treatment.

ASYMMETRY OF THE FACE.—The face is smaller on the side of the contracture. The corners of the eye and mouth are drawn down, the eye itself appearing smaller than that on the sound side, and of a different shape. The nose deviates slightly towards the affected side. This facial distortion may pass unnoticed in a baby, but becomes more obvious as the child grows older. It also becomes much more noticeable following treatment when the head is held straight, but gradually improves, and finally disappears. Parents should be reassured on this point. In young children it may right itself in a few months; in older patients it may take two or three years.

In bilateral cases, *both* sternomastoids are shortened. The head is then bent forward, and kyphosis is a complication. Such cases are, however, rare.

Principles of Treatment.—The *aims* of treatment are those of any postural deformity. Firstly the defective muscle must be lengthened so that the head and neck can be released from the deformity in which they are held. Secondly the child must be taught to control, and maintain, the corrected position. Physical measures, alone, are suitable only for cases in the very early stages, i.e., newborn babies and infants. In all other cases some form of surgical treatment is required before the physical treatment can be of benefit.

Treatment of Newborn Babies and Infants

Treatment should begin as soon after birth as possible and, if practicable, should be carried out two or three times a day. The baby should be placed on its back on a suitable plinth or table, with its head near the edge. The physiotherapist should stand or sit at the end of the plinth behind the child's head. A very low pillow should be placed under the head, which must be held in as correct a position as possible during treatment.

Massage is given to the neck to relax and stretch the contracted muscle, and the manipulations consist of stroking, finger-kneadings, and frictions, and picking up. The strokes should be firm but light, and performed with the tips of the fingers.

PASSIVE (FORCED) MOVEMENTS.—These form the most important part of the treatment, at this stage. The child is placed with the head beyond the edge of the table. It must be well supported by the physiotherapist's hands. An assistant should steady the child's shoulders during the passive stretching. In a *left torticollis*, the head must be *bent to the right*, and *rotated to the left*, being brought as far as possible towards an over-corrected position. The fact of the shifting of the head towards the sound side must not be forgotten, since this also requires correction, and a *lateral pressure away from the sound side should be exerted throughout the movement*. It is best to perform this part of the treatment expeditiously, and get it over. The baby will cry, and probably struggle, but it is much kinder to be quick and decisive than to endeavour to console the baby between movements.

As the child grows older, traction is sometimes applied to the neck. If so, it is best carried out manually, by placing one hand under the chin and the other beneath the occiput. A small child should *never* be placed in the head-suspension apparatus.

ACTIVE MOVEMENTS.—In very young infants these are impossible, but as soon as the child is old enough movement can be achieved by the attraction of toys or brightly coloured objects held in such positions that the head will be turned in the desired direction. The fascinating occupation of listening to a watch is helpful in inducing lateral flexion. During these movements the physiotherapist must be careful to see that the movement is really performed in the *cervical* region, and not merely produced by a *trunk* flexion or rotation. To prevent the latter, the shoulders must be fixed.

The child may also be turned over into the prone position. In this position, head extension can be more easily obtained, and the child may be persuaded to try to look back over her shoulder. The physiotherapist must, however, remember that in this position the movement must be *towards the affected side*, e.g., in a left torticollis the child looks back over the *left* shoulder.

Patients for whom treatment without operation is suitable are rarely old enough to be capable of performing resisted exercises, but if such are possible, they should be given to the unaffected side (this will not only strengthen the weaker, stretched muscle, but induce reciprocal relaxation in the contracted one) and to the extensors.

Older Children and Adults

These cases are more severe and may be acquired or due to neglected congenital torticollis. Massage and manipulation alone are insufficient, although a few of the acquired cases may yield to physical treatment. On the whole, they must be treated by operation if success is to be achieved.

SURGICAL TREATMENT.—The sternal and clavicular heads of the sterno-mastoid are divided close to their origins, and any contracted bands of fascia are also severed.

The head is then held in an over-corrected position until the stitches are removed in 10–14 days. Plaster, sand-bags, or some form of apparatus is used to maintain the correction.

PRE-OPERATIVE TREATMENT is sometimes ordered. It is designed to prevent atrophy during immobilization, and should include *all* the muscles of the neck, shoulder, and upper part of the back. Any active movements that are possible should be practised. Passive stretchings are less important in these cases, but they may be given if desired.

PHYSICAL TREATMENT is on the same lines as that for infants, the chief differences being in respect of the active exercises, and the position of the patient during the administration of massage and passive movements. For these patients the sitting position is usually best, the physiotherapist standing behind the chair or stool, but lying on a high couch, or half-lying, with the back of the plinth only slightly raised is suitable. The head must be supported in the corrected position by placing one hand under her chin.

The movements are the same as those used for infants, except that they will naturally be stronger and the presence of a scar must be taken into consideration. Head-suspension apparatus is also useful.

Active Movements form the most important part of the treatment and *it is necessary to fix the origin of the working muscle.* Both shoulders should be fixed, but it should be arranged that the shoulder on the affected side is a little lower than the other. Concentric and eccentric head-side-flexion, *away from the affected side, with rotations towards it*, should be given in the inner and middle range and head extension should also be practised. Free exercises should also be taught and practised several times a day at home, but 'home exercises', however conscientiously done, must not be made a substitute for attendance at the hospital, as these cases need careful watching. Self-correction before a mirror may be helpful. After-treatment should be continued for about 6 months.

CASES NOT TREATED BY OPERATION.—The less severe and acquired forms may be treated either by physical treatment alone, or by physical treatment in conjunction with some form of head support. This may consist of a collar arranged to keep the head corrected in side-flexion and rotation, or a head-band with shoulder straps. Massage, passive stretchings, and active exercise will be carried out as described above.

The Acquired Form.—We rarely see these cases, their origin begin psychological or inflammatory, and treatment must be directed to the causes. If physical treatment is ordered it follows the principles given above.

CHAPTER XVII

DISEASES OF THE RESPIRATORY ORGANS

Physiology. Effects of Disease. Principles of Treatment. I. Diseases of the nose and throat: Chronic nasal catarrh—Allergic rhinitis and hay fever—Chronic tonsillitis and adenoids. II. Diseases of the bronchi: Chronic bronchitis—Bronchiectasis—Asthma. III. Diseases of the lungs: Emphysema—Lobar pneumonia—Bronchopneumonia—Fibrosis of the lung—Tuberculosis. IV. Diseases of the pleura: Pleurisy—Empyema. V. Thoracic surgery. VI. Examples of breathing exercises.

PHYSIOLOGY OF THE RESPIRATORY SYSTEM

THE respiratory system is responsible for *external respiration* (the interchange of gases between the lungs and the capillaries surrounding them). The efficiency of this exchange governs the adequacy of *internal respiration* (the interchange of gases between the tissue cells and their capillaries), on which tissue health largely depends. Thus the respiratory system plays a major part in the maintenance of body health. It consists of air-passages and lung tissue, and may be divided into an upper and lower tract.

The *upper respiratory tract* constitutes the portion lying in the head and neck, the nasal passages, the pharynx, larynx, and trachea (*Fig.* 166), part of which lies in the thorax.

The *lower respiratory tract* constitutes the portion lying in the thorax, the bronchi, bronchioles, alveoli, and lung tissue (*Fig.* 167).

The whole of the tract is lined with ciliated epithelium until it becomes intra-pulmonary, i.e., as far as the small bronchi which end in bronchioles leading to the alveoli.

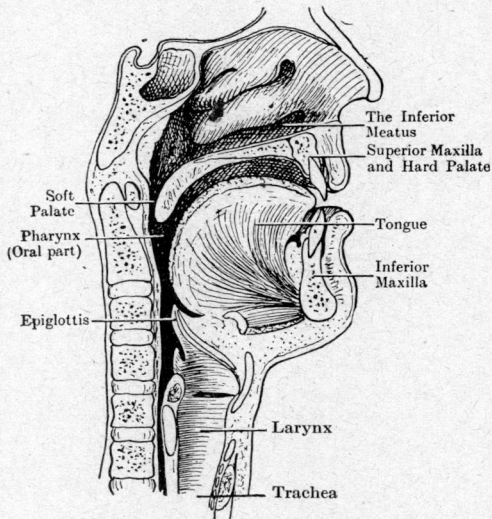

Fig. 166.—Showing respiratory passages. (*After Gray.*)

The lower tract contains smooth muscle and yellow elastic tissue in order to facilitate air entry and expulsion.

FUNCTIONS.—The upper and lower respiratory passages are responsible for the interchange of gases between the body and its environment, and for the warming and cleansing of the air before it reaches the lungs. The latter is achieved by means of lymphoid tissue in the nasal passages and pharynx, by the ciliated epithelium and by mucus secreted throughout the tract.

The lung tissue itself is responsible for the actual interchange of gases between venous and arterial blood.

EFFECTS OF DISEASE

Any part of the respiratory tract may become infected or diseased, and the consequences may have far-reaching results. As in any other part of the body the response to infection is an inflammatory reaction. The immediate result is hyperæmia and swelling which gives rise to difficulty in respiration and a degree of hypoventilation. If the condition becomes chronic, *fibrosis* may occur. In the respiratory tract, particularly in the lung tissue itself, this means a loss of elasticity, with a possible permanent decrease in ventilation. The oxygen intake is impaired and carbon dioxide accumulates. The tissues become

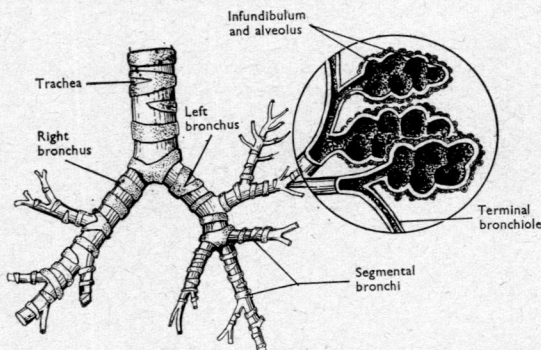

Fig. 167.—Diagrammatic representation of lower respiratory tract.

devitalized and the general health is affected. In particular the patient is easily fatigued, musculature is often weak, and posture is poor. If the lung tissue is affected the pulmonary capillaries may break down and the heart becomes strained through overwork.

In addition to the normal inflammatory reaction, mucus secretion is increased in the affected area. This adds to the effect of the swelling by blocking the air-passages. In certain conditions there is a danger of a plug of mucus forming in the lumen of a small vessel, in which case very serious changes may follow. Not only is ventilation decreased, but unless the blockage is removed, the portion of lung tissue below the obstruction collapses. *If immediate steps are not taken to regain expansion, the tissue ultimately fibroses and dies, permanently decreasing the power of ventilation.* In some cases suppuration occurs, and large areas of lung tissue may be destroyed in consequence.

PRINCIPLES OF TREATMENT

GENERAL PRINCIPLES.—Rest, fresh air, and good food are essential, and appropriate medical or surgical treatment will be administered.

PHYSICAL PRINCIPLES.—In all cases of respiratory disease there are two primary aims which *must* be achieved if the patient is to be restored to the fullest possible health:—

1. *To keep the respiratory passages clear.*
2. *To increase ventilation.*

METHODS.—

CLEARING OF AIR-PASSAGES.—In normal conditions the movements occurring during respiration loosen any excess mucus, which is carried upwards towards the main bronchus. This stimulates the cough reflex, and the mucus is forced into the mouth, whence it can be expelled. In cases where the mucus is thin and watery, respiratory movements are often sufficient to dislodge it, and the passages can then be kept free by teaching the patient breathing exercises and the correct use of the chest. In cases where the mucus is thick and sticky, i.e., the majority of chest infections, more vigorous measures are required to clear it. Percussion must be applied to the thorax (*chest-clapping, hacking*, and *vibrations*) and because of the complex structure of the bronchial tree, the body must also be positioned correctly for drainage to occur (*postural drainage*).

INCREASING VENTILATION.—This is partly achieved by clearing the air-passages, but breathing exercises are the principal means employed. *All parts of the lung must be fully used if maximum ventilation is to be achieved.* The chest is capable of movement in four directions: anteroposteriorly, laterally, upwards, and downwards. Lung tissue, like muscle tissue, is capable of hypertrophy when extra effort is required of it. Therefore, by means of breathing exercises even large areas of fibrosis can be compensated, and ventilation increased.

Any postural defects must, of course, be corrected, as they may seriously hamper movement of the thorax, and the mobility of the thorax must be maintained or improved. Any treatment which may be necessary in the interests of the patient's general health will, of course, be administered.

For purposes of description the conditions may be divided into diseases of the nose and throat, diseases of the bronchial tree, and diseases of lung tissue. With those of the upper respiratory tract we are little concerned, but in those of the bronchi and lungs physiotherapy plays a very important role.

When treating any chest condition the following points should be noted:—

1. *The Position of the Head.*—If there is any deviation from normal the state of the trapezius should be examined, as weakness of the upper fibres of one group may often lead to a postural deformity.

2. *The Mobility of the Shoulder-girdle.*—Elevation is the most important movement.

3. *Respiration.*—It is important to know the type of breathing, i.e., how the patient breathes (is it shallow, wheezy, or otherwise laboured?), where the patient breathes (i.e., does he fully use the chest?, does he use the diaphragm?, does he mainly breathe with the upper part of the chest?), and the rate of respiration.

4. *The Position of the Thorax.*—Is there any spinal or rib cage deformity?

5. *The Mobility of the Thorax.*—Can the chest move in all directions, or is there any rigidity or immobility?

6. *The State of the Muscles.*—Particularly of the rhomboids, erector spinæ, and trapezius.

7. *The Patient's General Posture and Physique.*

8. *Any Special Signs.*—E.g., cyanosis, breathlessness, clubbing of the fingers, the type and quantity of sputum.

When treating any chest condition for which the patient is confined to bed, the following rules must be scrupulously obeyed:—

1. *The patient's chart and case history must be examined,* and the former looked at before each treatment.

2. *No treatment should be given if there is any rise in temperature, or other untoward sign, without advice being sought as to the cause, and the suitability of continuing physiotherapy.*

I. DISEASES OF THE NOSE AND THROAT

CHRONIC NASAL CATARRH

A chronic inflammation of the nasal mucous membrane, with increased serous or mucopurulent secretion. The condition is either bacterial in origin or due to the inhalation of dust or other irritating substances.

Though not in itself dangerous to life it can be the cause of much ill health, especially as it often causes little inconvenience and is generally neglected. The patient's resistance to infection is lowered in consequence and it becomes a fruitful source of other troubles: (1) The very common 'catarrhal deafness' is caused by the extension of the inflammation to the Eustachian tube, which may later give rise to middle-ear infection. (2) Infection frequently spreads to the frontal and/or maxillary sinuses, giving rise to a painful sinusitis. (3) The infection may spread to the pharynx and larynx. In the latter the voice becomes husky and there may be periods when it is completely lost. (4) In some cases a general lowering of health takes place because of the hindrance to respiration and the inadequate oxygen intake.

Treatment.—Medical treatment consists of local applications of various kinds, given by means of sprays, nasal douches, etc., or of inhalations. In cases where adenoids, polypi, or defective septa are to blame, suitable operative treatment will be applied.

PHYSICAL TREATMENT.—This is usually directed towards the effects rather than the cause. The aims will be to improve the patient's general health, to relieve congestion in the membrane, and to assist in removing the mucous deposits. They are mainly achieved by electrotherapy and breathing exercises.

ELECTROTHERAPY.—Ultra-violet irradiation will raise the patient's general resistance. Initially, first degree erythema doses should be given daily, using a sectional technique. In about two weeks this should be changed to general suberythemal irradiation, treatment being given on alternate days. Local erythema doses may be given to the nasal mucosa by means of a special applicator. In some cases of middle-ear infection similar treatment may be given. Short-wave diathermy may be used to relieve pain and congestion in cases of sinusitis and middle-ear infection. It should be applied by the cross-fire method to give the best results. The dosage should be minimal to begin with and treatment should be given daily. If the patient is suffering from an acute exacerbation, twice- or thrice-daily treatment is advisable. Anodal galvanism or zinc ionization may also be administered for the relief of congestion, or the combating of infection. The nostril should be packed with tube-gauze soaked in saline or zinc sulphate. A special zinc or metal rod electrode is used, and a minimal current applied. If the infection is in the middle ear zinc ionization is applied in a similar manner.

BREATHING EXERCISES should include exercises for inspiration and expiration.

ALLERGIC RHINITIS AND HAY FEVER

These consist of an inflammatory condition resulting from sensitization from foreign protein, e.g., cat's fur, pollen, etc., which affects the nasal and pharyngeal mucosa and also the conjunctiva. The former usually becomes chronic, the latter is a temporary condition resulting, as its name implies, from exposure to pollen. It is, therefore, a seasonal condition.

Antihistamine drugs afford relief. Desensitization can often be achieved by injections of the offending protein. If physical treatment is required it will be on similar lines to those outlined above.

CHRONIC TONSILLITIS AND ADENOIDS

The conditions of adenoids and chronic tonsillar enlargement most frequently arise between the ages of 5 and 10 years. Although both are frequently found, either may exist alone. The adenoids are of various sizes, from "that of a small pea to that of an almond" (Osler). They are reddish in colour because of their numerous blood-vessels. Their presence is generally associated with that of nasal catarrh, and the inflammation may spread along the Eustachian tube to the middle ear. The tonsils are enlarged and may be red and inflamed. In long-standing cases sepsis may occur. The tonsils are filled with an extremely offensive matter containing pus, and small cavities may form in the tonsillar tissue.

Chronic tonsillitis is a condition of inflammation and enlargement of the tonsils themselves, and the patient generally suffers from frequent acute attacks of 'ulcerated' or septic throat. The term *adenoids* means overgrowth of lymphoid (adenoid) tissue in the vault of the pharynx, close to the openings of the Eustachian tubes. This overgrown tissue obstructs the passage of air.

SYMPTOMS.—

1. *Mouth-breathing.*—This is the most important symptom. Because of the obstructed pharynx and blockage of the nasal passages by mucous secretion, the child breathes almost entirely through his mouth, which he keeps continually open. The air thus inspired is insufficiently warmed and filtered, and the bronchi, or even the lungs, may suffer in consequence. The patient *snores at night*, and may even suffer from *dyspnœa*. There may be a troublesome cough.

2. *General Health.*—This is poor, the child suffering from *frequent colds* and *acute tonsillitis* or *bronchitis*. *Hearing, Taste, and Smell* may also suffer.

3. *Physical Signs.*—Growth may be stunted and changes in the shape of the chest are often very marked. The commonest form of thoracic deformity is '*pigeon breast*', in which the sternum is prominent, and 'Harrison's sulcus' (*see* RICKETS) is present. Less common are the '*barrel chest*' (*see* p. 383), which occurs in children subject to asthma, and the '*funnel chest*', in which the lower part of the sternum is drawn in during inspiration and finally remains fixed in that position.

4. *Mental Signs.*—The child may be backward, apathetic, and unable to concentrate on anything. Sometimes, however, the habit of keeping his mouth open gives an appearance of mental dullness, which is not, in fact, the case.

In some children the signs and symptoms are so slight as to pass unnoticed; but most, if not all, are subject to colds in the head, sometimes followed by troublesome coughs.

In cases of *chronic septic tonsillitis* the tonsils may be enlarged, or small and fibrosed. The breath is offensive, and the teeth are often decayed. The general health is poor and the patient is subject to recurrent attacks of pyrexia and 'sore throats'. If adenoids are also present, any or all of the above symptoms may be present.

Treatment.—Surgery provides the only effective cure.

The adenoids, and sometimes the tonsils as well,* are removed by the surgeon. If this is not done, the adenoids may dry up and disappear in time, but the damage will have been done, and the child may have been permanently injured in health.

PHYSICAL TREATMENT.—This is usually only requested *post-operatively*, the aims being *to teach correct breathing and to mobilize the thorax*.

Besides specific breathing exercises, these children need plenty of movement and activity.

It is a good plan to begin with some form of organized activity followed by '*Handkerchief drill*'. The children should be taught to clear the nasal passages, first by blowing down each nostril in turn while closing the other, and then down both together. This should be followed by a *breathing exercise*, the children breathing in through the nose with closed lips, and out through the mouth.

---

* Tonsillectomy was widespread at one time, being regarded somewhat in the nature of a cure for all ills. The tonsils, however, provide one of the principal body defences, and the modern trend is to remove them only when any useful function has clearly been destroyed. In cases of simple chronic tonsillitis removal of adenoids often effects a cure.

They should be able to breathe equally well through each nostril. If they cannot, the nose must be cleared.* Later, they must learn to breathe in and out through the nose. These patients should also be taught to breathe in all parts of the thorax, and to use their abdominal muscles correctly in breathing.

Other movements required, in addition to breathing exercises, are:—

1. *Exercises to increase the mobility of the thorax*—quick trunk-rotations, active trunk-rollings or circle-turnings, 'Sawing' side-bendings, etc.

2. *Balance exercises*, which compel attention and improve co-ordination besides helping to establish a correct postural reflex.

3. *Quick, active exercises*, such as marching, running, skipping, dancing, jumping, and games should be introduced into the class tables. These not only quicken the mental processes and rouse the apathetic child, but increase the range of breathing by making him slightly short of breath.

4. *Training in correct posture.*

The treatment outlined above can be adapted to individual treatments, and passive chest-liftings and mobilizing movements may be included.

Young children should have a short table of exercises which should be constantly varied. This applies to all tables for children, whether they are treated individually or in classes. It is often helpful to make use of balloons, windmills, light paper objects, cotton-wool swabs and balls, to interest small children in breathing exercises.

Children with barrel chests should not be allowed to make forced inspirations.

ELECTRICAL TREATMENT.—General ultra-violet radiation is very beneficial to children of this type. If available, the fluorescent tube or carbon arc should be used in preference to the mercury vapour arc.

II. DISEASES OF THE BRONCHI

CHRONIC BRONCHITIS

A chronic inflammation of the trachea and bronchi. It is the commonest disease of the respiratory tract.

AETIOLOGY.—

AGE.—Chronic bronchitis most frequently attacks people over 40 years of age and tends to recur every winter ('winter cough'). Children, however, are also subject to it, in which case it is generally associated with adenoids and enlarged tonsils. It occurs occasionally in young adults, sometimes after influenza (Osler).

SEX.—It is more common in men than in women.

CAUSES.—The causative organisms are the pneumococcus and the bacilli of influenza, or catarrh.

Predisposing Factors.—

1. Repeated acute attacks of bronchitis predispose to the chronic variety.

2. It is often associated with asthma, lung, heart, or kidney disease, or with such conditions as interfere gravely with venous return to the heart, and hence with the pulmonary circulation.

3. Infection may spread from nasal sinuses, throat, or tonsils.

4. A cold, damp, climate is favourable to its development.

5. Dust, gases, smoke, or fumes may contribute to, or aggravate, the condition.

---

* Once the habit of mouth-breathing has become established, it is most difficult to overcome, even though the obstruction which was its origin no longer exists, and much perseverance is necessary on the part of the physiotherapist.

PATHOLOGY.—

1. EFFECTS ON THE BRONCHI AND LUNG TISSUE.—The mucous coat of the bronchi may become thickened, or it may atrophy. In either case its cells and glands atrophy, and are finally destroyed. At first a thick viscid mucus is produced in the larger bronchi. It is copious to begin with, but as the cells degenerate it becomes less in quantity.

The fibres of the muscular coat atrophy and degenerate. The walls of the bronchi are thus weakened, and the tubes become dilated. This may lead to the condition known as 'bronchiectasis' (see p. 375). In any case, expiration is hampered. Because of difficulty in breathing and the constant coughing, the lung tissue may, in time, become stretched. This condition is known as 'emphysema' (see p. 381).

2. EFFECTS ON THE CIRCULATION.—

The Heart.—In the first place, the constant coughing puts a strain on this organ. Secondly, in a severe case where a certain degree of emphysema is present, many capillaries in the lung are obliterated, so that the right ventricle has to work very hard to pump the blood through the diminished number of vessels. This leads to dilatation and hypertrophy of the walls of that cavity.

The Portal Circulation.—As a result of the above, there may be back-pressure on the systemic veins, with subsequent congestion in the portal system.

SIGNS AND SYMPTOMS.—

1. The cough, which comes on in the winter ('winter cough'), becomes more and more severe and of longer duration each year, until finally it is present throughout the year. It is paroxysmal, usually being worst at night and in the early morning.

2. There is wheezing and tightness of the chest, especially early in the day, before the mucus deposits are loosened by coughing. Râles and rhonchi can usually be heard over the lower lobes.

3. The sputum may be scanty or considerable in amount (6–8 oz. at a time). It is often frothy, but may be mucopurulent or purulent if infection occurs in weakened or degenerate tissue.

4. Dyspnœa is a marked feature if the bronchitis is complicated by emphysema or by a strained heart. The patient becomes breathless on exertion, e.g., when walking fast or going upstairs. From the patient's point of view this is often the most distressing feature, and that which causes him to seek medical advice.

The patient's health may be quite good apart from the above symptoms— that is, if the bronchitis is uncomplicated. The patient may, however, be weak, and if the portal circulation is affected he may suffer from constipation and other abdominal disturbances. The symptoms of emphysema are described on p. 383. In advanced stages the patient becomes cyanosed (a bluish tinge on the skin, particularly noticeable in the lips and finger-nails), and the fingers become clubbed.

Treatment.—

GENERAL TREATMENT.—Warmth is essential but it is a great mistake for the patient to overload himself with heavy garments, or to remain in an overheated, stuffy atmosphere. He should have plenty of fresh air, regular exercise, and sufficient sleep. Food should be nourishing, and a special diet may be prescribed if the patient is overweight or underweight. Smoking and drinking are often prohibited. Medicines are prescribed to aid expectoration by day, and reduce coughing by night. Antibiotics and antispasmodic drugs will be given if required. The sufferer from chronic bronchitis should, ideally, live in a mild climate in winter, and avoid a dusty or smoke-laden atmosphere.

PHYSICAL TREATMENT.—The specific aims of treatment are as follows:—

1. To dislodge the mucus deposits from the walls of the bronchi, so that they may be expectorated.

2. *To assist respiration*, especially *expiration*.

3. *To improve the condition of the lungs and assist interchange of gases* by increasing the activity of their cells. The possibility of emphysema must always be taken into account in these cases, as its presence makes expiration even more difficult.

4. *To restore the mobility of the thorax*, or to preserve it should it be unimpaired.

If necessary, such complications as a weak or strained heart will also be treated (*see* Chapter XVIII).

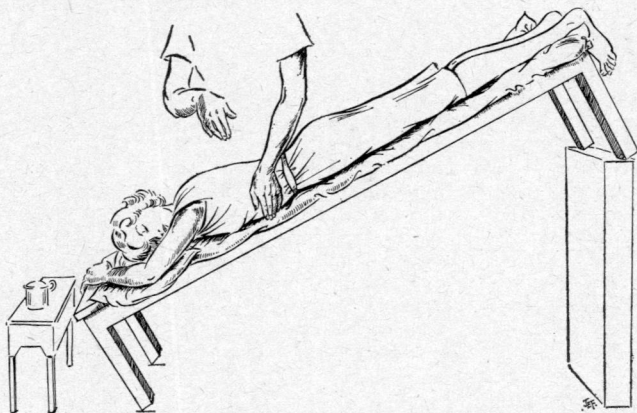

Fig. 168.—Postural drainage for bronchitis. Patient on plinth the foot of which is raised.
(*By kind permission of Dr. J. Cyriax.*)

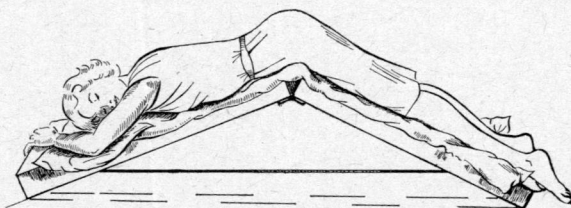

Fig. 169.—Tipping frame used instead of plinth.

For a case of chronic bronchitis with a tendency to emphysema, but without severe symptoms of the latter condition, the method of treatment may be as follows:—

POSTURAL DRAINAGE AND PERCUSSION.—Since the basal bronchopulmonary segments are most usually affected, it is often sufficient to place the patient on an inclined bed or on a tipping frame (*see* Figs. 168 and 169) in order to promote drainage. If more specific drainage is required the appropriate position must be adopted (*see* p. 377). The patient should be made quite comfortable by placing pillows under the hips and, if possible, she should lie in this position for ten minutes or so before treatment begins. *Chest-clapping*, *hacking*, and *vibrations* should then be vigorously applied for 10–20 minutes. The patient should be encouraged to cough up the loosened mucus, for which purpose a sputum mug containing a weak carbolic solution or similar disinfectant is provided. Rests, in the form of breathing exercises, may be given during this treatment. The patient is asked to *breathe out* as much as she can and *a normal inspiration* should then be taken. This should be followed by another prolonged and forceful *expiration*. This not only helps the patient to overcome difficulty in expiration, but also helps to stimulate the cough reflex and therefore aids expectoration. Vibrations may be given during expiration to help dislodge mucus and assist expectoration.

EXERCISES.—Breathing exercises and exercises for thoracic mobility follow postural drainage. General exercise may also be required, and should be adapted to the patient's age and strength.

Breathing Exercises.—These should make full use of the chest and special emphasis must be laid on *expiration. Posterior basal, lateral, apical,* and *diaphragmatic breathing* should all be taught, the most suitable starting position being crook-half-lying as this relaxes the abdominal muscles and prevents their fixing the thorax. In all these exercises, *natural* inspiration should be followed by a *full* expiration, *but neither movement should be forced.* (For further breathing exercises, *see* pp. 403–5.)

Exercises to Mobilize, or Preserve the Mobility of, the Thorax.—Danger lies in the thorax becoming fixed in a position of inspiration, but if complete expiration is practised this is not likely to happen. Breathing exercises mobilize the thorax, but free trunk-rolling, trunk-rotations, and side-bendings may also be given. For the latter, the patient's hand should be placed on the ribs in order to *localize the movement in the thorax,* otherwise it will mainly take place in the lumbar region. The pelvis should also be fixed, stride-sitting being a suitable starting position to ensure this.

General Exercises.—Besides the trunk exercises mentioned above, trunk-forward-bendings and abdominal contractions may be added, together with general arm and leg exercises. None of the trunk exercises should be very vigorous, since the majority of these patients are elderly and many have some degree of heart weakness* even if the latter is not serious. Most free trunk exercises of average strength, however, are suitable. Strong abdominal exercises like 2-Knee-updrawing and -down-pressing, 2-Leg-updrawing, and trunk-raisings which involve strong static abdominal exercises, are all unsuitable, not only because of the patient's age-group, but because they fix the thorax. Breathing exercises may be incorporated in most of these general exercises, if desired. Expiration can be considerably assisted by combining it with trunk forward flexion.

Electrical Treatment.—A course of general ultra-violet irradiation may be given to improve the patient's general health and, if necessary, raise his resistance to infection. Sectional or general technique may be employed, according to which is most appropriate. *If there is any suspicion of pulmonary tuberculosis, general ultra-violet irradiation must not be given.*

BRONCHIECTASIS

In this condition there is a permanent dilatation of the walls of the smaller bronchi and bronchioles, resulting in the formation of sacs in which mucus secretions lodge. These become infected and the disease is characterized by copious mucopurulent sputum.

AETIOLOGY.—

SEX.—Men are more often affected than women.

AGE.—The patients are generally between the ages of 20 and 40 years.

---

* The heart condition which often accompanies bronchitis (cor pulmonale) may require special precautions but, as a rule, the primary condition (bronchitis) should be treated. If the condition is really serious, the patient may have to be placed in an oxygen tent, with the foot of the be raised. He will then be treated primarily as a heart case (*see* Chapter XVIII).

CAUSES.—Bronchiectasis is almost invariably the sequel of some other disease of the bronchi or lungs, especially of:—

1. *Chronic bronchitis* and *emphysema*.—Coughing, and the constant effort to breathe out through obstructed tubes, further distends the already weakened muscular walls.

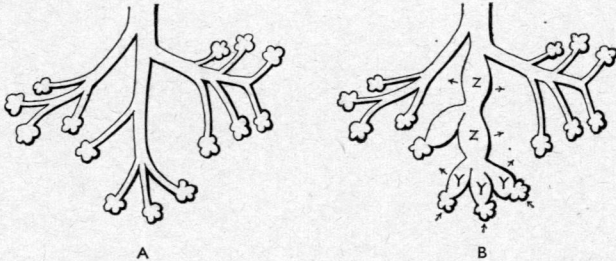

Fig. 170.—A, Normal terminal bronchiole showing alveolar ducts and alveoli. B, Effect of opposing forces brought about by fibrosis: Y, Fixed dilatation owing to pull of fibrosed tissue; Z, Dilatation resulting from pull of patent tissue against that of fibrosed tissue.

2. *Atelectasis* and *fibrosis* of the lung. The fibrous tissue contracts and forms a solid area in the lung. This pulls on the walls of the tube which are already weak because of the degeneration of the muscular coat, and holds them in a distended position. Thus, opposing forces are created between the fibrosed and the patent areas of lung tissue which pull in the opposite direction, leading to further dilatation (*see Fig.* 170).

3. *Tumours* or *aneurysm*, which compress and obstruct the bronchi.

4. *Bronchopneumonia.*

5. *Tuberculosis.*

Bronchiectasis sometimes follows *virus infections* in childhood and there is also a rare *congenital* form.

PATHOLOGY.—The muscular walls become weakened by disease, and later dilate from one of the above-mentioned causes. Mucous secretions collect in the pockets thus formed (*Fig.* 171), remain there, and decompose. This sets up an inflammation in the walls, leading to further softening and dilatation and, sometimes, to ulceration. The ciliated epithelium of the bronchi is replaced by squamous epithelium in places, so that the passage of mucus away from the lungs is still further hindered. The walls of the cavities become hyperæmic, and bleeding may take place. Bronchiectasis may involve any part of the lungs, but the lower lobes are most commonly affected. The mobility of the thorax is impaired, and in unilateral cases *scoliosis* may develop, with the *concavity* on the side of the affected lung.

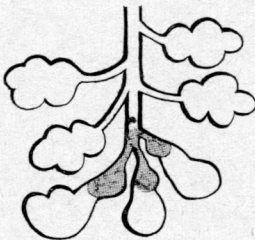

Fig. 171.—Diagrammatic representation of diseased and unaffected lung tissue. Note pockets in bronchiole and ducts in which mucus can collect.

SIGNS AND SYMPTOMS.—

(1) *Respiration is shallow* and *dyspnœa* (breathlessness) and *cyanosis* are often present. (2) There is a troublesome *cough* during which *hæmoptysis* (intra-pulmonary bleeding) may occur. It may even induce vomiting. (3) Large quantities of *highly offensive mucopurulent sputum* are usually coughed up, particularly on rising in the early morning. (4) The *breath*

is fœtid. (5) General health is often poor, the patient suffering from *lassitude* and *debility.* (6) There will be *radiological evidence* of the disease and there may be a *mediastinal shift.* (7) *Breath-sounds* may be altered and *percussion diminished.* (8) *The fingers and toes may become clubbed.*

In addition to the above symptoms, those of the causative condition may also be present.

PROGNOSIS.—The condition generally grows slowly worse, and advanced cases do not respond satisfactorily to medical and physical treatment alone. The condition may terminate in cor pulmonale or right-sided heart failure. If, however, the secretion is evacuated frequently and the cavities are kept drained, the general health improves, and the cough gives less trouble.

Treatment.—

GENERAL TREATMENT.—Rest, warmth, fresh air, hygiene, and nourishing food are essential.

MEDICAL TREATMENT.—Antiseptic inhalations are sometimes given to disinfect the cavities, and antibiotics are used to combat infection.

PHYSICAL TREATMENT.—This is similar in all respects to that described for chronic bronchitis. Since there is usually a certain degree of emphysema present, and since the primary aim of treatment is to clear the bronchial passages, emphasis is usually laid on *expiratory* rather than on inspiratory movements. It may sometimes be necessary, however, to attempt to gain *re-expansion* in collapsed areas of lung tissue, and in such cases specific *inspiratory* movements must be taught. Posture must be carefully checked and any faults corrected.

POSTURAL DRAINAGE AND PERCUSSION.—This is the most important part of the treatment. Breathing exercises can have little effect until the secretions are removed, and while these remain in the body, the general health is endangered. *Completely accurate drainage is essential,* not only to ensure clearance of the bronchial passages, but also *to avoid spreading the infection.* The position adopted by the patient depends on the part of the lung affected. He must be so placed that the diseased bronchi are directed *vertically downwards towards the main bronchus.* The force of gravity will then help to drain the secretions and infected matter from the cavities into the bronchus, whence it can be expelled by coughing. The positions suitable for all areas which may be affected cannot be given here.* The following, or some adaptation of them, are those most commonly used.

1. *For the Lower Lobes* (the most frequently affected).—The position adopted is the same as that described on p. 374, the upper part of the body being inclined downwards at an angle of 45°. If the patient's bed, or a plinth, is used, pillows should be placed under his hips, and the foot of the bed raised 14 in.

2. *For the Middle Lobes.*—The patient lies flat on his back, with pillows arranged to turn the body to left or right at an angle of 45° away from the affected side (e.g., for *right* middle lobe, 45° towards *left*). The foot of the bed is raised 12 in.

3. *For the Upper Lobes.*—Sitting upright.

It must be remembered, however, that the above positions may have to be modified according to whether the lesion is in an anterior, posterior, or lateral position in the lung. The position for draining *anterior parts* would be supine-lying; for *posterior parts,* prone-lying or lying tipped at an angle of 35° or 45°; for *lateral parts* side-lying on the sound side. The *exact site of the lesion must therefore be known,* in order to make an accurate decision as to the best position to adopt. If the condition involves more than one area, each must be drained in turn.

---

* For fuller details, *see* O. Guthrie-Smith, *Rehabilitation, Re-education and Remedial Exercises,* 2nd edition; and Gladys M. Storey, *Thoracic Surgery for Physiotherapists.*

The patient may be given an inhalation immediately before treatment, or while lying in the appropriate drainage position. The evacuation is greatly assisted by *chest-clapping, back-hacking,* and *vibrations,* administered during the drainage period.

Postural drainage should take place at least twice and, if possible, three times a day, for a period of about an hour at a time, beginning with a somewhat shorter period. The position for the lower lobes (tipping at an angle of 45°) should not, however, be maintained for more than half an hour at a time, ten minutes being sufficient to begin with.

The above treatment alone is suitable for slight cases and for inoperable bronchiectasis. In many cases, however, an operation is necessary.

SURGICAL TREATMENT.—Nowadays, operative measures are very often employed. These may be directed towards draining the cavities (*see* p. 395), but more usually consist of removal of the diseased areas of lung tissue either by: (1) *Lobectomy*—removal of the affected lobe or lobes; or (2) *Pneumonectomy* —complete removal of one lung.*

ASTHMA

In children and adults under 40 years old asthma, like hay fever, is an *allergic condition* consisting of intermittent attacks of acute dyspnœa, brought about by spasm of the muscles of the bronchioles, in response to irritation of the mucous membrane by substances to which the patient is peculiarly sensitive. It can, however, follow measles, whooping-cough, or an acute respiratory infection and in those over forty, it is more likely to be associated with bronchitis, or heart or kidney disease. Heredity, either in the form of asthma or an allied allergic condition, is commonly a factor. During the attacks *expiratory* movements are laboured and ineffectual.

AETIOLOGY.—

SEX.—Males are more often affected than females.

PSYCHOLOGICAL FACTORS.—Anxiety, worry, or protracted nervous strain may produce, or aggravate, the trouble. There is generally some physical factor present, but some cases appear to be pure, or almost pure, neuroses. In any case, the repeated attacks tend to engender fear of subsequent ones.

SUBSTANCES CAUSING ASTHMA.—These may be airborne or blood-borne. Among them are the pollens of various plants, grasses, and flowers; the emanations from various animals, e.g., poultry (feathers), cats (hair), and horses (dandruff); and various proteins taken in food—eggs, milk, meat, shellfish, etc.

PATHOLOGY.—During an attack there is *spasm of the muscles of the bronchioles,* and *swelling of the mucous membrane,* which increases secretion.

In chronic cases the chest loses its mobility and may become fixed in a position of inspiration, the muscles of forced inspiration being shortened.

PHYSIOLOGY.—In normal conditions, expiration is a passive act brought about by the elastic recoil of the lungs, once the difference in pressure on their inner and outer surfaces has been almost equalized (*see* p. 382). Air is thus pressed out of the lungs into the respiratory tract, whence it is exhaled.

In asthma the bronchioles are in spasm, and the lumen of the tubes is considerably reduced. Inspiration remains comparatively easy, but *expiration* is difficult. This apparent anomaly can be explained by the following facts. When, during inspiration, the thoracic pressure is low, the higher (atmospheric) pressure in the bronchioles tends to expand them, thus stretching their muscular fibres and reducing the spasm. During expiration, the pressure in the thorax rises. The bronchioles may even become compressed, but there is insufficient pressure

---

* *See* Section V, p. 398, for details.

between them and the lung to counteract the spasm. Much air, therefore, enters the lungs during an attack, but only a small amount of this can be expelled, until the spasm relaxes. The lungs therefore become more and more distended until a climax is reached. Signs of emphysema may be found, and the bronchioles may become the seat of chronic inflammation.

SYMPTOMS.—The attack generally takes place at night, the patient waking up with a feeling of *suffocation*. During the attack *expiration* is long and wheezing. *Inspiration* is short and shallow, and the face becomes pale and anxious. *The thorax is fixed in the position of inspiration*, and moves very little in spite of the patient's violent efforts. What breathing there is is costal, the diaphragm moving hardly at all. The patient very often tries to assist expiration by leaning forward and grasping some support in order to *fix the shoulder-girdle, enabling him to bring all the accessory muscles into play*. Despite this, his efforts are of no avail until a violent fit of coughing terminates the attack. The sputum is characteristic, being scanty and viscid to begin with, becoming more copious and watery later. The patient is exhausted at the end of an attack, whether it has lasted only a few minutes or continued for some hours. The length of the intervals between attacks varies in different individuals.

Some patients enjoy good health in the intervals, others show signs of bronchitis.

GENERAL SYMPTOMS.—As mentioned above, the chronic asthmatic patient tends to develop a 'barrel chest', with raised ribs, high shoulders, prominent anterior neck muscles, and an increased dorsal kyphosis. The face may have an anxious look. The chest may lose much of its mobility, and respiration may be shallow, the patient breathing almost entirely in the upper part of his chest. The lower part remains fully expanded and moves very little. The diaphragm is used only to a very slight extent, if at all.

PROGNOSIS.—In young people asthma tends to improve, or even disappear, especially if the particular cause can be discovered and the patient is appropriately treated. In older people in whom bronchitis or emphysema is present, the outlook is less encouraging.

Treatment.—

GENERAL AND MEDICAL TREATMENT.—The patient should have plenty of fresh air, and antihistamine drugs such as ephedrine may be used to ward off attacks. During an attack adrenaline affords relief. It may be injected or inhaled.

Patients whose trouble is caused by sensitiveness to a protein in food must avoid any dish which contains it, desensitization being of no avail in these cases. In cases caused by sensitivity to other proteins, desensitization may be achieved by means of injections of the particular substance.

PHYSICAL TREATMENT.—It is particularly important to allay the patient's fear of an attack, and to reduce the general tension of body and mind. The latter can be achieved by relaxation, the former by teaching breath control and the correct use of the chest. The specific aims, therefore, are as follows: (1) *To obtain relaxation of the whole body*, and particularly of the chest and shoulders; (2) *To educate the patient in breath control and the use of the diaphragm as a respiratory muscle*; (3) *To mobilize the thorax and help the patient to achieve full expiratory movements*; (4) *To correct posture*, and teach him to maintain it.

Besides relaxation and breathing exercises, treatment should include a short general table of arm, leg, and trunk exercises. These may be interspersed, or combined, with general breathing exercises as desired.

SPECIAL EXERCISES.—

1. *Relaxation.*—Treatment should begin with this. The most suitable position for the patient is half-lying or crook-half-lying, with pillows supporting the knees, head, and arms. Relaxation is then taught in the usual way. Particular

attention should be paid to head-rollings, to gain relaxation of the neck muscles; and to relaxation of the shoulder-girdle. It may also be helpful to teach the patient how to relax in his chosen sleeping position. Any faults of posture should be corrected in the relaxed position.

2. *Breathing Exercises.*—The emphasis must always be on *expiration*, no *deep* inspirations ever being allowed. Re-education in all types of breathing may be necessary, but it is important to teach *diaphragmatic breathing and control*, and *to re-establish lower costal breathing.*

a. Diaphragmatic breathing and control: Relaxation of the diaphragm is one of the most important factors in respiration. During this movement the central tendon is forced upwards and the lower ribs are drawn down and in, so that pressure is exerted on the lungs. We have seen that during an attack the diaphragm hardly moves at all, its movements being extremely restricted when the thorax is fixed in an inspiratory position. The patient should be taught the correct use of the diaphragm as a respiratory muscle, so that its action becomes an integral part of breathing. He should also be able to move it at will. In this way he may be able to maintain thoracic mobility when he feels an attack is imminent, and the knowledge that he has a measure of control over the situation considerably eases psychological (and, therefore, physical) tension. He must also be taught to use the abdominal muscles correctly in breathing, these being the most important muscles of expiration. To begin with the exercises should be taught in the crook-lying position, as this relaxes the abdominal muscles and allows them to be fully used. Later, the patient should be able to perform these movements in lying, half-lying, sitting, or standing positions.

b. Costal breathing: Dr. Hurst (of Guy's Hospital) taught us one of the best ways to accomplish this. The patient begins the exercise with an *expiration* (without a previous inspiration) and repeats this four or five times with *short* inspirations in between. The expirations should be as complete as possible, but should not at first be forced, as the chest must remain relaxed and not become fixed by the effort. The patient breathes out by the mouth, and it is recommended that he makes a hissing sound as he does so. The exercise should first be taught in crook- or half-lying, and later in sitting and standing. Vibrations may be given over the ribs to assist the expirations.

Miss Angrove, in her book *Remedial Exercises for Certain Diseases of the Heart and Lungs*, stated that the patient should himself be taught to perform these vibrations, so that he may be better able to practise the exercises at home. He will be wise to do so, as a precaution, for the rest of his life, even should apparent recovery take place. Miss Angrove also emphasized the importance of the development of new and correct posture.*

i. Lower costal breathing: To assist this movement, or when giving vibrations, the physiotherapist's hands are placed (α) at the *front* of the chest over the upper ribs; (β) At the *sides* of the chest over the lower ribs.

ii. Upper costal breathing: Rarely required. If given, the operator's hands are placed: (α) At the sides of the chest over the upper ribs; (β) On the front of the chest below the clavicles.

iii. Apical breathing: Hardly ever necessary. If required it may be performed as (β) above.

Importance of Teaching Breathing Control in all Circumstances.—It is most important to teach the patient to control his breathing in every possible position, and in all the circumstances of his daily life—and that in such a way as to attract no notice from others. Diaphragmatic breathing and shoulder relaxation

---

* Miss Angrove's book is still most valuable on this subject, and should be read by all students. She was one of the pioneers in the physical treatment of heart and lung diseases.

can be practised anywhere in sitting, standing, lean-sitting, or -standing. The patient may walk in time with his breathing, taking 2 steps for the short inspiration, 3 steps for the long expiratory phase, 1 step for the pause following it. He may establish a similar rhythm in going upstairs, or in performing any other routine actions.

3. *Mobility Exercises.*—In addition to breathing exercises, general exercises which mobilize the thorax and shoulder-girdle should be taught and practised at home.

The relaxation and mobility exercises in *Physical Exercises for Asthma*★ are most helpful. These should be studied by every physiotherapist. They consist of relaxation, mobility, and breathing exercises, elementary and advanced, as well as some specially suitable for children. Many of them are well-known remedial or educational exercises specially adapted for this condition, with directions as to technique, etc. The patient is instructed to perform them in the morning before breakfast, at night before retiring to bed, and at the first sign of an impending attack.

4. *Exercises to Correct the Posture.*—The defective position of the thorax must be rectified, and the patient must learn to depress the shoulder-girdle and draw in the abdomen. He must also learn to correct the kyphosis, by contracting the upper portions of the longitudinal back muscles. The head must be held erect and the 'tail tucked in'. This must be practised until the correct postural reflex is re-established. Head-extensions, abdominal contractions, and back-raisings should also be practised in order to strengthen postural muscles.

ELECTRICAL TREATMENT.—A course of general ultra-violet radiation is often beneficial.

III. DISEASES OF THE LUNGS

EMPHYSEMA

Loss of elasticity of the lung tissue, due to dilatation of the infundibula and alveoli.

VARIETIES.—Emphysema may be divided into two main varieties:—

1. INTERLOBULAR, in which, owing to a wound, or a rupture of many alveoli by coughing or straining, air has passed into the interstitial tissue of the lung. It is commonly known as 'Surgical emphysema' and generally resolves spontaneously.

2. VESICULAR, in which the alveoli have become distended and have lost their elasticity. There are three forms of vesicular emphysema.

a. Compensatory (inspiratory).—This occurs in one lung when the other is out of action owing to consolidation, fibrosis, etc., or in parts or lobules of a lung when other lobules are useless for similar reasons.

b. Atrophic.—This takes place in old age from atrophy of the lobules. The chest is small and shrunken.

c. Hypertrophic (expiratory).—This is the form with which physiotherapists are concerned. It is due to dilatation of the alveoli, with loss of their elasticity. Consequently there is difficulty in expiration.

CAUSES.—Hypertrophic emphysema may be due to:—

1. HEREDITY.—There is a congenital weakness or deficiency of the elastic fibres in the walls of the bronchioles, infundibula, and alveoli.

2. EXCESSIVE STRAIN ON THE ALVEOLAR WALLS, such as is produced by coughing and expiratory effort in bronchitis; by repeated attacks of asthma; or by

---

★ *Physical Exercise for Asthma*, published for the Asthma Research Council.

respiratory difficulty in children with adenoids. This overstrain may also be due to *occupations* which entail strong respiratory efforts, e.g., glass-blowing or playing a wind instrument, or to those so laborious as to impose continual strain on the respiratory apparatus.

In order to understand this condition it is necessary to consider the physiology of respiration, particularly that of expiration. It will be remembered that during quiet respiration *inspiration is a muscular act* brought about by the action of the diaphragm and intercostal muscles, whereas *expiration is a partly passive act.* The intake and outlet of the air is brought about by alterations in intra-thoracic and intrapulmonary pressure resulting from changes in the dimensions of the thorax and lungs. The thorax is an air-tight box, inside which lie the lungs, heart, œsophagus, great vessels, etc. The lungs are completely surrounded by the pleuræ, each consisting of two layers. The outer or *parietal layer* lines the chest wall and is reflected at the root of the lung onto the organ itself to form the inner, or *visceral layer*, which is closely adherent to the lung substance. The space between the layers is therefore a closed sac, having no communication with the parts outside it. The lungs, however, are in communication with the exterior by means of the trachea.

PHYSIOLOGY.—In the fœtus the thorax is a solid entity, but at birth the first inspiration leads to enlargement of the dimensions of the thorax, with a subsequent decrease in pressure. This creates a sub-atmospheric or negative pressure within the thorax and pleural cavities, known as *the negative pressure of the thorax.* This negative pressure is maintained throughout life, partly because no air can enter the thorax under normal conditions and partly because *the highly elastic lung tissue has a strong tendency to recoil*, which reduces the pressure on the parietal layer of the pleura. *The greater the stretch applied to the lung tissue, the stronger is the subsequent recoil*, as though the lungs were ever attempting to regain their pre-natal state. This state is never achieved, however, unless air gains access to the thoracic or pleural cavities,* because the lungs are prevented from collapse by being in communication with the atmosphere. The pressure within them (intrapulmonary pressure) remains more or less constant with that of the atmosphere, and is therefore higher than that within the thorax (intrathoracic pressure). At the end of expiration the thorax as much resembles the pre-natal state as is possible, the intrapulmonary pressure being atmospheric, while the intrathoracic pressure is only very slightly below it. When, however, the thorax is enlarged in *inspiration* the pressure within it falls. In other words, there is an 'increase of negative pressure'. The pressure in the lungs, which remains atmospheric, is now a good deal higher than that in the thorax and pleural cavities and the lungs therefore expand, by virtue of the fact that the infundibula and alveoli are highly elastic structures. This expansion of lung tissue *reduces the volume of the thorax*, but *increases the volume of the lungs. The intrathoracic pressure rises* (becoming less and less negative) as the lung tissue expands, while *intrapulmonary pressure falls* (becoming subatmospheric). Air therefore rushes into the lungs, until atmospheric pressure is again reached.

When *expiration* takes place the relaxation of the respiratory muscles reduces the dimensions of the thorax so that *the intrathoracic pressure continues to rise* until it almost equals that within the lungs. At the same time, however, *the elastic recoil of the lung tissue tends to reduce the volume of the lungs*, so that *the intrapulmonary pressure also rises* until it becomes higher than atmospheric pressure. Air therefore rushes out of the lungs until equilibrium is reached.

In emphysema, the elasticity of the lung tissue is lost, or considerably dimin-ished, and the lungs no longer tend to return to their original size. At the end of

---

* E.g., by a stab-wound, or surgical operation.

inspiration the atmospheric pressure in the lungs, unopposed by this elasticity, keeps the lungs expanded against the slightly lower pressure in the thoracic cavity, and expiration becomes difficult, forced expiration being necessary to expel all the air.

PATHOLOGICAL CHANGES.—

1. *The alveoli become stretched*, and the septa between adjacent cells are absorbed, so that they coalesce. The elastic fibres in their walls disappear, with the resultant difficulty in expiration explained above.

2. *The capillaries* passing over and between the alveoli *also become stretched*, and are finally obliterated. This tends to strain the right side of the heart, since it has to pump the same amount of blood through a smaller number of vessels.

3. Both these factors lead to an *imperfect interchange of gases* in the lungs and *hypoventilation*, so that there is interference with the general nutrition and metabolism.

4. Marked changes arise in the shape and mobility of the thorax. These will be described with the physical signs.

5. There may also be *abdominal congestion* resulting from fixation of the thorax in the inspiratory position. The consequent loss of mobility causes the respiration to be shallow, and renders the suction action of the thorax inadequate.

6. If, as is usual, bronchitis is also present, the bronchi are affected as in that disease.

SIGNS AND SYMPTOMS.—

1. *Dyspnœa* is the most marked symptom in the early stages. The inspiration is quick and short, the expiration very prolonged. At first this is only noticeable on exertion but later it becomes more and more pronounced, until it is continuous even at rest.

2. *Cyanosis* usually occurs in the later stages, owing to the defective interchange of gases. It may be very marked, yet the patient is able to get about.

3. The patient is very weak and fatigued, and heart symptoms may be pronounced.

PHYSICAL SIGNS.—The '*barrel-shaped thorax*' (*Fig.* 172) is characteristic of emphysema, the changes in form being as follows:—

1. *The anteroposterior diameter of the chest is increased*, the sternum being thrown forward; it may even be greater than the lateral diameter. The costal cartilages are prominent, and the intercostal spaces widened.

2. *The dorsal kyphosis is increased*, the back being rounded and the shoulders raised.

3. *There is a deep sternal fossa.* The clavicles are prominent and the neck appears to be shorter than normal, because of the elevation of the thorax and shoulders. *The neck muscles*, i.e., the muscles of forced inspiration, the scalenes, sternomastoid, etc., *are hypertrophied* and stand out prominently in the neck.

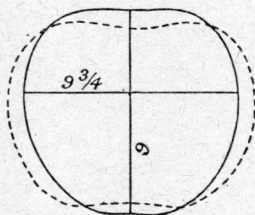

Fig. 172.—Horizontal section of an emphysematous chest showing barrel-shaped thorax. The dotted line indicates the natural shape. (*After French.*)

All this leads to *thoracic immobility*, so that the *range of inspiratory* as well as *expiratory excursion* is diminished. *Respiration is therefore shallow.*

PROGNOSIS.—This is poor. Bronchitis often complicates the condition and repeated attacks hasten the down-hill course. Death may occur from heart failure or pneumonia.

Treatment.—

GENERAL TREATMENT.—As for chronic bronchitis (*see* p. 373), the primary aim being to prevent this complication.

PHYSICAL TREATMENT.—This is similar to that required for bronchitis, the chief aim being to *mobilize the thorax* and *assist expiration.* How much we shall be able to do depends largely on the condition of the patient's heart. Those with *chronic bronchitis, slight emphysema,* and *no heart symptoms* may be treated as cases of mild bronchitis, but we must feel our way more carefully, and be content to advance more slowly. *Expiratory breathing exercises* are obviously of the greatest importance, but *specific exercises to mobilize the thorax,* and *graduated general exercises* are also essential. For those with *marked emphysema* and *definite heart involvement* much less can be done. They must be treated primarily as heart cases (*see* Chapter XVIII), but one should not expect the steady improvement that often takes place in a patient with, say, a mitral lesion. Careful chest vibrations, clapping, and expiratory exercises can generally be given with the physician's permission, but they must not be too forcible, and their effect on the patient must be watched. If there is any deterioration in his condition physical treatment should cease, or at least be greatly modified.

LOBAR PNEUMONIA

Inflammation of the lung tissue in one or both lungs, caused by invading micro-organisms. It sometimes occurs in epidemic form. Before the days of antibiotics the mortality-rate was high.

AETIOLOGY.—

AGE.—Lobar pneumonia is most common in children under 10 years of age and in elderly people, but it may occur at any age.

SEX.—In children the sexes are equally susceptible, while in adults men are more often attacked than women.

CAUSES.—The common causative organisms are the pneumococcus, but the staphylococci, streptococci, and influenza virus are sometimes responsible.

Predisposing causes: (1) Malnutrition, insufficient attention to hygiene, badly ventilated rooms, and overcrowding. (2) Debility from illness (measles, whooping-cough, etc.). (3) Alcoholism, or anything in fact which lowers resistance.

Exciting causes: (1) Cold, chill or exposure, or exhaustion following violent exercise may bring on an attack. (2) Lobar pneumonia is sometimes a post-operative complication, though bronchopneumonia is more commonly so.

PATHOLOGICAL CHANGES.—

1. Either or both lungs may be involved, and the disease may attack one or more lobes, or possibly the whole lung. If only one lung is affected it is usually the right.

2. The lung first becomes *congested* although it still contains air. Later the alveoli are filled with a solid, fibrinous exudate (*consolidation*).

3. Next follows *the stage of resolution,* or recovery. The fibrinous clot becomes liquefied by the action of enzymes which dissolve it.

Part of this fluid is expectorated, and part of it is absorbed and later excreted by the kidneys.

SYMPTOMS.—The *acute attack* begins with a shivering fit and a sudden rise of temperature to 103° or over. There is acute and agonizing *pain* in the side, due to accompanying pleurisy. It is increased by respiratory movements and by coughing, and to mitigate this the patient lies on the affected side. *Dyspnœa* is marked. *Respiration* is rapid and jerky (30–40 a minute in adults, 50–60 in children), but the *pulse-rate,* though raised, remains relatively slow. The patient has a *hacking or paroxysmal cough,* and the *expectoration is characteristic.* To begin with the sputum is scanty, being thick and mucoid. After 24 hours it becomes blood-stained owing to the presence of fresh blood in the alveoli. As this blood becomes stale it becomes rust-coloured ('rusty sputum') and more plentiful.

Course of Illness.—Recovery used to be described as being by *crisis*, which took place about the eighth day, the temperature falling in a few hours to normal or even below, the pulse- and respiration-rates falling with it. Sometimes, however, the illness terminated by *lysis*, i.e., a *gradual* fall of temperature, instead of by crisis. Both meant that the antitoxins of the patient's body had prevailed over the toxins of the bacteria. In fatal cases the temperature continued to rise and the patient generally died of heart failure.

These dramatic events are not seen nowadays, except in untreated cases, because the antibiotic drugs—penicillin or the sulphonamides—control the infection and bring about a fall of temperature in about 12–24 hours. The pulse- and respiration-rates fall also, and the other symptoms disappear in a few days. Old or debilitated patients sometimes fail to respond to treatment; the temperature remains high, and heart failure brings about a fatal issue.

Most cases of pneumonia recover completely in a short time and without after-effects, but a few suffer from *delayed resolution*. That is, the consolidation of the lung remains, and is very slow in clearing up.

COMPLICATIONS AND AFTER-EFFECTS.— These are rare. Pleurisy may continue. Empyema, lung abscess, endocarditis, and otitis media (inflammation of the middle ear) sometimes occur. Scoliosis, common after pleurisy, is rare after pneumonia.

Treatment.—

ACUTE STAGE.—Only medical treatment and efficient nursing are required.

CONVALESCENT STAGE.—Many patients make an excellent recovery, and need no special after-treatment. Some, however, recover slowly and are often benefited by physical treatment. This is especially true of the cases of 'unresolved pneumonia'.

PHYSICAL TREATMENT.—The aims of treatment are slightly different from those we have considered heretofore:—

1. We are primarily concerned with *re-expansion of the affected lung tissue*. We must, however, avoid over-stretching it in the early stages, since the tissue might easily be torn or injured.

2. It may also be necessary to prevent the development of scoliosis, and to improve the patient's general health.

The method of treatment in the early stage, with the patient still in bed, is as follows:—

POSITION OF PATIENT.—Half-lying, propped up with pillows. This is the correct position for all lung cases in the early stages because it decreases the pull of gravity on the thorax, and so facilitates breathing.

Before treatment the physiotherapist should inspect the patient's chart, in order to obtain information as to his general progress, noting particularly the temperature,* pulse, and respiration rates. She may herself take the pulse and respiration at the beginning and end of the treatment. *Breathing exercises* form the most important part of the treatment but chest-clapping and vibrations may be required.

BREATHING EXERCISES.—*Diaphragmatic* breathing is the most useful of all in re-expanding the base of the lungs, but *lateral costal* breathing should be practised assiduously, both in the lower and the upper parts of the thorax. *Apical* breathing should also be included in the programme.

---

* A rise in temperature contra-indicates treatment, and should be reported at once, as it may indicate empyema.

13

A difference of opinion exists as to the best way of localizing lateral costal breathing to obtain the maximum expansion of the affected lung. Some people believe that this is best achieved *by exerting pressure on the sound lung* in order to inhibit its action. Others feel that the movement should be completely bilateral, *slight resistance being offered to the movement on the affected side* in order to encourage expansion. To do this the physiotherapist places her hands on either side of the thorax, asking the patient to breathe in. As she feels the lungs expanding she increases the pressure on the affected side exhorting the patient to 'push into my hand'. Later, gentle side-bendings may be introduced. To assist expansion they should be combined with breathing exercises, the patient bending *towards the sound side on inspiration* and *re-assuming the upright position on expiration*. *Relaxed* alternate side-bendings may be used for mobility, as well as trunk rotations and relaxed trunk-rollings. These should not be too vigorous to begin with, but they may be progressed as the patient's condition improves. Posture should be checked and corrected if necessary. The use of mirrors may be useful in this respect.

LIMB EXERCISES.—While the patient is in bed a short general scheme of graduated exercises should be included in the treatment. This helps to maintain circulation and muscle power until such time as the patient is ambulatory.

BRONCHOPNEUMONIA

This is again an inflammatory condition of the lung tissue, *but it also involves the bronchioles*. Both lungs are involved, and the lesions are usually scattered throughout the lung tissue.

AETIOLOGY.—

1. AGE.—It is most common in early childhood and in old age.

2. Bronchopneumonia may be primary or secondary.

a. The Primary Form is the result of *pneumococcal infection*. It is seen only in children under 3 years of age.

b. The Secondary Form has causes similar to LOBAR PNEUMONIA. It occurs after the specific fevers (measles, scarlet fever, etc.) or in the form of 'aspiration pneumonia'. This is due to septic or otherwise noxious material being drawn down into the bronchi where it sets up an intense inflammation. For example, pus may drain into the bronchioles from an adjacent lung abscess, or vomit may be inhaled while the patient is unconscious.

PATHOLOGICAL CHANGES.—The inflammation starts in the smallest bronchioles, and spreads to the infundibula and alveoli which form the lobules into which the bronchus opens. These structures are *hyperæmic* and *swollen*. The bronchus and bronchioles are blocked with mucus, and the alveoli become filled with a mucous or mucopurulent exudate. This leads to *atelectasis** in the parts of the lung distal to the obstruction. Other lobules show signs of emphysema.

SYMPTOMS.—

1. In the *primary form* the onset, symptoms, and termination are similar to those of pneumonia, and the child recovers quickly. The prognosis is therefore good, and this form is rarely fatal.

2. In the *secondary form* the onset is gradual, the symptoms first resembling those of bronchitis, but as the air-cells become involved they assume a more serious aspect. There is a *painful cough, dyspnœa, intermittent fever, and a quick, weak, irregular pulse*. *The sputum is mucopurulent*.

---

* *Atelectasis*, or absorption collapse of the lung, occurs when a bronchus is blocked in any way, so that inspired air cannot pass beyond the obstruction. The air already present in the alveoli is absorbed into the blood, and the affected part of the lung shrinks and collapses, because its elastic recoil is unopposed by the pressure of air.

PROGNOSIS.—The condition is a serious one and antibiotics are less effective in this than in lobar pneumonia. The patient may die from exhaustion, heart failure, or asphyxia. In cases that recover, the termination is by *lysis* and convalescence is very slow. In some cases areas of consolidation remain unresolved for months.

COMPLICATIONS AND AFTER-EFFECTS.—Complications are rare, except for *heart failure.* (Such heart-failure, brought about by pathological conditions of the lungs, is known as 'Cor Pulmonale'.) In some cases a *lung abscess* may form, or whole areas of lung may become *gangrenous. Fibrosis* and *bronchiectasis* are common sequelæ.

Treatment during Convalescence

GENERAL AND MEDICAL TREATMENT.—It is necessary to increase the patient's resistance, combat the infection and prevent its spread, to get rid of secretions, and prevent atelectasis. Warmth is essential and the diet should be light and nourishing. Antibiotics are administered, and oxygen is also required. It may be given by means of an oxygen tent or mask. Inhalations may give relief and help expectoration.

PHYSICAL TREATMENT.—This is important, not only in alleviating the condition, but also in preventing fibrosis and bronchiectasis. The aims of treatment are as follows:—

1. *To clear the respiratory tract.* Before anything else can be done, *the exudate must be evacuated,* since it impedes respiration and its presence in the bronchioles may lead to bronchiectasis.

2. *To re-expand lung tissue.* The condition, being bilateral, will require *inspiratory exercises* to secure expansion of both lungs.

3. *To aid expiration.* Since this condition combines atelectasis with emphysema, *expiratory exercises* must also be given.

METHOD OF TREATMENT.—The patient's temperature must be carefully watched in the early stages. It may be advisable to take the pulse before and after treatment.

2. *Postural drainage and percussion* will be given as for BRONCHIECTASIS (p. 377).

3. *Breathing exercises* are essential. *Diaphragmatic breathing* is the most important of all, the damage being generally worst at the base of the lungs, but *costal and apical breathing* must never be neglected.

Inspiration is very important because the damaged lung tissue *must* be re-expanded, but emphasis should also be laid on expiration (*see* exercises for BRONCHITIS and ASTHMA, pp. 375, 379). Since the lesions are usually widespread and both lungs are involved, localized movements are not so necessary as in lobar pneumonia, but they must, of course, be given if there are any serious areas of collapse, particularly in the basal lobes.

4. *Mobility exercises* for the thorax may be added as the condition improves.

5. *A graduated scheme of general exercises* similar to that used in lobar pneumonia should be included. It must, therefore, be remembered that the patient is seriously ill and must on no account be overtired. General and local treatment should be continued when the patient is up and about again, but easy starting positions should be chosen and progressions will necessarily be slow.

FIBROSIS OF THE LUNG
(*Fibroid Lung; Interstitial Pneumonia*)

In this condition fibrous tissue replaces the lung tissue.

AETIOLOGY.—Fibrosis of the lung is generally secondary to some other inflammatory condition. It may follow atelectasis, unresolved bronchopneumonia, chronic pleurisy, or more rarely, lobar pneumonia; or it may be caused by tuberculosis* or tumours of the lung.   It may also be caused by the inhalation of irritating dust, and is common in miners and quarrymen.   The condition is chronic, and may continue from 15 to 20 years.

PATHOLOGICAL CHANGES.—

1. One or both lungs are affected, depending on the cause.

2. The lung tissue is replaced by fibrous tissue which presses on and obliterates the alveoli and the capillaries between them.   Moreover, the *muscular tissue in the walls of the bronchioles loses its contractility and becomes fibrous*.   Since fibrous tissue has not the resilience of muscular tissue the walls yield in places, giving rise to bronchiectasis (*see* p. 376).

3. The fibrosis may be local or diffuse.   In the former case there is often *compensatory emphysema* (*see* p. 381) in other parts of the same lung, since the areas of fibrosis are hard and contracted, and no air can enter them.   If one lung is entirely fibroid, the other lung is emphysematous.   The right ventricle of the heart becomes hypertrophied as a result of the strain entailed in pumping the blood through the reduced number of capillaries.

SIGNS AND SYMPTOMS.—Early symptoms are *cough, dyspnœa on exertion*, and sometimes *cyanosis*.   Otherwise the patient often enjoys good health.   The symptoms of bronchiectasis may be present.

In *unilateral* cases the affected side of the chest may be shrunken and the shoulder is drawn down, causing a *scoliosis, convex to the healthy side*.   The muscles of the shoulder-girdle on the affected side are atrophied.

Treatment.—Our principal aims are to *expand the affected lung* if possible, *to preserve the mobility of the thorax*, and *to prevent the establishment of scoliosis*.

PHYSICAL TREATMENT.—

1. *If the lung is completely fibroid*, it obviously cannot be made to expand.   In this case all we can do is to try to preserve as much thoracic mobility as possible, and prevent the development of a troublesome scoliosis as far as possible.   Treatment will therefore consist of a *general table of exercises* (passive or free) with special emphasis on *mobility* and *postural exercises*.   *Breathing exercises* must also be given, but these will need to be modified in accordance with the state of the lungs.

2. *If the lung is not completely fibrosed*, more may be done to improve matters.   We must then endeavour to expand it in much the same way as we should do in a case of pneumonia, although the active exercises can usually be more vigorous.   *Inspiratory exercises* should therefore be given, but since a degree of emphysema may be present, attention must also be given to expiration.

TUBERCULOSIS

Tuberculosis is a very widespread disease, affecting not only human beings but many species of animals.   Fortunately, however, it is becoming less prevalent owing to improved hygiene, better housing, and education of the public as regards the danger of infection and the importance of early diagnosis.

AETIOLOGY.—

AGE.—No age is exempt, but the old are less likely to suffer.   It may attack any part of the body.   Tuberculosis of bones, joints, glands, or membranes (peritoneum or meninges) is commonest in children; *phthisis* (pulmonary tuberculosis) is most often found in young people.

SEX.—The sexes are almost equally affected.

CAUSE.—The *Bacillus tuberculosis* is the actual cause.   Infection by this bacillus may take place in three ways: (1) *By inhalation*.   This is the commonest

---

* *Tuberculous Cases.*—Cases of fibrosis due to tuberculosis should not be treated by physical methods, as these might cause a quiescent infection to flare up.

way and it usually leads to pulmonary infection. Bacilli from the sputum of consumptives are blown about in the air and breathed in by others. (2) *By ingestion*, milk from a tuberculous cow being the usual vehicle of infection, the ensuing lesion generally being located in the intestine or tonsils. (3) *By inoculation*. This rarely happens, except to surgeons when performing operations or post-mortems. It generally produces a local lesion only.

PREDISPOSING CAUSES.—The two main ones are: (1) *Hereditary predisposition* (diathesis). The disease itself is not inherited but, rather, a certain liability to contract it. This may generally be counteracted by living a hygienic and well-regulated life which keeps the general health at a high level. (2) *Lowering of the body's protective forces* by unhealthy occupations, bad social conditions, weakening diseases, etc.

OCCUPATION.—Any occupation which lowers the resistance of the body predisposes to tuberculosis. People who work for long hours on scanty food; those who spend most of their time in ill-ventilated rooms; and those who are employed in trades which entail the inhalation of dust or irritating substances are all liable to this malady.

SOCIAL CONDITIONS.—Slum conditions of overcrowded, insanitary houses, coupled with malnutrition and insufficient clothing, are responsible for a high proportion of cases.

OTHER DISEASES.—Catarrh, specific fevers, exhausting diseases all predispose to the disease. Traumas, such as blows on the chest in the case of pulmonary tuberculosis, or injuries to bones, joints, or other parts may lead to its development.

PATHOLOGY (GENERAL).—

1. FORMATION OF THE TUBERCLE.—The tubercle bacilli, having invaded the tissues, spread and multiply there. An inflammatory reaction is set up and gathers round them, forming small, greyish, jelly-like bodies called 'tubercles', so that the bacilli lie in the innermost layer of cells.

2. CASEATION.—Partly because no blood-vessels pass into them, and partly because of the effect of the bacteria or their toxins, the tubercles degenerate. A number of them together form a soft cheesy mass.

3. TERMINATION.—This may occur by: (a) *Softening and liquefaction of caseated material* which is then absorbed and excreted in urine or fæces, or coughed up. This leads to the *formation of cavities*. Cavitation gives rise to conditions which are highly favourable to the growth of tubercle bacilli and, if this process continues, the result is fatal—unless, of course, the site of the lesion is one which can be dealt with surgically. (b) *Sclerosis* (encapsulation). In this case the normal process of healing occurs. Fibrous tissue forms round the tuberculous area, encapsulating the bacilli. There is always a danger that the fibrous capsule may break down with resultant flare-up of the living bacilli within it, but if all goes well the whole area may become calcified, or even ossified. The tubercle is then enclosed in a firm, hard structure, and cure supervenes.

Phthisis

(*Pulmonary Tuberculosis*)

Physical treatment is contra-indicated in cases of active tuberculosis because anything which increases metabolism, and therefore the respiratory rate, aggravates the condition. Breathing exercises in particular must be avoided as greater ventilation of areas of cavitation leads to a rapid increase in bacilli, with subsequent spread of infection. Physiotherapy is therefore only required in surgical cases but a little should be said about the disease itself. It may take one of two forms: (1) *The acute or miliary form* (popularly known as 'galloping consumption'), involving both lungs and very often the meninges and gastro-intestinal tract as well, which ends fatally in a few months; or (2) *The chronic form*, which is more common. The process generally starts in one lung, but may later involve both. The first point of attack is generally just below the apex of the lung, and the infection extends downwards along the anterior margin.

PATHOLOGY.—The changes are those described above, the alveoli and terminal bronchioles being attacked. Caseation and liquefaction take place, the cheesy material being absorbed or coughed up, so that cavities form in the lung. The process is sometimes divided for purposes of description into three stages.

1. INVASION, in which the bacilli settle down in the tissues.
2. CONSOLIDATION.—This is the stage of tubercle formation, and of caseation.
3. EXCAVATION.—During this stage the cavities form.

Thence the disease may progress to a fatal result, or healing may take place by encapsulation. It is always possible, however, for a quiescent tuberculosis to flare up again as the result of a breakdown in the encapsulating tissue, or of some infective condition elsewhere in the body.

SYMPTOMS.—The character of the *onset* varies. It may be insidious, the patient presenting vague ill-defined symptoms; or sudden, e.g., *hæmoptysis* (hæmorrhage from the lung due to the erosion of a blood-vessel) in an apparently healthy person. Whatever the mode of onset the following symptoms are characteristic: (1) *Lassitude and fatigue*; (2) *Loss of weight*; (3) *Anorexia* (loss of appetite); (4) *Night sweats*; (5) *Nocturnal pyrexia*.

Late symptoms include a *paroxysmal painful cough* with a *characteristic sputum*—the latter being copious and purulent and brought up in separate rounded lumps; *dyspnœa*; a *swinging temperature*; and *emaciation*, the cheeks being flushed and hollow, and the eyes bright and sunken. The *chest* may be long, narrow, and flattened, the anteroposterior diameter being short. The *ribs* become more vertical in direction than normal, making the costal angle more acute, and the *scapulæ* are often winged.

Treatment (Prophylactic).—

GENERAL TREATMENT.—The children of tuberculous parents, or those suspected of an hereditary predisposition to the disease, should pay special attention to hygiene. They should live in healthy surroundings, with plenty of fresh air and sunshine, spending as much time in the open as possible and avoiding sedentary work. They should not expose themselves to infection. Food should be nourishing and clothing should be light but warm. Children whose parents are suffering from active phthisis should preferably not remain with them.

PHYSICAL TREATMENT.—

EXERCISES.—These are sometimes, though rarely, requested *as a prophylactic measure*. The treatment consists of general exercises, given out of doors if possible, or at least in a room with wide open windows.

Breathing exercises are, of course, more important than any others. It is essential that all parts of the lung should be as fully aerated as possible, in order to improve pulmonary circulation, and to improve the nutrition of all the lung tissue. This not only makes for a healthy condition of the respiratory organs themselves, but increases the resistance of the patient's whole body to infection. In order to achieve full ventilation the lungs should be fully expanded, and the patient should therefore be taught to breathe in every part of the thorax, inspiratory and expiratory movements being equally important. The following should be practised:—

Exercises to Expand the Base of the Lungs.—
1. Half-lying Diaphragmatic breathing.
2. Half-lying lower Costal breathing.
3. The above two exercises combined.

Exercises to expand the Apex.—

*Half-lying Apical Breathing.—*The physiotherapist should place her fingers over the apices of the lungs, indicating to the patient the part she wishes him to expand. Some people suggest that if the patient finds this exercise difficult gentle pressure may be exerted on the lower ribs during inspiration so that expansion mainly occurs in the upper costal and apical regions only.

Should any symptom appear which might denote actual onset of the disease, treatment must cease at once. *Hæmoptysis is an absolute contraindication,* and no treatment must be given once it has occurred, nor may it be resumed other than at the request of the surgeon or physician in charge of the case.

Treatment of Hæmoptysis (First-aid).—Should an attack of hæmoptysis occur without any previous warning, the patient should be placed on a couch or a bed in the half-lying position, with the head and trunk well raised. If it is known from which lung the blood comes the patient is turned towards the affected side, but in the case of a first attack the patient will probably assume the position most comfortable to himself. Absolute rest and quiet are essential, and the patient should be reassured. (The hæmorrhage usually stops of itself unless a large artery has been eroded.) All tight clothing should be loosened, and the windows opened, so that the patient may have plenty of air, but he should be kept warm. Nothing should be given by mouth before the arrival of the doctor. Hæmoptysis may usually be distinguished from *hæmatemesis* (hæmorrhage in the gastro-intestinal tract) by the fact that in the former the blood is bright red and frothy, being mixed with air, whereas in hæmatemesis it is generally dark in colour, except, occasionally, in cases of gastric ulcer.

Treatment of Developed Tuberculosis.—

MEDICAL AND GENERAL.—Complete rest is essential for these patients. In a sanatorium good food, fresh air, and freedom from work and worry can be secured, but the patient's full co-operation is necessary to achieve success. Antibiotics such as streptomycin are given. If these measures fail, surgical operations may be performed.

SURGICAL TREATMENT.—The operations for tuberculosis of the lungs come under two headings.

(1) *Collapse operations,* designed to rest the affected lung tissue which is continually stretched during respirations, and thereby prevented from healing. The most important from the view of the physiotherapist is *thoracoplasty* (permanent collapse of lung tissue). Other operations which afford temporary collapse of lung tissue are *artificial pneumothorax* (introduction of air into the pleural cavity), *pneumoperitoneum* (introduction of air into the peritoneal cavity so that the diaphragm is raised and exerts pressure on the lung), *phrenic crush,* which leads to paralysis of the diaphragm. The last two are suitable only for cases of lower lobe lesions. Sometimes the two are combined. The collapse achieved by any of these measures is maintained for a period of 2–3 years or more, and sometimes a repetition of the treatment is required.

(2) *Resection operations,* which consist of removal of the whole of the affected area. This may be a whole lung (pneumonectomy), a lobe, or part of a lobe of the lung (lobectomy or segmental lobectomy).

PHYSICAL TREATMENT.—Post-operative treatment may be required following any of these operations, particularly following thoracoplasty, details of which are given in Section V, p. 401. In cases where temporary collapse has been undertaken, treatment may also be required to gain re-expansion of the collapsed area when the time comes, but *no attempt must be made to expand the lung before this.*

IV. DISEASES OF THE PLEURA

PLEURISY AND EMPYEMA

Pleurisy

Pleurisy is, as the name implies, inflammation of the pleuræ of one or both lungs. It most frequently affects the right lung.

AETIOLOGY.—Pleurisy may be: (1) *Primary*, that is, confined to the pleuræ and not following on any other disease or infection; or (2) *Secondary*—arising from a primary infection elswehere.

1. PRIMARY PLEURISY is always, or almost always, due to tuberculosis, though an attack may be precipitated by chill, cold, or exposure.

2. SECONDARY PLEURISY may be due to a number of causes, the foremost of which are pneumonia or other lung diseases, the infection spreading from the lung to the pleuræ. Less common causes are: (*a*) Specific fevers—scarlet fever, rheumatism, measles, whooping-cough, septicæmia; (*b*) Chronic disease in neighbouring structures—Bright's disease, pericarditis, carcinoma, etc.

The organisms responsible for the development of pleurisy are the pneumococcus, streptococcus, and tubercle bacillus.

PATHOLOGICAL CHANGES.—There are two varieties of pleurisy: (1) '*Dry*' *pleurisy*, and (2) *Pleurisy with effusion*.

1. 'DRY' PLEURISY.—The pleural membranes become hyperæmic and red in colour. Before long, fibrin is exuded and deposited on the membranes, giving them a rough, shaggy appearance, and forming adhesions between the visceral and parietal layers. These hamper the movements of the pleuræ and give rise to pain. In 'dry' pleurisy there are no further changes, and the trouble may clear up completely. Alternatively, organization may occur, with the formation of dense fibrous adhesions; or the fibrin exudate may be followed by a serous effusion.

2. PLEURISY WITH EFFUSION.—The following stages may be noted:—

Stage of Exudation.—The fluid is serofibrinous and varies in amount. If extensive it causes collapse of the lung, displacement of the heart and great vessels, and even, in very severe cases, of the liver and spleen. The movements of the diaphragm are much hampered in this case and breathing becomes very difficult.

Stage of Resolution.—The fluid is gradually absorbed but, whether the fluid has been great or small, adhesions form between the pleuræ. If it has been great, fibrosis may occur in the collapsed lung tissue.

Stage of Purulent Exudation.—The exudation, instead of being absorbed, may become purulent. The condition then arising is known as *empyema*. In some cases the fluid is purulent from the beginning. This often happens when empyema follows on pneumonia.

SYMPTOMS.—

1. 'DRY' PLEURISY.—The attack begins with *slight chills*, or shivering attacks, but not with a violent rigor like that which precedes pneumonia. The *temperature* rises to about 102° or 103°. There is malaise, headache, and a general feeling of illness. *Severe pain* is felt on the affected side and is increased when the patient coughs or takes a deep breath. This is due to the inflamed condition of the pleuræ which causes friction between them, and to movements which pull on the adhesions. *Respiration* is rapid and shallow. There is a *dry hacking cough*, but no expectoration. The patient leans towards the affected side to lessen the pain.

2. PLEURISY WITH EFFUSION.—The signs of 'dry' pleurisy are present to begin with, but the pain grows less as the exudation increases. *Dyspnœa* is a feature of pleural effusion, since the lung is compressed by the fluid and collapses wholly, or in part. Hence respiration becomes difficult or impossible on the affected side.

The *respiratory rate* is increased, and the patient again lies on the affected side—this time to allow freedom of movement in the sound lung. The *temperature* remains raised, and the pulse is quick. Again there is a *hacking cough*, but the expectoration is not increased, because the exudation is not in the bronchioles or infundibula. What sputum there is has no marked character, and is never 'rusty' as in pneumonia.

COURSE AND PROGNOSIS.—The temperature falls by *lysis*—that is, by a gradual decline. This happens as the fluid is absorbed—in from 7 days to 3 weeks or more, depending on the degree of effusion. The prognosis is good as a rule—better in the young than in the old. The greatest danger is that of cardiac failure.

AFTER-EFFECTS.—From the point of view of the physiotherapist, the most important after-effect is the formation of adhesions which prevent full expansion of the lung, and which tend to immobilize one side of the thorax. This may ultimately cause scoliosis in the form of a thoracic curve, with its convexity to the sound side.

Treatment.—'Dry' pleurisy often clears up entirely without after-results, and rarely requires physical treatment. If this is requested it should mainly consist of breathing exercises designed to expand the lungs as much as possible. By keeping the chest moving the pleuræ are continually stretched, and strong adhesions have less chance to form. In pleurisy with effusion *the most important treatment is that of the cause*, and some of the fluid is often removed to assist the diagnosis. If the fluid fails to absorb it must be drawn off, and a series of aspirations may be necessary.

PLEURISY WITH EFFUSION

The aims of physiotherapy are *to assist the absorption of the fluid* and to prevent the formations of disabling adhesions between the two layers of the pleura; *to obtain full expansion of the collapsed or partially collapsed lung*, and to increase ventilation; *to maintain or increase the mobility of the thorax*; and *to prevent the formation of scoliosis* by the maintenance of correct posture. Should adhesions have already developed before the patient comes under our care we must do all we can to lessen their effect on the respiratory system, and on bodily posture.

It must, however, be remembered that *the pleurisy may be tuberculous in origin, and such cases must not be treated except on express orders from, and under guidance of, the surgeon in charge of the case*. In any case, any increase of inflammation will add to the existing fluid, intensifying the danger of pressure on the lung and on the heart. Consequently, in the early stages of treatment, *great care must be exercised to avoid flaring up the inflammation or interfering with resolution*. A careful watch should be kept on the temperature, pulse, and respiration chart, and for any sign which might indicate a flare-up of the condition, such as a loss of mobility or increased difficulty with respiration. If there is a rise in temperature or pulse-rate, or any other unfavourable symptom appears, treatment should be discontinued at once and advice sought before it is resumed.

Empyema

This, as described above, is a condition in which the exuded fluid within the pleural cavity is purulent. In a *true empyema* the purulent fluid becomes thickened and localized and an abscess is formed, but a seropurulent or purulent pleural effusion is often loosely termed 'empyema'. Here we will deal with a true empyema. It is always secondary to pleurisy with effusion and to infection in an adjacent structure, usually the lung. The causes are the same as for pleurisy, the actual infecting organisms usually being the streptococci or pneumococci. Occasionally, the infection may be staphylococcal or influenzal. Empyema is, however, a more serious illness than simple pleurisy and the prognosis is worse. The fluid collects at the base of the lung, and may exert very dangerous pressure upon it, or upon other organs. Moreover, the patient's general condition becomes much worse and the strength of the heart is impaired, so that collapse from exhaustion is a possibility. This is especially the case when the empyema forms part of a general infection.

PATHOLOGICAL CHANGES.—In the early stages there is an acute pleurisy which later becomes a pleurisy with effusion. To begin with, the exudate may be serous, later becoming purulent, or it may be seropurulent from the beginning. This seropurulent exudate thickens and strong fibrous adhesions form round it, until the pus becomes encapsulated within them (*abscess formation*) (*Fig.* 173).

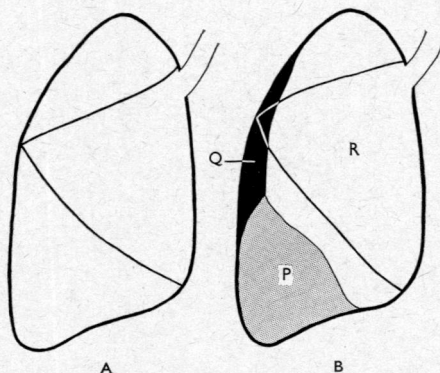

Fig. 173.—Diagrammatic representation of empyema. A, Normal lung; B, Changes occurring in empyema; P, Encapsulation of pus within limiting adhesions; Q, Increased pleural space resulting from fluid within the pleural diminished area; R, Patent lung tissue resulting from collapse of area behind abscess.

The lung tissue behind the abscess collapses, and there is a danger that the adhesions surrounding the abscess may become so dense and fibrous that they prevent re-expansion of the lung tissue.

SYMPTOMS.—In addition to those of pleurisy the following symptoms appear. The temperature rises and becomes *hectic* (remittent); that is, it rises and falls with several degrees' difference between the morning and evening temperatures, or between the temperatures at different times of the day. The patient suffers from *shivering fits*, and *night sweats* are common. The skin may be *pallid* or *hectically flushed* and there is usually some degree of *anorexia*. *Dyspnœa* may be marked, particularly if the empyema is very large in extent.

Radiological evidence reveals the presence of empyema, and blood-tests show *leucocytosis* (increase in the number of white corpuscles in the blood).

Treatment.—The aims of treatment are to control the infection, to evacuate the cavity, to gain re-expansion of the lung, and to prevent the formation of crippling adhesions which, besides diminishing the powers of ventilation, may also lead to scoliosis. Control of infection and evacuation of the cavity are the responsibility of the surgeon. *Re-expansion of the lung* and *the prevention of adhesions and postural defects* are chiefly the concern of the physiotherapist.

SURGICAL TREATMENT.—As soon as the presence of pus in the pleural cavity is confirmed antibiotics are administered, and the fluid is aspirated repeatedly, i.e., the pus is withdrawn by means of a syringe. An antibiotic may be instilled into the pleural space. These measures are often sufficient if the infection is slight, but if severe the thick pus in the abscess must be evacuated by operation under a general anaesthetic. A part of the 9th rib is resected, the cavity is cleared of pus, and a rubber tube inserted to maintain drainage. This is rarely undertaken before the third week, because the patient's general condition usually renders earlier operation unsafe.

Drainage in Empyema.—This may be by the open or closed method. *Open drainage* is used when the empyema is small and well localized, so that air cannot enter the rest of the pleural cavity and cause collapse of the lung (pneumothorax). The drainage tube is short and thick, its outer end being surrounded by a dressing and secured by a safety-pin fastened across its outer end to prevent it from slipping into the wound. *Closed drainage* is used when the empyema cavity is large, and the lung would collapse if air were allowed to enter the pleural cavity. A long tube is inserted into the cavity and fixed to the skin by means of a stitch. Its distal end is placed in a glass bottle, or jar, partly filled with water and attached to an underwater seal. The end of the tube must be kept under water so that *pus and air can pass out* of the cavity, but *air cannot pass in.* The jar is placed on the floor beside the bed so that gravity assists drainage. Another method is to attach a suction apparatus to a catheter which is introduced into the pleural cavity between two ribs. Thus "a slow drainage of pus continues simultaneously with expansion of the lung" (Angove).

PHYSICAL TREATMENT.—The importance of physiotherapy cannot be over-emphasized. The aims are the same as in pleurisy but when considering the possibility of adhesions we have to remember that these may form, not only between the two layers of the pleura, but also in the more superficial tissues at the site of the wound—muscles, fascia, and skin. If such a scar forms and contracts, it may cause irreparable damage in the form of limitation of thoracic and shoulder mobility. In post-operative empyema, the patient's body leans *away* from the affected side so that the *shoulder is lowered on the affected side.* At the same time *the hip on this side has been raised.* This causes a scoliosis *convex to the sound side.* A compensatory curve may develop in the cervical region, and sometimes a kyphosis may also develop. As well as preventing these deformities, we hope, in the early stages of treatment, to assist drainage and prevent the pus from 'pocketing' in any locality.

Empyema is a far more satisfactory condition to deal with, from the physiotherapist's point of view, than is pleurisy with effusion, since in empyema there is free drainage from the pleural cavity; also the patients generally progress extremely well.

Treatment should begin as soon as possible after the patient's return from the operating theatre.

CONDITION OF PATIENT.—It must be remembered that the patient is still very ill, and due allowance must be made for this. Great care and consideration are necessary in dealing with anyone who has not yet fully got over the shock of an operation, but in thoracic cases it is even more important, since success depends so much on the patient's co-operation which will not be given if he is roughly handled or tactlessly dealt with initially.* Even if he has had pre-operative treatment (*see* Section V, p. 399) he may be nervous, and afraid of moving or being touched. Much persuasion and encouragement may, therefore, be necessary. In any case he will tire very easily and the guiding precept should be 'little and often' in the early stages.

---

* Even if a satisfactory course of pre-operative treatment is impossible, because of the patient's general condition, the physiotherapist should endeavour to see the patient, even for a few minutes, before his operation. In this way, she will not be an entire stranger to him, and this is a great help later.

If the short type of drainage tube is being used it will be found sloping rather downwards in the wound. The safety-pin across its end is wrapped in gauze to prevent it hurting the patient by coming in contact with the wound. Over the tube are placed several layers of gauze, and above these a large pad of cotton-wool. Nowadays the dressing is usually kept in place by adhesive strapping, but in some cases a many-tail bandage may be used. The patient lies propped up with several pillows, in which a hollow is arranged to avoid pressure on the wound.

REMOVAL OF BANDAGES.—If a many-tail bandage is used it is useless to try to obtain chest expansion with the bandage on, as it constricts the chest. If open drainage is employed it may be desirable to remove the tube during treatment if it makes the patient cough or causes undue pain. *The ward-sister's permission must, however, be obtained for this and it must only be undertaken by a qualified nurse.*

The bandage should be unfastened in front—it need not be entirely removed—and, if necessary, the tube is taken out, washed, and sterilized, so as to be ready for insertion after the treatment. Meanwhile, the wound must be kept covered with a pad of sterile gauze and another of wool, which may be secured by one or two strips of the bandage pinned *loosely* across the chest, or by strips of adhesive plaster.

If the drainage tube is closed, the jar must be put on a chair or stool, so that there is no tension on the tube and there is no danger of the tube coming out of the water. Great care must be taken to see that the tube does not become blocked and to this end a watch must be kept on the fluid fluctuations. If blockage occurs the fluid in the bottle ceases to fluctuate as the patient breathes. Should the tube become blocked it must be 'milked' (*see* Section V, p. 401) and if it leaves the water it must be compressed until the matter can be rectified.

MASSAGE AND EXERCISES.—The early treatments will be similar to those given following any thoracic surgery (*see* Section V, pp. 401–3), and should not last longer than fifteen minutes at most. The patient's chart must be looked at before each treatment.*

With regard to breathing exercises, *to exert slight pressure on the sound side* will result in increased inspiratory efforts, and thereby increase the range of thoracic movement on the affected side, but *obviously the sound lung must not be gravely hampered while the other remains incompletely expanded.* For this reason it is probably better to use slight pressure on the *affected* side, to indicate where special effort is required. In the later stages it is permissible to put the sound lung partially out of action, in order to encourage full expansion of the thorax and lung on the affected side, but even then, it must not be forgotten that the patient has two lungs, and *for full ventilation both must be used equally.* The patient should therefore be taught to breathe in all parts of both lungs, though the affected side needs special attention throughout. *Diaphragmatic* and *lower costal* breathing are most important, since they expand the base of the lung on which, in empyema, there has been most pressure; but *apical* breathing should also find a place in the patient's scheme of exercises, since this is the part of the lung

---

* In empyema, should the patient's temperature suddenly rise having been normal for a time, it will probably be because the drainage is not satisfactory, and pus is collecting somewhere within the pleural cavity. It is generally held that physical treatment should be continued in spite of the fever, as active work increases the amount of pus, and often causes it to be discharged by breaking down the adhesions that kept it in. Advice on this should, however, be sought. If the temperature remains raised for more than 24 hours and the pus does not escape of itself, it must be liberated by the surgeon. In this way empyema differs from pleurisy with effusion, when physical treatment must be stopped immediately if the temperature rises, as there is no drainage.

where tuberculosis is most likely to develop and complete aeration of the part lessens the risk. Chest-clapping and back-hacking may be given if required, but the area of the scar should be avoided.

Before the physiotherapist leaves the patient, she should be careful to see that the pillows are arranged in such a way that he is in a good position, with the back straight and the chest unhampered. Those in attendance on him should be asked to see that this position is maintained, and that the thorax does not become compressed by the patient's slipping down in bed. Treatment should be given twice or thrice a day. Exercises will progress according to the rate of progress in the patient's general condition. Provided the patient maintains full elevation of the shoulder-girdle arm exercises can be tapered off, but leg exercises should be increased in preparation for walking.

PROGRESSIONS.—The following are a few suggestions for altering and progressing the exercises as the patient improves.

1. *Breathing Exercises.*—

a. When giving side-bending, the arm on the affected side may be placed in *neck-rest* and later in *stretch position.* The side-bending may be carried a little further each day.

b. Later, the patient may lie flat on his back, with legs and body bent towards the sound side ('*Whiting position*'). This position facilitates full expansion of the affected lung, while limiting movement on the healthy side.

c. Alternatively, he may lie on the unaffected side with a large cushion under him. This exerts pressure on the sound side and so obliges him to use the affected lung. This is an advanced exercise, and, in any case, the respiration in the sound lung ought not to be hampered to any great extent until the wound is healed.

In connexion with this last point, one is often asked by students whether the lung on the affected side can expand while the wound remains open. Of course, it cannot do so as long as there is communication between the pleural cavity and the outer air, since the intrapleural pressure will then be atmospheric, and will equal that in the lung. If the lung is to expand, intrapleural pressure must be negative. It has been seen, however, that open drainage is never undertaken if there is a risk of air entering the pleuræ and the closed drainage method is designed to *prevent* air entering the cavity, so that to all intents and purposes, the wound is *not* open. It must be remembered that even when the lung is incompletely expanded, the affected side of the *thorax* can still be enlarged by the muscles of inspiration. Therefore, breathing exercises preserve the mobility of the thorax, thus preventing contracture of scar tissue at the site of the wound, and also draw the parietal layer away from the visceral layer. Since the parietal layer is attached to the chest wall and the visceral layer to the collapsed lung, the movement between them tends to stretch any adhesions which have formed and prevents the formation of strong adhesions. Any air left in the pleural cavity after the wound has healed is gradually absorbed, and the intrapleural pressure falls until it is again slightly negative. Once this happens the lung begins to resume its function, and if treatment has been efficiently administered it will be unhampered by contractures and adhesions.

2. *Active Work.*—This may be advanced—

a. By giving harder exercises.

b. By increasing the number of times each exercise is to be done.

c. By adding resistance.

d. By adding trunk exercises, beginning with trunk-rotations and back-raisings. These may be combined with breathing exercises. *Exercises which impede respiration*, e.g., strong abdominal exercises, *should not be given at any time.*

V. THORACIC SURGERY*

The most common operations performed for diseases of the lung are: (1) *Lobectomy*—removal of a lobe or a segment of a lobe (*Segmental lobectomy*); (2) *Pneumonectomy*—removal of the complete lung; (3) *Thoracoplasty*—permanent collapse of the lung tissue by thoracic reconstruction.

Lobectomy and *pneumonectomy* may be performed for pulmonary tuberculosis; malignant growths; purulent conditions such as bronchiectasis; and fibrosis which may occur following pneumonia, lung abscess, empyema, etc. Whenever possible lobectomy is performed, it being desirable to leave as much remaining lung tissue as possible. The general term *thoracotomy* is used to cover any incision in the thorax for purposes of removal of pleural or mediastinal contents. The basic principles of treatment apply to any thoracotomy.

Thoracoplasty is only used in cases of pulmonary tuberculosis, or when it is desired to obliterate a cavity.

THORACOTOMY

The commonest incision is a *posterolateral* one, following the line of a rib from the vertebral border of the scapula to the anterior angle or costal margin.

Lobectomy.—This consists of *rib resection* and *removal of the whole, or part, of a lobe, the incision usually being made through the bed of the 7th or 8th rib.* During the operation *the trapezius, latissimus dorsi, rhomboids*, and *serratus anterior* are cut.

Pneumonectomy.—This consists of *rib resection* and *removal of the complete lung.* The technique is the same as for lobectomy but *the incision is usually made through the bed of the 5th rib.*

PRE-OPERATIVE TREATMENT.—It is usual for the patient to be admitted to hospital a week or ten days before the operation.† During this time any necessary pre-operative treatment will be given to ensure that the patient is as well as possible before undergoing surgical treatment, and the physiotherapist may be called upon to give intensive postural drainage and breathing exercises, particularly in cases of bronchiectasis. Even if this is not required, she should use the time to prepare the patient for post-operative treatment and to gain his confidence and trust, without which she cannot hope for the co-operation which is so essential to success. She should explain her role as fully as she can, and should teach him exactly what will be required post-operatively. Having explained and taught the patient how the chest works and the importance of using it fully and clearing secretions, she should go on to explain the importance of posture and shoulder elevation.

For thoracotomy patients a full post-operative routine should be practised each day, the patient being put into the drainage position if possible.

For thoracoplasty patients the primary concern must be postural correction of the head. Breathing exercises must be kept to a minimum, if allowed at all, but an effort must be made to teach diaphragmatic control or abdominal contractions pre-operatively.

Provided adequate pre-operative treatment has been given the patient and the physiotherapist may look forward to the post-operative period with confidence, both knowing that everything has been done to ensure a speedy and uncomplicated recovery.

---

* *See* Olive F. Guthrie-Smith, *Rehabilitation, Re-education, and Remedial Exercises*, Chapter XV; Lois Caink, *Physiotherapy in the Treatment of Pulmonary Tuberculosis by Thoracoplasty*; Gladys M. Storey, *Thoracic Surgery for Physiotherapists*; and Hester S. Angove, *Remedial Exercises for Certain Diseases of the Heart and Lungs.*

† Cases awaiting thoracoplasty may be admitted much earlier.

POST-OPERATIVE TREATMENT.—The patient returns from the theatre with a closed drainage tube inserted, as no air must be allowed to enter the thorax. Drainage is usually continued for 3–7 days, somewhere between the 3rd and 5th day being the most usual time for its removal. The patient is nursed in the upright position, the pillows being arranged to avoid kinking or blockage of the tube (*Fig.* 174).

In thoracic work, perhaps more than any other, the surgeon, nursing staff, and physiotherapist should work as a team. There is much work involved in the nursing routine and the physiotherapist should co-ordinate her work with that of the nursing staff.

Fig. 174.—Arrangement of pillows in post-operative chest conditions. Four or five banked on each other. Two divergent side pillows allow the tube to lie in the hollow thus formed and to pass out behind one of them.

PRINCIPLES OF PHYSICAL TREATMENT.—Following any operation involving a general anæsthetic, there is an increase in the amount of secretions in the respiratory tract, and these must be removed in order to avoid the risk of post-operative atelectasis resulting from blockage of a small bronchus or bronchiole. Following thoracic surgery there is, in addition, a collection of blood and tissue fluid in the space formerly occupied by lung tissue. Because the scapular and shoulder-girdle muscles have been cut there is a grave risk of adhesions forming, which could seriously limit both shoulder and thoracic mobility. As in empyema there is the same risk of scoliosis and, as in any operation, there is a risk of thrombosis, although this is less likely following thoracic surgery than following abdominal or pelvic operations.

AIMS OF TREATMENT.—

1. *To promote drainage.* The drainage tube will drain the actual cavity but mucus and a certain amount of blood must be cleared from the remaining lung tissue via the respiratory tract.

2. *To increase ventilation.* The area of lung tissue having been decreased by the operation, a resultant decrease in ventilation will occur. In *lobectomy* there is also a certain amount of *collapse in the lung tissue adjacent to the operation site* which must be re-expanded.

3. *To maintain shoulder-girdle and thoracic mobility* and thereby prevent the formation of limiting adhesions.

4. *To maintain correct posture* and thereby prevent the formation of post-operative scoliosis.

5. *To prevent the occurrence of thrombosis.*

6. *To progress treatment to the final rehabilitation.*

METHODS OF TREATMENT.—

These will include *massage*; *postural drainage* and *percussion*; *breathing exercises*; *arm* and *leg exercises*; and *postural correction*.

POST-OPERATIVE ROUTINE.—The first treatment should begin as soon after the patient's return from the theatre as possible and treatment should be given twice or thrice daily.

The same basic routine can usually be followed in any case of thoracotomy:—

1. *Preparation.*—Before seeing the patient the physiotherapist should familiarize herself with details of the operation and with the patient's chart. She will receive any special instructions regarding the patient, or the treatment, from the ward sister.

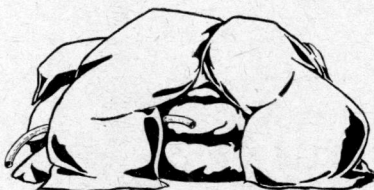

The first part of the treatment should be given in the drainage position, the patient having been lifted down the bed and placed in side-lying. Before this is done the precautions regarding the drainage tube described on p. 396 will be observed. Next the pillows are removed, and two people lift the patient down the bed and turn him onto his side. *A shoulder lift is precluded* because of the site of the wound and *a sacral one* should be used.

Drainage positions: In *Lobectomy* the patient should lie on *the sound side*, it being necessary to clear the remaining lung tissue on the operation side, i.e., in a *right lobectomy* the patient *lies on his left side*.

In *Pneumonectomy*, however, the patient lies on *the operation side* it being essential to clear the remaining lung, i.e., in *right pneumonectomy* the patient lies *on his right side*. What is perhaps of greater importance than the clearance of the lung is the fact that *if the patient were to lie on his sound side whilst there is fluid in the operation cavity, it would be free to drain into the remaining lung and the patient might, quite literally, drown.*

2. *Treatment in the Drainage Position.*—In this position massage is given to the shoulder-girdle and to the area around the scar, avoiding the scar itself. There is a great tendency to guard the scar by holding the arm rigidly to the side and massage helps the patient to relax. He is then more willing to move the shoulder and arm. *Chest clapping and vibrations* may be given over the thorax to assist in loosening the mucus and to stimulate the cough reflex, but in the early days some authorities prefer to roll the patient gently from side to side rather than to give percussion. *Breathing exercises* are also given, with the emphasis on expiration to promote coughing. Coughing is encouraged by the physiotherapist holding the thorax gently but firmly with both hands. The psychological help given by the knowledge that the scar is supported is tremendous and assistance may then be given in the form of vibrations if required. It is desirable that the patient should cough at least once while in this position, but *it is of great importance that the patient should not be exhausted.* Treatment should therefore be kept to a minimum and the novice should not despair if, despite all her efforts, the patient has not coughed; very often the effect of returning the patient to the sitting position produces the desired result.

In order to avoid causing fatigue and unnecessary upheaval to the patient, washing and attention to pressure-points can be carried out by the nursing staff while physiotherapy is being given.

3. *Treatment in the Upright Position.*—After about 5 minutes of treatment in the drainage position, the patient should be returned to the upright position. The physiotherapist places her arm behind the patient's shoulder in such a way as to support the head and lift him forwards and up into a sitting position, whilst the pillows are re-arranged. Two people then lift him back against them. Breathing, arm, and leg exercises are now given and posture checked and, if necessary, corrected.

Breathing exercises: Diaphragmatic, Lateral costal and Apical breathing must all be given, all parts of the chest being used as fully as possible. Stress must be laid on any area which requires expansion, and coughing is again encouraged.

Arm exercises: It is of the utmost importance that *full elevation of the shoulder is achieved immediately after the operation and maintained until the danger of adhesions is past.* It will be found helpful if the patient uses his sound arm to support the other, giving assistance on the upward movement and taking its weight as the arm is returned to the side. Other arm exercises may be given if desired, but *one full range of elevation must be achieved at each treatment.*

Leg exercises: Foot exercises, quadriceps drill, and knee bending and stretching are given from the beginning.

Postural correction: As in empyema the patient tends to lean away from the drainage tube, producing a curve *convex to the sound side*. To correct this it is essential to see that the weight is taken evenly on both buttocks, and that the shoulder-girdle and head are in alinement. As a rule correction of the pelvis is automatically followed by correction of the shoulder-girdle and head.

4. *Final Measures.*—Before leaving the patient the drainage bottle is returned to its position on the floor and the fluctuations in fluid level checked. If these have ceased it indicates a blockage, either from kinking of the tube, pressure on the tube, or a barrier to flow within the tube. The first and second are easily remedied, the third may be remedied by 'milking' the tube, i.e., holding it gently but firmly into the wound with one hand and applying suction by squeezing and pulling along its length with the other, until fluctuations recommence.

The patient is usually allowed up between the third and fifth days and thereafter a scheme of progressive exercises may begin. Active trunk exercises can be started as soon as the tube is removed, but care must be taken not to stretch the scar until the wound is truly healed. As the patient progresses he must learn to walk a little further each day and to climb stairs without any respiratory distress. The absence of respiratory distress indicates compensatory hypertrophy of lung tissue, and governs the rate of progress towards final rehabilitation.

THORACOPLASTY

This is only undertaken in cases of pulmonary tuberculosis, or when cavities in the lung can only be closed by permanent collapse of the whole, or part, of a lung.

The operation consists of resection of a varying number of ribs, leaving the periosteum in position. From four to ten ribs may be removed, depending on the desired effect.

The operation is usually carried out in two or three stages, with a two- or three-week interval between each. At the first operation the first three ribs are removed completely as far as their costal cartilages. At subsequent operations the requisite number of ribs is resected, a little more of each rib being left as progress is made down the thorax. The incision is a J-shaped one running down the posterior angles of the ribs before curving along the line of the 6th, 7th, or 8th rib.

COMPLICATIONS.—The removal of the first rib leaves *the scaleni* without their distal attachment. The scapular and shoulder muscles are cut as in thoracotomy, and there is danger of serious deformity occurring.

DEFORMITY.—The following changes are liable to occur:—

1. *The head and neck are displaced towards the sound side* owing to the unopposed pull of the undamaged scaleni. The head may also 'poke' forwards.

2. *The trunk leans towards the affected side*, to balance the displacement of the head.

3. *The shoulder is raised on the affected side* in consequence, *but it also tends to rotate medially* because of the interference with the rhomboids and middle fibres of trapezius.

If steps are not taken to correct these postural deformities, a permanent and unsightly S-curve may develop as a result of contractures. Here it should be said that a *slight* scoliosis is inevitable. Although the ribs will in time regenerate, since the periosteum is left, the latter will by then have sunk in towards the underlying soft tissues and the thorax will remain permanently smaller on the affected side. This deformity should not, however, be disabling and should be scarcely noticeable.

Paradoxical Respiration.—In order to understand this the student should revise the mechanism of normal respiration. *See* p. 382. Normally the stability of the thoracic cage resists any sucking inward of the chest wall during inspiration. After several ribs have been removed the chest wall in this area is flaccid and unstable, so that when air is sucked in *the unstable part of the wall is sucked in also*. The lung becomes smaller, and air is forced out of it. This impure air is drawn into the sound lung, together with the entering atmospheric air, as inspiration proceeds. During expiration, *the rising pressure in the lungs forces the soft part outwards, thus enlarging the lung on that side*, and air, including that leaving the sound lung, is sucked into it (*Fig.* 175). This, of course, reduces the pulmonary ventilation, some of the de-oxygenated air being breathed in again instead of being driven out; *also infected material from the diseased lung may be carried over to the sound one*. To prevent paradoxical respiration, a special strapping may be put on over the soft part of the chest. One wide piece (or two rather narrower ones) is applied over the shoulder from back to front, a 4-in. pad of cotton-wool being placed beneath the clavicle, and two or three pieces are applied from back to front beneath the axilla. The strapping must not extend to the sound side. Heavy external splintage may also be applied in the form of sand-bags or lead shot, but a more modern method is to pack the thorax with polythene balls or similar material.

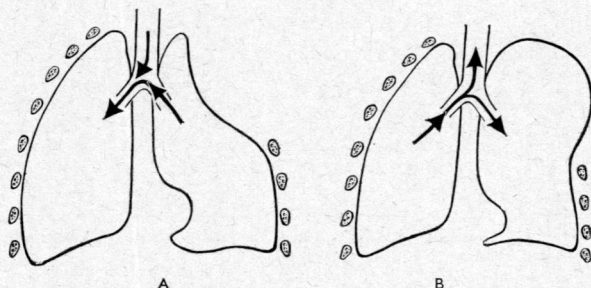

Fig. 175.—Diagrammatic representation of paradoxical breathing. A, Sucking in of chest wall on inspiration with transference of air, and possibly infected material from affected lung; B, Transference of air from sound to affected lung during expiration, with inflation of weakened chest wall.

A more recent form of thoracoplasty is performed in one operation. The first rib is left in place. The second, third, and fourth ribs are removed, and sewn across the top of the rest of the ribs to make a bony roof for the thoracic cage. This has the advantage of causing less deformity, and also of leaving intact the attachments of the scaleni anterior and medius, thus avoiding the troublesome displacement of the head to the sound side. Also there is less tendency to paradoxical respiration.

Treatment.—

POST-OPERATIVE TREATMENT.—The patient may return from theatre with an open drainage tube inserted but this is usually removed within 24 hours. He is nursed in the upright position but to begin with he may be inclined slightly towards the affected side, a more upright position being achieved each day.

PHYSICAL TREATMENT.—This can generally be given after each stage of the operation, and usually begins at once, but it must be emphasized that *because these patients are usually tuberculous cases no hard-and-fast rule can be laid down*, and the greatest co-operation is needed between the surgeon and all who deal with the patient. There may well be an active lesion in the other lung which will necessitate modifications in treatment. An outline of the general principles of treatment is given below together with *the basic differences in techniques*.

Aims.—These are the same as those applying in thoracotomy but they have a different emphasis. They may be summarized as follows:—

1. *To prevent post-operative atelectasis.* This is not the contradiction in terms which it appears. Although the aim of thoracoplasty is to collapse the lung, *it is of vital importance to prevent collapse in the remaining lung tissue.* Besides the hazard of post-operative increase in secretions, two grave dangers may arise as the result of paradoxical breathing. One has been mentioned (the hypoventilation and sucking in of air and secretions from the affected lung). The other is that *paradoxical breathing renders it difficult for the patient to build up sufficient pressure to cough and evacuate the sputum.*

2. *To correct posture and prevent the development of fixed deformities.*

3. *To teach the patient to use the chest as fully as posssible* in order to establish full ventilation.

4. *To relieve pain and spasm* in order to enable the patient to use the arm and thorax more fully.

5. *To prevent thrombosis.*

6. *To rehabilitate the patient.*

Methods.—*Massage* to the arm and shoulder-girdle, *percussion, breathing exercises, arm and leg exercises,* and *postural correction* are given as for thoracotomy with the following differences in technique.

1. *The key to the prevention of atelectasis lies in the control of paradoxical breathing.* This may be achieved in two ways.

a. *By early institution of diaphragmatic breathing.*

b. *By firm manual pressure over the damaged chest wall during breathing exercises, and particularly when the patient coughs.*

Postural drainage is not given as a rule, unless at the express wish of the surgeon in charge of the case, but the patient may lean forwards over supporting pillows to allow vibrations and percussion to be given.

2. *The key to postural correction lies in head control.* The patient should be given *resisted movements for the scaleni,* pressure being applied over the temporomandibular joint. The chin must be kept 'tucked in' during the movement. The weight must, of course, be taken evenly on both buttocks, but since the deformity stems from the displacement of the head, the emphasis should be placed on correcting this. Mirrors are often a valuable help.

3. *Breathing Exercises.*—Diaphragmatic breathing is of vital concern, although other exercises may have to be modified considerably.

In other respects treatment is given as for thoracotomy cases. Progress will, however, be very much slower. Convalescence may take nine months or more, and the patient may be kept in bed for three months after the operation. The abdominal muscles may be used as a substitute for the diaphragm if a phrenic crush has been performed.

VI. EXAMPLES OF BREATHING EXERCISES

EXERCISES ESPECIALLY FOR INSPIRATION

GENERAL EXERCISES.—

Free Exercises.—

1. Crook-lying, half-lying, sitting, or standing-Deep-breathing.

The starting position is chosen according to the strength and condition of the patient. The breathing, in many cases, is at first commanded, that is, the operator gives the commands 'Breathe in' and 'Breathe out'. Later the patient breathes in his own time. Heart cases should not breathe too deeply and, as a rule, the breathing is not commanded at any stage.

2. Lax-sitting Chest-lifting and relaxing.

Similar to a free back-raising vertebra by vertebra. There should, however, be no movement in the hip-joints, but only in those of the spine, which is completely relaxed during expiration, the patient letting the breath escape audibly through the mouth, as a deep sigh. Inspiration is taken on the upward movement, followed by relaxation with expiration.

The movement may also be given in knee-sitting.

3. Sitting (or standing), 2-Arm-raising sideways, with breathing. Greater relaxation may be obtained during expiration in the sitting position.

4. Standing (or sitting) 2-Arm-rotation-out, with breathing.

5. Standing (or sitting) 2-Arm-raising to shoulder level plus rotation out, with breathing.

6. Yard-standing (or sitting) 2-Arm-rotation-out plus Head-extension, with breathing.

The patient starts with the head bent slightly forward and the palms of the hands downwards. He then turns the palms upwards and carries the head backwards, a little beyond the upright position. A full head-extension must not be made, nor should the spine be lordosed.

7. Lax-stride-sitting Chest-lifting and relaxing plus 2-Arm-raising to shoulder level plus rotation out (plus Head-extension). This consists of No. 2 combined with No. 3, or No. 5 and No. 6.

8. Sitting (or standing) 2-Arm-circling with breathing.

The arms are carried forward and upward, then outward and downward. It is not advisable that they should be carried quite up to the vertical, as this almost invariably produces lordosis. This can only be prevented by strong contraction of the abdominals which, of course, impedes respiration.

9. Sitting (or standing) 2-Arm-parting with breathing.

LOCALIZED EXERCISES.—

1. DIAPHRAGMATIC.—Crook- (or half-) lying Diaphragmatic breathing. The physiotherapist places her own, or the patient's hand on the diaphragm in the costal angle, telling him to push away her hand when breathing in. He is told to draw in the abdominal muscles when breathing out.*

2. COSTAL.—Crook- (or half-) lying, or sitting-Deep (costal) breathing. The physiotherapist places her hands over the lower or upper ribs, at the front or sides of the body, thus indicating to the patient which she wishes him to expand. Later, he may place his own hands on the part, to appreciate the movement fully.

3. DIAPHRAGMATIC AND COSTAL COMBINED.—The patient places the palms of the hands on the thorax with the fingers resting lightly on the diaphragm. On inspiration he pushes into his hands. Co-ordination is not easily acquired, however, and much patience may be required.

4. APICAL.—Crook- (or half-) lying Apical breathing. The physiotherapist, standing behind or beside the patient, places her fingers over the apices of the lungs just above the clavicles, asking him to 'push out here' as he breathes in.

5. PECTO-APICAL.—This corresponds to the upper lobe of the right lung, and a similar area of the left lung. The hands may be placed just below the clavicles, to indicate the area where expansion is required.

6. PRESSURE EXPANSION EXERCISES.—These may be given for costal breathing in any part of the thorax. The physiotherapist places her hands on the patient's ribs, and *resists* as he pushes out. A webbing belt encircling the chest may also be used to apply resistance.

---

* Many patients make the mistake of thrusting the chest out and drawing in the abdominal muscles, under the impression that this is diaphragmatic movement. A demonstration of diaphragmatic breathing by the physiotherapist is often helpful, and the physiotherapist must persevere with the teaching of this method of breathing until the patient has completely mastered it.

EXERCISES ESPECIALLY FOR EXPIRATION

GENERAL EXERCISES.—

FREE EXERCISES.—

1. Lax-sitting (or knee-sitting) Chest-lifting and relaxing, with short inspirations and long expirations.

The 'lifting' is minimized, and the 'relaxing' emphasized.

2. Free breathing, with emphasis on expiration.

3. Special exercises in *Physical Exercises for Asthma* (*see* p. 381).

4. Wing- (or lax-) stoop-stride-sitting Back-raising (vertebra by vertebra) with breathing. Emphasis on relaxation and expiration as in 1.

LOCALIZED EXERCISES.—

1. DIAPHRAGMATIC.—Crook- (or half-) lying Diaphragmatic breathing, given as described above, but the inspirations must be short and the expirations long.

2. COSTAL (Upper and lower).—For description, *see* ASTHMA (p. 380).

EXERCISES FOR INSPIRATION AND EXPIRATION

All the free exercises given above in the list of inspiratory exercises may be used for this purpose, equal emphasis being laid on each respiratory phase. Nos. 3, 4, 5, 6, 8, and 9 should be given in sitting rather than in standing, since relaxation is easier in this position. The patient may be directed to draw in the abdominal muscles during expiration.

UNILATERAL BREATHING EXERCISES

These promote breathing especially, or only, in one lung.

TO EXPAND THE BASE OF ONE LUNG.—

1. Half-lying Diaphragmatic breathing. The patient may bend very slightly to the sound side. The arm on this side may be held close to the body with the forearm across the chest, the physiotherapist supporting it in this position. The exercise is then taught in the usual way.

2. Half-lying Costal breathing. The patient's position is as above. The physiotherapist places her hand on the ribs of the affected side and tells the patient to push it away.

3. Half-lying Diaphragmatic and Costal breathing. The above two exercises combined. All these exercises may later be done in sitting or standing.

4. Pressure expansion exercises. As LOCALIZED EXERCISES, No. 6 (*see* p. 404), but pressure applied to the lower or upper costal, or pecto-apical regions of one side, the hands placed on the *exact* part where expansion is required.

5. Half-lying Side-bending (e.g., to the left if the right lung is affected) with breathing.

The arm on the affected side to be (*a*) at the patient's side, (*b*) in neck-rest, (*c*) stretch. The same exercise may later be done in stride-sitting and standing.

6. Stride-sitting Side-bending, combined with Diaphragmatic breathing.

7. Side-lying Deep breathing. The patient lies on the sound side (he need not at first lie quite flat). The patient's arm, or a soft cushion, is kept between the thorax and the bed or plinth on which he lies, in order to put the sound lung more or less out of action. The position of the arm on the affected side is as in the previous exercises (Nos. 5 and 6).

8. 'Whiting position'. Costal breathing.

9. Half-wing-half-stretch-stride-standing Side-bending.

10. Half-wing-half-neck-rest (later, -stretch) high-ride-sitting Side-bending with breathing.

11. Half-wing-half-neck-rest (later, -stretch) high-ride-turn-sitting Side-bending with breathing.

CHAPTER XVIII

DISEASES OF THE HEART

The normal heart. Anatomy and physiology: I. Pathological conditions—Medical conditions—Coronary thrombosis—Cardiac failure and valvular lesions. II. Cardiac surgery: General principles—Types of operation and conditions treated—Pre- and post-operative treatment.

DISEASES of the heart fall into two categories—*medical* and *surgical* conditions—but before considering the pathology of the heart, the student should be familiar with the anatomy and physiology of the normal heart. A brief description only will be given here, but it is a subject which *must* be thoroughly studied by all who have to deal with these cases.

ANATOMY.—It will be remembered that the heart is a hollow, muscular organ divided into four chambers, and enclosed like the lungs in a two-layered, sero-fibrous sac (pericardium). It is lined with a delicate membrane (endocardium) from which the valves are formed. The two upper chambers (right and left atria) are divided by the interatrial septum and the two lower chambers (ventricles) by the interventricular septum. Atria and ventricles connect with each other by means of the tricuspid valve on the right, and the mitral valve on the left. Venous blood enters the right atrium from the great veins, and leaves the right ventricle by the pulmonary artery. Oxygenated (arterial) blood enters the left atrium via the pulmonary veins, and leaves the left ventricle via the aorta and coronary arteries.

PHYSIOLOGY.—

THE CONTRACTION OF THE HEART.—It will be remembered that the impulse of contraction of the heart passes in a wave-like manner from base to apex, originating in a mass of specialized tissue known as the 'sinu-atrial node', situated in the right atrium at a point near the mouth of the superior vena cava. From this sinu-atrial node, which has been called the 'pace-maker' of the heart, the impulse passes downwards over the walls of the atria to another mass of specialized tissue called the 'atrioventricular node' ('A-V node'). Thence it is carried to the ventricles by way of a bundle of muscular tissue, the atrioventricular bundle or bundle of His, which runs down the ventricular septum before dividing into two parts, one of which is distributed to each ventricle. If this bundle is injured or destroyed by disease, some or all of the beats of the atria are *blocked* and do not pass on to the ventricles (heart block).

THE CARDIAC CYCLE AND THE ACTION OF THE VALVES.—The *cardiac cycle* is the name given to the sequence of events which takes place during a single beat of the heart. The heart beats about 70–75 times a minute and each occupies about $\frac{8}{10}$ second. The contraction of the atria, known as *atrial systole*, lasts for $\frac{1}{10}$ second, and the contraction of the ventricles or *ventricular systole*, for $\frac{3}{10}$ second. For the remaining $\frac{4}{10}$ of the cycle the whole heart relaxes and is at rest, this period being known as *total diastole*. (*See Fig.* 176.)

1. *During atrial systole*, the contraction of the atria closes the mouths of the great veins (the superior and inferior venæ cavæ, coronary sinus, and pulmonary veins) so that no blood enters the heart. At the same time, the rising pressure in the atria forces open the atrioventricular valves (tricuspid and mitral) and the blood pours through into the ventricles.

2. *During ventricular systole* the atria relax, and the blood again begins to enter the heart from the great veins. The rising pressure in the contracting ventricles closes the tricuspid and mitral valves and at the same time opens the semilunar valves of the aorta and pulmonary artery, so that the blood is pumped into these vessels. The first heart-sound (lubb) occurs during ventricular systole and is caused by the contraction of the ventricular walls and the vibrations of the chordæ tendineæ which, by their tension, prevent the rising pressure in the ventricles from forcing the tricuspid and mitral valves backwards into the atrium. Disease of either of these will therefore alter the nature of this sound.

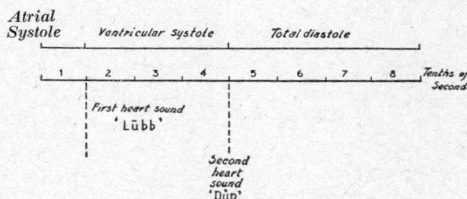

Fig. 176.—Diagram of cardiac cycle.

3. *During total diastole* the whole heart relaxes. The aortic and pulmonary valves close, because the pressure in the great vessels now becomes higher than that in the relaxing ventricles. They remain closed until the beginning of the next ventricular systole, thus preventing regurgitation of the blood. The atrioventricular valves open as the ventricular pressure falls, so that the blood trickles from atria to ventricles, as well as from the open mouths of the great veins into the atria. The second heart-sound (dup) takes place at the beginning of diastole and is caused by the closing of the aortic and pulmonary valves. This sound is altered, or absent, in disease of either of these valves.

CAUSATION AND REGULATION OF THE HEART'S BEAT.—The heart contracts because of the inherent property of cardiac muscle, and not as a result of impulses from the central nervous system. *The rate of contraction,* however, is controlled by the autonomic system through the vagus and sympathetic nerves. The heart-rate is *decreased by the vagus nerve,* and *increased by the sympathetic nerves.* Adrenaline (the secretion of the medulla of the adrenal glands) stimulates the sympathetic system, and its secretion is increased in emergencies, especially in such as occasion the emotions of fear or anger. This, if the heart is not sound, involves a risk of overstrain and failure, because among the results of this increased secretion are (1) an increase in the heart-rate, and (2) constriction of the arteries, the vasoconstrictors of which are supplied by sympathetic nerve-fibres which raise the blood-pressure. The heart, therefore, not only beats more quickly but has to work harder to drive the blood through the narrowed vessels. Hence the danger of undue excitement in a patient with heart disease.

EFFECT OF MUSCULAR EXERCISE ON THE HEART.—When muscular exercise is taken, more blood is carried back to the heart. Two main factors concerned in this are the deepened respiratory movements, which increase the suction action of the thorax, and the pressure of the contracting muscles on the veins, which further assists venous return. The heart, therefore, being better filled during diastole, can pump out more blood during the ventricular systole, because cardiac muscle, like other muscles in the body, works more strongly when it has been stretched. Because the heart's impulse is more forcible, and the volume of blood pumped out is greater, the blood-pressure is raised. By a local reflex action, vasodilation occurs in the arterioles in the working muscles, and the blood is therefore taken to the parts where it is most needed.

The work of the heart is thus increased by *emotion*, and by *muscular exercise*. The normal heart, however, has a certain amount of *reserve force*, upon which it is able to call in emergencies. When the need for an increased blood-supply ceases, the heart soon returns to its normal rate and strength of work. The unhealthy heart, however, may be obliged to use all its reserve force merely to maintain the circulation during rest and has nothing left to fall back on in emergencies. Hence a *sudden* demand upon it may produce serious or fatal results, as we shall see later.

Diseases of the heart may be divided into: (1) *Medical conditions*, (2) *Surgical conditions*.

MEDICAL CONDITIONS

Under this heading come inflammatory conditions (pericarditis, endocarditis, and myocarditis); degeneration of the myocardium (heart muscle), either from disease or from blockage of the coronary arteries (coronary thrombosis); and valvular lesions. With the former we are not greatly concerned, except in so far as pericarditis may so restrict the action of the heart that general heart symptoms ensue, and endocarditis* may affect the valves, so that they become stenosed, or incompetent.

Valvular lesions are now treated largely by surgical means, but, as will be seen later, they may give rise to heart failure. The two medical conditions with which we are primarily concerned are *coronary thrombosis* and *heart failure*.

CORONARY THROMBOSIS

In lay terms this is probably the most well known of heart conditions, being commonly called a 'heart attack'. It may prove immediately fatal, but if the patient survives for 24 hours the case is hopeful. If he survives for 7–21 days the prognosis is usually good. An attack may result from some extra effort, such as running for a bus, or may occur at rest or during normal activity.

AETIOLOGY.—It is commoner in men than women, and generally occurs from early middle age upwards.

CAUSES.—

1. Arteriosclerosis, leading to narrowing of the coronary arteries, with consequent diminution of the arterial blood-supply to the heart.

2. Embolism, the embolus lodging in one of the coronary arteries, causing obstruction and subsequent necrosis of the heart muscle supplied by the occluded arteries.

SYMPTOMS.—

1. PAIN.—In cases caused by arteriosclerosis, the patient has probably had previous attacks of angina—pain over the region of the heart (precordial pain) and radiating down the arm. The angina is caused by cramp of the heart muscle, due to the lack of arterial blood-supply, and therefore of oxygen.

On the other hand, the pain may be a severe crushing pain in the region of the heart.

2. SWEATING.

3. NAUSEA.

4. COLLAPSE.

Treatment.—

GENERAL.—This consists of complete rest in bed for a period of 3–6 weeks, depending on the severity of the attack, and the age and general health of the

---

* Endocarditis, which results from rheumatic fever, is in fact one of the commonest causes of valvular disease.

patient. Suitable medication will be administered, and the patient may require oxygen. Alcohol and tobacco are usually prohibited, and a fat-reduced and salt-free diet is prescribed.

PHYSICAL TREATMENT.—This will begin at the physician's discretion, and will follow that described below (*see* Cardiac Failure).

The usual time for recovery in an initial or moderate attack is 3 months, and young patients can usually return to work at the end of this period. If the attack has been severe, and/or the patient is elderly, a further period of 3 months off work, or on light duty, may be required. It should be stressed when dealing with young patients that a coronary attack does not necessarily mean a life of invalidism, unless, of course, a large area of heart muscle is involved. In fact, if one considers the physiology of the heart, it will be realized that moderate activity strengthens the heart muscle, and many coronary cases continue to enjoy an active, healthy, and useful life long after the initial attack.

COMPLICATIONS.—As in any heart lesion, there is a danger of ultimate heart failure, subsequent attacks leading to further involvement of the heart muscle, and reduction in its compensatory powers.

CARDIAC FAILURE AND VALVULAR DISEASE

Cardiac failure is the result of myocardial degeneration, the heart being unable to meet the demands made on it. Heart failure may be right-sided or left-sided, but there is usually a certain amount of failure on both sides. Despite the somewhat ominous sound of its name, it should be realized that heart failure does not necessarily mean the final stage of heart disease, and many cases respond well to treatment.

CAUSES.—As has been said, heart failure is due to degeneration of the myocardium, but this may result from a variety of causes:—

1. Chronic overstrain of the heart, which in turn results from valvular disease or peripheral arteriosclerosis.

2. Coronary thrombosis (*see above*).

3. Disease of the muscle itself, either from inflammatory conditions such as rheumatic fever, other toxins, or fatty degeneration of the myocardium.

Since the results are the same whatever the cause, the condition can best be understood by considering valvular disease.

Valvular disease leads to deformity of one or more of the valves of the heart, preventing them either from opening fully (stenosis) or from closing completely (incompetence or insufficiency). The mitral, aortic, tricuspid, or pulmonary valves may all be affected.

AETIOLOGY.—The commonest causes of valvular disease are:—

1. ENDOCARDITIS, which is generally the result of acute rheumatic fever, though it may result from other toxic conditions.

2. ARTERIOSCLEROSIS.—This leads to hardening of the valves, especially of the aortic valve, with curling or puckering of their segments, causing incompetence.

PATHOLOGICAL CHANGES.—

1. The endocardium is inflamed, this condition being most marked in the valves.

2. Small growths appear on the *atrial surface of the mitral valve* or on the *ventricular surface of the aortic valve* (the so-called '*warty vegetations*'). They are at first composed of little masses of fibrin and corpuscles, and are sometimes only attached to the valves by very thin stalks, so that they are easily detached. Later, they become organized into connective tissue. *They are commonest on the mitral valve; hence the greater danger of embolism in mitral disease.*

3. The valves themselves may become thickened, deformed, and puckered, so that the cusps no longer meet, this state of things being known as *insufficiency*, or *incompetence*; or the edges of the cusps adhere to each other, so that the valve

will still not open fully, this condition being called *stenosis* (Greek *stenos* = narrow). Stenosis and insufficiency are often combined, the valve neither opening nor closing completely.

RESULTS OF VALVE LESIONS.—

BACK PRESSURE.—To explain exactly what is meant by this term, it will be easiest to take a concrete example. Let us suppose the *aortic valve* to be incompetent. *When the left ventricle relaxes after its systole, some of the blood flows back into it from the aorta*, which is no longer completely sealed off. The ventricle becomes over-full, since it has to hold not only the blood sent on into it by the left atrium, but that which has regurgitated from the aorta. It therefore has to work harder in order to pump on this extra blood, i.e., *to overcome the back pressure on it*. The left ventricle *dilates* in order to accommodate the increased amount of blood, and *hypertrophies* as the result of the extra work. If, however, too much strain is put on the heart, *the dilatation exceeds the hypertrophy*, and, owing to this excessive dilatation, *the atrioventricular orifice* becomes larger, so that the cusps of the mitral valve can no longer meet across it. This is called *relative incompetence*. There is therefore a *back-flow of blood into the left atrium* when the ventricle contracts, i.e., *back pressure on the atrium*. This chamber now becomes over-full and, in its turn, dilates and hypertrophies. *The atria, however, are not capable of any great degree of hypertrophy* and the dilated and engorged condition of the left atrium soon forms an obstruction to the entrance of blood from the lungs. There is therefore *back pressure on the pulmonary circulation*. The resulting congestion causes *back pressure on the right ventricle* which, like the left ventricle at an earlier stage, dilates and hypertrophies. The same process which we noticed on the left side of the heart is now repeated on the right. *The tricuspid valve becomes relatively incompetent.* The right atrium, capable of but little hypertrophy, dilates and becomes engorged with blood, and a condition of *back pressure on the systemic circulation is set up*, since the return of the blood from the body by way of the superior and inferior venæ cavæ is obstructed. This leads to serious symptoms due to venous congestion in the body, and especially in the abdominal cavity.

COMPENSATION.—A patient with valves injured by disease may, notwithstanding, live long and enjoy fair health, *provided that he does not subject his heart to sudden strain, or undertake violent exercise*. This is because the heart muscle, if it is healthy, is able to accommodate itself to the changed conditions; in other words, to *compensate* for the valvular deficiency.

As we have already seen, the heart has a certain amount of reserve force which it does not use in the ordinary way of life, but upon which it is able to draw in times of emergency. *In valvular disease, an increased amount of force is required, even when the body is at rest, to drive the blood through the narrowed opening in stenosis, or to pump out both the oncoming and the regurgitating blood in insufficiency.* The heart, therefore, has *less force in reserve for emergencies*. However, as we have seen, the increased work strengthens the heart muscle to a certain degree and causes its fibres to hypertrophy. Comparatively, therefore, it has *more power* than the normal heart, but this is required to maintain its normal work. It therefore has *less in reserve*, and a *sudden* demand upon it will cause symptoms of exhaustion long before they would occur in the normal heart. In other words, *the compensation breaks down*. The heart of the patient with diseased valves is always much nearer to breaking point, and it is of the utmost importance to remember this when treating such cases.

It must also be borne in mind that 'compensation' is a relative term. A patient's heart may, for instance, be sufficiently compensated for the requirements of the body at rest in a recumbent position but not for sitting; or it may be compensated in sitting but not in standing. That is to say, the patient may be comfortable while he sits in a chair but show signs of distress if he tries to walk about.

If, for any reason, the heart is *incapable of hypertrophy* and its total strength is only just sufficient to maintain the circulation during rest, cardiac failure takes place suddenly on the least extra exertion with fatal results. This is very liable to happen when there are degenerative processes in the muscle-fibres themselves.

GENERAL HEART SYMPTOMS.—The symptoms of all types of heart disease are similar. It will be most convenient, therefore, to summarize them here.

1. CYANOSIS.—Owing to the slow circulation, and the interference with gaseous interchange due to pulmonary congestion, a relatively large amount of oxygen is given off to the tissues and an extra quantity of CO_2 is collected. Cyanosis is most apparent in the face which is often purplish in colour, the lips having a bluish tinge. In other cases the skin may be pale, owing to poor arterial supply to the part.

2. DYSPNŒA.—There is interference with respiration owing to engorgement of the blood-vessels in the lungs.

3. ŒDEMA.—Again, because of the slow circulation, the vessels dilate and, their walls being thinner, an abnormal amount of lymph is exuded from the vessels. It is most often seen in the extremities, but in very severe cases, e.g., tricuspid insufficiency, there is marked œdema in the abdominal cavity. This is known as *ascites*, or dropsy.

4. PAIN occurs in some types of lesions (Angina pectoris, *see* p. 408).

5. PALPITATION.—This consists of quick, strong, irregular beating of the heart perceptible to the patient. (Such action when *not* perceptible to the patient does not constitute palpitations.) It is due to the heart's efforts to drive on the blood while working at a disadvantage.

6. THE PULSE.—The character of this varies with the nature of the lesion. *Hypertrophy* produces a *strong slow pulse*. In *failing compensation* the *pulse* becomes *weak, rapid,* and *irregular*.

7. CEREBRAL SYMPTOMS.—These are generally found in aortic disease. They consist of syncope (faintness) due to anæmia of the brain; and often of mental symptoms such as irritability and depression. Cerebral hæmorrhage may occur.

8. ABDOMINAL SYMPTOMS.—Venous congestion in the abdomen may cause constipation, indigestion, etc.

AORTIC DISEASE

AORTIC STENOSIS.—This is rare and is often combined with incompetence, but it is a far less serious condition than *Aortic Insufficiency*.

AORTIC INSUFFICIENCY.—This is the most dangerous of all valvular lesions, particularly if it arises from arteriosclerosis.

EFFECT OF INSUFFICIENCY.—In *aortic insufficiency*, some of the blood which has been pumped into the aorta by the left ventricle regurgitates through the incompetent valve during ventricular diastole, with the result that less blood is pumped out into the body, under a lower pressure. The arterial circulation throughout the body becomes deficient, which means that the coronary circulation is also reduced. If arteriosclerosis is the cause, the coronary vessels may themselves be affected, which further reduces the blood-supply to the heart. Another grave danger in aortic disease is that an embolus may break off the damaged valve and lodge in one of the nearby coronary vessels. This may completely deprive the myocardium of its blood-supply, with fatal results.

Compensation.—In *aortic insufficiency* this is brought about by dilatation and hypertrophy of the left ventricle. Compensation in *aortic stenosis* is brought about in the same way, but the dilatation and hypertrophy are not so great, the ventricular hypertrophy being greater in aortic insufficiency than in any other valvular lesion.

Symptoms.—These are caused by *poor arterial supply* to all parts of the body. Despite compensation the systemic circulation is diminished, and the symptoms therefore closely resemble those of anæmia. *The pulmonary circulation does not suffer, however, unless the mitral valve is also involved.* The symptoms are more marked in regurgitation than in stenosis. The most important are:—

1. *Pallor* of the face due to the poor blood-supply.

2. *Precordial pain,* or angina pectoris, is a frequent and early symptom in these patients. It is caused by the ischæmic condition of the myocardium itself.

3. *Cerebral symptoms* are marked; headache, faintness, and giddiness occur. The patient may sleep badly, or suffer from actual insomnia, and is often irritable and depressed.

4. *Palpitations* commonly occur.

5. *Œdema* is not marked, and only occurs late in the course of the disease.

6. *Dyspnœa* may be a feature, but it is less troublesome than in mitral disease, as are all the pulmonary symptoms.

7. *Abdominal symptoms,* if present, are slight.

Sudden death is common in aortic insufficiency. This may be due to occlusion of the coronary blood-supply, to syncope, or cerebral hæmorrhage, the frequency of the last being due to arteriosclerosis of the vessels of the brain.

MITRAL DISEASE

Mitral insufficiency may be the result of rheumatic disease of the valve itself, or it may be a *relative insufficiency,* due to extreme dilatation of the left ventricle. *Stenosis and incompetence usually coexist.*

EFFECTS.—When the left ventricle begins to contract, some of the blood regurgitates through the mitral valve into the left atrium, which becomes over-full, having to hold both incoming blood from the lungs and regurgitated blood from the ventricle. It therefore dilates and hypertrophies, in order to accommodate the extra volume of blood and drive it into the left ventricle. That cavity, therefore, also dilates in order to accommodate the extra blood, and hypertrophies in order to drive it on into the aorta. Thus the systemic circulation is maintained, despite the fact that some of the blood regurgitates into the left atrium.

Meanwhile, *the dilatation of the left atrium obstructs the return of the blood through the pulmonary veins, producing venous congestion in the lungs.* In order to overcome the resultant back pressure, the right ventricle also dilates and hypertrophies.

COMPENSATION.—This is achieved by the following series of events: (1) Dilatation and hypertrophy of the left atrium; (2) Dilatation and hypertrophy of the left ventricle; (3) Dilatation and hypertrophy of the right ventricle. Should the right ventricle fail to compensate the lesion, the tricuspid valve becomes relatively incompetent.

In *mitral stenosis alone* the changes are similar, but the left ventricle does not hypertrophy. The reason for this is that, although the left atrium dilates, the narrowness of the valve prevents any great quantity of blood reaching the ventricle.

SYMPTOMS.—Whereas aortic valvular disease affects the arterial blood-supply, *mitral lesions affect the venous supply.* The symptoms are therefore those of *venous congestion,* which appears first in the *pulmonary,* then in the *systemic* vessels. The principal symptoms are as follows:—

1. *Cyanosis,* especially noticeable in the face.

2. *Dyspnœa* is a very marked feature, owing to the congestion of the lungs. The patient may be troubled by a cough, and hæmoptysis is not uncommon.

3. *Œdema* is marked owing to the venous congestion throughout the body. It is particularly noticeable in the extremities, and ascites may follow later.

4. *Palpitations* are a feature of the disease.

5. *Abdominal symptoms* are much in evidence because of the back-pressure on the systemic and portal circulation.

6. *Emboli* are common in mitral disease. They may reach the brain and cause hemiplegia, or may lodge in one of the coronary arteries, so endangering life.

7. *Cerebral symptoms* are not marked.

8. *The pulse* may be very irregular in advanced cases.

Despite the occurrence of emboli sudden death is rare in mitral lesions. The heart more often gives out gradually than as the result of an embolus.

PULMONARY STENOSIS

This is a congenital deformity consisting of narrowing of the pulmonary valve.
SYMPTOMS AND PATHOLOGICAL CHANGES.—Insufficient blood passes into the lungs; there is dyspnœa, cyanosis, fatigue, and sometimes syncope. The right ventricle hypertrophies.

TRICUSPID INSUFFICIENCY

Tricuspid insufficiency cannot be compensated for long because the right atrium is incapable of much hypertrophy. Once the compensation fails there is back pressure on the whole of the systemic circulation. Tricuspid insufficiency is more often the result of a left-sided heart lesion than of diseases of the valve itself.

SYMPTOMS.—These result from back pressure and are similar to those of the late stages of mitral disease, namely: extreme *cyanosis, dyspnœa,* marked *œdema* with *ascites,* and serious *abdominal congestion.*

TREATMENT OF ORGANIC HEART LESIONS
(Heart Failure and Valvular Lesions)

PRINCIPLES OF TREATMENT.—
In treating any case of organic heart disease it must be remembered that the primary aim is *to establish compensation.* Whether one is considering the case from a medical, nursing, or physical point of view, three great principles have always to be kept in mind.

1. *The heart must be rested and relieved* as much as possible. This is most essential, especially in the early stages when compensation begins to break down.

2. *The supply of oxygen to the body must be increased.* In most cases the patient suffers respiratory embarrassment and is therefore unable to take in enough oxygen, or to breathe out enough carbon dioxide. In addition, the interchange of gases in the lungs may also be inadequate owing to the congested condition of these organs. Unless this state of things can be remedied, the metabolic processes will be adversely affected and all the tissues of the body, including the heart muscle itself, will become weak. This is a very important factor which should be kept in mind at all stages of the disease.

3. *Hypertrophy, as we have seen, is Nature's compensation. This must therefore be assisted as much as possible.*

These three principles form the chief basis of treatment, and we shall apply these first to general and medical treatment, and then to physical treatment.

GENERAL TREATMENT.—
RELIEF OF THE HEART.—Rest is essential and the patient is confined to bed and complete rest. The foot of the bed may be raised to help venous return. If there is difficulty in breathing the patient will be propped up with pillows; otherwise he will lie flat. The diet must be light and digestible, and he may be kept on a milk diet in the early stages. Suitable drugs will be administered and surgical

treatment may be used later. Any measures which may be necessary to improve the patient's general health and strength will be taken.

INCREASE OF OXYGEN SUPPLY.—The patient may require the use of a ventilator.

PRODUCTION OF HYPERTROPHY.—This is a natural phenomenon, but we know that it can be assisted by carefully increasing the demands made on the heart. The patient will, therefore, gradually assume more and more activity until compensation is established.

WHEN COMPENSATION IS ESTABLISHED.—The patient must lead a quiet and regular life free from worry or over-exertion. He must take as much exercise as his health allows and carefully follow any directions given by his doctor with regard to diet or other matters. It is particularly important to avoid putting on weight, as this leads to further strain on the heart. Very hot baths are dangerous, and excessive smoking or drinking is also injurious.

PHYSICAL TREATMENT.—The three principles enumerated above may be applied as follows:—

1. RELIEF OF THE HEART.—To bring about this result, we must endeavour to decrease the peripheral resistance in the vessels by assisting venous return to the heart. This may be done by:—

a. Massage and Passive Movements.—The former should be rhythmic and rather slow. Effleurage, and kneading with the palms of one or both hands, are the best movements. The limbs are treated, and the back may sometimes be included. The latter should be *true passive movements*, and should again be rhythmical and rather slow. This treatment may also be used to treat œdema, if present.

b. Breathing Exercises.—These help venous return by increasing the changes in pressure in the thorax (*see* p. 382), thereby exerting a suction effect on the inferior and superior venæ cavæ. Inspiratory and expiratory exercises may be given, but *forced respiratory movements must be avoided*, since they tend to raise the blood-pressure and therefore strain the heart. In mitral disease, especially, the patient should not breathe too deeply, because to do so would increase the congestion in the already engorged lungs. Most physiotherapists prefer to instruct the patient to breathe freely in his own time, without commands, seeing that he breathes adequately but not too deeply.

2. INCREASE OF OXYGEN SUPPLY.—The mobility of the patient's thorax must be maintained, or increased by suitable exercises. It is also important that his posture be corrected if faulty, since a bad posture interferes with respiration, as well as with other bodily functions. Should any secretion be present in the lungs or bronchi, it may be necessary to give a modified form of postural drainage (*see* Cardiac Surgery, p. 423). The oxygen intake can then be increased by appropriate breathing exercises. Vibrations and gentle squeezing can usually be given over the thorax, to assist in loosening the secretions.

3. PRODUCTION OF HYPERTROPHY.—Hypertrophy, as we have seen, is brought about by *graduated* activity. It is the job of the physiotherapist to provide a suitable scheme of graduated exercises, and she has need of all her skill and judgement if the case is to progress uninterruptedly to a successful conclusion. She has to give the heart *just enough work to strengthen it, but not enough to cause another break-down*. The progression must be steady but gradual. If at any time it becomes evident that the patient has attempted too much, the amount of active work must be reduced for the time being.

When beginning a course of exercises for the patient whose heart is compensated in lying or half-lying, movements will only be given to the wrists, feet, and ankles. Each movement will be given four or five times on the day of its introduction, and increased by one or two each day. Progression is made by adding movements of the knee and elbow, daily increasing the number of times they are to be performed, and later those of hip and shoulder. The effect on the patient of each progression must be carefully watched. Finally, easy trunk exercises are added, *provided that they do not hamper the breathing*, as do concentric back-risings and free trunk-rotations. All the exercises chosen must, of course, be suitable for the patient while still in bed. When the doctor allows him to get up the strength of the exercises may be increased and he rhould begin to practise walking. To begin with a walk of only a few yards will be attempted, but the distance should be increased daily. Throughout the treatment the physiotherapist should always keep in mind the necessity for *gradual* progress.

In order to know whether the patient is doing enough, but not too much, active work, a careful record should be kept of its effects on (1) respiration, (2) the pulse, and (3) the general appearance.

1. *Respiration.*—The exercise should be hard enough to increase slightly both the range and rate of respiration, *but the patient should not be made breathless.* Furthermore, respiration should have returned to its normal rate two minutes after ending the exercises (Hunt).

2. *Pulse.*—This is the principal test. As to how much it is permissible to raise the pulse, the late Dr. Hunt,* of Guy's Hospital, gives the following figures:—

a. In early cases, *at the beginning of treatment*, the pulse should not be raised more than 6 beats by any exercise.

b. After 10 *days'* treatment, it should not be raised more than 8–14 beats.

c. After 3 *weeks*, not more than 12–16 beats.

d. After *the patient gets up*, not more than 16–20 beats.

In any case, the pulse should have returned, or almost returned, to its *resting* rate, that is, to what it was before the exercise began, at the end of two minutes.

At this stage (when the patient is up), Dr. Hunt used what he called the '*pulse ratio*' to test the patient's capacity for work. A certain exercise in the scheme—the hardest—is chosen. The patient's pulse is taken before beginning it. Immediately on its completion, the pulse is counted for two consecutive minutes. The pulse after exercise is then divided by the 'resting' pulse, the result being the 'pulse ratio', e.g.:—

```
Pulse before exercise ..      ..      ..      ..      ..      80
Pulse after exercise:—First minute   ..      ..    ..   100
                      Second minute  ..      ..    ..    85
                                                        ----
                                                        185
```

Ratio = 185 ÷ 80 = 2·3

```
Pulse before exercise ..      ..      ..      ..      ..      80
Pulse after exercise:—First minute   ..      ..    ..   105
                      Second minute  ..      ..    ..    90
                                                        ----
                                                        195
```

Ratio = 195 ÷ 80 = 2·4

The ratio in valvular disease should not as a rule exceed 2·3 at this stage, and in muscular disease 2·1. If it is used at a slightly earlier stage of valvular disease, it is safer not to let the ratio be above 2·2.

A ratio of 2·3 means, roughly, that the pulse is not raised more than about 20 beats, and has returned to its resting rate, or within a few beats of it, by the end of two minutes.

3. *General Appearance.*—Obviously no pain or distress ought to be caused, and this should not occur if the pulse and respiration are carefully studied.

* *Guy's Hospital Reports.*

RECORD OF OBSERVATIONS AND PROGRESSION.—The importance of keeping an accurate record of the progress of these patients cannot be over-emphasized. It should include:—

1. *The Work Done.*—The exercises performed should be noted down, with the number of times each was done, and the amount of resistance, if any. Later, the distance the patient has walked, and at what rate, will be entered. Unless this record is carefully kept, a proper graduation of the exercises is impossible.

2. *The Pulse-rate.**—The pulse at the beginning and at the end of the whole series of exercises may be recorded. The hardest exercise in the table consti-tutes the test of the patient's ability to do active work. The pulse is taken for 1 minute before it is begun, and immediately after its termination the patient is placed in a relaxed position, and the pulse counted for 2 minutes. The pulse ratio is taken, in the manner described above, and recorded (*see* specimen of record). In earlier cases the pulse may simply be taken during the first quarter of a minute after exercise, and multiplied by 4. By comparing the result with the resting pulse, we may ascertain as nearly as possible the exact number of beats it has been raised by the exercise, e.g.:—

$$\begin{aligned}
\text{Pulse before exercise} &= 90 \\
\text{Pulse during first quarter-minute after exercise} &= 25 \\
25 \times 4 &= 100
\end{aligned}$$
Pulse is therefore raised 10 beats by exercise.

Any remarks concerning respiration, the general condition, etc., should be added if necessary. If this chart is conscientiously kept, the physiotherapist has ready to hand a complete record of her patient's progress, on which she may base her future treatment, and from which a colleague can work in an emergency.

DETAIL OF TREATMENT.—

Early Stage

The patient is in bed and compensation has been established in half-lying.

1. When treating the patient for the first time, *look at his chart*, and notice the average speed of the pulse. *The chart should always be consulted before treatment*, so that any alteration in the pulse-rate may be observed. (The physiotherapist need not allow herself to be alarmed by sudden *isolated* rises of the rate, as there is often a perfectly natural explanation—as a rule, the patient has been agitated, startled, or suddenly awakened from sleep.)

2. *Take the pulse, and record it*, but put the patient at his ease as far as possible before doing so, because if he is nervous or worried his pulse-rate will rise. After placing the fingers on his wrist allow a half-minute or a minute to elapse before beginning to count.†

3. At first the scheme of treatment, in a serious case, consists only of massage, passive movements, and breathing. Early treatment should be very short— not lasting for more than fifteen minutes at most. Pulse and respiration will be taken again at the end of the treatment. Until active work is added, it should be the same as, or lower than, it was at the beginning.

Progression.—Gradually add passive movements to elbow and knee, and shoulder and hip.

---

* It should be stated here that many authorities disapprove of so much pulse-taking on the ground that it concentrates the patient's attention too much on his heart, and it is often confined to the test exercises.

† In some cases, especially if the pulse is irregular, it is better to take it over the apex of the heart and not at the wrist. But this should not be done if it alarms the patient. These points are specially important at a first treatment, and until the patient is used to the physiotherapist. While taking the pulse note the respiration rate.

As the patient improves—generally in a few days, or after a somewhat longer period if progress is slow—active movements are substituted, beginning with those of small joints.

PROGRESSION.—The amount of work done may be increased in the following ways:—

1. *Increase the number of times each movement is to be performed* (one more each day). When the patient is stronger the movements may be done *at a certain rate*, which is also increased daily. For instance, 2-Arm-bending and -stretching upward and downward may be done so many times a minute for two minutes. Let us suppose the patient performs the movement 6 times a minute for 2 minutes, and continues until he can do 16 times a minute (32 times in all). He may then try, say, 12 times a minute for 3 minutes (i.e., 36 times in all). (This is, of course, a fairly advanced exercise, and will probably be the 'test' exercise for some time.)

2. *Let the movements be performed in larger joints*, e.g., add successively exercises for the elbow and knee, for the hip and shoulder, and for the trunk. A new movement should never be done more than 6 times at first in the case of extremity exercises, or 3 times in that of trunk exercises. Do not alter both the arm and leg exercises to harder ones on the same day.

3. *Resisted exercises may, in part, replace the free ones.* The resistance may be given by the physiotherapist or, in certain arm exercises, the patient may hold small weights in his hands (first 1 lb., then 2 lb., etc.). When resistance is added, the number of times the movement is performed is *reduced*, and gradually increased again, e.g., if he has been doing free 2-Arm-bending and -stretching upward 15 times a minute for 3 minutes and he is now made to hold a 1-lb. weight in each hand, he will go back to 6 times a minute for 3 minutes. If his pulse rises unduly, the work will be even further reduced.

Later Stages

The patient is now allowed up.

Walking Exercise generally takes the place of the leg exercise, the patient's daily walk being regulated in some definite way. For instance, as far as the end of the bed next to his own and back; the next day the exercise may be 'two bed-lengths'; later, half the length of the ward, etc. The same method will be used when he comes to the physiotherapy department.

'*Stepping*'* is the final test exercise suggested by Dr. Hunt. A small platform or stool about 12 inches high is provided, and the patient steps up on to it and off again (backwards) a given number of times, beginning with 6 times a minute for 3 minutes. The pulse is taken before and immediately after the exercise, and the ratio calculated in the usual way. The exercise must be stopped at once if the patient shows signs of becoming breathless. Those unused to this method are often surprised to find that a 'heart case', after some practice, can step on and off that stool considerably quicker, without getting breathless, than they can themselves!

By this time the patient will almost be ready for discharge. (The course of treatment, in most cases, lasts some months.) Younger men or women may sometimes do class-work at this stage.

Some patients suffer from periodical break-down of compensation, generally as the result of overwork. They then require rest and possibly a further course of graduated exercises.

---

* This exercise is sometimes used as an *exercise tolerance test* before the patient begins treatment. The physician should in this case be consulted as to its advisability, and his advice obtained as to details.

I4

CARDIAC SURGERY

The introduction of the 'heart–lung' machine, which allows the cardiac and pulmonary chambers and vessels to be by-passed whilst maintaining the body's circulation, has led to one of the major advances in modern surgical techniques —that of cardiac surgery, and surgeons are now able to perform operations on the heart itself which were hitherto impossible.

Although no student, or physiotherapist, should attempt to treat post-operative heart cases, or indeed any serious heart condition, without adequate training and experience, either in her training school or at a special chest unit, it is felt that this important subject should be included in a general text-book. It should be stressed, however, that the following brief description of the conditions dealt with by surgical means and their pre- and post-operative care, should be regarded merely as an introduction to the subject.

Cardiac surgery is undertaken in cases of valvular disease and congenital abnormalities. Whenever possible surgery is performed before the symptoms become marked. Medical treatment is generally applied before deciding to operate, in order to improve the patient's general condition, and, in the case of severe symptoms, to enable the patient to withstand surgery. Ideally the patient is admitted about 5 days before the operation, unless a long period of medical treatment is envisaged.

GENERAL PRINCIPLES OF SURGERY

The operations may be *closed* or *open*. In the former, although the heart muscle is incised, the incision is a small one and the heart need not be drained. In open operations the incision is a large one and the chambers are drained. A few years ago hypothermia was generally employed to reduce the body temperature, and thus the oxygen requirements of the body, during open-heart surgery, but nowadays perfusion is the method of choice. The patient can remain on perfusion for a maximum of 4 hours, which reduces the risk of brain damage from oxygen lack during lengthy operations.

Whenever possible a mediasternal* incision is made, but if the approach has to be through the pleura, a thoracotomy is performed.

Conditions treated by surgical means fall into two categories: *congenital conditions* and *acquired lesions*.

CONGENITAL CONDITIONS.—These consist of Fallot's tetralogy; transposition of the great vessels; atrial and ventricular septal defects; stenosis of the pulmonary artery; coarctation of the aorta; and patent ductus arteriosus (*Figs.* 177–182).

1. FALLOT'S TETRALOGY (*Fig.* 177).—This is the commonest of the congenital lesions and consists of the following:—

a. Pulmonary stenosis.

b. A defect in the interventricular septum, so that the ventricles connect with each other.

c. A displacement of the aorta to the *right*, so that it has its origin over the defect in the intraventricular septum, and thus receives blood from both ventricles.

d. Hypertrophy of the right ventricle, in consequence of the effort required to pump blood through the narrow pulmonary valve.

The result of these defects is that during ventricular systole, the right ventricle cannot pump sufficient venous blood into the lungs and, moreover, as the ventricles contract, they *both* pump blood into the aorta, that from the right ventricle being

---

* The incision may also be known as a 'median sternotomy' or a 'median split'.

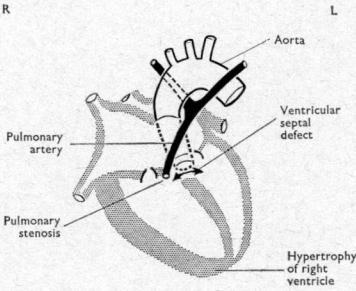

Fig. 177.—Fallot's tetralogy: As a result of the stenosis, the pulmonary artery is small. The right ventricle hypertrophies as a result of the effort required to pump blood through the narrow lumen of the pulmonary artery.

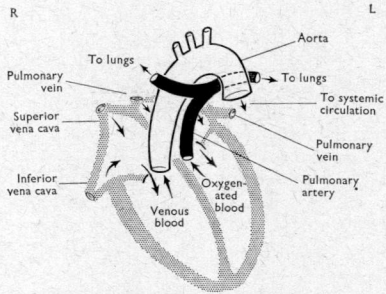

Fig. 178.—Transposition of the great vessels: The aorta, arising from the right ventricle, carries impure venous blood. The pulmonary artery arising in the left ventricle shuttles oxygenated blood from heart to lungs.

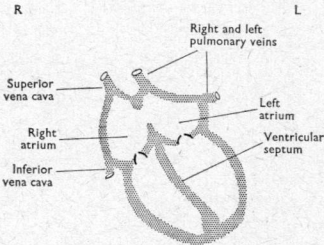

Fig. 179.—Atrial septal defect.

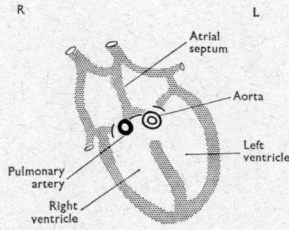

Fig. 180.—Pulmonary stenosis.

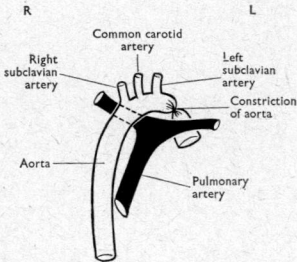

Fig. 181.—Contraction of the aorta.

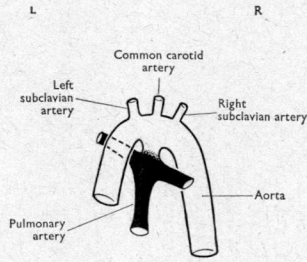

Fig. 182.—Patent ductus arteriosus.

Figs. 177–82.—Diagrammatic representation of congenital heart lesions.

impure venous blood. Because of the last two symptoms, the child tends to adopt a squatting position, in which he finds breathing easier (*Fig.* 183).

In infancy the operation known as Blalock's operation is usually performed. This consists of an anastomosis of the right or left pulmonary artery and the corresponding subclavian artery, so that blood from the subclavian artery, where pressure is higher, passes into the pulmonary artery and so to the lungs. Later this operation is followed by total repair of all the defects, either at one operation or in stages, depending on the condition of the patient. In any case of Fallot's tetralogy, the operation is an *open* one.

2. TRANSPOSITION OF THE GREAT VESSELS (*Fig.* 178).—This is a congenital abnormality in which the aorta and pulmonary artery are reversed, the aorta arising from the right ventricle and the pulmonary artery from the left. In effect this gives rise to two closed circuits, the systemic circuit carrying nothing but impure blood and the cardio-pulmonary circuit carrying the oxygenated blood. In order to overcome this, a funnel is made to connect the pulmonary veins with the aorta, the most usual operations being Mustard's or Blalock-Hanlon's. Again the operations are *open* ones.

3. ATRIAL OR VENTRICULAR SEPTAL DEFECTS (*Figs.* 177, 179).—In these cases there is an opening in the interatrial or interventricular septum ('hole in the

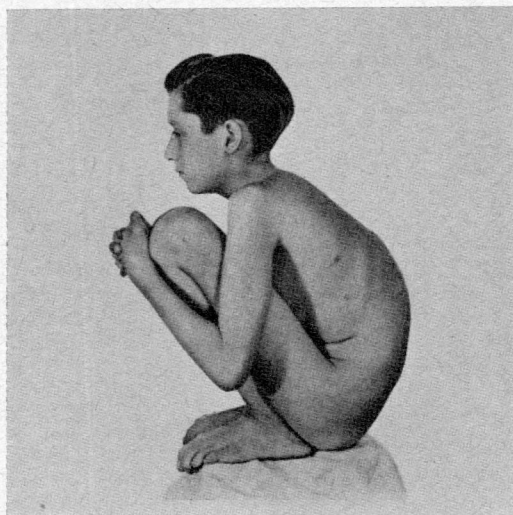

Fig. 183.—Fallot's tetralogy—squatting posture. (*Reproduced by kind permission from 'Physiotherapy', 1960, Vol. 46, p. 195.*)

heart') so that blood passes between the two chambers. Repair consists of 'patching' the defect with a piece of teflon or, if the defect is a small one, stitching it together. Again the operations are *open* ones.

4. PULMONARY STENOSIS (*Fig.* 180).—In any case of valvular stenosis, the cusps become adherent and the opening narrowed. In the case of pulmonary stenosis, insufficient blood passes to the lungs and there is dyspnœa, cyanosis, and fatigue. A pulmonary valvotomy is performed, the adherent cusps being separated by means of a dilator or the surgeon's finger. The operation is *closed*.

5. COARCTATION OF THE AORTA (*Fig.* 181).—This consists of a narrowing of the vessel just below the origin of the left subclavian artery. The blood-pressure is high in the upper part of the body (that supplied by the vessels given off above the constriction), but low in the lower part of the body, and the circulation is poor.

There is hypertrophy of the left ventricle. At operation the restricted portion is removed, the divided ends being joined together. Sometimes an arterial graft is put in. The operation is a *closed* one.

6. PATENT DUCTUS ARTERIOSUS (*Fig.* 182).—In foetal life the ductus arteriosus connects the aorta with the pulmonary artery. It normally closes soon after birth but sometimes fails to do so. As the pressure is higher in the aorta than the pulmonary artery, extra blood passes into the latter and is carried through the lungs a second time. This alone would not produce serious symptoms but it gives increased work to the heart and may, eventually, lead to cardiac failure. Ligature of the duct is therefore performed as soon as possible, the operation being a *closed* one.

ACQUIRED CONDITIONS.*—These are mainly the result of rheumatic fever (*see* pp. 409–10) and consist of mitral stenosis, in which case a mitral valvotomy is performed (*see above*, Pulmonary Stenosis); mitral stenosis and incompetence; tricuspid incompetence; and aortic incompetence.

In cases of valvular incompetence, surgery consists of *repair* or *replacement of* the damaged valves, and the operation is an *open* one. Replacement may be by homograft, or artificial means. A homograft involves excision of the diseased valve and replacement by a healthy valve taken from a cadaver. Since it must be a perfect fit there are certain obvious disadvantages and it is more usual to do an artificial replacement using a 'Starr-Edward' valve. This consists of a steel, or other inert metal cage, containing a teflon ball which rides up and down thus performing the function of a valve.

In cases where the valve is repaired the cusps are extended by tissue taken from the patient's body. A thin strip of tissue is taken from the fascia lata (fascia lata repair), or from the pericardium. The latter is avoided if possible, it being necessary to preserve as much of the heart tissue as possible. In cases of repair a drainage tube will be inserted into the area from which the graft was taken. Fascia lata is always taken from the *right* groin, the heart–lung machine being attached through the left groin to the left femoral artery (*perfusion*).

All these operations constitute very major surgery and may last from 6 to 10 hours or more. *The first* 24–48 *hours post-operatively are the most crucial*, though the risk of post-operative complications exists from 3 to 7 days or longer. The longer the operation (and therefore the lengthier the perfusion) the greater will be the risk. The chief dangers are *heart failure* and *hepatic* or *renal congestion*.

Following any form of cardiac surgery, the patient is returned from theatre to a special reception ward (Intensive Care Unit), where he remains from 2 to 5 days, though in some cases it may be as long as 3 weeks. During this time he receives intensive medical and nursing care, and a careful watch is kept on blood-pressure, pulse and apex beat, E.C.G. recordings, temperature, and respiration, all of which are recorded on his chart. *But most important of all are the body-fluid balance and the chemistry of the blood.* If there is any sudden alteration in blood-pressure, the patient becomes jaundiced, or the blood ceases to drain, action must be taken immediately if the patient is to survive. Although the responsibility for this lies in the hands of the nursing and medical staff, the physiotherapist must be aware of the risks and danger signals. She must study the chart before beginning treatment *and should keep a constant watch on the E.C.G. recording during treatment*. If she is at all worried, advice should be sought as to the desirability of treatment.

Before considering the physical treatment, a word should be said about the tubes and drains which can be expected.

---

* For the effects of valvular incompetence, *see* pp. 410, 412. It should be noted that valvular lesions may be congenital.

DRAINAGE TUBES.—It is standard practice for the patient to return from the theatre with the following:—

1. Pericardial and mediastinal or pleural drains, depending on the nature of the incision, as in any thoracotomy.*

2. If the operation has been a repair there will be a right groin or pericardial drain, depending on the site from which the tissue was taken.

3. For the first 24–48 hours there will also be a drainage tube in the left groin where the heart–lung machine was attached.

4. A catheter will have been inserted pre-operatively and will remain for 24–48 hours.

5. A Ryle's tube is also inserted and remains for a similar period.

6. Saline and glucose drips will be inserted in the arm.

As well as this somewhat formidable array the patient will be receiving oxygen through some form of humidifier; electrodes from the E.C.G. machine are attached to the leg; and in addition an endotracheal tube or tracheotomy tube may have been inserted, and the patient may be on a respirator (*see Fig.* 184 E).

The length of time for which a patient is on a respirator depends on the O_2/CO_2 ratio of the blood, which is tested daily. It is discarded as soon as possible, the patient being weaned from it by increasing periods without it, starting with 10 minutes. Radiographs are taken daily while the patient is in the Intensive Care Unit, and will, of course, be continued if necessary after the patient has been transferred to the general ward. The drains are generally taken out before the patient leaves the Intensive Care Unit and the stitches are removed in 14–18 days.

PRINCIPLES OF PHYSICAL TREATMENT

OPEN OPERATIONS.—As has been said, these are performed in cases of Fallot's tetralogy, transposition of the great veins, interseptal defects, and valve replacement or repair. The aims are basically the same as for any thoracic surgery, the most important factors being *to prevent post-operative atelectasis* and *to increase ventilation*. It should be stressed that methods vary slightly depending on the views of the surgeon, and that the physiotherapist works *only* on his instructions.

PRE-OPERATIVE TREATMENT.—As in thoracic surgery, the pre-operative time is spent in preparing the patient for the post-operative routine. Since the patient will see a great deal of his physiotherapist, the reason for this should be fully explained, together with the importance of his co-operation. General and localized breathing should be taught and the importance of postural drainage and coughing made clear. It is interesting to note that, whereas thoracic cases are inhibited through fear, cardiac cases seem to lose the ability to cough. He should thoroughly understand the work the physiotherapist will require of him. It is also extremely important that he should be told about the routine in the Intensive Care Unit and the various tubes and attachments with which he will be encumbered, otherwise he may well become frightened and jump to conclusions that things have gone wrong. This is not necessarily the physiotherapist's job but she should make sure that it has been done.

POST-OPERATIVE TREATMENT IN THE INTENSIVE CARE UNIT.—Hyper-sterile precautions are taken in this unit and all who enter the ward must wear gowns.

It is generally 24 hours from the time of the operation before treatment begins, although the physiotherapist may have seen the patient earlier.

* Tubes vary in number from one to four, depending on the views of the surgeon and the site of the incision.

Day 1.*—The patient is turned† and treatment is given four times during the day. It should be remembered that these patients should not lie flat and in the Intensive Care Unit the head of the bed is adjustable so that the patient can be lowered to a degree compatible with his comfort. Pillows are placed to support the head and shoulders and two people turn the patient, one taking the hips and one the shoulders. They can stand side by side or facing each other. It should be stressed that *turning should never be hurried* and *great care must be taken not to disturb the drainage tubes and drips.* For the first four treatments the patient is *turned to one side or the other at alternate treatments.* Since the left lung is the one most likely to collapse, the first position is onto the right side. If possible the patient remains turned for 10 minutes, *but he must not be allowed to become distressed.* With the patient in the turned position, simple local and general breathing exercises are given, followed by gentle percussion or vibration to encourage coughing. If a tracheotomy tube is in use, or the patient is unconscious, the secretions are cleared by 'bag-squeezing'.‡ The anæsthetist disconnects the patient from his respirator and inserts a connexion to a sterile anæsthetic bag, by means of which he manually inflates the chest. While he is doing this, the physiotherapist squeezes and vibrates the chest and produces a simulated cough. The nurse then removes the secretions with the suction apparatus. Again it should be stressed that extra sterile precautions are taken with regard to the bag and suction tubes.

When the patient has been returned to the upright position, simple passive and active, or active-assisted, movements are given to the feet and legs. At the next treatment the patient is turned on the left side and the above routine carried out. At the third treatment he is turned to the right again and at the fourth, to the left. *The arm is put through one full range of movement each day.*

Days 2–5 or 7.—Treatment continues as above, whether in the Intensive Care Unit or general ward, but the patient is only turned three times, being turned on both sides at each treatment. (For the first 5 days it is better to turn the patient onto the other side from the lying position, but after the fifth day he finds it more comfortable to come up to a sitting position before being turned to the other side.) It cannot be overstressed that *great care must always be taken of the tubes and attachments, and in particular there must be no interference with the main drainage.*§ *Treatment should never be rushed* and, whilst aiming at a minimum of 10 minutes in the turned position, *the patient must not be allowed to become distressed.*

A distinction must be made, however, between discomfort and distress. In order to avoid the former it should be possible to co-ordinate physical treatment with the administration of routine analgesics. This is particularly important in cases where there is a chest complication, or in which the risk of one is high, as it enables the physiotherapist to give more vigorous percussion. (It should be noted that percussion can be better tolerated if given over a blanket, or the physiotherapist's hand.)

COMPLICATIONS.—Besides the specific risks attendant on cardiac surgery listed above, the usual risks in thoracic surgery of pulmonary œdema (which the patient may well have had before the operation), post-operative atelectasis, and deep-vein thrombosis are also present. These fall more specifically within the physiotherapist's province—especially thrombosis, which may well pass

---

* Day 1 is taken to be 24 hours post-operatively.

† Turning varies in different hospitals. Some surgeons like the patient to be turned at the first treatment, others never turn for 48 hours.

‡ *See* Hamilton, D. E. (1964), 'Case of the Unconscious Patient', *Physiotherapy*, **51**, 12.

§ In thoracic surgery it is quite usual to clamp the main drainage tube. In cardiac surgery surgeons forbid this owing to the vastly increased drainage which is brought about by movement of the patient.

unnoticed by the nursing staff, the patient hesitating to 'worry' them with yet another 'minor' pain. Another factor which may add to the patient's discomfort is the tendency to severe bed-sores, particularly on the buttocks. These are presumably occasioned by the length of time the patient lies inert on the operating table, but if care is taken to pad vulnerable areas in the theatre, and the patient is nursed on a ripple mattress this should be overcome. Oil and spirit massage is given routinely and again this can often be combined with the physiotherapist's treatment times. It cannot be overemphasized that in the Intensive Care Unit there is much to pack into one short day and medical, nursing, and physiotherapy staff work together as a team in order to avoid exhausting the patient and to make things easier for themselves. The physiotherapist, of course, adheres strictly to the surgeon's wishes.

POST-OPERATIVE TREATMENT IN THE GENERAL WARD.—The exact date on which the patient is transferred to the general ward depends on many factors—chiefly on how soon he can manage without a ventilator, and the progress he makes towards recovery from the operation. Again the routine will vary slightly in different hospitals but a common procedure is for the morning treatment to follow the routine given in the Intensive Care Unit. For the first 5–7 days the patient is turned twice a day (turning to each side at each treatment) and for the second 5–7 days he is turned once a day in the same manner. Afternoon treatments consist of a ward class in which breathing exercises, arm and leg exercises, and simple trunk and abdominal exercises are given, the work suited to each patient being carefully assessed. On the eighth day the patient sits in a chair for half an hour. From then on he gradually progresses to longer periods out of bed, walking graduated distances, and managing stairs. He is usually ready for discharge in about 2 weeks. He attends the hospital for routine checks on his heart condition, but physiotherapy is not usually required after discharge.

There is a tendency for mitral stenosis to recur within 10 years, and a second or even third operation may be undertaken in perhaps 10 per cent of cases.

CLOSED OPERATIONS.—These are undertaken in cases of valvotomy, coarctation of the aorta, and patent ductus arteriosus. The principles are the same as in open operations, but the patients generally progress more quickly. If blood-pressure and apex beat are satisfactory, and there have been no complications, treatment begins 4 hours post-operatively. The routine is the same as for open surgery, the patient being turned at the first treatment if his condition permits. Breathing exercises are given in lying and side-lying, and the usual foot and leg exercises are performed. These patients are usually transferred to the general ward within 24 hours and are discharged about 2 weeks after the date of operation.

CARDIAC ARREST

Before closing this chapter, a word should be said on this subject. The term 'cardiac arrest' means cessation of an adequate circulation. It may prove fatal, but in many cases is a temporary phenomenon which can be reversed. Since the brain can only survive for 3 minutes without oxygen, *the sooner resuscitation commences the higher the chances of recovery.*

SIGNS AND SYMPTOMS.—There is a sudden deterioration in the patient's condition, marked by four cardinal signs:—

1. Unconsciousness.
2. Apnœa or cessation of breathing.
3. Absence of pulse—and in the case of patients who have had cardiac surgery the E.C.G. shows a flat line.
4. Dilatation of the pupils.

Treatment.—It is essential to provide an artificial circulation of oxygenated blood. This can be achieved by *external heart massage* and *artificial respiration* (*Fig.* 184 A–E).

CARDIAC MASSAGE.—The patient must lie absolutely flat. The heel of the hand is placed on the lower half of the sternum with the other hand placed on top. With straight arms, and using body weight, the sternum is depressed and released 60–80 times a minute (*Fig.* 184 A). In this way, the heart is compressed between sternum and vertebræ and its blood-content ejected. After compression, the chest *must* be allowed to expand fully in order to allow venous return to take place. Care must be taken to avoid pressure other than on the sternum, because of the danger of fracturing a rib.

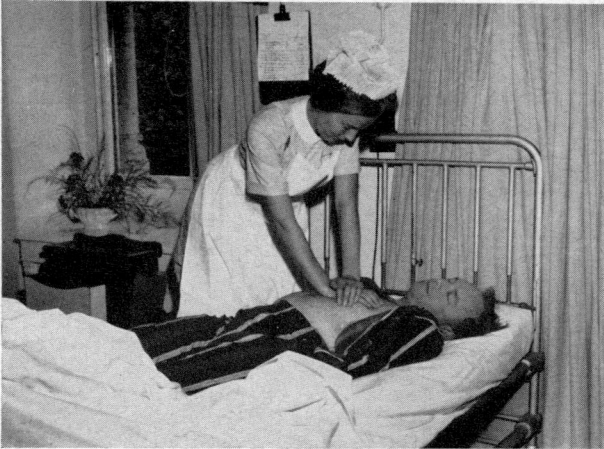

A, The bedclothes are thrown back, the pillows pushed out, and the patient pulled flat. Kneeling on the bed the nurse places her hands one on the other over the lower half of the sternum and starts external massage with a quick but firm compression.

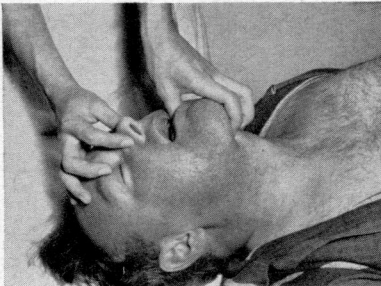

B, Mouth-to-mouth respiration. The head and neck are extended and the position is maintained by a hand on the forehead which also pinches the nostrils. The thumb of the other hand is placed in the mouth and the jaw grasped between fingers and thumb to pull it forward and hold the mouth open.

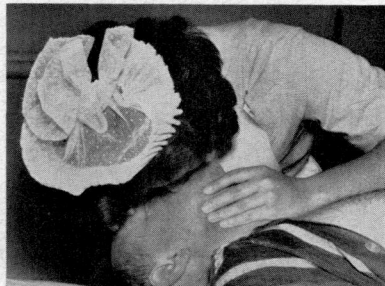

C, Ventilation is performed by placing the nurse's mouth completely over that of the patient and obtaining an airtight fit. The mouth is removed to allow the patient to exhale.

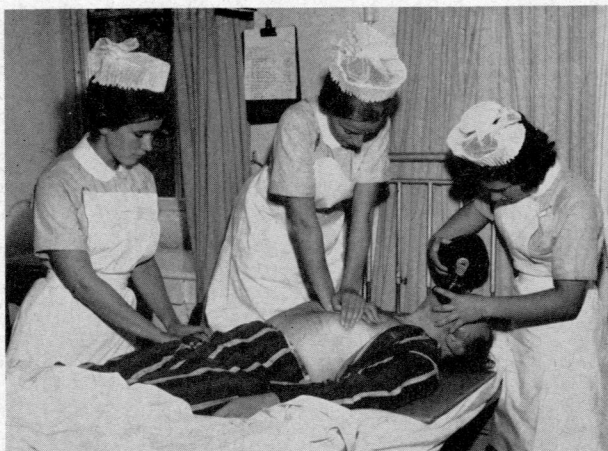

D, Simultaneous external cardiac massage and artificial ventilation.

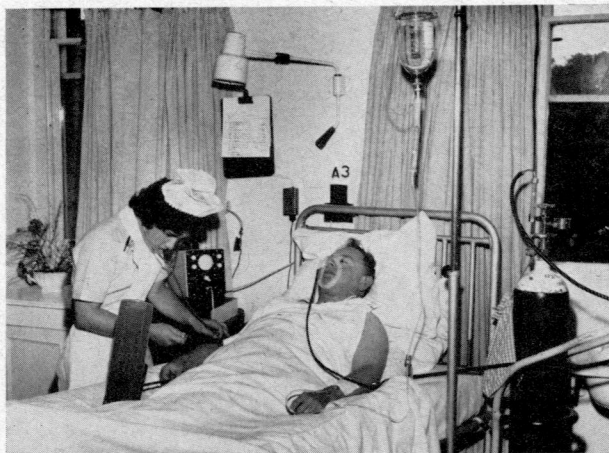

E, After-care: continuous monitoring of pulse, blood-pressure, and E.C.G. Oxygen is administered by mask and a nasogastric tube passed. The urinary catheter is not seen, nor the electrodes to the E.C.G. machine. If this were a 'post-operative' case he would also have right and left femoral, and pericardial drains. The oxygen tubes would be replaced by a ventilator.

Fig. 184.—The treatment of cardiac arrest.
(*Reproduced by kind permission from 'Nursing Times', November, 1965.*)

Artificial Respiration.—Before this can begin the respiratory passages must be free from obstruction. To facilitate this, the head is extended and the jaw drawn forward, a position which must be retained throughout the treatment (*Fig. 184 B*). If available, a ventilator may be used, or the mouth-to-mouth method ('kiss of life') employed (*Fig.* 184 C). With either method, *it is essential to see that the patient's mouth is completely covered and that the chest really expands.* Success is denoted by the return of the pulse and shrinkage of the pupils. If two people can give first aid, heart massage and respiration can be given simultaneously (*Fig.* 184 D). If only one person is available, the two must be given alternately.

With the arrival of the medical staff, resuscitation, if still required, is taken over by them, and an endotracheal tube inserted, together with drips for appropriate medication. Oxygen will be administered, and pulse and blood-pressure charted ¼-hourly until full recovery has occurred (*Fig.* 184 E).

It cannot be overstressed that prompt action on the part of those nearest the patient at the time can make the difference between life and death.

CHAPTER XIX

DISEASES OF BLOOD AND LYMPH-VESSELS

I. Diseases of the arteries: Arteriosclerosis—Aneurysm—Thrombo-angiitis obliterans (Buerger's disease)—Raynaud's disease—Chilblains. II. Diseases of the veins: Phlebitis—Thrombosis —Phlegmasia alba dolens ('White-leg')—Varicose veins. III. Obstruction of lymphatics (Œdema).

IT will be remembered that arteries and veins have three coats: the *tunica adventitia*, or outer coat of connective tissue; the *tunica media*, or muscular coat, composed of unstriated muscle-fibres running circularly around the vessel; and the *tunica intima*, or inner coat, formed of epithelial cells. The tunica media is thick and strong in the arteries, whereas it is thin in the veins. The structure of each set of vessels is otherwise similar.

I. DISEASES OF THE ARTERIES
ARTERIOSCLEROSIS
(Atheroma)

It is unlikely that we should be called upon to treat this condition as such, but since it is likely to be a factor in cardiac cases and patients referred for treatment of some other complaint, a brief description will be given here. Arteriosclerosis is a condition of chronic inflammation of the innermost coat of the arteries, leading to degenerative changes which spread to the two outer coats.

It is more common in men than in women. The larger arteries are most affected, especially the aorta. This is because the blood-pressure is higher in these than in the smaller vessels. The whole length of the arteries is affected.

AETIOLOGY.—Hardening of the vessels is always present to some extent in old age, as the result of the wear and tear of the arteries during life; but it may supervene in middle age from various pathological causes: (1) Hereditary predisposition; (2) Very laborious occupations, which cause continual strain on the arteries, by keeping the blood-pressure high; (3) Any other conditions producing high blood-pressure, e.g., poisoning by lead or alcohol, which brings about changes in the blood which make it flow less easily through the vessels; kidney disease, too much nitrogenous food, etc.

SYMPTOMS.—*Superficial arteries* (e.g., the radial), if affected, may be felt to be *hard and thickened*, even when the pulse is obliterated by pressure. The *blood-pressure* is high and the *pulse* tense. Some patients suffer from *coldness and numbness of the feet*, or *cramp* in the legs. *Intermittent claudication* (*see* p. 430) may sometimes occur as a late symptom. *Discoloration of the skin*, and *œdema in the lower extremities*, are sometimes present.

The *heart*.—The left ventricle is hypertrophied, because of the hard work entailed in pumping blood through the unyielding arteries. *Sclerosis of the coronary arteries* (cardiosclerosis) may lead to angina pectoris, to sudden death from thrombosis, or to fibrous degeneration of the heart. If dilatation takes the place of hypertrophy, owing to failure of the reserve force (*see* pp. 410, 411) the symptoms will be similar to those of valvular disease.

RESULTS.—As the result of arteriosclerosis, there may also be: (1) *Aneurysm* (*see below*), especially in the arch of the aorta; (2) *Thrombosis* due to clotting of the blood over the degenerate patches on the arterial wall; (3) *Rupture of an artery* from some trivial cause such as a slight blow or injury, or a sudden rise in blood-pressure. If this causes a cerebral hæmorrhage, hemiplegia may follow.

PRECAUTIONS.—Arteriosclerotic patients, other than cardiac cases, requiring physical treatment for some other disability should be treated with great caution. Exercises must be very carefully chosen, and nothing be attempted which would raise the blood-pressure to any extent. *Over-exertion must be avoided at all costs. Buerger's exercises (see* p. 431) may be required in cases where severe symptoms are present in the legs or feet.

ANEURYSM

An aneurysm consists of a dilatation of the wall of an artery, forming a sac in communication with that vessel. Again the physiotherapist is more likely to treat a patient with aneurysm for some other condition than for the aneurysm itself. When dealing with these patients it is of vital importance to avoid any treatment which might raise the blood-pressure. Should treatment be specifically requested the aim would be to relieve the heart by assisting venous return.

AETIOLOGY.—Aneurysm is most common in men between the ages of 30 and 45 years and the most usual causes are syphilis, acute infections, or specific fevers which result in damage to the vessel walls, but there is sometimes a traumatic origin.

PATHOLOGY.—The vessel wall is weakened, and in some forms of aneurysm the two inner coats rupture altogether and blood passes between them (*dissecting aneurysm*). The large arteries, or those near the joints, are most often affected—aneurysm of the thoracic aorta being the most common of all. The cause is usually syphilitic.

PROGNOSIS.—The prognosis depends on which artery is implicated. Rupture of the aneurysm, or pressure on some vital organ or nerve (e.g., vagus or phrenic) may cause death. The patient may, however, live for many years, but is always in danger. Spontaneous recovery occasionally takes place, either because the aneurysm presses on the artery and occludes it altogether, or because clotting takes place within the sac. In the former case occlusion of a small vessel causes the blood to flow through the collateral vessels, and in the latter the clot becomes organized so that the aneurysm remains as a mere fibrous body on the arterial wall.

SYMPTOMS.—These are caused by pressure on the structures in the neighbourhood of the tumour, and depend on which artery is implicated, but the following may occur:—

Intense pain (pressure on the vertebræ or on the chest wall).

Paraplegia (pressure on the nerve-roots or the spinal cord).

Angina (involvement of the beginning of the aorta and the coronary arteries).

Œdema of the arm (pressure on the subclavian vein or superior vena cava).

Cough, dyspnoea, loss of voice (pressure on the respiratory organs, or on the nerves that supply them).

Difficulty in swallowing (pressure on the œsophagus), etc.

Treatment.—Operations are sometimes undertaken to induce clotting in the sac. In some situations the aneurysm can be *excised*, sometimes with a graft inserted to connect the two ends of the vessel until union takes place.

Post-operative physical treatment is given as for any cardiac case.

THROMBO-ANGIITIS OBLITERANS
(*Buerger's Disease*)

A disease of the arteries, generally occurring in the lower extremities. The cause is unknown, but it appears to have some connexion with cigarette smoking.

The substances present in tobacco damage the walls of blood-vessels in certain people hypersensitive to them, and thus render the vessels liable to attack by some bacteria of unknown origin. There may be an hereditary factor. It is almost invariably found in young men, and is said to be particularly common in Jews.

PATHOLOGY.—Certain segments of the arteries are affected, not the whole length as in arteriosclerosis. All three coats of the vessels are attacked and become inflamed. Because of the inflammation in the tunica intima clots are formed which obstruct the lumen of the artery, and the affected vessel may ultimately degenerate and turn into a mere fibrous cord. The adjacent vein and nerve are often involved, and all the structures may become bound together in fibrous tissue. Pressure on vasomotor nerves may cause spasm. As in ordinary thrombosis, small vessels may ultimately grow through the clot.

SYMPTOMS.—

Early Stage.—The feet are cold, and there may be vasomotor symptoms like those in Raynaud's disease (*see below*).

Later Stage.—In some cases there are red and tender spots over the superficial veins, as in thrombophlebitis. The two principal symptoms are *intermittent claudication* and *gangrene*.

Intermittent claudication consists of *pain which comes on in the calf or foot while the patient is walking, and which passes off when he rests.* It is due to ischæmia in the limb, the diminished blood-supply being sufficient for resting, but not for working, muscles. As the disease progresses the pain gets worse, comes on sooner with exercise, and subsides more slowly on rest.

Gangrene.—Trophic changes take place in the leg. There may be ulceration, and gangrene develops, making amputation necessary. The pain associated with the onset of gangrene is extremely severe.

COMPLICATIONS.—Coronary or cerebral thrombosis may occur due to an embolism.

PROGNOSIS.—The disease is generally progressive, though there may be remissions.

Treatment.—

GENERAL AND MEDICAL TREATMENT.—Smoking is forbidden because it causes vasoconstriction. There is no *specific* medical treatment since the cause is unknown, but the physician will administer suitable vasodilator and analgesic drugs.

PHYSICAL TREATMENT.—The *aims* are *to improve the circulation* in order to increase the blood-supply to the affected limbs, thus delaying the onset of gangrene; and *to relieve pain*. The circulation may improve by assisting the collateral circulation and, possibly, by reducing spasm in the arteries, if present. Since the disease is progressive, treatment is mainly palliative.

Massage may remove waste products from the tissues, and relieve spasm. The leg is slightly elevated during treatment, unless this increases pain. The best movements to use are gentle effleurage and kneading, but the former may be painful owing to the drag on the skin. If so, kneading only is indicated, the physiotherapist being very careful to keep the hand stationary on the skin, and to lift it and replace it when moving from one area to another (Angrove). Any painful area must be avoided. In some cases, *connective tissue** massage has been used with success.

EXERCISES.—*Buerger's exercises* may be given, especially in cases of intermittent claudication without gangrene.

---

* A specialized technique of German origin. It cannot be described here. "Massage of Reflex Zones", L. Mahoney, *J. chart. Soc. Physiother.*, March, 1957; "Connective Tissue Massage", M. Ebner and B. Reymann, *Ibid.*, July, 1955.

Buerger's Exercises

The patient lies flat on a bed or couch. The legs are raised 45° and supported in that position until the skin blanches (about two minutes). The patient then sits with his legs over the side of the bed for three minutes, i.e., until the skin becomes congested, after which he again lies flat, until the colour of the limbs becomes normal. The process is repeated four or five times about three times a day. It stimulates the sluggish circulation, and brings about changes of pressure in the peripheral vessels. In some cases the times have to be shortened, as the required positions, especially the dependent one, may be too painful. Sometimes only half a minute each way is possible. The exercises are usually preceded by heat (*see below*).

These exercises may be ordered for various vascular diseases affecting the legs.

HEAT AND ELECTRICAL TREATMENT.—Heat is generally applied to the *abdomen* or *thighs*, although some authorities prefer to irradiate the *lumbar region*. The warm blood from this area passes to the vasomotor centre, depresses its action, and causes relaxation and vasodilation of all the blood-vessels in the extremities. Short-wave diathermy may be given by means of an induction coil, or by a co-plane technique, but radiant heat is equally effective. *Heat must never be applied to the feet or lower legs only, or in cases where the spasm cannot be relieved, as this only produces a local vasodilation which, without an increased blood-supply, damages the tissues.* Contrast baths, cathodal baths, or sinusoidal baths for the limbs have also been tried.

Indolent ulcers are very liable to form, and care must be taken to avoid damaging the skin. Any ulcerated areas should be treated in the usual way by local doses of ultra-violet light, massage, etc. (*See* Chap. V, pp. 96–9.)

SURGICAL TREATMENT.—*Lumbar sympathectomy* (removal of sympathetic ganglia) is sometimes performed to bring about relaxation of the artery walls, and thereby increase the blood-supply to the extremities.

POST-OPERATIVE TREATMENT.—Routine post-operative treatment will be given to lessen the risk of post-operative thrombosis or chest complication. Buerger's exercises may also be given.

Amputation of some part of the leg may be necessary to save the patient's life in cases of gangrene. (For post-operative treatment, *see* pp. 111–15.)

RAYNAUD'S DISEASE

This is a *syndrome* rather than a disease. The patients are unduly sensitive to cold which, even in a mild degree, causes excessive contraction of the arteries. It is particularly noticeable in the hands and fingers, but the toes, lobes of the ears, or tip of the nose may also suffer.

AETIOLOGY.—The cause of this condition is not fully understood. Raynaud's own view was that it was due to abnormal activity of the vasoconstrictor nerves, probably caused by some irritation of the vasomotor centre in the medulla, or of the sympathetic nerves themselves. In some cases it appears to be due simply to increased susceptibility to cold, producing a local effect on the unstriated muscle-fibres of the arterioles of the fingers. Pressure on, or occlusion of, an artery may, of course, cause it, and it may be seen in patients who have a cervical rib, atheroma, arteriosclerosis, or Buerger's disease.

The condition is more common in women than in men, and generally appears in young people or in early middle life.

SYMPTOMS.—These vary in different patients, and with the severity of the conditions, but two definite patterns emerge.

1. The parts affected become white and 'dead'. Sensory changes such as tingling, dulling of sensation, or numbness occur. The attack may last from a

few minutes to several hours. Pain and tingling accompany the return of the circulation to normal.

2. There is much local congestion, or almost complete stasis, in the part and the affected areas are blue, or even black, in colour. If the area is compressed a white mark appears, which disappears slowly when the pressure is released. There is swelling, stiffness, intense pain, and sometimes anæsthesia.

Both patterns may occur in the same person, or only one variety may appear. Either may end in:—

LOCAL (SYMMETRICAL) GANGRENE.—This is, as a rule, limited to a small part of the area affected. It varies in severity from a mere peeling of the skin, or a blister which bursts and leaves an ulcer, to necrosis of finger or toe bones. The latter is, however, rare.

PROGNOSIS.—Slight cases may remain stationary, but serious ones may get worse until the condition becomes more or less permanent. These are the cases in which symmetrical gangrene is likely to occur.

Treatment (between attacks).—

PHYSICAL TREATMENT.—Massage may be given to the thighs and/or back for the purpose of improving the circulation. Connective-tissue massage may, again, prove effective. Active exercises may also be given to increase the general circulation.

ELECTRICAL TREATMENT.—Radiant heat or short-wave diathermy may be given as for intermittent claudication, but *heat must never be applied during an attack*. Sinusoidal or galvanic baths are often effective, and patients may benefit from a course of general ultra-violet radiation. Calcium ionization is sometimes effective, since it relieves spasm due to irritability of nerves.

CARBACHOL IONIZATION.*—This treatment has been tried with success in many cases of Raynaud's disease. Choline ions produce dilatation of the blood-vessels through their effect on sympathetic nerve-endings. Ideally it should begin before the cold weather aggravates the symptoms of the disease.

Method.—For the lower extremity, a large cathodal pad may be placed on the lumbar spine or beneath the buttocks. A layer of lint soaked in carbachol solution is placed on the dorsum of each foot—or wrapped round the foot—at the level of the roots of the toes, and a saline pad of the usual number of layers placed over it. The two electrodes are attached to the positive pole. For the upper extremity the cathodal pad is placed on the thoracic spine between the shoulders, and the anodal pads on the backs of the hands, or wrapped round them at the level of the roots of the fingers, prepared as described above.

Dosage.—Since there may be considerable local and general effects, it is advisable to begin with a small dose, which should be increased gradually. Some authorities start with 3 mA. for five minutes, increasing to 10 mA. for 10 minutes. Others assess the dosage on 1 mA. per square inch and increase the time to 20 or 30 minutes. The result to be expected is reddening of the area under the pad, and of the fingers and toes.

Systemic Reactions.—The physiotherapist must watch carefully for these, and the patient must not be left unobserved during treatment. The patient should be warned of the possibility of a systemic reaction, in order that he may report anything untoward. The main symptoms are *a feeling of heat*, with *sweating* and *flushing of the face*. This may sometimes be followed by nausea, abdominal cramp, faintness, palpitations, diarrhœa, and vomiting. At the first sign of any of these symptoms, the current should be turned off at once.

---

* *See* article on the subject of carbachol ionization in the *J. chart. Soc. Physiother.*, June and December 1945.

Treatment is generally given three times a week, but it is sometimes prescribed daily for a week, and thrice weekly after this. Because of the unpleasant side-effects, it is more usual nowadays to use *amechol* or *priscol* by which the systemic effects are considerably reduced.

SURGICAL TREATMENT.—In some cases, *cervical sympathectomy* or removal of the superior cervical ganglion is performed, in order to bring about reduction of vasomotor tone in the upper extremity. Impulses pass from this ganglion to join the spinal nerves of the upper part of the body. These are the vasoconstrictor nerves which bring about constriction of the blood-vessels. If the ganglion is removed, the vessels dilate.

CHILBLAINS

This condition is a localized inflammation of the superficial tissues. The toes, heels, hands, and fingers frequently suffer, and occasionally the ears or even the nose.

CAUSES AND PATHOLOGY.—The cause of this troublesome affection is obscure. It is commonly ascribed to 'bad circulation', but since chilblains are so common in children and young people, many of them in robust health, and with their circulation apparently satisfactory, there must surely be some other cause. There may be a deficiency of some substance in the blood, or a disorder of calcium metabolism. The condition may possibly amount to a slight degree of Raynaud's disease, cold having the effect of producing spasm of the muscles of the arterial walls, which later results in a reaction producing the congestion which is so marked a feature of chilblains.

SYMPTOMS.—The part is *red* and *congested*; at first, *irritation* is intense; later, *pain* may follow. Chilblains on the heels may make walking almost impossible, the pressure of the shoe on the inflamed part causing intense pain. If the part is not adequately protected, the skin over the chilblain may break.

Treatment.—

ELECTRICAL TREATMENT.—Galvanic or sinusoidal baths are beneficial, and calcium or iodine ionizations may be helpful. Local treatment by ultra-violet radiation is also given to stimulate calcium metabolism. Carbachol ionization may be tried, but this is not usual. Contrast baths are a useful home treatment.

A *broken chilblain* should be dressed with ointment spread on lint. Penicillin ointment is often prescribed. Finger-kneadings should be given round it, and ultra-violet light or zinc ionization may be given to prevent sepsis and promote healing.

II. DISEASES OF THE VEINS

PHLEBITIS

Inflammation of the wall of a vein.

CAUSES.—

1. Injury of the vessel; pressure exerted upon it either by tumours in its course, or by constriction due to tight garters or other garments.

2. Varicose veins (*see* p. 437).

3. Inflammatory or septic cases arise by extension of infection from tissues round the vein, e.g., from septic wounds.

4. Sometimes no definite cause can be found.

PATHOLOGICAL CHANGES.—The inflammation may involve only the tunica intima, or may spread to the tunica media and adventitia as well. In simple cases a clot forms, which becomes organized (*see* THROMBOSIS). The inflammation may even spread to surrounding tissues, and an abscess may form (Hey Groves).

SYMPTOMS.—Phlebitis is most common *in the veins of the leg*, e.g., in the femoral vein. *Pain is felt in the line of the vein*, with a hard, cord-like swelling. In the case of a superficial vein, the skin over it is *dark in colour and œdematous*.

If the large, deep, main vessels of a limb are affected, there is much lymphatic obstruction, the slowed venous circulation involving a greatly increased exudation of lymph. *Œdema*, similar to that described as following the removal of the axillary glands, will make its appearance. *The superficial veins may be seen to be increased in size*, in order to carry on the collateral circulation, and so compensate for the block. In septic cases *abscesses* may develop round the inflamed vessel.

General symptoms: The patient has fever and shivering fits; these symptoms are more pronounced in infective cases.

Treatment.—
The treatment of phlebitis is so similar to that of thrombosis that the two will be considered together.

THROMBOSIS

Blocking of a vein by the formation of a blood-clot.

CAUSES.—

1. Injuries to the vessels, e.g., in fractures, or through compression by forming callus.

2. Phlebitis, or extension of inflammation from surrounding structures.

3. Degeneration of the vessel walls; varicose veins.

4. Any conditions that produce abnormal slowing of the circulation: heart or lung disease, anæmia, debility.

PATHOLOGICAL CHANGES.—If there is an inflamed area on the vessel wall, it acts as a source of irritation, like a foreign body, and fibrin is deposited upon it by the blood, a clot being thus formed. If the circulation is very slow, the blood sometimes becomes stagnant behind the valve cusps and clots there, especially if the vein is dilated and the valves do not close. The clot may completely fill the lumen of the vein, preventing any flow of blood through it.

Thrombosis may terminate by:—

1. RESOLUTION.—The clot may be removed by the leucocytes, in which case the circulation through the vessel again becomes normal, although this rarely happens.

2. ORGANIZATION.—New connective tissue is laid down until the clot becomes a fibrous mass, completely blocking the vein. New blood-vessels grow into the fibrous clot, and to a certain extent re-establish the circulation by forming passages through it.

3. EMBOLISM.—The thrombus, or part of it, may become detached from the vessel wall, and be carried away by the blood-stream. This free body circulating in the blood is known as an *embolus*, and is a source of considerable danger.

4. DISINTEGRATION.—The thrombus—generally a septic one—may dissolve and be carried away by the blood, spreading infection through the body. Abscesses may form elsewhere, or the patient may die of *pyæmia* (general poisoning).

THE COLLATERAL CIRCULATION.—It must be realized that even should a main vein be completely blocked, the circulation is not entirely stopped in that area. If that were so, the arterial circulation would also cease, no new blood could reach the part, and gangrene would set in. This does not happen because the branches of veins anastomose very freely. The blood, therefore, is able to return to the heart by way of these branch veins, which form what is known as the *collateral circulation*.

SYMPTOMS.—*A definite tender point* can be felt at the site of the thrombus. The patient complains of *pain, resembling cramp*, in the surrounding tissues. There is marked *swelling* in the area below the thrombus, and the power of moving the limb is much impaired. *Marked enlargement of the collateral veins* can be observed. The patient's temperature may rise.

EMBOLISM.—Emboli may be *simple* or *infective*. The amount of damage that can be done by an embolus depends on its nature, and on the position in which it finally lodges. If it occludes an artery which forms the only blood-supply of an important organ, the results are likely to be fatal, since the part thus deprived of its blood-supply degenerates and dies. A septic embolus causes the formation of an abscess in the area where it lodges.

The most usual situations in which an embolus may lodge and give rise to serious danger are:—

1. The *pulmonary artery* (causing sudden death, because all outflow from the right side of the heart is stopped).

2. One of the *coronary arteries* which may also cause sudden death, as these are 'end-arteries'. They do not anastomose with other arteries, or to any extent with each other, so that that part of the heart which is deprived of its blood-supply is unable to work at all.

3. The *brain*, generally in the middle cerebral artery. Softening of the area supplied follows, with resulting hemiplegia.

4. One of the *vessels of the lung*, causing pain, dyspnœa, or hæmoptysis.

Treatment of Phlebitis and Thrombosis

GENERAL AND MEDICAL TREATMENT.—Rest and immobilization of the thrombosed area are essential. The patient is kept in bed with the limb raised. Belladonna applications, or kaolin poultices, may be used to relieve pain. In phlebitis, injections of an anticoagulant drug may be given to reduce the tendency to thrombosis.

SURGICAL TREATMENT.—In recurrent cases of phlebitis in superficial veins, the latter are sometimes excised. For post-operative treatment, *see* VARICOSE VEINS, p. 438.

PHYSICAL TREATMENT.—*This is contra-indicated in the acute stage*, but it may possibly be ordered in the late stages. The condition may well arise post-operatively, post-partum, or following trauma, in a patient already receiving physiotherapy. *It is of the utmost importance that the physiotherapist should be aware of this possibility*, and the following points must always be borne in mind: (1) *In phlebitis there is the danger of clot formation.* (2) *In thrombosis, that of dislodging an imperfectly organized thrombus, and so setting free an embolus which may bring about a serious, or even a fatal, result.*

Should any of the symptoms of thrombus arise in a patient already receiving physiotherapy, the treatment must be discontinued immediately, and the matter reported at once. The physiotherapist must then await instructions from the physician or surgeon in charge before resuming treatment.

In a case of phlebitis, treatment may be allowed to continue fairly soon, *but nothing must be done which could possibly increase the inflammation*, and *the area of the diseased vein should always be given a wide berth.*

In a case of thrombosis no treatment must be given until it is firmly organized, and it is for the doctor to decide when this has taken place.

METHODS OF TREATMENT.—

THROMBOSIS.—*Acute Stage*:—

Massage.—Many authorities feel that massage should be avoided at all costs, but if it is to be given, the most useful manipulation will be effleurage, since the purpose of treatment is to assist venous and lymphatic circulation. It should be given very lightly, carefully avoiding the area of the vein in which the organized clot is situated, that is, the strokes may be given around, but not over it. If the thrombus is situated in one of the deep veins of the leg, e.g., in the posterior tibial vein, massage may be given to the thigh, and also to the front and outer side of the leg. If the femoral vein is affected, the inner side of the thigh must be avoided, especially Scarpa's triangle. If the popliteal vein is affected, the popliteal space must then be avoided. A few days later, if all goes well, gentle kneadings may be added.

Movements.—Provided care is used, these are generally allowed from the beginning. They should start as *passive movements*, and progress through *active assisted* to *active movements.** They are first given to the foot and gradually incorporate the other joints.

Movements will assist venous return by exerting pressure on the vessels, but since such pressure must of necessity fall on the affected vein, as well as on others, the physiotherapist must make certain that all possibility of embolism has disappeared.

Buerger's Exercises.—These may also be given and should be practised three times a day, or even, in some cases of severe obliterative thrombosis, every two hours. The patient can often only tolerate the modified form—half a minute up and half a minute down—the dependent position being too painful if continued longer.

Breathing Exercises.—These will also assist venous return, but the patient must not be allowed to breathe too deeply, because this might produce a pulmonary embolism.

When allowed to walk, the patient should begin by doing a very little at a time. It must not be forgotten that the lack of exercise will predispose to weakness and eversion of the foot. In both acute and chronic cases a supporting bandage, or an elastic stocking, should be worn when the patient is out of bed.

Chronic Stage.—In long-standing cases, where a *firmly organized* thrombus is giving rise to lymphatic congestion and severe œdema, effleurage and kneading may be given *deeply and firmly*, as described on p. 440. The position of the patient before and during treatment should be the same as that for VARICOSE VEINS (*see* p. 438).

PHLEBITIS.—Similar treatment can be given, but the area of the inflamed vein should be given a very wide berth.

PHLEGMASIA ALBA DOLENS
('*White-leg*')

This troublesome condition is seen following childbirth. It generally arises two or three weeks after delivery. If it occurs it consists of a phlebitis, or thrombosis, of the femoral vein, due either to sepsis, or to thrombosis in the vein near Poupart's ligament. In this locality the circulation is always slow, and is especially so when the patient re-assumes the erect position after her time in bed, the vasomotor system not having had time to adapt itself to the change of attitude. It is seen less frequently today than formerly, owing to improved ante- and postnatal care, and the shorter time for which the mother is confined to bed.

SYMPTOMS.—The first signs are generally *fever* and *chill. General symptoms* then arise—constipation, gastric and intestinal symptoms, loss of appetite, and vomiting. The patient complains of a feeling of *weight* and *stiffness in the leg*, and sometimes of *pain in the calf*. There may be tenderness along the course of the femoral vein, and some of the more superficial veins may be similarly affected. There is *sudden and intense swelling of the leg*, generally beginning at the foot and spreading upwards. The limb becomes so hard from venous and lymphatic

---

* *See also* Miss Angrove's method of treatment in her *Remedial Exercises for Certain Diseases of the Heart and Lung*, p. 93.

congestion, that the stretched skin does not pit on pressure. The *left leg* is more often affected than the right, but both may be successively involved.

Treatment.—

GENERAL TREATMENT.—As in the case of ordinary thrombosis the patient is kept in bed, with the leg well raised.

PHYSICAL TREATMENT.—As in THROMBOSIS, all massage or movements must be deferred until the thrombus is organized, because of the danger of embolism (p. 435). When treatment is begun, it consists of slow, deep effleurage, and rhythmic kneading with hand and fingers; later, of passive movements and careful active movements. The area of the affected vein, especially in Scarpa's triangle, is to be avoided. The treatment, in fact, resembles that for ŒDEMA (*see* p. 440), with precautions as for THROMBOSIS.

VARICOSE VEINS

A condition in which the veins become dilated, lengthened, and tortuous, with incompetent valves. Superficial varicose veins are noticeable through the skin.

CAUSES.—

1. Heredity is sometimes a factor.
2. Occupations necessitating constant standing predispose to this condition. It is often found in nurses, shop assistants, etc. The veins are continually over-extended, because the force of gravity tends to keep the blood in the lower parts of the body. In *walking*, however, the pressure of the muscles on the vessels, and the deepened respiration, cause increased changes of pressure in the thorax which helps venous return, and so prevents this congestion.
3. Anything, therefore, which hinders respiration or limits its range will for the same reason predispose to the disease.
4. Any condition which raises pressure in the abdomen and so impedes the return of blood from the legs, e.g., pregnancy or tumours, will have the same effect; also tight corsets or garters.

PATHOLOGICAL CHANGES.—

1. The saphenous veins are most often affected. The veins of the rectum also suffer (hæmorrhoids).
2. The veins dilate and lengthen, owing to the increased pressure of blood in them. They become twisted and, because of the dilatation, the valves are drawn apart and become incompetent. A vicious circle is set up, the ineffectual valves permitting regurgitation, and the increased amount of blood thus left in the veins still further dilating them and drawing the valve-cusps still farther apart. Thrombosis may occur.
3. The walls of the veins degenerate. The muscular coat atrophies, while the outer coat is hypertrophied.

SYMPTOMS.—The patient complains of *pain, aching*, and *fatigue* in the legs. There may also be *gastrocnemius cramp* if the dilated veins lie deeply among the muscles. The *appearance* of the veins is as described above. There is *congestion* and *œdema* in the limb, due to the engorgement of the dilated veins and the abnormally high pressure in the capillaries, which results in increased exudation of lymph. Owing to faulty nutrition, the musculature becomes weak and the skin is devitalized. Because of the flabbiness of the muscles, they no longer give support to the veins and a vicious circle is thus established.

COMPLICATIONS.—

1. Eczema and varicose ulcers occur in neglected cases. The latter heal slowly or not at all (*see* p. 94). Hæmorrhage may follow rupture of a varicose vein.
2. Thrombosis or phlebitis.

Treatment.—

GENERAL TREATMENT.—

1. REST.—Periods of rest are required, the patient being recumbent with the legs raised. If the patient's occupation necessitates much standing, a change is advisable, if possible.

2. SUPPORT.—When the patient is up, elastic stockings or firm supporting bandages should be worn. The latter are preferred by some authorities, as the pressure from the former may be excessive (Angrove). These should be put on before the patient rises in the morning, and should not be removed until he goes to bed at night.

PHYSICAL TREATMENT.—In any case of venous or lymphatic congestion the principal aim of treatment is *to assist fluid return*. This can best be done by *elevating the limb* so that gravity will assist drainage, by *massage*, and by *movement*.

POSITION OF PATIENT.—Lying or half-lying, with the legs well raised. The bandage is removed in this position, and it should be reapplied before the patient rises. If possible this position should be assumed for about a quarter or half an hour before treatment, so that the effect of gravity may be made use of well before treatment begins. The limb should remain in the elevated position during the whole of the treatment.

MASSAGE.—Rarely does a patient come for treatment for varicose veins alone. More often they have to be taken into account when dealing with other ailments, or with varicose ulcers. The aim, as in phlebitis and thrombosis, is to help the collateral circulation. The manipulations used are: *effleurage, kneading, squeezing kneading*, and *picking up*. Since the aim is to relieve congestion as well as to improve the collateral circulation it is essential *to decongest the proximal drainage channels before any attempt is made to relieve the more distal areas.*

If, for instance, the short saphenous vein is affected, effleurage and kneading should first be given to the thigh, then the anterior tibial group of muscles and the calf. Careful effleurage is permissible alongside, but not over, the dilated vessel. In severe cases it may be better not to treat the lower leg at all.

The author does not personally consider it wise to carry the manipulation *over* affected superficial veins, though massage may be given *above* and *around* them. A varicose vein might quite easily become inflamed, or a thrombus might form, and it does not seem justifiable to risk such an accident.

EXERCISES.—These are perhaps a more satisfactory form of treatment if we are only dealing with varicose veins. Anything which helps venous return will be useful.

1. *Breathing exercises* should be used freely.

2. *Passive movements*, such as Foot-rolling, Knee-bending and -stretching, and Leg-rolling may be given quickly but not too vigorously.

3. *Active movements* for all joints of the lower limb should be practised, in lying or half-lying. Few, if any, exercises should be given in standing. If they are given at all in this position, the patient should wear the bandages while doing them. In slight cases, however, exercises which entail constant use of the muscles of the legs and feet are useful, *but the patient must not stand about between exercises.*

SURGICAL TREATMENT.—*Severe cases*, or those in which it is essential that the patient should be able to continue an occupation involving much standing, may be treated by operation, which consists of removal, or ligature, of the offending veins. Other cases are now treated by certain kinds of injections.

POST-OPERATIVE TREATMENT.—Firm bandages are applied to the leg or legs, and early movement is essential. Vigorous exercises should be given to the foot and ankles, and to the knee and hip. Bandages should be worn during the exercises, to add to the pressure exerted on the veins by the contracting muscles. The patient is usually allowed to walk a short distance on the second or third day after the operation but, again, it is essential that he does not stand about or remain on his feet for long at a time.

EMERGENCY TREATMENT OF A BURST VARICOSE VEIN.—Rupture of a varicose vein may occur as the result of a slight injury, the weakened walls giving way easily; or by the erosion of the wall by an ulcer. The hæmorrhage may be very severe, and measures must be taken to stop it at once. The blood escapes from both the proximal and distal ends of the vein, the incompetent valves being unable to prevent regurgitation.

Should such an accident occur, the patient should be placed in the lying position with the limb well raised. A pressure pad consisting of several thicknesses of gauze or linen should be placed on the wound and bandaged firmly into position. If this does not stop the bleeding, narrow bandages should be applied to the limb, both above and below the site of the injury. The patient should remain in this position until the arrival of the doctor.

Varicose Ulcers
(*See* Chapter V, pp. 94–9)

III. OBSTRUCTION OF LYMPHATICS (ŒDEMA)

All 'swelling' is œdema, since the latter consists of the presence of an excessive amount of lymph in some part of the body. This may arise as the result of an inflammatory process, when slowing or stasis of the blood circulation causes excessive fluid exudation from the capillaries. On the other hand it may arise from obstruction of the lymphatic vessels or glands, the exuded fluid being unable to escape from the part.

Œdema due to venous stasis has been considered in connexion with the special conditions in which it arises. We have now to consider those œdematous states which are due to actual damage to, or interference with, the function of lymphatic vessels or glands. The commonest condition of this kind is the intense œdema of the arm following *radical mastectomy* (amputation of the breast).

ŒDEMA OF THE ARM AFTER REMOVAL OF THE AXILLARY GLANDS IN CASES OF CARCINOMA OF THE BREAST

Carcinoma (cancer) of the breast generally occurs in middle-aged women. It begins in the mammary glands and spreads to the skin, fascia, and muscles in the chest. Later, the lymph-glands themselves may become diseased. Lymphatic spread is rapid, and more remote parts of the body may also become involved.

Treatment.—

SURGICAL TREATMENT.—The operation consists of removal of the mammary gland, with part of the pectoralis major, and of the skin and fascia of the chest. Either to avoid further lymphatic spread of the disease, or because they are already involved, the axillary glands on the affected side are also removed.

POST-OPERATIVE CONDITION.—The removal of the axillary glands destroys most of the channels by which the lymph returns from the arm. There is, therefore, an intense lymphatic congestion which causes the arm to be *œdematous, hard, tender,* and *painful.* The joints are stiff, and movement is difficult. There may also be swelling over the front of the chest and the back of the shoulder. The œdema persists until the lymph has forced new channels for itself through the axilla to the subclavian glands or, if these have also been removed, to the thoracic or right lymphatic duct.

SUPPORT.—Post-operatively, the arm may be kept bandaged to the side, supported on a pillow, or slung in elevation, depending on the views of the surgeon.

PHYSICAL TREATMENT.—The start of this also depends on the surgeon's views. Some allow no physical treatment for 10 to 14 days at least, in order to allow the wound to heal. Others allow gentle massage and movements at once. The aim of treatment is to force on the lymph, thereby relieving congestion in the arm, and assisting in the formation of new drainage paths by raising the pressure in the lymphatic vessels. The methods of treatment are the same, whether it is begun at once or later in convalescence.

POSITION OF PATIENT.—The patient should lie down with the arm in elevation, so that gravity can assist the lymphatic flow. The arm should be comfortably supported by pillows and, as in varicose conditions, it is a good plan for the patient to lie with the arm thus raised for 15 to 20 minutes before treatment.

MASSAGE.—The most important manipulation is *slow, deep effleurage*. This should first be given to the upper part of the arm, so as to empty the lymphatics in that area. The part immediately below this should next be treated, to press the lymph on into the vessels above, after which a return should be made to the upper region. The physiotherapist should continue working on the principle until the whole length of the arm has been treated. *Slow, deep kneadings* and *picking up* may also be given, and *frictions* should be used round the joints. The arm should be considerably reduced in size by the end of the treatment, but the physiotherapist must not be disappointed to find it is as bad as ever next day. Indeed, some degree of residual œdema is inevitable, since a certain amount of organization occurs, but much can be done by physical means to soften the tissues and keep them pliable.

Similar manipulations may also be used if the swelling is present over the patient's chest, back, and side, *provided care is taken not to stretch or damage the wound*, but the effleurage must accurately follow the direction of the lymphatics in these parts.

MOVEMENTS.—*Passive and active movements* should follow the massage, to assist the venous and lymphatic flow and prevent permanent stiffness in the joints. *Abduction, elevation*, and *external rotation* are particularly important. Treatment may well be required for many weeks after the operation.

ELECTRICAL TREATMENT.—*Faradism under pressure* is a valuable method of treatment. The arm should be bandaged with elastic bandages. The active electrode may be applied under the bandage, or the nerve-trunk may be left exposed for stimulation. The bandages restrict the direction of movement of the muscle-fibres, and pressure is therefore exerted on the veins and lymphatic vessels as the muscles contract.

LATER TREATMENT.—As has been said, a certain amount of residual œdema is inevitable, and many patients suffer considerably from this. If organization has occurred, it may be necessary to stretch adhesions in order to regain the movements of the arm. The stretching must be gradual and not too forcible. Care must be taken to see that the active exercises chosen do not produce too violent a drag on the tissues, but at the same time it is necessary to regain full mobility in the shoulder-joint. *If there is the least sign of an increase in swelling or pain, all treatment must cease until the surgeon has seen the patient.* Recurrence of the original trouble is unfortunately not uncommon, even after several years. Medical advice should always be sought before attempting massage in the immediate neighbourhood of the scar.

CHAPTER XX

CONSTITUTIONAL DISEASES

Acute and sub-acute rheumatism—Chronic rheumatism of joints (chronic villous arthritis)—Panniculitis—Rickets—Gout—Diabetes mellitus—Obesity.

ACUTE AND SUB-ACUTE RHEUMATISM
(*Rheumatic Fever*)

THIS condition has no connexion with infective arthritis or rheumatoid arthritis and should not be confused with them, though, from the point of view of physical treatment, it is very similar, and the precautions necessary are the same. It is characterized by *fever* and *arthritis* and the heart is usually involved. There appears to be a connexion between rheumatic fever and chorea.★

AETIOLOGY.—

AGE.—Acute rheumatism is commonest in *children* at the school age, in *adolescents* and *adults* between the ages of 15 and 25 years. In adults the sexes are about equally affected; in young people, girls are more liable to the disease than boys.

THE ACTUAL CAUSE is unknown, but it appears to be connected with streptococcal infection. It is a disease of temperate climates and manifests itself amongst the poor. It is perhaps not so much a constitutional, as an infective disease, but bad housing, over-crowding, and under-nourishment are predisposing causes.

SYMPTOMS.—The onset is gradual, generally beginning with a *sore throat*, followed by a *sudden rise in temperature* (102°–4° in an adult) and *tachycardia* (quickening of pulse-rate). *Pain and swelling in the joints* appear soon after. The temperature then falls gradually, but is liable to rise again suddenly at any stage of the disease. *Relapses*, in fact, are a danger until recovery is complete. Other symptoms are a *raised blood sedimentation-rate, profuse sweating*, sometimes leading to skin eruptions, *pronounced anæmia, leucocytosis, scanty and highly coloured urine*, and *cardiac changes* (pericarditis, myocarditis, or endocarditis). These are most frequent in children.

THE ARTHRITIS OF ACUTE RHEUMATISM

PATHOLOGICAL CHANGES.—The *synovial cavity* of the joint is distended with fluid, and the inflammation often spreads to the tendon sheaths in the neighbourhood. *There is never any tendency to suppuration*, however intense the inflammation. The *fibrous tissues* round the joint are swollen and slightly œdematous. The inflammation may extend to the *muscles* and the *skin* over the joint. "So rapid are the changes in acute rheumatism that a joint which exhibits the most intense inflammation one day may appear perfectly normal next morning."†

SYMPTOMS.—Many joints are involved. *The arthritis develops very rapidly, and subsides with equal suddenness.* It begins in certain joints, and then spreads

---

★ For the connexion of chorea with rheumatism, *see* p. 351.
† M. B. Ray, *Rheumatism in General Practice*.

to others, while the first ones show signs of recovery. It most often affects the larger articulations; as a rule *one or both knees* are first attacked, and shoulders, wrists, ankles, and elbows may suffer in succession. The smaller joints are rarely involved. In appearance the joint is *swollen and œdematous*, and the *skin* over it may be red. In some cases there are multiple pea-like nodules under the skin. The *muscles are tender and painful*. Pain in the joints themselves may be intense, a characteristic feature being that *it flits from joint to joint*. The pain is much increased by movement or jarring, and even the weight of the bedclothes may be unbearable. In severe cases the patient may be quite helpless. There is nearly always some *myocardial involvement*.

In *sub-acute cases* the changes are slower, and fewer joints are involved. The severity of joint changes varies greatly in different cases of acute and sub-acute rheumatism. "There may be no objective signs of inflammation, but merely pain on movement, and the patient may be able to drag himself about" (Ray).

Treatment.—

GENERAL AND MEDICAL TREATMENT.—*The main danger in this disease lies in its effect on the heart and the possibility of valvular disease arising from it.* The patient is kept flat in bed to avoid possible heart complications, or at least to mitigate their severity. Bed-rest may be continued from 6 weeks to 6 months or longer, according to the severity of the illness. Great care has to be taken because of the danger to the heart, and activity must be very gradually resumed. A period of convalescence may be necessary.

The joints may be wrapped in cotton-wool, and sometimes a light splint affords relief. A cradle should be placed under the bedclothes. The patient should lie between blankets because of the excessive sweating. Various liniments may be used and salicylates administered, the chief of which is salicylate of soda, or aspirin. As regards the administration of cortisone, *see* p. 146.

No physical treatment is given at this stage.

SUB-ACUTE RHEUMATISM

As we have seen, this may be a condition in itself, or it may follow the acute stage. Various joints may be involved, and although the infection is no longer active—demonstrated by a completely normal pulse, temperature, and blood sedimentation-rate—they may still show signs of swelling, and the patient may complain of pain and aching.

Treatment.—

GENERAL.—It is essential that the patient's home conditions should be hygienic, and that he should receive nourishing food.

PHYSICAL.—Whether the condition follows the acute stage or is a manifestation in itself, physiotherapy can now be employed. The *aims* of treatment are *to relieve pain* and to *regain mobility and muscle power*.

HEAT AND BATHS.—*Hydrotherapy*, if available, is of great value and various forms of *baths* are employed in treatment. Ideally the patient should have a period of residence at a suitable spa. *Wax baths, radiant heat or infra-red rays*, and *short-wave diathermy* may also be used to advantage.

MASSAGE.—It must be remembered that the condition is a bacterial one, and that the patient may be subject to sudden exacerbations of the illness at any stage of the disease. A more or less quiescent inflammation may suddenly flare up, swelling may increase, and pain become intensified. This may be due to injudicious treatment, some indiscretion on the part of the patient, or some altogether unknown cause, but for this reason physical treatment must be most carefully administered. Massage is rarely used, but if it is, gentle effleurage and kneading only should be given to the muscles of the affected limb. The effleurage may be carried over the affected joint, and the surrounding muscles gently kneaded with hand or fingers. *Frictions should not be given to the joint*—in fact, except for the above-mentioned effleurage, the joint itself should not be touched, though finger-kneading may be given above and below it.

EXERCISES.—

Passive Movements.—Only *relaxed* movements should be given. They must be administered very gently, but *the physiotherapist should aim at putting each joint through one full range of movement daily.* Very careful assisted active movements may also be given.

Free active movements are most important but they require extreme care at first. The patient should practise the movements on his own, increasing the range as improvement takes place. These patients must be content to progress slowly. If the patient is able to walk, he should be given foot-drill in the sitting position (*see* exercises in sitting, pp. 314–15). His footwear should receive attention and, if necessary, transverse arch supports or valgus wedges should be worn (*see* p. 316). Re-education in walking may be required.

ELECTRICAL TREATMENT.—Anodal galvanism or ionization with salicylates or analgesics is sometimes used. Faradism may be used to strengthen muscles at a later stage.

CHRONIC RHEUMATISM OF JOINTS

(*Chronic Villous Arthritis*)

In this condition the peri-articular structures, rather than the actual joint surfaces, are affected. The condition appears most frequently in middle-aged or elderly people, especially as the result of long-continued exposure to cold and damp, and men and women are both affected.

THE ACTUAL CAUSE is probably a toxic one, the toxins being due to the presence of bacteria; or to some derangement of the metabolic processes of the body.

PATHOLOGICAL CHANGES.—

1. The *synovial membrane of the joint is inflamed*, but exudation, though present, is slight.

2. The fibrous tissues round the joint are most affected. There is *inflammation*, and consequent thickening, of the *ligaments*, and also of the *tendons* or *aponeuroses of the muscles* attached close to the joint. There is, however, little or no muscle wasting. The patient not infrequently suffers from fibrositis as well as arthritis. Bony changes are not marked.

SYMPTOMS.—The main features are *pain*, *stiffness*, and sometimes *slight swelling of the joints* with enlargement of surrounding tissues. *Crepitus*, or *creaking* in the joint is noticeable on passive movement. The pain, which is of a dull aching character, is generally worse at night, or when the patient has been at rest for a long time. He is often very sensitive to changes of weather. *Many joints* are affected, but the knees and shoulders most frequently suffer.

CLIMACTERIC ARTHRITIS.—An arthritis of the above type is common in women at or near the time of the menopause.* The onset is gradual, and it chiefly affects the knees. The synovial membrane becomes congested, especially the ligamenta alaria, which protrude on either side of the patella, and later the membrane becomes thickened and fringed, but there is little exudation. The symptoms are similar to those described above. There is some *swelling* and *tenderness at each side of the patella* and over the *internal lateral ligament*, possibly because the patient strains it by walking with everted feet. The swelling may

---

* Some authorities consider, however, that it has no actual connexion with the menopause, as a similar, or identical, arthritis occurs in middle-aged men. (*See* Cyriax, J., *Text-book of Orthopædic Medicine*, I.)

increase later, and the bursæ round the knee become distended. If neglected, bone and cartilage may become involved, and the condition may then have the appearance of a true osteo-arthritis.* The patient may otherwise be in good health. In some, however, there may be signs of thyroid insufficiency—obesity, thinning of hair and eyebrows, etc.

Treatment.—The aims and methods of treatment are very similar to those described in OSTEO-ARTHRITIS, pp. 148–9.

PANNICULITIS

This inflammatory reaction is situated in the subcutaneous tissues—superficial fascia and fat. The disease, though occasionally found in men, is commonest in women at or near the menopause. It is found in connexion with obesity, rheumatism and fibrositis, gout, anæmia or other circulatory disorders, and debility.

THE EXCITING CAUSE may be *chill*, or *strain*. *Infection* may contribute to the condition, or there may be an *endocrine factor*.

PATHOLOGICAL CHANGES.—The nature of the changes is obscure but the areolar tissues undergo hypertrophy. In thin individuals this hypertrophied tissue is fairly evenly distributed, and the skin feels bound down to underlying structures. The deeper layers of the dermis may be affected, in which case the skin becomes very tender. Later small pea-shaped bodies, which can be rolled under the finger, make their appearance. Where more fat is present, the fat itself is liable to become hypertrophied in the vicinity of the inflamed fibrous patches, and small, very tender, fibro-fatty nodules appear.

It is stated in Dr. Copeman's book that "it is generally assumed that it is the collagen or fibrous tissue which is affected in this condition"; Copeman believes, however, that the underlying mechanism of the pain lies in a shift of extracellular body fluid into the fatty tissue cells in these regions, causing pressure on the local nerve-endings from the resulting distension.†

SYMPTOMS.—While this affection may be found in almost any part of the body, it is *most common* in the neck and shoulders, the deltoid region and inner side of the arm, the abdominal wall, the gluteal region and the upper parts of the backs of the thighs, and at the back of the knees. The patients, like those with fibrositis, are generally very sensitive to cold, and sometimes complain of *numbness* or some form of *paræsthesia*. The affected area is *very tender*, and all pressure over it is painful. The symptoms are generally increased during exercise, since the contracting muscles press on the subcutaneous fat and areolar tissue. *Bruising* takes place very easily, and the patient has a feeling of *general stiffness*. *Thickenings* in the superficial tissues are numerous and easily felt. There is *aching* and *pain*, which is sometimes neuralgic in character; if the region of the neck is affected, *headaches* are frequent.

Treatment.—

MEDICAL TREATMENT.—Any septic foci will be removed, or the metabolic disturbance treated. Obesity will be dealt with by means of suitable diet, exercise, or hormones. It is important to promote skin activity.

PHYSICAL TREATMENT.—The treatment is much like that for fibrositis, except that the massage need not, and, indeed, often cannot, be given so deeply.

HEAT may, or may not, be effective, and some authorities consider it harmful.

---

* Or occasionally of the *rheumatoid* type of arthritis.
† W. S. C. Copeman, *Textbook of the Rheumatic Diseases*, Chapter XV. For another view, *see* J. Cyriax, *Text-book of Orthopædic Medicine*, 18, 501.

RICKETS

(Rachitis)

Rickets is a disease of disordered calcium metabolism occurring in infants and young children, the most characteristic changes taking place in the bones. It was at one time a very common disease amongst the poor, but with the improvements in social conditions and standards it is fortunately rare now.

AETIOLOGY.—

AGE.—The disease generally appears between the ages of six months and two years. 'Late rickets', occurring at puberty, may be a recurrence of slight infantile rickets, or it may start at this period.

CAUSE.—The disease *is due to a deficiency of vitamin D*, a substance found in some, but not all, of the same articles of food as vitamin A. For instance, both vitamins are found in cod-liver oil, but many fats which are rich in vitamin A contain little vitamin D, e.g., cow's milk. The chief action of vitamin D is to bring about the absorption of calcium from the intestine and *without this vitamin, the calcium salts and phosphates in the body*—which are not themselves necessarily deficient—*cannot be used to produce ossification of the bones. An ill-balanced diet,* especially one containing an excess of carbohydrates and a deficiency of fats, *aggravates the condition.* An excess of cereals is especially injurious, because cereals provide calories which cause the child to grow quickly but the calcification of the skeleton is unable to keep pace with this growth. Cereals, moreover, contain an acid which *decreases* the absorption of calcium in the intestine.

PATHOLOGICAL CHANGES.*—The most marked changes are found in the bones, the process of ossification being delayed and irregular.

In a normal bone, the process of ossification begins from one or more centres, and spreads outwards from these in a regular manner. In the case of a long bone, e.g., the humerus, the first centre to appear—early in fœtal life—is in the middle of the diaphysis (i.e., the shaft). The centres in the epiphyses make their appearance much later. If such a bone were examined microscopically, it would be found to consist of regular zones, each at a different stage of development. Next the centre would be a ring of true bone, clearly marked off from the zone beyond, where calcification would be far less advanced; then there would be a zone where there was merely a re-arrangement of cartilage cells preparatory to ossification, and beyond this, again, an area of unchanged cartilage.

In the rickety bone the ossification is irregular, the zones no longer being marked off from each other. Small portions of ossifying bone are found among the cartilaginous parts, and groups of cartilage cells in the bony layer. Moreover, the deposit of calcium and phosphates is insufficient and the bone remains too soft. It does eventually harden when the acute stage of the disease is over, and it then becomes very hard and ivory-like. The increase in length is arrested for a time, while the disease is active, so that the bone never grows as long as it should have been, while growth beneath the periosteum is excessive, making it abnormally thick. The changes are very marked at the epiphysial junction, which is swollen, hyperæmic, and increased in thickness. This condition is often very noticeable in such situations as the wrists and ankles.

SYMPTOMS.—*Sweating of the head* and throwing off the bedclothes at night are usual symptoms. The child has a slight *fever*, and sometimes cries from discomfort or pain when handled, though tenderness is not always marked. He is generally *pale* and may be *thin and wasted*, or *fat and flabby*. The *muscles* suffer as well as the bones, and are *hypotonic, weak*, and *badly developed*. The

---

* The student is advised to revise carefully the process of normal ossification.

nerves are usually *hyperexcitable*. The patient does not learn to walk until long after the normal time, or ceases to do so if he has already begun.

The general health suffers, and the child is subject to such complications as bronchitis, catarrh, or convulsions. *The abdomen is distended and prominent*, partly because the spleen and liver are enlarged, partly from flatulence. The patient often suffers from constipation or diarrhœa. *The teeth appear late* and are generally defective. Ossification of the bones of the skull is much delayed, and the sutures are late in uniting. The fontanelles, especially the anterior one, do not close until long past the normal period.

Bending of the long bones takes place, and *deformities* tend to develop.

THE DEFORMITIES OF RICKETS.—These are due partly to muscular and ligamentous weakness, and partly to the softness of the bones.

1. THE SKULL.—

The flat bones of the cranium, especially the frontal and parietal bones, are much thickened, so that the head becomes square in shape, and appears abnormally large. This is the more noticeable because this over-development does not take place in the bones of the face, which appears very small in comparison to the vault of the cranium.

2. THE SPINE.—The most common deformity is *kyphosis*, consisting at first of one long curve backward, involving both the thoracic and the lumbar region. Later, when the child walks, a lumbar lordosis may develop, owing to the prominent abdomen with its weak muscular wall.

3. THE THORAX.—Alterations in the shape of the thorax are marked because the ribs are very soft (*Fig.* 185). The following are the most usual:—

a. Pigeon Breast.—The thorax is compressed at the sides, and is therefore elongated from before backwards; its posterior aspect is flattened, and the sternum is thrust forward.

b. Vertical Grooves.—These are found on either side of the sternum, where the ribs are joined to their costal cartilages, and also at the mid-axillary lines, where they are farthest from their fixed points.

c. Harrison's Sulcus.—This is a transverse groove found along the insertion of the diagram, caused by the pull of the diaphragm on the softened ribs.

d. The ' Rickety Rosary'.—This consists of bony enlargement at the junction of the ribs with the cartilages—at which point growth is very active at the age when rickets occurs. The overall effect is that of a chain of beads.

4. THE LOWER EXTREMITIES.—Besides shortening of the bones and consequent dwarfing of the patient, almost any kind of distortion may take place, e.g., coxa vara, genu varum or valgum, bow-legs or forward curving of the tibiæ, flat-foot (talipes vulgus), etc.

5. THE UPPER EXTREMITIES.—Deformities of the upper limbs are uncommon, and only occur if the child puts weight on his arms in crawling.

6. THE PELVIS.—The pressure of the femoral heads, as well as other factors, tends to decrease the size of the true pelvis. This may have serious consequences in women, with regard to pregnancy and childbirth.

PROGNOSIS.—In untreated cases the disease may go on for several years, the child generally beginning to walk during its third year, at which time the deformities of the lower extremities develop. These, and other deformities, tend to spontaneous improvement as he grows, but traces always remain, and the child's growth is stunted if the rickets has been severe. Respiratory infections and gastro-intestinal troubles are the most common complication of rickets. Anæmia may also be a feature.

Treatment.—

PRINCIPLES OF TREATMENT.—The primary aim of all forms of treatment is *to restore normal calcium metabolism*. As we have seen rickets is not caused so much by an actual calcium lack as by a deficiency of vitamin D, which prevents the absorption of calcium and phosphates from the gastro-intestinal tract. It is essential, therefore, *to make good the vitamin-D deficiency.* By doing this a major part of the battle is won, but it may also be necessary to improve the general health, muscle strength, and posture, and to correct any deformities which may exist.

GENERAL AND MEDICAL TREATMENT.—

The *diet* is all-important. Since the deficiency of vitamin D is at the root of the trouble, measures must be taken to see this is made good. For infants, the food will be chiefly milk, and it is important that this should be of the best quality. If the baby is still being nursed by its mother, attention to her food is necessary. In older children, the diet should contain plenty of protein and

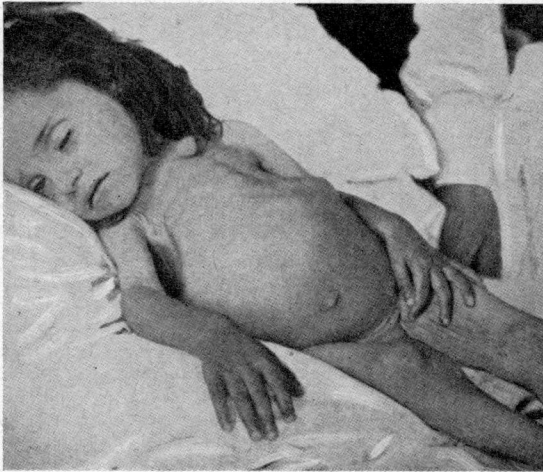

Fig. 185.—Rickets. Severe deformities of chest, clavicle, and long bones.

fat, and the amount of starchy food should be restricted. There must also be a proper supply of the other vitamins—A, B, and C. Cod-liver oil, or halibut-liver oil, will be ordered for the child, as these are rich in vitamins D and A. Ergosterol, which has been subjected to the action of ultra-violet rays, is also used in treatment. Ergosterol, besides being present in the human body (*see below*), is obtainable from yeast, ergot of rye, etc. Calcium will also be administered if required. Besides attention to diet the patient should spend as much time as possible in fresh air and sunlight.

PHYSICAL TREATMENT.—Much can be done by ultra-violet irradiation to make good the vitamin-D deficiency. Sebum contains two substances of great importance here—ergosterol and an impurity, cholesterol. The latter, when irradiated with ultra-violet rays, is changed into vitamin D. Thus *ultra-violet irradiation is one of the most important forms of treatment.* Today one rarely sees a case of rickets, and even in such as do occur one does not meet the frightful deformities of former days, but it may be necessary to take steps to prevent deformity pending improvement in ossification of the bone, and to improve muscle tone and strength.

ULTRA-VIOLET IRRADIATION.—The rays in natural sunlight which bring about the formation of vitamin D are those with wave-lengths between 3300 Å and 2900 Å (the antirachitic band). The whole body is exposed to the rays of the lamp, a general technique being used, the dosage being suberythemal. The carbon arc lamp is preferable to the mercury vapour arc since it more nearly resembles the spectrum of sunlight. The treatment is given about three times a week, and usually continues for about two months.* Further courses may be required at intervals.

BREATHING EXERCISES.—These are important and should be taught from the beginning if the child is of a suitable age, in order to prevent thoracic deformity and to increase the intake of oxygen, thereby improving general health and reducing the risk of chest infections. Inspiration is especially important.

ACTIVE MOVEMENTS.—These should also be practised. Movements of the limbs should be given if, or when, the child is able to understand what is required of him. To begin with they should be given without weight being taken on the limbs. They will, of course, be free movements, and, in small children, can be given in the form of play.

Because of improved conditions and better knowledge of the subject and its treatment it is unlikely that the modern physiotherapist will meet a severe case of rickets but if deformities are likely proper support must be afforded to the bones while they are still soft, as a prophylactic measure.

GOUT

Gout is a disorder of metabolism, due to the presence of an excess of uric acid and other purine bodies in the blood. It chiefly affects the joints, but often produces other constitutional disturbances as well. It may be *acute* or *chronic*. It is most frequent in men over the age of 40 years.

PATHOLOGY.—It is not necessary to go in detail into this very difficult subject. The actual cause of gout is, as stated above, an excess of purine bodies, among which is uric acid. Purine bodies result from the breaking down *of nucleins,* complex chemical substances containing protein, phosphorus, etc. These nucleins may be forming part of the tissues of the body itself, or may be taken in in the food. In either case, they may be broken down to form uric acid and other purine bodies and for some reason certain people cannot easily get rid of these purine bodies (Osler).†

The Joints are chiefly affected, the metatarsophalangeal joint of the big toe suffering most frequently and most acutely. A deposit of biurate of soda takes place, affecting first the articular cartilage, then the synovial membrane and the ligaments. The changes are similar to those of arthritis—erosion and final destruction of the cartilages, thickening of the membranes, and enlargement of the bone-ends round their articular surfaces. The deposits also appear in the structures round the joints, forming small hard nodules known as 'chalk-stones' or 'tophi'. They are common in the hands at the metacarpophalangeal joints, and in this position may actually work their way out through the skin. They are sometimes found also in the ear-lobes or in other cartilaginous structures in the body. *The Kidneys* may contain similar deposits, causing inflammation (nephritis), and *arteriosclerosis* is often associated with gout. This puts a strain on the heart, and may cause *myocarditis*.

---

* E. H. and W. K. Russell, *Ultra-Violet Radiation and Actinotherapy.* It must be realized, however, that authorities differ a good deal as to the exact times and methods of exposure in this and other conditions.

† "The uric acid and purine bodies circulate in the blood in an abnormal form, and the kidney is unable to separate and eliminate uric acid from this combination. Uric acid salts consequently accumulate in the blood."—H. L. Tidy, *Synopsis of Medicine.*

SYMPTOMS.—Gout may manifest itself in various forms. It may chiefly affect the joints, as described above, or it may cause symptoms quite unconnected with the joints, e.g., cerebral, cardiac, gastric, etc. The acute attack is often heralded by *twinges of pain* in the joints of hands or feet, by *an attack of dyspepsia*, or by *restlessness* and *irritability*. The attack itself generally begins at night, with agonizing pain in the big toe which is acutely inflamed, hot, red, and very tender. The skin is shining in appearance and rapid swelling takes place, sometimes extending upwards over the foot. The patient's temperature rises to about 103°. The pain decreases towards morning only to return the next night. This may go on for a week or more, the patient being comparatively free from pain during the day, but always worse at night. The patient should refrain from alcohol and rich foods, and should drink water freely. The doctor will prescribe the medical treatment, the drug most commonly used being colchicum.

PHYSICAL TREATMENT.—It is only very rarely, if at all, that these cases are sent for treatment, and during the crises of acute pain nothing can be done, as the patient cannot bear to be touched. *Lithium ionization* may sometimes be requested between attacks. Lithium forms a *soluble lithium urate* in place of *insoluble sodium urate*.

DIABETES MELLITUS

Diabetes is a disease of metabolism characterized by the presence of an abnormal amount of sugar in the blood, and by its excretion in the urine. It is due to a deficiency of the internal secretion of the 'Islets of Langerhans', to which the name of *insulin* has been given. It is produced in the pancreas. It is very unlikely that any physiotherapist would now be required to treat a case of diabetes *as such*, but diabetics, as well as other people, are subject to accidents or intercurrent diseases and the physiotherapist should, therefore, understand something of the condition.

AETIOLOGY.—

Diabetes is generally a disease of middle life, appearing between the ages of 40 and 60 years but an acute form occurs in children. In middle life women are more often affected than men.

PHYSIOLOGY: CARBOHYDRATE METABOLISM.—In studying this subject we have to take into consideration the activities of three of the endocrine glands.

1. THE PANCREAS.—As well as its external secretion the pancreatic juice, this organ secretes *insulin* which is one of the prime factors in the regulation of blood-sugar, converting it into glycogen which is capable of being stored.

2. THE PITUITARY BODY.—The secretions of this gland, particularly those of its *anterior lobe*, act in an antagonistic manner to that of the pancreas and *inhibit* the storing of sugar in the tissues. If these hormones are deficient, the individual is able to ingest abnormally large amounts of sugar without its appearing in the blood or in the urine. *If insulin is absent, the action of the pituitary secretion is unopposed*.

3. THE ADRENALS (suprarenal glands), the medulla of which secretes the substance called *adrenaline*. Among other functions, this hormone has that of converting glycogen stored in the liver into glucose. *It also depresses the action of insulin*.

In diabetes there is no doubt that the trouble is due primarily to disease or exhaustion of the cells of the islets of Langerhans. Glucose is not converted into glycogen, nor can it be burned up in the tissues, and it consequently remains in the blood in large quantities. Its excretion in the urine is Nature's attempt to get rid of a substance which, necessary and valuable in its proper quantity, is a deadly poison when in excess.

15

This disorder of carbohydrate metabolism leads, moreover, to disorder of the metabolism of *fats*, which cannot be fully oxidized in the tissues in the absence of carbohydrates. Hence certain acids are formed, the products of incomplete oxidation, which appear in the blood and urine causing *acidosis*. This may produce very serious symptoms such as *diabetic coma*, which is a very serious condition which may end in death.

With proper diet and treatment these patients can live an active, normal life. The administration of insulin is now the feature in the medical treatment. It is given by means of injections, since if taken by the mouth it is destroyed by pepsin and trypsin, and so never reaches the blood-stream.

OBESITY

"In present-day Britain obesity is more common, and gives rise to more ill-health, than any other nutritional disorder." (Davidson.) There are various types of obesity but that with which we are most concerned is caused by *excess of food, insufficient exercise,* or both. It may occur at any age, but is commonest in middle-aged people, both men and women, who have begun to lead a less active life than they have done hitherto and have not modified their diet accordingly.

SYMPTOMS AND COMPLICATIONS.—These patients suffer from a feeling of weight and heaviness, and become fatigued on slight exertion. They feel the heat very much, perspire profusely, and easily become breathless. The condition may be complicated by panniculitis, a weak heart, varicose veins, or other cardio-vascular diseases. The increased weight may lead to arthritis of hips or knees, and to flat-foot.

Treatment.—

GENERAL TREATMENT.—The *diet* should be prescribed by the patient's physician, and will vary according to his ideas and the patient's general condition. Broadly speaking all starchy foods, sugars, and fats are reduced, and some are forbidden. Protein is allowed freely and the patient is usually required to drink a lot of water, hot or cold, especially about half an hour before meals. The patient *must* obey the doctor's instructions as to diet, otherwise treatment will be useless. Many authorities consider that regulation of the diet is the only useful form of treatment and that exercise (or exercises) makes little difference. Others consider physical treatment to be a useful adjunct to dietary or medical measures. In any case, the patient *must* be prepared to render strict obedience to the diet. The patient should be weighed at least once a week, so that progress can be gauged.

PHYSICAL TREATMENT.—It was the custom in the past to rely very much on massage for the treatment of obesity. All too often the result was an exhausted masseuse, and a patient who lost weight very slowly if at all. It has been said that over the door of every physiotherapy department should be written: "We cure nobody here; we help people to cure themselves." In no condition is this more applicable than in that of obesity; the patient *must* help herself, or the work of the physiotherapist will be wasted. Many a patient would prefer 'having massage' to exerting herself or restricting her diet, but it can be stated categorically that massage (particularly general massage) is neither necessary nor desirable for this type of patient.

EXERCISES.—Three points have to be considered:—

1. The patient's need of oxygen to assist in the combustion of the body-fats.

2. The necessity of vigorous muscular work to set free energy and break down the fat. Static work should be avoided. It is of no value to the patient and only produces fatigue.

3. The extra weight the patient has to carry and the possibility of straining the heart.

With regard to the first point, it is obvious that *breathing exercises* must figure prominently in the treatment. They should be given at the beginning and the end of the table, and several times during its course. Any deep breathing exercises are useful and diaphragmatic breathing assists in obtaining full expansion of the lungs, and also increase the work of the abdominal muscles. If the patient is inclined to become breathless during the scheme several deep breaths should be taken between each exercise.

As regards the second and third points, it should be realized that a large amount of exercise is necessary to obtain any considerable reduction in weight, and this is generally beyond what the patient is willing, or indeed able, to manage. She must, however, be prepared to do the best she can. A table of *home exercises* must be given and these *must* be performed faithfully and regularly.

The actual exercises must be vigorous, but not too numerous, especially at the beginning of the course. Resisted exercises may be given if desired, but we have to remember that the extra weight of the patient's body and limbs does constitute a resistance in itself, and, moreover, that the muscles may be weak and hampered by fatty deposits between their fibres.

CHAPTER XXI

ABDOMINAL AND PELVIC CONDITIONS

I. Abdominal conditions: Chronic gastritis—Dilated stomach—Gastric and duodenal ulcer—
Appendicitis—Inguinal hernia. II. Pelvic conditions/Inflammatory conditions—Pregnancy
and the puerperium—Prolapsed uterus.

I. ABDOMINAL CONDITIONS

THE general conditions described in this chapter are mostly met with post-operatively, and physical treatment is rarely required for the conditions themselves. At one time abdominal massage was considered beneficial but is now thought to have little or no effect.

CHRONIC GASTRITIS

Chronic inflammation of the stomach, of which *faulty habits or unsuitable food* are the principal causes, but it may also be associated with cancer of the stomach.

The mucous membrane of the stomach becomes irritated and inflamed. It becomes hyperæmic, and there is an excessive secretion of mucus which blocks up the mouths of the tubular glands which secrete the gastric juice. The *cardiac* glands, which produce not only pepsin but hydrochloric acid, are mainly affected. At a later stage ulceration may occur. Finally, the whole mucous membrane may be destroyed.

Treatment.—

Physical Treatment is only required in ulcerative, or malignant, conditions for which an operation has been performed. Routine post-operative treatment is then given (*see* p. 453).

DILATED STOMACH

This is a rare but dangerous condition which sometimes follows abdominal operations but is mainly caused by obstruction of the pylorus by ulcers, tumours, etc. Food does not leave the stomach, and fermentation therefore takes place, resulting in the formation of gases which give rise to gross abdominal distension. Large quantities of liquid and undigested food are vomited, and the patient may collapse.

Treatment.—

SURGICAL TREATMENT.—The stomach must be left free of food. A Ryles tube is passed and the stomach emptied by continuous suction. Nothing may be taken by mouth, so rectal or intravenous drip feeding will be employed. If the cause is an obstruction surgical measures will be undertaken.

PHYSICAL TREATMENT.—Routine post-operative treatment will be given, breathing, foot, and leg exercises being of the utmost importance in the early days. Later a progressive scheme of exercises may be given.

GASTRIC AND DUODENAL ULCER

Gastric ulcers are most common in young women between the ages of 15 and 25. *Duodenal ulcers* are commoner in men, and occur at a later age, generally between 30 and 50. The exact cause is unknown but, since the ulcers only occur in areas in which gastric juices are present, it is probable that the mucous membrane is in an unhealthy or weakened condition, and that this is aggravated by the acid gastric juice. The gastric ulcer is generally situated at the pyloric end of the stomach, or on the lesser curvature. As it heals, the scar tissue may shrink to such an extent as to cause serious deformity of the organ ('hour-glass stomach'), which may bring about obstruction. Other dangers are *hæmatemesis*, or *perforation* of the ulcer leading to *peritonitis*.

SYMPTOMS.—The onset may be insidious or the condition may assume a serious form without any very marked early symptoms—perforation or hæmorrhage being the first definite signs. The following are the most common symptoms:—

GASTRIC ULCER.—

1. *Pain*, in the epigastric region, coming on immediately after a meal. This is because the ingestion of food causes an outpouring of gastric juice, the acid of which irritates the ulcer.

2. *Vomiting* after food. This generally relieves the pain. Because of the pain which results the patient may be afraid to take food, although the appetite is usually good.

3. *Hæmatemesis.*—The vomited blood may be dark in colour (i.e., typical of hæmorrhage from the stomach) but this is not always so as vomiting may occur before blood has been changed by the action of the gastric juice, or mixed with food particles.

DUODENAL ULCER.—

1. The *pain* in this case is in the right hypochondriac region, and *comes on two to four hours after food*, that is, when the acid chyme begins to pass from the stomach into the duodenum. It is relieved by eating, as the taking of food reduces the acidity of the stomach content and the pyloric sphincter remains closed.

2. Hæmatemesis is not common, but there may be *passage of blood from the bowel* (melæna).

PERFORATION.—There is a sudden attack of intense pain, the abdominal muscles go into spasm, and the patient becomes faint and exhibits signs of shock. The patient must be admitted to hospital at once.

HÆMATEMESIS (First-aid).—Should an attack take place without warning, the physiotherapist should lie the patient down at once, with the head and trunk well raised. No attempt should be made to move the patient before the arrival of the doctor. The windows should be opened, and the patient's clothing loosened, but he should be disturbed as little as possible. *Nothing should be given by the mouth.*

Treatment.—

SURGICAL TREATMENT.—*Partial gastrectomy* is usually performed. This consists of removal of that part of the stomach in which the ulcer is situated, but in some cases *total gastrectomy* may have to be undertaken.

PHYSICAL TREATMENT, other than post-operative treatment, is contra-indicated in these cases.

PRE-OPERATIVE TREATMENT.—This should be given whenever possible, in order to acquaint the patient with his physiotherapist and the post-operative routine (*see* Chapter XXII).

POST-OPERATIVE TREATMENT.*—This is usually begun 24 hours after the operation. *Breathing exercises* are given in crook-half-lying. The patient must be encouraged to cough, and as he does so the physiotherapist should support the wound by placing her hand over it. Vibration and gentle clapping may be given to assist expectoration. Foot movements are important since they help to keep

---

* For rationale, *see* Chapter XXII.

the circulation active, and to prevent thrombosis. They should be performed vigorously and resistance may be given if desired. If the patient is having a blood transfusion or saline drip the apparatus must not be disturbed.

From the second day onwards the treatment is gradually advanced. Leg, arm, and trunk movements are added, and after a few days the patient is usually allowed out of bed for a gradually lengthening period. If all goes well the patient should leave hospital in about 3 weeks.

COLLAPSE OF THE LUNG.—Should this occur as the result of blockage of the bronchioles by mucus, *postural drainage* with *percussion* must be carried out as described for post-operative lobectomy cases. The treatment should not continue for more than 5–10 minutes, but may be given several times a day. The patient must try to expand the affected part by breathing exercises.

Similar surgical treatment is carried out in the case of a duodenal ulcer. but it is usual to by-pass the duodenum by suturing the stomach to the jejunum. *Physical treatment* is carried out in the same way as for partial gastrectomy.

APPENDICITIS

Inflammation of the vermiform appendix caused by bacterial infection is most common in young people, especially in those under the age of 20.

PATHOLOGICAL CHANGES.—The disease may be acute or chronic. It may consist simply of inflammation of the appendix, or may go on to ulceration or even gangrene of that organ. In the ulcerative form there is danger of perforation, and if this occurs it may infect the peritoneum and set up *peritonitis*. In the chronic form the appendix becomes bound down by adhesions to the surrounding intestines (ileum and cæcum) and this may result in *obstruction*.

SYMPTOMS.—The symptoms of the attack consist of: *severe pain*, first right across the front of the abdomen and later in the region of the appendix itself; *fever* (100°–102°); *furred tongue, constipation*, and *vomiting*. Slight cases may recover completely in a short time, but the attack is liable to recur.

Treatment.—

SURGICAL TREATMENT.—Appendicectomy is now the recognized form of treatment, since even a mild type of appendicitis may become dangerous at any time, and recurrence is the rule. In serious cases the patient's life may depend on early operation. If perforation occurs and peritonitis sets in the chances of recovery may be small. The operation is generally performed within thirty-six hours or so of the onset in acute cases.

PHYSICAL TREATMENT.—Pre- and post-operative treatment should be given as described for GASTRECTOMY. *Abdominal exercises* should be included in the post-operative treatment, both to *assist the passage of the intestinal contents*, especially in the region of the cæcum and ascending colon, and to *strengthen the abdominal muscles*. The weakness of the abdominal wall in the area of the incision must, of course, be taken into consideration. *For the first few days*, while the wound is still unhealed, gentle abdominal contractions only are permissible but as the wound heals gentle abdominal exercises may be added. Crook-half-lying and Crook-lying are the most suitable starting positions. Stretching of the right side of the abdomen should be avoided for some time. Arch positions and exercises which entail very strong static contractions of the abdominal muscles should be avoided. If the patient suffers from flatulence it may sometimes be relieved by stroking and kneading of the colon, particularly the descending portion. If massage is given to the ascending colon great care must be taken to avoid any drag or pull in the region of the scar.

TREATMENT OF THE SCAR.—If the scar becomes adherent to the deeper tissues, *gentle frictions* may be given around it once healing has occurred, the movement being towards the scar. It may also be held between the physiotherapist's fingers while the patient contracts the abdominal wall. In this way it can sometimes be freed from the underlying tissues.

INGUINAL HERNIA

In this condition some of the contents of the peritoneum protrude through the abdominal wall in the inguinal region. Herniation occurs more frequently in men than in women. The descent of the testes, and the position of the spermatic cord in the inguinal canal, predisposes to weakness of the abdominal wall in the inguinal region. Inguinal herniæ are almost always due to a congenital defect or weakness, although they are often not apparent until later in life, the condition being aggravated by weakness of the abdominal wall.

VARIETIES.—Inguinal hernia may be direct or indirect.

Direct.—This takes the form of protrusion of peritoneum through the posterior wall of the inguinal canal. It is due to defective musculature.

Indirect.—This is due to the persistence of the *Processus vaginalis*, the embryonic pouch of peritoneum which precedes the descent of the testes. Normally this closes before birth, but if it fails to do so it forms a congenital sac into which the abdominal contents may fall.

SYMPTOMS.—These consist mainly of discomfort. The hernia can be felt and the protrusion is increased during activities which strain the abdominal wall.

Treatment.—

GENERAL AND MEDICAL TREATMENT.—The patient must avoid heavy lifting and strenuous activities which strain the abdominal wall. In slight cases a truss may be worn, the object being to retain the hernia and force it back into position.

SURGICAL TREATMENT.—

Indirect herniation may be repaired by removal of the peritoneal sac.

Direct herniation requires repair of the inguinal sac. This may be done by means of *a nylon darn* uniting the conjoint tendon to the inguinal ligament behind the spermatic cord, *by fascial strips* to strengthen the weakened tissue, or *by taking a flap from the rectus sheath* to close the gap.

PHYSICAL TREATMENT.—In all cases intensive abdominal exercises are required. Pre- and post-operative treatment is given as for appendicitis, special attention being paid to the abdominal muscles.

OTHER VARIETIES OF HERNIA.—Herniation may sometimes occur through the femoral ring (*femoral hernia*), or the umbilicus (*umbilical hernia*). The latter requires repair similar to that used for inguinal hernia. Umbilical hernia may be congenital, in which case it usually reduces as the infant develops, or due to divarication of the recti following parturition. Surgical repair is necessary. The principles of pre- and post-operative physiotherapy are the same in all cases.

II. PELVIC CONDITIONS

INFLAMMATORY CONDITIONS
(*Salpingitis and Pelvic Abscess*)

The two most common inflammatory conditions met in physiotherapy are *Salpingitis* (inflammation of the Fallopian tubes), and *Pelvic Abscess*. The latter may arise from salpingitis, or may exist on its own. The former may be acute or chronic.

CAUSE.—Infection may result from unhygienic habits, or may follow parturition or abortion. In some cases it is gonococcal.

PATHOLOGY.—The usual inflammatory reaction follows infection, the mucous membrane becoming hyperæmic and swollen. In the case of salpingitis the neighbouring ovarian fimbria may become closed by adhesions. Pus may then collect in the enclosed area and an abscess form.

SYMPTOMS.—There is *pain* and acute tenderness in the region of the pelvis. *The temperature is raised* and may be of the swinging variety. *Amenorrhœa, dysmenorrhœa,* or *menorrhagia* may occur. There is usually a *vaginal discharge* which may or may not be purulent.

Complications.—Adhesions may form which give rise to chronic pain and disturbance in menstruation.

Peritonitis may result from rupture of an abscess and may lead to *septicæmia.*

Treatment.—

GENERAL AND MEDICAL.—Rest and scrupulous attention to hygiene are essential. Antibiotics will be administered.

PHYSICAL TREATMENT.—In the acute stage the aims are *to control infection, to relieve congestion and pain,* and *to prevent the formation of adhesions* in so far as this may be possible.

In chronic cases it may be possible to soften the thickened tissues by improving the circulation.

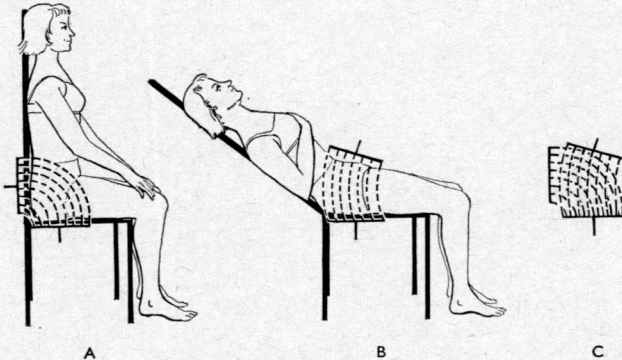

Fig. 186.—Short-wave diathermy using the cross-fire method. A, Patient in first position; B, Patient in second position; C, Diagrammatic representation of field showing concentration of heat on the pelvic organs.

ELECTRICAL TREATMENT.—In the acute stage *short-wave diathermy* may be given twice, or thrice, daily. The cross-fire method of application is the one of choice, as this ensures thorough treatment of the pelvic organs (*Fig.* 186). The treatment is divided into two halves. During the first half the patient sits over an electrode with another over the sacral region: during the second half the patient lies back and the sacral electrode is placed over the abdomen (*Fig.* 186). The dosage should be subthermal, or just thermal. The treatment may usually be given for 5 minutes each way to begin with. The dosage is gradually progressed to 10 minutes each way. Soiled dressings should be discarded before treatment and a clean dry one applied.

Ultra-violet irradiation may also be given. If the patient's health is poor a sectional technique should be employed, otherwise general treatment can be given.

Chronic cases are treated in a similar manner, but short-wave diathermy need not be given more than three times a week and the dosage can be stronger.

PREGNANCY AND THE PUERPERIUM

This is a most important subject from the point of view of the physiotherapist. While it is true that pregnancy and childbirth are physiological and not pathological conditions, it is also true that during the former period many inconveniences arise among women of the civilized races which are not found, or are found to a much lesser extent, among savage or less advanced peoples. Also, after the birth of the child, ill health may supervene because of a weak and stretched abdominal wall or pelvic floor. Much can be done, by means of pre- and post-natal physiotherapy, to overcome these difficulties.

PHYSIOLOGY.—

When the developing ovum reaches the uterus it embeds itself in the mucous membrane of its wall. The fœtus then becomes surrounded by a sac filled with fluid, and is nourished by the maternal blood through a body called the placenta. The placenta is formed partly from these membranes forming the sac, and partly from the tissues of the uterine wall. Meanwhile, the uterus enlarges to hold the growing fœtus, and its muscular wall becomes hypertrophied. For the first three months it still lies within the pelvis. At the end of the third month it rises above the pelvic brim, and at the end of the fifth and sixth months it is, respectively, just below and just above the umbilicus. It gradually reaches its highest level, that of the ensiform appendix, at about eight and a half months. Meanwhile, the vagina becomes softened, and the ligaments of the pelvic joints (sacro-iliac and pubic) become slightly stretched. The breasts enlarge and increase in weight.

2. LABOUR.—Reflexes arise within the uterine muscle, which set up contractions in the muscular walls of the organ. In time the vagina dilates, and the child passes down it and is expelled, together with its covering membranes and the placenta.

3. THE PUERPERIUM.—This is the period following the birth of a child, during which the organs gradually return to their normal condition. The function of *lactation* also becomes established.

Involution of the Uterus.—After delivery, the uterus reaches to about the level of the umbilicus, and weighs about 2 lb. Its upper part (fundus) is tightly contracted, and this contraction of the muscular fibres renders the uterus anæmic, less blood being able to pass into it. This brings about a rapid disappearance of the excess muscular tissue developed during pregnancy, the hypertrophied muscle-fibres returning to their normal size. In the first few days after delivery the process takes place very rapidly, but after this it continues more slowly, because the uterus becomes more relaxed and the blood can circulate more freely through it. The level of the fundus diminishes by about three-quarters of an inch daily, and it disappears below the pelvic brim in 10 days or less. At the same time, the mucous lining of the organ is renewed, the dead tissue being thrown off. During this process, a discharge known as the 'lochia' takes place. It ceases in about a fortnight.

Meanwhile, the other stretched structures, the peritoneum and the muscles of the abdominal wall and pelvic floor, are gradually returning to their normal condition. The recovery of the muscles may not, however, be complete, in which case they remain stretched and weakened.

Lactation.—The mammary glands consist of a number of lobes divided into lobules. Each lobe has a duct which ends in a small opening at the nipple. The milk is secreted by the cells of the lobules, and passes along the ducts to the nipple. The secretion of true milk does not begin for two or three days after the birth of the child, but during pregnancy, and for these first few days after delivery, a yellowish fluid called 'colostrum' can be obtained. The stimulus to the secretion of milk is the suction on, and emptying of, the breast by the baby.

Physical Treatment.—Physiotherapy has an important part in ante- and post-natal cases.

ANTENATAL TREATMENT.—

Many of the much-vaunted "difficult labours" of which our mothers and grandmothers were so proud, were needlessly occasioned by fear and ignorance, which prevented the mother from relaxing and co-operating with the medical staff concerned in her delivery. Today much light has been shed on the subject and the dark days of hushed voices and hints of travail are mercifully over. However, far too many women still face their first pregnancy in ignorance and fear, and there are still helpful friends and relatives who rush to tell the expectant mother of the "terrible time" they had.

Much help is now given pre-natally by lectures, discussion groups, etc., held in the maternity departments of our hospitals, and the importance of physical training is widely recognized.

AIMS OF PHYSICAL TREATMENT.—It is important that the mother should look forward to the actual birth of her child and recognize it for what it is—a hard physical feat requiring much muscular effort. The *aims* of physical treatment are twofold:—

(1) *To assist in establishing a healthy psychological approach to the birth.* (2) To *teach the patient to relax* in order that she may really rest between uterine contractions and thus conserve her energy.

The Psychological Aspect.—This is largely in the hands of the medical and nursing staff. It may, however, be the task of the physiotherapist to instruct the patients in the elementary physiology of labour. She should therefore be thoroughly conversant with this, and should in any case explain to the mothers the importance of relaxation, and the reason for the exercise. She should also be prepared to answer simple questions the mothers may ask.

Relaxation.—The patient is usually most comfortable in lying, with her knees slightly flexed; or in side-lying, with the opposite arm and leg slightly flexed. She must be warm and well supported by pillows. Instructions should be given in a low monotonous voice, and the patient should breathe deeply and rhythmically. Besides relaxation, the treatment sessions include *breathing exercises*, gentle *abdominal* and *pelvic floor contractions*, and *pelvic rocking*. It has been found that during the first stage of labour, deep slow breathing is most helpful. As the second stage approaches, some form of deep breathing, followed by quicker, shallower breaths, helps to raise the pain threshold as a contraction reaches its peak,* and diaphragmatic breathing (panting) prevents premature bearing down.

During the second stage, diaphragmatic breathing and controlled abdominal contraction augment the bearing down until the head is crowned.

At one time elaborate exercises to 'stretch the muscles of the pelvic floor' were taught, but it is now recognized that they serve little useful purpose, and may even lead to increased tension in the muscles. By teaching simple pelvic floor contraction and relaxation, it is hoped to make the patient aware of her ability to contract and *relax* the muscles at will, so that she is better equipped to relax them fully during a contraction.

Foot exercises (see flat-foot, pp. 314–15) should be taught, to mitigate the effect of the increasing weight, and *postural correction* may be necessary, it being particularly

---

* There has perhaps been a tendency in the past to claim that these preparations can lead to 'painless child-birth'. What we really do is teach the mother techniques with which she can *control* the pain. The term *uterine contraction* is now properly used instead of 'labour pain'—but the student can perhaps guard against over enthusiasm by this salutary tale. An 18-year-old mother in the post-natal ward when chided by the others for the 'awful noise you made', replied, 'Well nobody told me it was going to *hurt*'!

important to prevent lordosis which leads to backache and also throws an added strain on the abdominal wall.

SYMPTOMS ARISING DURING PREGNANCY.—Pregnancy is a normal physiological process but, as has been said, various inconveniences and minor disorders are liable to occur in expectant mothers of civilized races. Some of these may be relieved by physical treatment.

Among such troubles may be headaches, insomnia, or other neurasthenic manifestations; œdema of the feet, varicose veins, and hæmorrhoids due to pressure of the fœtal head on the pelvic veins; vomiting, constipation, cramps in the legs; pains in the back; and flat-foot due to the patient's increased weight. Treatment may be required also for the breasts if they are poorly developed, or have badly formed or retracted nipples. Preferably this should begin during pregnancy.

FLAT-FOOT.—Ordinary foot-drill should be practised (*see* pp. 314–15) and faradic foot-baths may be given.

ŒDEMA AND VARICOSE VEINS receive the usual treatment. The patient's legs should be kept higher than the body during treatment, and she should rest as much as possible with the pelvis and legs elevated.

THE BREASTS.—If these are badly developed, the mother should be taught to massage them, stroking from the periphery to the nipple. Alternate hot and cold sponging, and the use of olive oil rubbed in during the massage, are to be recommended. If the nipples are retracted, an attempt should be made to draw them gently outward. For the technique of breast massage, *see* p. 460.

THE PUERPERIUM

The following remarks refer to a *normal puerperium* only. The principal aim is *to strengthen the abdominal and pelvic muscles* and the patients are usually eager to co-operate.

It was, at one time, customary for a woman to remain in bed for many weeks after the birth of her child but it is now the practice for the mother to be allowed up for short periods on the second or third day after delivery. Ideally she is still kept in bed for 7 to 10 days, but is allowed up for longer periods each day. Unfortunately many mothers have to be discharged on the second or third day, owing to the acute shortage of hospital beds, but it is necessary to ensure that she still has adequate rest. The mother who straightaway plunges into household chores makes too many demands on her strength and this diminishes her supply of milk, besides making her tired and irritable, both of which adversely affect the baby. Whether at home or in hospital she should spend some part of each day resting, preferably in bed or on a couch.

EXERCISES.—*Breathing exercises, pelvic floor contractions*, and *foot and leg exercises* are given from the beginning.

On the second day *pelvic rocking* may be added. The patient is usually allowed to sit out of bed or do her exercises on top of the bed from the third day onwards. Thereafter selection may be made from the following exercises:—

1. Stride-lying Alternate trunk-rotation, with arm flexion across the chest.
2. Lying Alternate hip-updrawing.
3. Lying Alternate side-flexion.
4. Lying Head- and shoulder-raising.
5. Prone-kneeling Abdominal contractions.
6. Prone-kneeling Alternate side-flexion.
7. Prone-kneeling Alternate trunk-turning, with or without arm-flinging.
8. Sitting Back-raising (vertebra by vertebra).
9. Sitting (or standing) Trunk-flexion; Trunk side-bending; Trunk-rotation.

Postural correction is very important when the mother gets up, and *foot-drill* should not be neglected.

It is useless to give the mother a long table of exercises for home use, but most are anxious to get their figures back. Two exercises the author believes invaluable are *gluteal, perineal,* and *abdominal contractions with ankles crossed* and *pelvic rocking with pelvic contractions.* Both can be done in lying or standing, so can be practised after a rest period, or while doing the washing-up.

PRECAUTIONS.—

1. *Patients who have had a perineal tear* for which stitches have been inserted must avoid any movements which pull or drag on these. If the tear is a third-degree tear (extending through to the anus) treatment is contra-indicated.

2. Patients who have been delivered by Cæsarean section should be treated as post-operative cases for the first few days, breathing exercises being of particular importance. Steps must be taken to clear the respiratory passages of mucus, and should post-operative atelectasis occur, re-expansion must be gained by the usual methods.

3. *Arm exercises* should not be given to patients in whom there is a tendency to engorgement. Vigorous arm exercises should be performed by those in whom lactation is poor.

COMPLICATIONS.—

1. *Sepsis.*—If this occurs in a stitch *infra-red radiation, radiant heat,* or *ultra-violet light* may be applied. Otherwise physical treatment should be discontinued until the infection is controlled.

2. *Hæmorrhage.*—Physical treatment should be discontinued and medical advice sought before it is resumed.

3. *White-leg.*—See p. 436.

4. *Divarication of Recti.*—No outer-range abdominal work should be given. Carefully graduated inner-range work is permissible and the muscle should be manually supported during treatment.

TREATMENT OF THE BREASTS DURING THE PUERPERIUM.—Two difficulties may arise in connexion with the establishment of the function of lactation. (1) On about the third day after the child's birth the lobules of the breasts may become engorged, owing to some obstruction of the ducts, or because the child cannot suck sufficiently strongly to empty the breasts. This causes considerable pain, and the patient's temperature may rise. (2) The mother may not have sufficient milk to feed the infant. This may be the result of a poorly developed gland, or it may be due to the inability of the child to apply the suction stimulus strongly enough. Nowadays treatment is largely the prerogative of the nursing staff and cupping is frequently used, but the physiotherapist may be called upon to give the following treatment.

1. *Treatment for Engorged Breasts.**—The patient lies on her side, warmly covered up, only the part to be treated being exposed. Her garments and the bedclothes are carefully protected by macintoshes and towels, and a 'receiver' or kidney tray is placed beneath the breast. The physiotherapist, having washed her hands, bathes the breast with very hot water for about ten minutes. Alternatively, a clean cloth which has been wrung out in hot water may be applied to the breast before treatment. Soap and oil massage is then given. Squeezing, stroking movements should be applied from the circumference of the breast towards the nipple, the breast being supported by one hand if it is very heavy. After this, careful frictions with the fingers or thumb may be given over any hardened lobules, the treatment finishing with a repetition of the squeezing, stroking movements. The breast is then dried with a clean towel. The hot bathing is sometimes repeated after the massage. The patient then turns over

---

* In this connexion the student will do well to read the description in *Training for Childbirth* by Miss Randell.

and the other breast is treated in a similar manner. Great relief is often afforded in this way.

2. *Treatment to Increase the Flow of Milk.*—The technique is similar to that described above but, in this case, *alternate hot and cold bathing* is given in order to stimulate circulation through the gland, by bringing about alternate constriction and dilatation of its vessels. By increasing the circulation the activity of the gland is also increased. The massage manipulations employed are similar, but they can be applied more vigorously and should be followed by arm movements.

PROLAPSED UTERUS

The condition arises following childbirth, usually in women who have had several pregnancies. It results from a weak pelvic floor, and the fact that the uterus is in a flaccid state following parturition. Because the pelvic floor is weak, the uterus, when it resumes its normal state, contracts down into the vagina, where it remains, giving rise to discomfort and pain. It is frequently accompanied by stress incontinence, due to stretching of the urethral sphincter by the weakness of the pelvic floor.

THE MUSCLES OF THE PELVIC FLOOR AND THEIR FUNCTION.—The muscles of the pelvic floor, sometimes called the pelvic diaphragm, are *the levatores ani* and *the coccygei*. Besides their special function connected with defæcation, they have the task of supporting the pelvic viscera from below. The levatores ani arise from the inner surfaces of the sides of the true pelvis and meet in the middle line, being attached to the apex of the coccyx. They are inserted into the sides of the rectum and vagina, which pass through them. The coccygei have their origin at the ischial spines, and are inserted into the sides of the coccyx and lowest part of the sacrum, their anterior borders lying beside the posterior borders of the levatores (*Fig.* 187). If these and other muscles of this region become weak or atonic, there is a downward displacement of the pelvic organs.

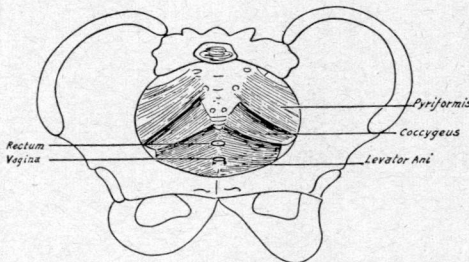

Fig. 187.—Diagram of muscles of pelvic floor.

Treatment.—

SURGICAL TREATMENT.—In many cases the uterus can be replaced manually under anæsthetic, and may thereafter be retained by means of a ring. In some cases a partial hysterectomy may have to be performed.

PHYSICAL TREATMENT.—The most important aim is to strengthen the muscles of the pelvic floor. This may be done by exercises such as static pelvic floor and gluteal contractions, crook-lying pelvic rocking, and lower abdominal wall contractions. Faradism may be given to the pelvic floor, a large indifferent pad being placed on the sacrum and a special electrode being inserted into the vagina. Abdominal exercises should be included in the treatment, as many as possible being done in the lying or crook-lying position to avoid strain on the pelvic floor. Posture should be carefully checked, and corrected where necessary.

CHAPTER XXII

PHYSIOTHERAPY IN SURGICAL CONDITIONS

I. Principles of surgery: Types of anaesthetic—Post-operative complications. II. Principles of physiotherapy. III. Operations commonly encountered. IV. More specialized operations.

So far, relevant surgical treatment, together with the appropriate pre- and post-operative physical treatment, has been briefly described as and when the need arose. Before ending this book it is felt that more should be said on the subject of physiotherapy in relation to general surgery. It is now widely recognized that physiotherapy can play an important part in hastening the patient's recovery, and in preventing some of the complications which were, at one time, common operational hazards. For this reason, pre- and post-operative treatment forms a large part of the work of the modern physiotherapist.

I. PRINCIPLES OF SURGERY

Surgery is undertaken for the following reasons:—

1. *To Remove Diseased Tissue.*—In the case of an *organ or gland* the operation is referred to by the suffix *-ectomy*, e.g., *pneumonectomy* (removal of a lung), *mastectomy* (removal of a mammary gland), *hæmorrhoidectomy* (removal of hæmorrhoids (rectal varicosities)). The removal may be partial or complete in most cases. In the case of a limb the removal is known as an *amputation*. Removal of a breast is sometimes referred to as a *radical amputation*, it being an external organ.

2. *For Purposes of Repair.*—In these cases the suffix *-orrhaphy* is applied, e.g., *herniorrhaphy* (repair of a hernia), *colporrhaphy* (repair of a lacerated perineum).

3. *For the Purpose of Procuring an Artificial Opening.*—In such cases the suffix *-otomy* or *-ostomy* is applied. The most common forms are *gastrostomy* or *gastrotomy* (an opening being made in the stomach for the purpose of feeding or evacuating the stomach), *colostomy* (an opening made in the transverse or sigmoid colon for purposes of evacuation), and *tracheotomy* (an opening made in the trachea for breathing). Any of these may be temporary or permanent.

4. *For Purposes of Inspection.*—If a speculum or some form of viewing apparatus is passed the suffix *-oscopy* is applied, e.g., *cystoscopy* (inspection of the bladder), *sigmoidoscopy* (inspection of the sigmoid colon). If the area is opened up for inspection or exploration the suffix *-otomy* is again used, e.g., *laparotomy* (inspection or exploration of the abdominal contents).

Pre-operative Treatment.—Ideally the patient is admitted 24 hours or more before operation. This enables the patient to become acclimatized to hospital conditions and to meet those who will be responsible for his treatment. The diet can be attended to, a light diet being required pre-operatively. The operation site can be prepared, pre-medication given, and sedatives administered if required.

If any specialized treatment, tests, or investigations are considered necessary the patient will, of course, be admitted several days, or even weeks, before the operation.

Post-operative Treatment.—Post-operatively, the trachea must be kept patent and free from obstruction until the patient regains consciousness. For this purpose an air tube is placed between the patient's lips. The patient is nursed flat in bed in a side-lying position until he regains consciousness. If the patient is shocked, treatment is given in the form of a saline drip. Sedatives will be administered if necessary. Normal micturition must be re-established as soon as possible, a catheter being passed if necessary to prevent retention and the possibility of bladder infection. After certain abdominal operations it will be necessary to rest the stomach and gastro-intestinal tract. The diet will be a fluid one administered intravenously, and the contents of the stomach will be evacuated by means of suction apparatus. The suction apparatus will have been inserted in the theatre, as will any drainage apparatus which may be required. In cases other than abdominal operations it is better to re-establish bowel action as soon as possible and even if a fluid diet is required it will be maintained for as short a time as possible. *It is essential to keep a careful watch on the patient's chart as any alteration in temperature, pulse-rate, or respiration may herald post-operative collapse, hæmorrhage, infection, or embolism.*

TYPES OF ANÆSTHETIC

Many of the former operative risks and complications arose from the methods of anæsthesia used at that time. Today great strides have been made in this field. This not only enables patients who would formerly have been unsuitable operation candidates to undergo and withstand surgery, but it also enables surgeons to perform hitherto undreamed-of operations.

The following methods are commonly used:—

1. *General Anæsthesia.*—This is used for most major operations, it being necessary to render the patient completely unconscious. The anæsthetic may be administered by inhalation or intravenously. Whereas chloroform and ether were previously used, the modern drugs, such as pentothal, are easily broken down and excreted from the body. This avoids much of the nausea and vomiting common in former days, together with many post-operative risks.

2. *Deep Freezing.*—This is a recent innovation which renders operation possible on patients who could not otherwise tolerate anæsthesia. The temperature of the body is gradually reduced and in this way consciousness is lost.

3. *Regional Anæsthesia.*—The anæsthetic is injected into a plexus in order to anæsthetize the whole area served by the plexus.

4. *Spinal Anæsthesia.*—The anæsthetic is injected into the subarachnoid space, inducing anæsthesia up to the desired level of the cord.

5. *Local Anæsthesia.*—Minor operations and certain eye operations are performed with this technique. The anæsthetic is introduced into the appropriate nerve, the effect being very localized.

POST-OPERATIVE COMPLICATIONS

Despite the modern advances in anæsthetics, certain complications do still arise which can, in part, be attributed to the anæsthesia. The chief of these, at least from the physiotherapist's point of view, are *post-operative chest conditions* and *deep-vein thrombosis.*

POST-OPERATIVE CHEST CONDITIONS.—As stated in Chapter XVII, one of the effects of anæsthetics is to dry and thicken the mucous secretions in the respiratory tract. The mucus is difficult to dislodge and therefore remains in the air-passages. Plugs of mucus may form, and the bronchi and bronchioles are in danger of becoming blocked.

Several conditions may arise:—

1. POST-OPERATIVE ATELECTASIS.—This is due to blockage of a bronchus or bronchiole. The subject has been fully discussed in the chapter on chest conditions. Here it suffices to say that this is by far the most common of the post-operative chest complications. The basal lobes are most often affected. In severe cases a whole lung may collapse, but this only occurs if the main bronchus is occluded. *High abdominal, thoracic, and mediastinal operations carry a higher risk of atelectasis than do lower abdominal or pelvic operations* because of the proximity of the lung tissue to these regions. Atelectasis usually occurs between the first and third day after operation.

2. BRONCHITIS.—The presence of static mucus in the respiratory tract may act as an irritant. The mucous membranes then become inflamed and the secretions are increased. Thus a vicious circle is established, the inflammation further blocking the air passage and the increased secretions acting as further irritants and increasing the inflammation. Bronchitis usually appears about 3 days after the operation.

3. PNEUMONIA.—If the mucus plugs in the former, and mucous secretions in the latter, are not removed there is an added risk of pneumonia with its attendant dangers (*see* pp. 384–6).

In all post-operative cases, therefore, it is essential to clear the respiratory passages and to maintain full ventilation.

DEEP-VEIN THROMBOSIS.—The exact cause of this is not fully understood. It may be due to pressure on a vein while the patient is unconscious and thus completely inert. It may be that in some way the anæsthetic causes abnormal platelet disintegration, leading to liberation of thrombokinase. Certainly handling of abdominal or pelvic viscera seems to predispose the condition and *the risk is therefore higher in low abdominal and pelvic operations* than in others. The fact that the circulation is reduced post-operatively, while the patient remains in bed, may aggravate the condition. *The great danger lies in the fact that a small fragment (embolus) may break off the clot and travel in the blood-stream until it lodges in a small vessel.* If this occurs in a coronary or pulmonary vessel the condition is very serious indeed and may prove to be fatal (*see* p. 435). The condition usually arises 10 to 14 days after the operation.

OTHER COMPLICATIONS which may arise are: *pressure sores* which are largely due to the patient remaining static during the operation, or lying inert in bed. Pressure is exerted on the tissues, which become ischæmic, and the skin becomes devitalized and breaks down. Once this occurs the ulcer may be very slow to heal; *bladder infections* chiefly caused by retention of urine; *sepsis* caused by micro-organic invasion; and *general muscular weakness and loss of joint mobility.* The muscular weakness may result from a lengthy or debilitating illness, coupled with confinement to bed. Loss of joint mobility arises mainly from adhesions in the region of the scar.

II. PRINCIPLES OF PHYSIOTHERAPY

AIMS.—The primary aims of physical treatment are: (1) *To prevent post-operative complications,* (2) *To assist in overcoming the effects of the anæsthetic* as quickly as possible, (3) *To maintain full muscle power and joint range.*

METHODS.—

PREVENTION OF POST-OPERATIVE COMPLICATIONS.—

1. *The Prevention of Chest Complications.*—The physiotherapist must take two other factors into consideration besides the effects of the anæsthetic on the secretions in the respiratory tract. One is that *pain causes reflex inhibition of the diaphragm* and breathing is therefore difficult. The other is that *in any operation involving the abdominal muscles the patient tends to avoid using them,*

partly through fear of damaging the wound and *partly because of pain.* Respiration is therefore hampered by this, as well as by factors already mentioned.

It is most important that the lungs should be fully ventilated and that mucus should be loosened and cleared from the respiratory tract.

a. Breathing exercises should be given to all parts of the chest, *diaphragmatic breathing* being the most important movement of all. Emphasis should be laid on *expiratory movements* in order to help loosen the mucus and to stimulate the cough reflex. *Deep breathing not only helps in the prevention of complications, but also helps in overcoming post-anœsthetic nausea and vomiting, and in breaking through the post-operative pain reflex.*

b. Coughing must be encouraged. Partly through fear and partly through pain, many patients try to clear the mucus by a genteel clearing of the throat. This is quite useless and only serves to tire the patient. In order to help the patient to achieve a worthwhile cough, the physiotherapist should support the wound while the patient coughs. It is often helpful if the patient bends the knees and leans slightly forwards.

c. Percussion can be used to assist in loosening the mucus and in stimulating the cough reflex. Gentle *back-clapping and -hacking* should be used and *vibrations* may be given in conjunction with expiration. It is often sufficient to let the patient lean forward over a pillow supported on the knees but, if the condition is serious, appropriate postural drainage may be required. *Should post-operative atelectasis occur steps must be taken to regain expansion as soon as possible.* The methods used are fully described in Chapter XVII, pp. 385–6, 400.

d. Postural drainage may also be required for bronchitis. *Should pneumonia occur, the physiotherapist must abide by the surgeon's wishes regarding physical treatment.*

2. *The Prevention of Thrombosis.*—*Adequate movement in bed is essential* in the prevention of this condition. Rest in bed tends to reduce circulation, and the lower extremities suffer most in this connexion. Also many patients tend to lie completely inert in bed, and this increases the risk. It is necessary therefore to ensure that the patient *moves his whole body* in bed. He must be encouraged to move around in bed, to get what he wants from his locker or bed-side table for himself, and to be as independent as he can.

Exercises: Besides the use of a general scheme of exercises, particular attention must be paid to foot and leg movements. *Full range movements must be given to the foot and ankle.* They should be performed vigorously and resistance may be given if desired. This increases the work of the muscles, which therefore exert more pressure on the underlying vessels. This in turn increases venous return and therefore assists the general circulation. *Quadriceps contractions* and *knee-bending and stretching* should also be given. *If the patient has an intravenous drip inserted into a lower limb, or if there is any form of pelvic drainage, leg movement must, of course, be modified.* In the case of the former, leg movements must not be given whilst the drip is in position. In the case of the latter, any movements which might interfere with the drainage should be avoided, or considerably modified.

Massage: Some people advocate massage of the legs to assist circulation and decrease the risk of thrombosis. There is always a possibility, however, that massage may detach an embolism from a hitherto unsuspected clot, and that the first one knows of it is the occurrence of a pulmonary or coronary embolism. To many the possible benefits do not outweigh this risk. If massage *is* given great care should be exercised, particularly in the region of femoral vessels.

Should deep-vein thrombosis be suspected, treatment must cease immediately and should not be resumed until further instructions are received from the surgeon (*see* pp. 435–6). The presence of an intravenous drip sometimes causes a *superficial phlebitis and cellulitis*. *Heat* is sometimes prescribed for this. It is usually administered in the form of infra-red radiation, or radiant heat.

3. *The Prevention of Pressure Sores.*—Again the chief factor in preventing these is movement.

Exercises.—A general scheme of bed-exercises should be given to prevent the patient from lying inert in bed, a factor which may be responsible for this condition. The nursing staff will apply spirit or soap and oil massage, to increase the skin resistance in any areas likely to be subjected to pressure, i.e., buttocks, sacrum, shoulders, and elbows. *Should pressure sores arise* the area should be treated as an open wound (*see* p. 192).

4. *The Prevention of Sepsis.*—This is not the concern of the physiotherapist but if the wound does become septic local doses of *ultra-violet light, infra-red radiation*, or *short-wave diathermy* may be required. If the sepsis is internal, treatment may have to be discontinued until the infection is controlled. Thereafter appropriate physical treatment may be required in addition to the resumption of normal post-operative treatment.

5. *The Prevention of Bladder Infections.*—Again the physiotherapist can do little to prevent this occurrence, which is usually caused by retention of urine. Catheterization may be necessary but this is not the physiotherapist's province. By teaching the patient to contract the abdominal wall she may perhaps help towards complete emptying of the bladder, which will prevent stagnation of residual urine.

6. *The Prevention of Muscle Wasting and Joint Immobility.*—By giving a simple scheme of bed-exercises and by ensuring that the patient uses his joints in full range, these complications are avoided (*see below*).

OVERCOMING THE EFFECTS OF THE ANÆSTHETIC.—The chief of these are *nausea and vomiting*. Deep breathing exercises can help considerably.

MAINTENANCE OF MUSCLE POWER AND JOINT RANGE.—With regard to *muscle power* the following factors must be taken into consideration when planning post-operative treatment:—

1. Certain muscles waste very quickly during a period of inactivity. This applies particularly to large, coarse-fibred muscles, e.g., the glutei and quadriceps.

2. The patient may have suffered a long and debilitating illness prior to the operation, and the general musculature may be poor.

3. Any muscles which have been interfered with during the operation will be sore and painful, and the patient will be disinclined to move them. They will soon suffer from disuse atrophy and, in the case of the abdominal muscles particularly, this can have serious consequences. It should also be remembered that the patient's postural sense may be affected, and this may also have far-reaching results.

With regard to joint mobility the following must be considered:—

1. If disuse atrophy is allowed to occur, joint mobility will be affected. Pain is an important factor here, as it leads to reflex inhibition, which predisposes to disuse atrophy.

2. Adhesions may form in the region of the scar and, if this involves joint structures, mobility will be impaired.

Exercises.—Early movement is essential. This is covered by the use of a general scheme of exercises. In addition, any special exercises must be given and any joint which might become involved in adhesions must be put through its full range of movement daily, e.g., special abdominal exercises will be required following abdominal operations, and the shoulder-joint must be put through its full range after thoracic operations.

Besides being of use in preventing many post-operative complications, it should be realized that early movement helps to break through the pain reflex, and thereby adds to, rather than detracts from, the patient's general comfort.

DANGER SIGNALS.—A very careful watch must always be kept on the patient's chart. It is necessary, however, that the physiotherapist should know what she is looking for.

THE CHART.—*A rise in temperature* may presage any of the post-operative complications. *A swinging temperature usually indicates sepsis.*

Alteration in pulse-rate and/or respiratory rate and depth may indicate respiratory or circulatory complications, shock, or hæmorrhage.

SPECIFIC SIGNS AND SYMPTOMS.—*It is in no way the job of the physiotherapist to diagnose.* It is helpful, however, if she has sufficient knowledge of the meaning of certain signs and symptoms to be able to act intelligently on her suspicions.

Post-operative Atelectasis.—The chart will indicate a *rise* in temperature (about 101°), pulse-rate (100 or more), and respiration. In addition the patient is usually *flushed and feverish* and may complain of a feeling of *tightness* and *discomfort* on the affected side. There is *poor chest expansion* on the affected side; the percussion sounds are flat and there are adventitious sounds. X-ray reveals the collapse.

Bronchitis.—The chart reveals a *slight rise* in temperature; there is a *cough and copious sputum*; and the mucus *bubbles and rattles* in the respiratory passages.

Bronchopneumonia.—The chart reveals a *rise* in temperature, pulse, and respiration, and the *patient's colour is usually bad.*

Thrombosis.—

Deep: The chart reveals a *rise* in temperature. In addition the patient complains of *pain in the leg* (usually in the groin or behind the knee). *Later* the *leg may be swollen* and the *hard, cord-like* vein may be palpable.

Superficial: The site is painful and swollen and the skin is red and shiny.

Embolism.—In serious cases the chart reveals a *rapid rise* in temperature, pulse, and respiration. The patient's *colour is bad* and he complains of *severe pain in the chest*. Death may ensue within a few minutes. If he survives the patient will be very ill for some time.

In less serious cases the chart reveals a *rise* in temperature, pulse, and respiration. The patient complains of a *sharp stabbing pain* in the side of chest. To all intents and purposes he has pleurisy. In 2–3 days the *sputum becomes bloodstained* and the condition begins to subside.

Pressure Sores.—The skin is sore and red. It ultimately breaks down and an ulcer forms.

Sepsis.—The chart reveals a *high temperature* (probably swinging). If the sepsis is superficial, e.g., stitch abscess, the surrounding area is red and tender. Later the skin breaks down and the pus discharges. If deep, e.g., lung abscess, the chart reveals *a high swinging temperature* and a rapid pulse. The patient has a *toxic appearance* and *loses his appetite*. X-ray reveals a solid shadow.

PRE-OPERATIVE ROUTINE

Whenever possible the patient should be given pre-operative treatment. Ideally treatment should be given daily, several days in advance of the operation. This is not always possible, but even in cases where the patient is only admitted the previous day, the physiotherapist should make an effort to see him so that she can introduce herself to him, and explain and teach as much as possible of the post-operative routine.

The following routine should be followed:—

1. Meet the Patient and talk to Him.—During this time the physiotherapist should explain her work in relation to the patient, and should answer any questions truthfully and simply. *She should not, however, take upon herself the responsibility of discussing the patient's condition or the operative procedure.* This cannot be over-emphasized, and much harm can be done by a physiotherapist who cannot confine herself to her own subject.

If the relationship between patient and physiotherapist is to be a happy and successful one, and if she is to gain his confidence and trust, she must put over the following points:—

a. The importance of deep breathing and the way in which the chest works: Her explanation should be simple but she should emphasize that deep breathing is most helpful in overcoming post-operative nausea and vomiting, should these occur.

b. The importance of coughing: Without alarming the patient, it should be explained that an effect of the anæsthetic may be to increase mucus secretion which must be got rid of. It must be emphasized that although coughing will hurt to begin with, *it will not damage the wound or the stitches*. The physiotherapist should show the patient how to cough whilst giving the support she will give after the operation. If it is thought advisable, i.e., if the patient is likely to need it, postural drainage and percussion may also be demonstrated.

c. The importance of movement: This can be explained quite simply as a need to maintain circulation, the rate of which tends to decrease when a person is in bed for some time.

2. Teach the Post-operative Routine.—Having talked to the patient and explained what will be required of him post-operatively, the physiotherapist then teaches the post-operative routine:—

a. Breathing exercises: All movements must be practised—*basal, lateral costal, apical*, and *diaphragmatic*—particular attention being paid to the latter.

b. Any special exercises or techniques which will be required: For example, abdominal contractions must be taught where they are particularly required; full arm movements should be practised if the scar is likely to involve the shoulder-joint; elevation and massage of the arm should be explained to a patient awaiting mastectomy.

c. Foot, and ankle movements, and quadriceps contractions should be taught.

The general exercises, which will be added as the patient improves, need not be taught at this stage. It is sufficient to incorporate them in the treatment as it progresses.

POST-OPERATIVE ROUTINE

Before treatment begins the physiotherapist should see the ward-sister and inquire if there are any precautions which must be taken, or if there are any special instructions regarding the patient or the treatment. She should read the notes, to familiarize herself with details of the operation, and should look at the patient's chart.

The routine treatment is then given, unless any modifications or alterations are required. The following is usually suitable for the first day:—

Position of the Patient.—Crook-half-lying or Half-lying.

Breathing Exercises.—Some people like to give basal, lateral costal, apical, and diaphragmatic movements before moving on to other exercises—others prefer to intersperse the treatment with breathing exercises. Certainly *basal* (or lateral costal) and *diaphragmatic movements* should be given at the beginning, *emphasis being laid on expiration*. Vibration may be given during expiration and the patient must be encouraged to cough.

N.B.—The physiotherapist should always place her hands on the patient's chest. In this way she can guide and encourage movement; she can note any inequality in expansion, and feel any mucus in the chest. Care must be taken not to disturb a drip.

Abdominal Contractions follow naturally on diaphragmatic breathing. If it is thought advisable to keep the treatment to a minimum, in order to avoid tiring the patient, they may be combined with breathing.

Foot and Leg Movements.—*Dorsi- and plantar flexion, inversion and eversion,* and *foot circling* should be performed vigorously. *Toe* movements and *quadriceps contractions* should also be given.

A second series of breathing exercises, or any special movements such as full elevation of the arm, may be interposed between the foot movements and the quadriceps contractions.

Final Breathing Exercises.—Diaphragmatic breathing and lateral costal or basal movements should conclude the treatment.

Before leaving the patient, the physiotherapist should check the patient's posture and position, making any necessary corrections, and should see that all is well regarding drips, drainage tubes, or any other apparatus in use.

On the Second Day such simple exercises as Lying head-raising; Lying Alternate arm flexion across the body to the opposite shoulder; Half-lying knee-bending and -stretching may be added.

Thereafter, simple arm and trunk exercises can usually be added each day until a full scheme is being given.

The Physiotherapist's Manner.—In all her dealings with the patient, particularly post-operatively, the physiotherapist should be quiet and confident. She should talk as little as possible (without being churlish or unkind), and her directions and explanations should be clear and concise.

Precautions.—No treatment should be given without first consulting the ward-sister or her deputy. If for any reason the physiotherapist is worried by the patient's symptoms, the matter should be reported, and it may be advisable to discontinue treatment until further instructions have been received. The treatment must be kept to a mimimum, care being taken not to over-tire the patient. No treatment should be given which might adversely affect drainage, intravenous drip, etc.

Should the physiotherapist inadvertently displace any apparatus, or suspect that she may have done so, she should report the matter at once.

III. OPERATIONS COMMONLY ENCOUNTERED

It is not proposed to deal at length with any specific operations, but many surgical cases can be somewhat frightening to the novice. For this reason a brief résumé is given below of operations commonly encountered by the physiotherapist, together with any special points which may prove helpful.

MASTOIDECTOMY.—Here the balance of the ear may be temporarily upset and the patient may suffer considerably from nausea and giddiness. Treatment may therefore be given on similar lines to that for fenestration cases (*see* Section IV). The posterior neck muscles may require attention.

LARYNGECTOMY is performed for malignant growths. A tracheotomy tube is inserted. There is usually a great deal of mucus, some of which the patient may be able to cough up, but which, in the main, must be removed by means of suction apparatus.

CHOLECYSTECTOMY (removal of the gall-bladder) is frequently met in middle-aged women. A high abdominal incision is required and there is considerable risk of post-operative atelectasis. A drainage tube is inserted, the method of drainage being closed, and remains in situ until the drainage of bile ceases. The patients often suffer considerable discomfort from flatulence. Breathing exercises, particularly diaphragmatic and lower costal, and abdominal contractions require special attention. The patient is usually allowed to get up before the drainage is removed.

COLOSTOMY.—Operations on the intestines usually involve the large intestine and are generally performed for malignant or other obstructive conditions, and ulcerative conditions. In most cases a *colostomy* is necessary for fæcal evacuation. This may be permanent or temporary, closure then being undertaken at a later date. It is important to get the colostomy working as early as possible and the patient must therefore move about as much as possible. He is usually allowed up on the second or third day after the operation, and post-operative treatment should be fairly vigorous. Foot and leg exercises are important, there being a slightly higher risk of thrombosis than of atelectasis in these cases. The dressings are massive, however, and these may restrict lower costal and diaphragm movement. Breathing exercises must therefore be practised assiduously. Abdominal exercises are also important from the point of view of the colostomy.

PROSTATECTOMY is performed in cases of an enlarged prostate gland. It is a common condition in middle-aged and elderly men. Catheterization and drainage is necessary for four or five days after the operation, and care must be taken when giving leg movements to see that there is no interference with the drainage.

IV. MORE SPECIALIZED OPERATIONS

THE CENTRAL NERVOUS SYSTEM.—Various operations may be performed on the brain and spinal cord, usually for tumours and malignant conditions. Many of the cases are complicated by neurological symptoms such as spasticity which must receive appropriate treatment (*see* pp. 185–8) in addition to general post-operative treatment. Following head operations the patient's balance may be considerably upset and the patient may suffer from giddiness, nausea, and vomiting. Treatment given as for fenestration (*see below*) is often helpful in overcoming this. In the early days, however, the patient may be nursed flat in bed and very little movement is allowed. Breathing exercises must be practised assiduously, and massage and passive movements of the legs may be given.

EYES.—Following operations on the eye itself (e.g., for removal of cataract) the patient must remain perfectly still in bed for a week or ten days. Breathing exercises, massage and passive movements may sometimes be required. All must be given very gently and great care must be taken not to disturb or excite the patient. Since the patient's eyes are bandaged the physiotherapist's manner and approach are most important, the patient relying on hearing and touch to form an opinion of her.

EARS.—Apart from mastoidectomy, two fairly common ear operations are *Fenestration* (the making of a new 'window' in the vestibular portion of the inner ear) and *Labyrinthectomy* (removal of the inner ear). The former is undertaken for otosclerosis and Ménière's disease. The latter may also be undertaken for Ménière's disease, or for chronic conditions affecting the middle and inner ear. The labyrinthine balance mechanism is upset in both cases, the patient suffering severe vertigo, nausea, vomiting, and giddiness. The post-operative treatment is most interesting and aims at re-establishing the labyrinthine pathways, or at achieving compensation through over-activation of the remaining balance mechanism. Everything is done with a view to further upsetting the patient's balance, in order to achieve these ends. Treatment may usually begin on the third day post-operatively in the case of labyrinthectomy and on the fifth day in the case of fenestration. Simple head exercises are performed until the patient is allowed up (on the fifth and seventh days respectively). Thereafter, trunk exercises may be added. The exercises are first performed slowly, then quickly, with the eyes open and with the eyes shut. Flexion and extension, head-turning and circling, should all be included from the beginning. Once the patient is up exercises are done in sitting and later in standing. It is important to see that *the head moves with the body, and that the eyes move with the head.* The same principle of performing the movements slowly and quickly, and with the eyes closed and open is followed. Re-education in walking is required and should not only be given as a simple walking exercise, but should include walking combined with head movements, walking with the eyes shut, turning, walking on slopes and up stairs. Much use can be made of ball exercises and ball games in treating these cases. As has been stated above, this method of treatment is most helpful in certain cases of head injury and in some nervous diseases.

Experience is the most valuable teacher in all surgical cases. Each case must be treated on its merit, the patient's general condition and the surgeon's views and wishes concerning physiotherapy being the guiding principles, but the aim of this chapter is to give the student a basis from which to work.

CHAPTER XXIII

CLASS-WORK. CHILDREN'S CLASSES. TREATMENT OF AGED AND CHRONIC PATIENTS. SPECIAL METHODS

I. Class-work: Advantages; Selection and grading of patients; Size of class; Relation of physio-therapist to class; Place for class; Apparatus and accessories; Dress and assembly; Arrangement of class; Choice and progression of exercises; Examples of class schemes in ward and gymnasium. II. Children's Classes. III. Treatment of Aged and Chronic Patients. IV. Special Methods: Suspension Therapy; Pulley Exercises; Medicine-ball Exercises.

I. CLASS-WORK

REFERENCE has been made in previous chapters to the treatment of patients in groups or classes. Class-work used at one time to be associated almost entirely with educational gymnastics—those suffering from any disability almost invariably received individual treatment. But for many years now, especially since the increasing number of patients in physiotherapy departments and large clinics has made it necessary to treat as many as possible in the time available, it has become more and more the practice to group patients into classes; and this has since been found to have other advantages than the mere saving of time.

Some physiotherapists like this type of work; others prefer dealing with individuals separately. This is largely a matter of temperament, but whatever a physiotherapist's personal preference, it is necessary that he or she should at least be able, if and when required, to organize small classes and that, while obtaining the advantages of group work, she is able to do justice to all the individuals composing that group.

Advantages of Class-work.—

1. Since so much time is saved by this method, it becomes possible to accept and deal with more patients than would otherwise be possible. This is a great gain, and does away, in some degree at least, with the distressing weeks, or even months, of waiting before the patient's treatment can begin. Moreover, it is far more satisfactory thus to group patients, than to take each separately, and be forced to shorten his or her period of treatment for lack of time. If, say, twelve patients exercise together for half an hour under one physiotherapist, there should be time for some of them to have, in addition, heat, massage, special manipulations, or any other form of treatment prescribed, whereas if the physio-therapists in the department had to give each of these patients half an hour's exercise alone (occupying in all 6 hours) there would certainly be no time for any other kind of treatment.

2. The patient is stimulated by the element of competition present in class-work. He is encouraged by the progress of others to do his best, and to expect improvement in himself, ceasing to think of his own difficulties as insurmountable. There is also a very definite pleasure in carrying out movements in a rhythmic manner in company with others. In *children*, the spirit of play can be encouraged, and the work can thus be made thoroughly enjoyable. They will be less apt to think of themselves as exceptional, or inferior to other children, and their competitive spirit can be stimulated. Any antagonism to the treatment in general, or the physiotherapist in particular, caused by unwise parents, teachers, or companions, can often be better overcome in class than by

individual treatment. It must be remembered, however, that certain children may react most unfavourably to class-work, becoming over-excited or seeing in it a chance to show off and incite others to follow suit.

Selection of Patients.—However great the advantages of class treatment, it *must* be realized that it is not suitable for every patient.

1. There *are* patients who are too nervous, sensitive, or self-conscious to profit from class-work, although they may be physically capable of it. This applies especially in the early stages of their treatment, and often arises in connexion with postural or 'general' classes. There are patients, especially children and young girls, who are hypersensitive about their disabilities or their physical peculiarities, and who think that they will be objects of comment or ridicule if they work with others. Another unsuitable group consists of difficult, resentful patients who feel that they are not receiving enough attention, or that 'the hospital doctor' does not understand them. Their spoken, or unspoken, comment is: 'I could do all that at home without bothering to come to hospital. My doctor at home said I should have massage and radiant heat.' Such patients require tactful handling, for their co-operation must be gained if treatment is to have any beneficial effect. They must be treated with sympathy, patience and consideration, and if their dislike of class-work cannot be overcome by these means, they must be treated individually, at least for a time. A patient who hates or dreads the treatment is unlikely to make progress, and it becomes a waste of time for all concerned. Fortunately, these patients are a small minority, but they do exist.

It should also be realized that the patient who requires a lot of encouragement, or 'pushing' on the part of the physiotherapist, is rarely suitable for class-work, his temperament rendering him unable to achieve much for himself without more constant supervision than the class allows. The patient who uses his 'illness' to evade work, or for 'compensation' purposes, will also find a class gives ample scope for his peculiar talents.

2. There are also patients whose disabilities render them unsuitable for class-work. For example, patients needing re-education following peripheral nerve injuries need individual attention, especially if the hand is affected; and there is little likelihood—except, perhaps, in special hospitals for nervous diseases—of others being at the same stage of recovery as themselves. Elderly patients with systemic nervous diseases are rarely suitable except for ward classes consisting of breathing exercises and very easy movements. Indeed, any case of organic nerve lesion must be *very* carefully considered before admission to a class. Hospitals, or departments which specialize in nervous diseases, often include class-work in the treatment schemes, but this is a different matter from the class-work now under discussion. Such classes demand special skill, much organization, and more time than is usually available in average general hospitals. Medical cases are generally better treated individually, although many respiratory cases do very well in classes, e.g., asthmatic or bronchitic patients, and those requiring more general breathing exercises. There is always, of course, a danger of putting patients into classes *at too early a stage*, when, for physical or psychological reasons, they are most unlikely to derive benefit from this type of work. In the early stages of treatment, most patients need special instructions and more detailed correction than can be given to the members of a class.

Grading of Patients.—As a general rule the members of a class should be so graded that they can *all* do the same exercise. It *is* possible to tell certain patients to 'fall out' for particular exercises, or even to drop out of a class at a specified stage and watch the other patients for the rest of the time, but it is better to have them graded into separate classes if at all possible. Differentiation is often done in Ward Classes (*see below*), but in the gymnasium it is a troublesome method and needs skilful organizing. Matters should not be made too complicated for the physiotherapist in charge of the classes, especially if she is unused to this type of work, when mistakes can easily be made. If this method *must* be adopted, the patients who do not do the full scheme should be distinguished by some physical means, e.g., coloured arm-bands (*see* WARD CLASSES).

Patients suffering from different disabilities can often join the same class, provided that the exercises chosen are of suitable strength for all. For instance, patients who have sustained spinal fractures may be able to work with those who have been operated on for a displaced intervertebral disk, because both need exercises for the back extensors. This does not, however, mean that all patients suffering from a disability in some particular part of the body should *necessarily* work together. One would not, for example, bring all 'foot cases' together—pes planus, cavus, varus, or valgus—and expect them to do the same exercises, whether appropriate or inappropriate. This comment may seem so obvious as to be unnecessary, but such things have been known to happen! Of course, patients may sometimes practise certain exercises together (e.g., mobility and postural exercises) and each may, in addition, be given special exercises designed to benefit his particular disability. Patients with various types of spinal curvatures may, and as a rule should, join a general★ or posture class, provided that the structural cases also receive any special treatment they may require.

Size of Class.—Classes should not, as a rule, exceed twelve patients at most, six or eight being the optimum. General posture classes *may* be a little larger, but it is not desirable to have them as large as an educational class. The fact that patients all do the same exercises does not ensure that they will all do them equally well, all make the same mistakes, or all need the same amount of encouragement or correction. *The physiotherapist must remember that they are individuals, and that she is treating patients, not classes.* A careful watch must be kept on each, and it must be remembered that the slowest and least intelligent patient has as much claim on the physiotherapist's attention as has the brightest and most responsive. If a patient does not make the progress which may be reasonably expected of him, the physiotherapist should have no hesitation in removing him from the class and substituting individual treatment, either temporarily or permanently.

Relation of the Physiotherapist to the Class.—The physiotherapist's manner and bearing is most important, and has often been subjected to criticism. Many students, and sometimes qualified physiotherapists, automatically adopt a 'stimulating' and 'hearty' manner simply because they are taking a class. This is excellent at the right time and for certain types of class; but there *are* times when a quieter bearing and a gentler approach is better, whether we are dealing with classes or individuals. Patients recovering from a severe illness or operation, and those who are weak, debilitated, tired, or nervous, do not respond well to aggressive cheerfulness, and the physiotherapist must not run the risk of antagonizing her patients by what appears to them to be hardness, and lack of understanding of their difficulties.

★ For purposes of description, a '*general*' class is taken to mean one suitable for patients of poor physique, with weak muscles, defective co-ordination or control of movement, minor faults of posture or gait, bad breathing habits, etc. An individual with a major disability (e.g., a *structural* scoliosis) may participate in such a class, but should have special exercises as well. A '*special*' class is one in which patients with a definite disability or weakness are made to concentrate on its improvement, e.g., a stiff joint or joints, due to injury or disease (fracture, arthritis, spondylitis); a lung disease (asthma, empyema); or a state of weakness of certain muscles. Some general exercises may or may not be included.

It goes without saying that, as mentioned above, all patients in a class should receive an equal share of their instructor's interest and attention. No patient must feel himself ignored, or made to feel clumsy or ridiculous. Good-natured chaff may be well received, but must be used with discrimination.

Place for Class.—Classes may be held in a *ward*, in a large or small *gymnasium* or other suitable room, in a *courtyard*, or on a *lawn*. In a ward, the patients are generally still in bed, or only just beginning to get up, it being better, as a rule, for the stronger ward-patients to attend the hospital gymnasium for their class-work. A gymnasium or large room is indispensable for more advanced classes, for final rehabilitation and strengthening classes, or when more than one class must be held at the same time. Provided it is secluded, a courtyard or lawn is excellent for general and posture classes and, in suitable weather, for patients with respiratory difficulties. It is also ideal for advanced games, for kicking footballs, throwing medicine balls, etc.

Apparatus and Accessories.—The following are desirable:—

1. *The Ordinary Apparatus of the Well-equipped Gymnasium.*—Rib-stalls, boom, balancing forms, stools, plinths, trestle table for knee, hand, and forearm exercises, straps, etc. Delorme boots and weights, pulleys and springs, rowing- and wrist-machines, stationary bicycles, etc., are useful for individuals and, if sufficiently numerous, for classes also. For the rehabilitation of men who are to return to heavy work, educational apparatus will be required, such as vaulting horses, ropes for hanging and climbing exercises, etc.

2. *Small Mattresses, Pillows or Small Cushions.*—For exercises in lying.

3. *Blankets.*—For relaxation classes.

4. *Miscellaneous Apparatus.*—Balls, small and large (for medicine balls, *see below*); footballs, small celluloid balls, and balloons for 'blowing' exercises; bean-bags or small sand-bags; netball apparatus; poles and rods; dumb-bells or other weights. Indian clubs are effective, but may be dangerous if dropped, unless the class is very well disciplined. Sand trays and plasticine are useful for hand classes. A selection of shorts, gym-shoes, and bodices will be most useful.

5. *Music.*—This is often helpful for general, postural, or advanced classes of any sort, since it promotes rhythm, timing, and control of movement, but it must not be allowed to become an end in itself (the same applies to singing exercises for children). It is not suitable for a class of unequal abilities, because the tempo will almost certainly be too quick for some, while others have no sense of time at all. This will give them a hopeless feeling of being continually out-distanced, and having 'lost their place' by some mistake, and being unable to regain it, they will continue helplessly, out of time and out of rhythm, until the music stops and they come to an undignified halt in the middle of the movement before last! Music is rarely suitable for special classes, but can often be used to advantage in relaxation classes and other specialized classes.

Dress and Assembly.—The patient's clothing must allow free movement, and patients in posture or spinal classes may need special dress. Ideally, shorts, short skirts, or knickers should be worn with upper garments which allow the back to be seen (*see* p. 348). Gym-shoes should always be worn. Instructions as to dress should be faithfully followed by the patients, and compliance should be insisted upon, unless there is a very good reason to the contrary. The patients should not, therefore, be required to wear anything they are unlikely to possess, or which they cannot obtain easily or cheaply. Suitable places should be provided for changing and leaving clothes. Patients should arrive punctually, and should wait or rest as instructed. They should not be allowed to play or lounge about the department, but the latter should not be enforced too strictly in the case of elderly patients.

Arrangement of Class.—In small classes, patients take their places, sitting, standing, or lying, as instructed. *They should be so spaced that everyone has room for unimpeded movement and all can be seen by the physiotherapist,* who must also be *visible* and *audible* to all. Elderly patients who are short-sighted, or hard of hearing, should be placed well forward. Larger classes, e.g., posture classes, consisting of children or young people, are perhaps better begun, like educational classes, with some form of controlled activity, e.g., marching or a team game. This produces a feeling of discipline and a sense of co-operation. Difficult or unruly children should be kept in view, and prevented from settling in the rear ranks.

Choice of Exercise.—In a *general class,** exercises should be chosen to improve the whole body. Any good medical or educational system of arrangement may be adopted. There must be exercises to promote good carriage and correct faults of posture; exercises to control and co-ordinate movement; activity exercises to improve circulation, to increase the rate and depth of breathing, and to provide general stimulation; relaxation or mobility exercises, and respiratory exercises. Naturally the difficulty of the work must be adapted to the age, strength, and capabilities of the individuals composing the class. Equally, any special disabilities of any of its members must also be taken into consideration. In a *special class,** time should not be wasted on general exercises, no more being given than are necessary to provide the patients with rests. On the whole general exercises can be omitted, provided the patients are allowed proper intervals between exercises. Obviously, too many exercises imposing heavy work, or special strain, should not be given consecutively.

Progression of Exercises.—It is most essential that a patient, in the course of his rehabilitation, should not remain too long at any one level of attainment, but should advance gradually from one stage to another. If he is being treated individually, the exercises will be changed from time to time—each one being discarded after it has been completely mastered, and has become too easy, a more advanced movement being substituted. In class treatment, orderly progression is equally important. It may be obtained by various methods.

1. 'Junior' and 'Senior' classes may be held, and the patient is transferred from one to the other as he progresses. There may be easy, medium, and advanced classes for the same condition, or classes 'without weight-bearing', 'with partial weight-bearing', and 'with full weight-bearing'. Some hospitals and clinics have a series of five or six set schemes for each special disability, and the patient progresses from one to the other until ready for discharge.† The classes may or may not be taken by the same physiotherapist.

2. An individual physiotherapist may keep the same patients throughout their course, increasing the amount of work done by some, or all, according to their requirements and progress. The exercises are altered or varied as she sees fit, but are not confined to set schemes. This is more often the method used in smaller institutions. The first method makes it easier to gauge and record the patient's progress; the second makes, perhaps, for more initiative in the physiotherapist, and avoids monotony. In some cases the two methods are combined, the patient passing from one class to another, but the exercises in each are varied to some extent, although the general standard of attainments is maintained.

Ward Classes.—It should be realized that many patients in the wards require individual treatment, and that some will never be suitable for class-work at all. Equally, in hospitals devoted to specific conditions ward classes as well as gymnasium classes must be planned on special lines. In small wards, all suitable

---

* *See* footnote, p. 474.
† J. Colson, *The Rehabilitation of the Injured,* Vol. II.

patients can exercise together. They must, of course, be graded according to their disabilities and stage of progress. In large wards, some division of patients into groups must be made. Sometimes the beds are so arranged as to facilitate this, but this cannot always be done. The physiotherapist must then be prepared to exercise ingenuity, rather than disturb the arrangements or routine of the ward.

Fractures and Other Injuries.—The patients may be in plaster, or some form of traction. The method of fixation may limit certain movements, or debar some patients from performing certain exercises, but static contractions of the muscle can usually be used to replace the actual movement. If the scheme is too long for any individual he should perform only certain selected exercises.

SURGICAL CASES.—As we have seen it is now customary to give exercises to all surgical cases, both before and after operation. The pre-operative exercises should be taught to each patient individually, especially in thoracic and cardiac cases. Post-operative general surgical cases can often be treated in a class, but again, unless the unit is a specialized one, thoracic and cardiac cases require individual attention. The following is the routine general treatment in one of our great London hospitals.

Before Operation.—All patients are taught breathing and foot exercises.

After Operation.—*First day.* Special breathing exercises are given three times a day to the patients individually, if there are no complications. After this they take part in the group treatment. Certain patients continue with special individual treatment for a time, but join the group as soon as possible.

Group Treatment and Progression.—All patients take part in this unless there are definite contra-indications. Four progressive tables are given. Coloured bands are placed at the end of each bed to show which stage the patient has reached. The temperature and pulse charts are inspected, and the progression for each patient is discussed with the staff on duty in each ward.

POST-NATAL EXERCISES.*—Here it is certain that the physiotherapist will have to deal with patients at many different stages. She must therefore be able to adapt her schemes so that no patient does *more* than is good for her, while ensuring that all patients do *enough*. Since these patients do not remain long in hospital, the physiotherapist cannot expect beds to be moved about to suit her convenience. She must adapt herself as best she can, making it clear to each patient which exercises she is to do, and which to omit. It is important that the patients should be kept warm while exercising. *Coloured bands* may be used as for surgical ward cases.

II. CHILDREN'S CLASSES

Children are generally treated in hospital classes, or school clinics, for poor posture, for deformities of the spine or feet, or for defective breathing, as in asthma, or removal of tonsils and adenoids. If they are to be dealt with satisfactorily, they *must* be carefully graded into age-groups. It is most unsuitable for a child of eight or nine to be required to work with adolescents performing

---

* The physiotherapist must remember that some maternity patients may not be suitable for immediate inclusion in a class. A nervous or delicate patient, or one who has had a long and difficult labour, is not always fit for this until she has had a fairly long rest. The same may apply to a patient of difficult temperament, to an elderly primipara (one who is having her first child), to a tired woman who has worked hard up to the last moment before her confinement, to one suffering from emotional stress (e.g., an unmarried mother, or one who has lost her baby). Such patients need tact, patience, and sympathy. There have been complaints (whether justified or not) by mothers in hospital, of want of consideration on the part of the physiotherapists, and it is better to lose one day's exercise than the patient's co-operation. The ward-sister should always be consulted before a class begins, and the physiotherapist should be prepared, if necessary, to treat the patient by herself until she is ready to take her place with the others.

exercises far in advance of his years. Equally, a child of the same age who has been put among 'kids' of six or seven, to the great detriment of his self-respect, will become bored, and most probably obstreperous. Generally speaking, 'infants' under 6 years are not suitable for classes, whereas children from 6 to 8, 8 to 10, and 10 to 12 or 13 years respond well (though the latter may need a firm hand). Again, it must be remembered that certain children are not, and never will be, suitable members of a class. Some children are shy, restless, or very self-conscious; others may resent criticism, or expect an inordinate amount of attention; while others may simply be 'bad mixers'. It is far better to treat a difficult child individually, than to let him upset the discipline of a whole class, or, alternatively, keep himself in the background and do as little work as possible.

The majority of children, however, enjoy class-work provided that it is interesting, and includes plenty of movement and variety. The following points must be remembered in arranging a children's class.

1. The work must be suitable for the children's age-group, as well as for their disabilities.

2. The exercises, especially for children under eight, must be simple—complex movements, with difficult co-ordination, being avoided. Children should not be required to stand still for long at a time, and there should not be a great deal of static work in the table. There must not be intervals of inactivity, or exercises needing lengthy explanations, both of which encourage the children to drop into bad postures, or to become bored and to begin to fidget. The schemes must not be too long, and the exercises must be changed frequently.

3. Full play must be given to the children's imaginative faculties. There should be at least one game in all general tables, but for little children the whole scheme should be a game, or a series of games, perhaps bound together by a story (see below).

4. The movements should be free, rhythmic, and as graceful as possible, but they must be really effective, and not merely 'pretty'. If the children are being treated for deformities, or respiratory difficulties, the exercises *must* be such as will improve these conditions, and all must perform them as correctly as they can. It is possible for a class of small children to go through a table of exercises *looking* perfectly charming—and yet not a single exercise is likely to do them any good, except perhaps in so far as it entails *some* activity.

For little children of six or thereabouts, the whole scheme, as mentioned above, can be a game. 'Here we go round the mulberry bush' can be made into quite an effective table, the movements being such as are required for stretching when waking up in the morning, washing face and hands, brushing hair, washing and wringing out clothes and hanging them up to dry, riding a bicycle to school, crossing a bridge (the balancing form), playing ball or football, picking flowers, etc., with the final relaxation of going to bed and to sleep. Or the children can imitate animals: 'This is the way the pussy goes . . . the kangaroo goes . . . the bunny goes'; Back-raising may be the hedgehog unrolling itself, expiration the snake hissing or the bee buzzing, inspiration the pouter pigeon, etc.

Alternatively exercises may be embodied in a continuous story, e.g., of a visit to an old woman living in a cottage in a wood. Some of the old fairy tales could be adapted in the same way.

III. TREATMENT OF AGED AND CHRONIC PATIENTS

No patient, of whatever age, should be considered 'finished with' until he (or she) has obtained the maximum improvement of which he is capable. It should be stressed, however, that if treatment is likely to be prolonged (e.g., in cases of arthritis, poliomyelitis, and other nervous diseases), there is a great danger of the patient's becoming 'hospitalized' if treatment continues for too long at a time. In such cases it is often better to break the treatment up into definite periods to which a time limit is attached, than to let treatment continue *ad infinitum*, to the detriment of both the patient's and the physiotherapist's interest.

Formerly, old or 'chronic' patients were, all too often, left on one side because the results of treatment were neither so brilliant nor so complete as with younger patients, whose powers of recuperation are greater. The strength of the elderly declines rapidly in sickness and their recovery is slow. Much can be done for these patients, however, and the importance of geriatric treatment is now widely recognized. If they could always be treated by correct physical methods from the beginning of their illness, there would be much less permanent disability among them and much less deterioration, both physical and mental. Even patients who have suffered long periods of neglect may improve, markedly, under treatment.

The Bedridden.—It takes a very short time for an elderly patient to become bedridden. "It has not been realized in the past that even as short a period as 10 days of such inactivity [in bed] may lead to permanent bedfastness."* Immobilization may easily lead to the development of contractures—the joints become stiff, the muscles waste, and permanent deformities may arise. The lungs are particularly vulnerable, and bed-sores often occur. Unless physical activity is encouraged, the bedridden patient's mind, like his body, may become inert. He tends to give up hope of recovery, feels himself useless and unwanted, loses his self-respect, becomes apathetic, querulous, and unco-operative. He may become careless about personal cleanliness, or even incontinent, although there may be no pathological reason for this. This does not make for happy domestic relationships, and often none of these things need have happened at all. Many such patients might have been sent home from hospital completely restored to health (or at least enabled to be useful and amiable members of their families) had proper attention been paid to their physical and mental needs, during their stay in hospital.

The Psychological Aspect.—This is all-important in the rehabilitation of elderly or chronic patients. Much *tact*, *sympathy*, and *patience* are necessary. Some patients are co-operative; others—for a wide variety of reasons—are the reverse. Some patients feel they cannot face the world again, after their stay in hospital; others dread becoming a burden to their relatives. An anxiety state, or even a form of hysteria, may develop as an escape from unbearable social conditions. Even with the most willing and co-operative patients, progress is often very slow, and none is possible unless the co-operation and confidence of an unwilling patient have first been gained. A different, though similar, set of problems arises where the patient is in his, or her, own home. The presence of a helpless invalid in a busy household does add enormously to the housewife's burden. As a result, all sorts of unfortunate reactions may arise between the members of the family. If the invalid can be made even a little less dependent on others, the situation may be definitely relieved. Should he be enabled to get about by himself (even with difficulty), to feed himself and attend to his own toilet, the improvement in his physical and mental health, and of everyone's tempers, will be a result infinitely worth having.

THE ELDERLY PATIENT IN HOSPITAL

Treatment.—

GENERAL TREATMENT.—As in the case of younger patients, the rehabilitation of the elderly should begin when he enters hospital. As soon as he

---

* G. S. Crockett and A. N. Exton-Smith, "Physical Medicine in the Treatment of the Aged Sick", *Brit. J. phys. Med.*, April, 1950.

has recovered sufficiently from the primary illness, he should be allowed up. Old patients are liable to be kept in bed too long. They are less trouble in hospital—or at home, for that matter—if they do not have to be dressed, got into chairs or to the dining table, and later undressed and returned to bed again. While the patient is in bed, care must be taken to see that he does not develop secondary disabilities. Apart from the avoidance of chest or bladder infections, his position should be constantly changed, to avoid the development of bed-sores from pressure on the skin. The mattress should be firm but comfortable, and rubber rings, or cushions, used where necessary. The pillows should be care-fully arranged so as to maintain a good posture, it being particularly important to avoid forward flexion of the head, constriction of the chest, or rounding of the back. The lumbar spine should be supported by a pillow, but *pillows or bolsters under the knees should be avoided*, as they tend to produce permanent flexion of hips and knees. The bedclothes should not be tightly tucked in over the patient, as this may prevent movement and put pressure on the feet. A cradle should be placed over the latter, or they should be protected in some other way. Elderly patients should not be kept waiting for bedpans or urinals. (This may seem purely a nursing problem, but, apart from the distress caused to the patient, the incontinence to which this neglect contributes may later be a serious handicap to the physiotherapist undertaking his rehabilitation.)

The late Dr. Neligan* emphasizes the importance of attractive food, pleasant surroundings, entertainments, and interesting occupations for this type of patient. Reading, listening to the radio or television, conversation, and suitable games with other patients should be encouraged.

THE PATIENT IN BED.—The patient should be encouraged to do as much as possible for himself—to feed and wash himself, to get what he wants from locker or bedside table. He should be shown how to move his limbs, and encouraged to put his joints through as full a range as possible. If he cannot move freely, the physiotherapist should put each joint through its complete range of move-ment at least once daily, unless the patient's condition contra-indicates this. Even if very weak, he can generally be given some simple exercises, and persuaded to practise them constantly. Suspension exercises are useful at this stage (*see* pp. 481–5). They promote relaxation, reduce resistance to movement, and interest the patient. Spring exercises may be added gradually. All parts of the body should receive attention, and breathing exercises should be carefully taught and practised.

During this period the patient may be ordered special treatment for the relief of pain or stiffness, or for the improvement of the general circulation. Such treatments as infra-red, or radiant heat, ultra-violet radiation, paraffin-wax baths, ionization, short-wave diathermy, or massage may be required as well as the medical treatment. In addition to their direct effect, these will have the indirect advantage of keeping the patient interested and hopeful of recovery.

THE PATIENT IN THE WARD.—As soon as the physician or surgeon permits, the patient should get up. He may require a wheel-chair at first, but its use should not be continued for longer than is absolutely necessary. He must be taught to stand, and walk, as soon as possible, and must be encouraged to help himself to do so. He can, for instance, pull himself up to a standing position by holding the end of his bed, or the uprights of a suspension frame. If necessary he should be instructed in the correct use of a walking machine, crutches, or sticks. The former should, however, be avoided if possible, as it often tends to make the patient less, rather than more, independent. He should wear suitable boots or

---

* A. R. Neligan, *Brit. J. phys. Med.*, **10**, 38, March–April, 1947.

shoes, and the possible need for chiropody must not be forgotten. Posture also requires careful attention.

Group Exercises in the Ward.—It is very good for these patients to exercise together, if this can be managed. If their numbers are sufficient, they may be grouped according to their disabilities (e.g., hemiplegia, rheumatoid arthritis, etc.). Otherwise they may do simple general and breathing exercises together, special exercises being given individually as required.

THE ELDERLY PATIENT IN THE GYMNASIUM

Group Exercises and Games in the Gymnasium.—These patients often derive a good deal of advantage merely from being able to get out of the ward into a different environment. There they will meet and talk with other people, and will compete with others in exercises. Often a healthy rivalry develops, which can do much to encourage the depressed and enliven the apathetic. The exercises should be as interesting as possible. Bean-bags and light balls or balloons may help to vary the programme, and in some cases games such as darts, quoits, or a form of bowls may be played.

A Course of Occupational Therapy, suited to the patient's ability, often contributes greatly towards his recovery. As well as helping to loosen the joints and strengthen the muscles, it gives him an interest in life, and does away with that most depressing feeling of uselessness and frustration. In some cases it may even be the beginning for him, or her, of a new trade or means of livelihood. Both physiotherapist and occupational therapist must, however, be careful to see that an enthusiastic patient does not overdo things, especially at first, and close co-operation should exist between the two.

IV. SPECIAL METHODS

SUSPENSION THERAPY

By the Late Mrs. Guthrie-Smith, M.B.E., F.R.S.P. (Hon.)

(St. Mary's Hospital, W.2; formerly Principal of the Swedish Institute, London, S.W.7)

Suspension therapy offers a new approach to many physiotherapeutic problems. The three cardinal principles underlying the method can be shortly described as: (1) *Physiological*—the increasing of bodily function by carefully graded exercise; (2) *Psychological*—in that the work done is usually self-operated, though under supervision; (3) *Mechanical*—in so far as weight and friction are under control and that *graded* resistance or assistance can be arranged as desired.

Weightless Exercise.—By suspending a body or limb we obtain a type of exercise that is *active*—yet the easiest possible to perform because the weight of the body is transferred to the apparatus and counterbalanced. Nearly all friction can be abolished with accurate technique by arranging the supporting positions of the ropes. Weightless exercises are in fact exercises of 'minimal activity', as they are tuned to match the weakest of human muscle efforts. Moreover, there is *rhythm* in the movement induced by suspension, pulley, or spring work which is valuable in assisting muscle actions.

When an arm is lifted over the head, eight, ten, or more pounds of actual weight is lifted against the force of gravity; to this is added the weight of clothing, or the resistance of tight sleeves. Yet so great is normal muscle power that the effort is not noticed. But if muscle power is *not* normal, the matter is very different. (All students of physiotherapy must try to realize the terrible weakness of paresis or paralysis.)

16

Therefore, in attempting to restore voluntary function in tissues grossly damaged (from whatever cause), we must eliminate the mechanical forces of gravity and friction which are an obstacle to movement in the early stages. Also, we must be acutely aware of the factor of *fatigue*. The fatigue factor is brought much more under control of the operator by the use of suspension, as the slightest variation of the muscle's output of strength can be detected by palpation. Periods of rest and effort can thus be interposed as required.

The psychological effect of movement *actually visible to the patient*, while he realizes that it is being made under his own power, is an immense help in nearly every condition, but of surpassing value in cases of paralysis.

Grading of Exercises.—Up-grading is applied by gentle progression, using movement *controlled* against the pull of gravity, as in holding a limb out of the vertical position—to counting or 'halting'; then by *swinging* the limb (or even the whole body) and holding it out of the vertical by muscle power. This latter method is much employed for paraplegic patients, to produce hypertrophy in arm and chest muscles; then the body is swung from side to side while the patient holds on to the suspension frame with his arms.

In other cases *resistance* is applied, either *manually* in eccentric or concentric muscle action, or by means of a *pulley and weight* applied at right angles to the suspended limb, the weight in this case being a measured quantity (*Fig.* 188). Variable resistance is obtained with high tension *springs*. These springs, if suspended above the body in a vertical position, act as a resistance in one direction (if pulled downwards) and also by their recoil assist the limb to return upwards against the force of gravity (*Fig.* 189). If they are applied horizontally they offer resistance to the moving part; but if attached below the body their force is greater, as it acts in the same direction as that of gravity.

Apparatus for Total Suspension.—A steel frame is required for this purpose (*Fig.* 190). The patient is supported by ropes and canvas slings. Resistance may be applied in several ways: manually; by springs graded by poundage; or by pulleys and weights.

The frame makes a portable gymnasium available for a patient in bed or in the department: also, in any circumstance, the apparatus constitutes a *labour-saving device*, definitely relieving the operator of the very heavy work entailed in supporting the body or limbs of a patient, and setting the hands free for more important tasks, such as palpation, resistance, or assistance.

Chief Uses.—Suspension therapy is applied to those cases in which—though their pathology may be widely different—the common denominator is loss or weakness of voluntary movement. It is specially applicable to the following types:—

1. *Spastic cases*, where the teaching of relaxation is of supreme importance, accompanied by co-ordination exercises of a weightless character.

2. *Flaccid conditions*, any condition in which skilled *re-education of muscle* (i.e., active work of certain muscles or muscle groups) is required—for example, early or severe anterior poliomyelitis.

3. *Those requiring corrective manipulations and mobility exercises*, such as kyphosis, scoliosis, and spondylitis.

4. *Orthopædic conditions*, such as the after-care of fractures, arthroplasty of the hip, and other cases which may be in heavy plaster casts; and for muscle training required in disk cases to strengthen the erector spinæ after removal of the intervertebral cartilage, or the quadriceps after excision of the meniscus.

5. *Rheumatic conditions*, e.g., osteo-arthritis to increase joint movement and assist muscle tone.

6. *Geriatric Cases.*—Here simple suspension and oscillatory exercises with springs applied bilaterally do much to limber up stiff joints and restore function to aged patients.

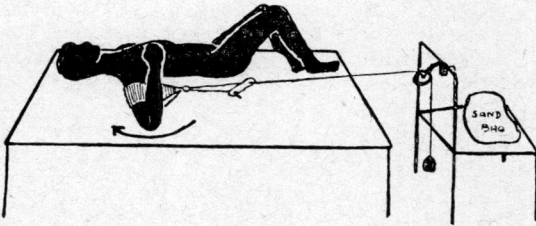

Fig. 188.—Abduction of shoulder resisted by pulley and weight.

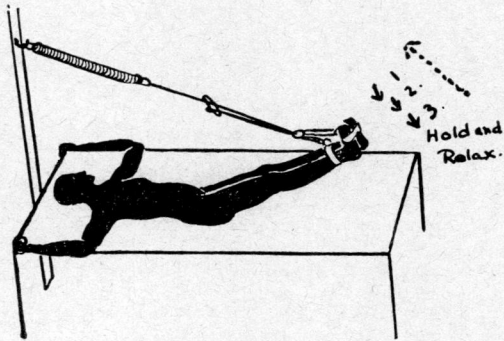

Fig. 189.—Oscillation and resistance combined.

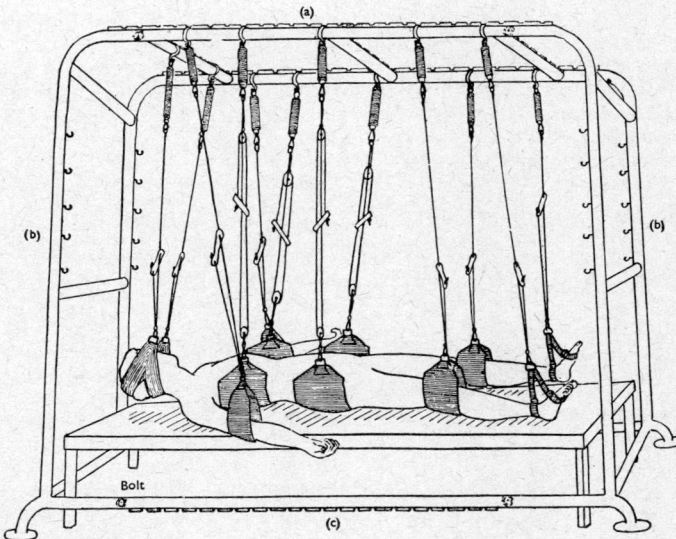

Fig. 190.—Suspension apparatus. The frame is constructed of light-gauge steel tubing of $1\frac{1}{2}$ in. diameter. It is made in five parts, viz.: (a) the top (roof unit), (b) two side units, and (c) two loose bars which unite the latter near the feet. The eight necessary connexions are secured by bolts and nuts; the position of these is shown in the figure.

Cases requiring Relaxation.—Complete relaxation is a necessary preliminary to most types of treatment. It can be more quickly obtained if adequate physical support is provided, because by this means a feeling of confidence and a plastic condition of mind can be induced. Lying in a hammock is a reposeful experience most of us have tried and found successful. Remedial suspension in comfortable supports is likewise conducive to this reposeful state, and tends to remove spasm or tension of any kind. The firm steady support of the slings is reassuring to the patient, and the required mental and physical condition should follow if the operator knows the technique of relaxation.*

For cases of *fracture*, the joints are stabilized by mechanical support of the injured part in the correct position, instead of by muscle activity; the muscles are therefore left free to act more easily on the levers of the body—that is, to move the joints—in smooth and regular pendulum rhythm. Only simple apparatus is required to take the weight of the splinted limb. The movements are always performed in the horizontal plane, the patient's position being varied to suit the required action. Space does not permit of a technical detailed exposition of the treatment of fractures on these lines, but the following is an example of a single case. To encourage movement in the knee-joint after an old *fracture of the patella* the patient is placed on the sound side; the injured leg, being the uppermost one, is suspended in supports above and below the knee-joint, the operator steadies the thigh against her own body, while the patient alternately flexes and extends the knee. After a while the pace of movements will increase till he is able to perform 'kicking' movements briskly the and with confidence, thus restoring normal function to the joint, and tone to the quadriceps.

Corrective Manipulation.—It is evident that corrective manipulations can be carried out if intelligent use is made of suspension, the counter-effect of gravity being then applied over the maximum point of the deformity. Long-continued stretchings can thus be administered without risk, accompanied by willing and intelligent relaxation or 'letting go' on the part of the patient. This technique is immediately followed by small voluntary and oft-repeated localized muscle contractions by the patient. It is an accepted principle that we must try to work stretched muscles in shortened positions. If we employ the above method of correction in suspension, the patient is *held* in the corrected position, and has only to concentrate on muscle contractions to complete the treatment.

For instance, in severe kyphosis the patient lies on his back, and one sling is placed exactly under the maximum convexity of the curve. He is then raised up three, four, or more inches by means of the adjustable ropes, attaching the sling to the overhead bars, while the rest of the body and the head are at a lower level, resting on the couch. In this 'span-bending' position the force of gravity is used to correct the deformity, and the patient should be encouraged to relax in this position, the arms being outstretched at shoulder level, and supported by two more slings. (Deep breathing should accompany relaxation.) Thus passive stretching can be safely given and kept up for quite a long period, and, if necessary, the upward traction of the 'convexity sling' can be increased till a maximum correction is obtained. The operator should now sit behind the patient's head, and putting her hands below the sling, lightly touching the muscles of the patient's back, should direct and encourage him to make localized contractions. *Small, active, and often-repeated efforts* are required to get results which may be considered to constitute a permanent cure.

---

* *See* details in *Rehabilitation, Re-education, and Remedial Exercises*, by O. F. Guthrie-Smith, 2nd edition (Chapter VI, also *Fig.* 79).

Poliomyelitis.—The fact that the weight of the limb is transferred to the apparatus, and that the two opposing forces of gravity and friction are removed, allows every tiny muscle effort to have free play, and gives rise to visible movement. Moreover, the movement has a natural rhythm, thanks to the swing induced; and with a little practice it will be found that the weak muscle contractions can be 'timed' to take place at the best possible moment, in harmony with this swing.

Such 'floating' movements are not unlike movements given in water, and have been termed 'dry water treatments'. The chance of the swing becoming mechanical must be fully realized by an ever-watchful operator; she must prevent this by introducing 'halts', purposeful movements (as kicking at a ball for knee movements), or manual or weight resistances—so that the patient is compelled to use his brain, and thus to co-operate in his own treatment, being in this way encouraged to progress from strength to strength, in a proper gymnastic manner.

PULLEY EXERCISES

By the Late Mrs. Guthrie-Smith, M.B.E., F.C.S.P. (Hon.)

(*St. Mary's Hospital, W.*2; *formerly Principal of the Swedish Institute, London, S.W.*7)

Some very useful exercises can be carried out with the assistance of a single pulley block (fitted with patent sheaves for choice), four yards of good rope,

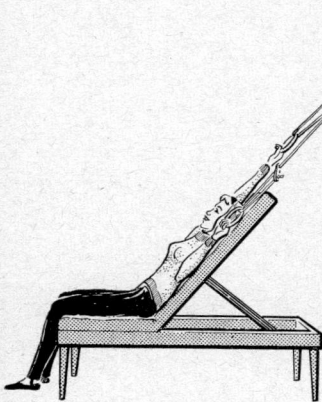

Fig. 191.—Pulley exercises for stiff joints.

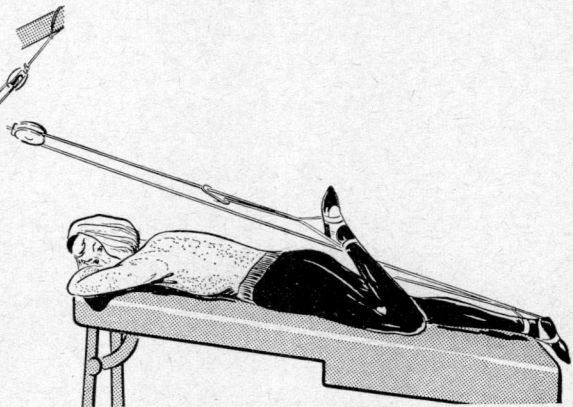

Fig. 192.—Pulley exercise adapted to knee case, giving good exercise for weak quadriceps (bilateral method). Note sloping position of couch; this makes the exercise much more effective. The foot must be over the edge of the couch.

and wooden adjustment cleats, foot straps, and handles. *Figs.* 191, 192 show such an outfit in action.

The physiotherapist must have a clear therapeutic *aim* as to the result she desires to obtain, and must see that the exercises are carried out in a proper manner, with due regard to the starting position. It is essential that the height and position of the pulley and the tension of the rope should be correct for each individual patient, otherwise he will perform the wrong movements. The movements are always double-sided, and are carried out in alternate directions by the limbs, which are in a circuit with the ropes working through a fixed point (the pulley block). The ropes are tightened with wooden cleats, and must be made taut in the starting position, so as to allow of movement and yet be capable of exerting traction.

The best primary position for the arms is for the *sound* arm to be in full *stretch*, while the *injured* one is in flexion or *bend position (see Fig.* 191); then when the movement takes place the position of the arms is reversed, and a powerful stretching is obtained in the joints of the injured limb. If *elevation* is aimed at, it is best to hang the pulley block from an overhead bar, away from walls, and place the patient directly under it; if *backward* traction is the required movement, it should be behind and above him. All sorts of movement can, in fact, be obtained by thinking out the positions, including excellent rotation exercises.

The movements can be performed in three ways, giving respectively, *passive, gentle rhythmic active,* or *energetic active* movement to the injured side. In the first case the good arm does all the work, pulling up the injured limb; the latter then returns by its own weight, supported and controlled by the sound arm in the rope circuit. Although this is a most useful exercise in some conditions, it is a mistake to limit the utility of the apparatus to this kind of movement alone. The physiotherapist should next direct the patient to move both arms alternately up and down in a *rapid rhythmic manner,* even if the full range of movement is not obtained. For 'functional' conditions this rapid alternate movement is most useful, as it tends to confuse the patient, and there will therefore be less inhibition of movement, so that it is easier to detect the real disability. *Energetic active* movements should now follow, with the command '*Up* and *up*'; the '*up*' should be emphasized while the injured arm is thrust upward. With time and practice the correct innervation will be obtained.

For stretching adhesions in joints this method has most obvious advantages, as the pain, if any, is self-inflicted and absolutely under the patient's control; yet 'self help' is encouraged to the utmost, and by the assistance of the 'pulley and purchase' much additional power is obtained.

The apparatus is cheap, reliable, and efficient, and if prepared under skilled supervision provides a valuable help to the physiotherapist in giving exercises.

MEDICINE-BALL EXERCISES*

Medicine balls are large balls with covers of leather, rubber, or canvas. They can be obtained in a variety of weights. Rubber balls vary from 1 lb. to 9 lb., and are cheaper than the leather-covered ones, which vary from 4 lb. to 9 lb. The leather ball is easier to control and is used for throwing and catching exercises; the rubber ball can, in addition, be bounced. An old football may be used, if suitably stuffed. (Ordinary footballs *can* be used, but they have—in hospital departments, at least—an unfortunate property of vanishing without trace!)

Medicine-ball exercises can be used for many purposes, and their effects can be briefly summarized here. They bring into play large groups of muscles in all parts of the body, providing resistance according to their weight. They also help to mobilize joints, the weight and momentum of the ball producing the overstretch. For instance, throwing the ball behind the body after a quick turning movement of the trunk will mobilize the vertebral joints and strengthen the trunk rotators. They improve co-ordination and neuromuscular control, since concentration and quickness are required in throwing and catching a ball. The patients usually enjoy these exercises, which can be used as the 'game' in

---

* E. Major, *Medicine-ball Exercises and Games.*

ordinary tables; or, in suitable circumstances, the whole or part of a table may be composed of them. As with Indian clubs care must be taken in throwing them, especially when many patients exercise together, though they are less likely to cause harm than the wooden clubs. Patients in class should be under strict orders not to pick up dropped balls while others are still exercising in order to reduce the risk of accident. Obviously, precautions as to windows or other breakable objects must be taken.

Medicine balls may be used for a patient working alone, for two patients as partners, or for classes. Competitive team games can be organized if the class is large enough.

Lighter balls may effectively be used in the treatment of nervous diseases.*

---

* See K. Hern's *Physical Treatment of Injuries of the Brain and Allied Nervous Disorders.*

489

INDEX

PAGE

ABDOMINAL conditions - - - - 452
— exercises in lordosis - - - - 362
— reflex - - - - - 174
— symptoms of heart disease - - 411
Abduction fractures of ankle - (Fig. 25) 44
— — neck of humerus - (Fig. 7 C) 20, 21
— transcervical fracture - (Fig. 17 A) 35
Above-knee amputation - (Figs. 50, 51) 110
Abscess(es) - - - - - 99
— formation complicating Pott's disease 165
Acetabulum, abnormal, in congenital dis-
    location of hip - - - - 295
— fracture of, complicating dislocated hip 62
Achilles tendon reflex - - - - 173
— — rupture of - - - - 83
— — shortening of, in pes plano-valgus - 311
— — tenosynovitis of - - - - 156
Achillodynia - - - - - 158
Acid burns - - - - - 101
Acromioclavicular joint, dislocation of
    (Fig. 30) 55
— — exercises for - - - - 118
— — subluxation of - - - 55, 56
Acromionectomy for ruptured supraspina-
    tus tendon - - - - 80
ACTH therapy in rheumatoid arthritis - 147
Adduction fractures of ankle - - - 44
— — neck of humerus - (Fig. 7 B) 20, 21
— transcervical fracture - (Fig. 17 B) 35, 36
Adenoids - - - - - 370
Adhesion(s) causing stiff joints - - 116
— — — manipulative treatment for 133
— complicating fracture - - 12, 13
— — lower limb fractures - - - 31
— due to pleurisy - - - 392, 393
— following joint injury - - - 54
— — formation - - - - - 6
— in joints, pulley exercises for (Fig. 191) 485
— in osteomyelitis, treatment for - 163
— prevention of, in dislocation - - 55
— — empyema - - - - 397
— — following shoulder dislocation - 57
— — in knee injuries - - - 63
— — rupture of gastrocnemius - - 83
— — scapular fracture - - - 20
— — sprains - - - - 73
Adolescent coxa vara - - - 300, 301
— genu valgum - - 302, 303, 304
— idiopathic scoliosis - - - 346
— kyphosis - - - 357, 360
Adrenal glands and diabetes - - - 449
Adrenaline secretion increasing heart-rate 407
Afferent neuron lesions, symptoms and
    principles of treatment of - 237
After-effects of injury, treatment for
    (Figs. 53–59) 116–133
Age factor in rheumatoid arthritis - - 139
Aged and chronic patients, treatment of - 478
Aids and appliances, use and care of - 7
Air-passages, clearing of - - - 368
Albee's operation - - - - 292
Alcohol injection, spinal, in intractable
    spasticity - - - - 199
Alcoholic neuritis - - - - 280
Allergic rhinitis - - - - 370
Allergy causing asthma - - - 378
Ambulatory plaster - - - - 34
— — for foot fractures - - - 46
— — Pott's fracture - - 44, 45

PAGE

Amphiarthrosis - - - - 68
Amputation(s) - (Figs. 50–52) 109
— phantom pain following - - - 114
— in thrombo-angiitis obliterans - 430, 431
— of tuberculous joint - - - 155
Amyotonia congenita - - (Fig. 121) 286
Amyotrophic lateral sclerosis - (Fig. 89) 213
Anæmia, neuritis due to - - - 280
Anæsthesia, dissociated - - - 176
— — in syringomyelia - - - 222
— — due to injury of tracts in cord - 176
— — nerve injury - - - 240
— — peripheral nerve injury (Fig. 75) 175
— — transverse myelitis - - 234, 235
— in femoral paralysis - - - 258
— general - - - - - 463
— of hand in ulnar paralysis - - 246
— in Klumpke's paralysis - (Fig. 114) 257
Anæsthetic, overcoming effects of - 466
— types of - - - - - 463
Anaphylaxis, theory of, in rheumatoid
    arthritis - - - - 143
Aneurysm - - - - 428, 429
Angina pectoris - - - 408, 412
Angulation of fracture - - (Fig. 1 B) 10
Ankle dislocation - - - - 68
— dorsiflexion, maintenance of, in frac-
    tured limb - - - - 17
— exercises, free - - - - 127
— sprained - - - - - 74
Ankle-clonus - - - - - 174
— in hemiplegia - - - - 186
Ankle-jerk - - - - - 173
Ankle-joint, dorsiflexion of, in talipes
    calcaneus - - - - 323
— fractures round - (Figs. 25, 26) 43
— irreparably damaged, in Pott's fracture 45
Ankylosing spondylitis - (Figs. 67, 68) 151
Ankylosis, fibrous and bony - - - 138
— — — in osteomyelitis - - 162, 163
— — — of tuberculous joint - - 154
— of toe in hammer toe - - - 337
Annulus fibrosus, rupture of - (Fig. 34) 70
Antenatal treatment - - - - 458
Anterior horn cell(s) activity, loss of,
    treatment for - - - - 179
— — degeneration in progressive
    muscular atrophy
    (Fig. 88) 211, 212
— — large and spindle-circuit
    (Fig. 155) 340
— — lesion, disabilities due to 178, 179
— — in poliomyelitis - (Fig. 84) 199,
    (Figs. 86, 87) 208
Anteroposterior curves of spine
    (Fig. 157) 342, 344
Antibiotic control of pneumonia - - 385
Antibodies - - - - - 4
Aorta, coarctation of - - (Fig. 181) 420
Aortic aneurysm - - - 428, 429
— disease - - - - - 411
— incompetence causing ventricular hy-
    pertrophy - - - - 410
— insufficiency - - - - 411
— stenosis - - - - - 411
— valves - - - - - 407
Aphasia due to cerebral hemiplegia
    189, 191, 194
— in hemiplegia - - - - 183

498 INDEX

NOTES

NOTES